BIOCHEMICAL AND MOLECULAR
ASPECTS OF SELECTED CANCERS

VOLUME 1

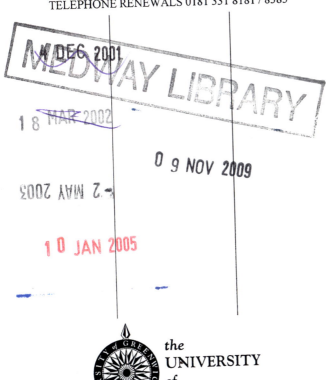
the
UNIVERSITY
of
GREENWICH

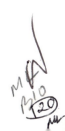

Biochemical and Molecular Aspects of Selected Cancers

EDITED BY

THOMAS G. PRETLOW II AND THERESA P. PRETLOW

Institute of Pathology
Case Western Reserve University
Cleveland, Ohio

VOLUME 1

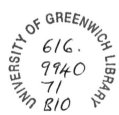

ACADEMIC PRESS, INC.

Harcourt Brace Jovanovich, Publishers

San Diego   New York   Boston   London
Sydney   Tokyo   Toronto

Copyright © 1991 by ACADEMIC PRESS, INC.

All Rights Reserved.

No part of this publication may be reproduced or transmitted in any form or by any means, electronic or mechanical, including photocopy, recording, or any information storage and retrieval system, without permission in writing from the publisher.

Academic Press, Inc.
San Diego, California 92101

United Kingdom Edition published by
Academic Press Limited
24–28 Oval Road, London NW1 7DX

Library of Congress Cataloging-in-Publication Data

Biochemical and molecular aspects of selected cancers / edited by
    Thomas G. Pretlow II and Theresa P. Pretlow.
        p. cm.
    Includes bibliographical references and index.
    ISBN 0-12-564498-1
        1. Cancer--Molecular aspects.   2. Cancer--Genetic aspects
    3. Cancer--Pathophysiology.   I. Pretlow, Thomas G.   II. Pretlow,
    Theresa P.
        [DNLM: 1. Genetics, Biochemical.   2. Molecular Biology.
    3. Neoplasma.   QZ 200 B6138]
    RC269.B49   1991
    616.99'4071--dc20
    DNLM/DLC
    for Library of Congress   91-17195
                                                                    CIP

PRINTED IN THE UNITED STATES OF AMERICA
91 92 93 94   9 8 7 6 5 4 3 2 1

Contents

1. Tumor-Suppressor Genes and Human Neoplasia

GARY R. SKUSE AND PETER T. ROWLEY

2. Protein Kinase C in Neoplastic Cells

SUSAN A. ROTENBERG AND I. BERNARD WEINSTEIN

3. HER-2/*neu* Oncogene Amplification and Expression in Human Mammary Carcinoma

D. CRAIG ALLRED, ATUL K. TANDON, GARY M. CLARK, AND WILLIAM L. McGUIRE

4. Extracellular Matrix Interactions with Tumor-Progressing Cells: Tumor versus Cell Type-Specific Mechanisms

LLOYD A. CULP, ROBERT RADINSKY, AND WEN-CHANG LIN

5. Structural and Functional Characteristics of Human Melanoma

ULLRICH GRAEVEN, DOROTHEA BECKER, AND MEENHARD HERLYN

6. Glutathione Transferases in Normal, Preneoplastic, and Neoplastic Tissues: Forms and Functions

KIYOMI SATO AND SHIGEKI TSUCHIDA

7. Steroid Hormones and Hormone Receptors in Neoplastic Diseases

CLARK W. DISTELHORST

8. Patterns and Significance of Genetic Changes in Neuroblastomas

GARRETT M. BRODEUR

9. Colonic and Pancreatic Mucin Glycoproteins Expressed in Neoplasia

YOUNG S. KIM AND JAMES C. BYRD

10. Pyruvate Kinase in Selected Human Tumors

G. E. J. STAAL AND G. RIJKSEN

11. Biochemical Basis for Multidrug Resistance in Cancer

MICHAEL M. GOTTESMAN, PATRICIA V. SCHOENLEIN, STEPHEN J. CURRIER,
EDWARD P. BRUGGEMANN, AND IRA PASTAN

12. Role of p53 in Neoplasia

MOSHE OREN

13. Chromosomal Markers of Cancer

SANDRA R. WOLMAN AND ANWAR N. MOHAMED

Preface

Our goal in the two volumes of this treatise is to provide an overview of important topics and prototypes in cancer research for the investigator with little prior specialized expertise in this area. From E. V. Cowdry's "Cancer Cells," published in 1955, one could obtain a degree of familiarity with most major areas of cancer research, and its excellent bibliography could be used as a source for more specialized reading. J. Greenstein's "Biochemistry of Cancer," published in 1954, provided a more biochemically oriented source. The progress of science since these books were published has led us to believe that a readable, truly comprehensive treatise on the biochemistry of cancer is no longer feasible. The biochemistry of cancer has become interwoven with tumor biology, cytogenetics, molecular genetics, immunology, etc., and the impact of these formerly separate disciplines is being felt increasingly even in the clinical arena as they affect both diagnosis and the choice of therapy.

This growth of knowledge has resulted in a much higher degree of specialization than was common two or three decades ago, which has resulted in many researchers who no longer see cancer research as a tenable area of interest. Instead, interests are much more highly focused, i.e., "molecular oncologists" or "cancer nutritionists." Tragically, many cancer researchers do not even become well versed in the biomedical sciences. One encounters investigators who work with "normal 3T3 cells" who are unaware that 3T3 cells were derived from unidentified embryo cells, are not "normal," and are tumorigenic under some circumstances. The potential tumorigenicity of "normal 3T3 cells" was first demonstrated by Boone (1975): "The Balb/3T3 mouse embryo cell line has been frequently used in cancer research as representative of nontumorigenic cells with the characteristic *in vitro* properties of postconfluence inhibition of cell division, low saturation density, and anchorage dependence." Mice that he "subcutaneously inoculated with an average of 15,400 Balb/3T3 cells attached to two glass beads . . ." all developed malignant tumors of blood vessels. These tumors killed transplant recipients in six weeks. More recently, Fridman *et al.* (1991) made the important observation "that NIH 3T3 cells suspended in Matrigel induced tumors when these cells were injected into athymic mice. . . ." Perhaps more importantly, when some scientists are made aware of these important facts that characterize the system with which they work, they are undisturbed, since they are more interested in "transformation" or in other phenotypes than in the broad biological significance of their work.

This two-volume treatise emphasizes topics relevant to cancers in humans. Cancers in experimental animals differ substantially from those in humans. For example, many cancers in animals can be caused by viruses; moreover, some of these are polyclonal in contrast to most human tumors. Cancers in inbred animals can more commonly be transmitted by viruses. The link between human cancers and viruses is more tenuous; in fact, although there are some associations between viral infections and a small number of human cancers, there is no conclusive proof that a virus is a sufficient cause for any human cancer. This is true despite the fact that, since the 1960s, there has been a large proportion of our national cancer research budget spent in the effort to prove a viral etiology for human cancer. As another example of differences between cancers in experimental animals and cancers in humans, most humans are exposed to carcinogens for ten to fifty years before cancers develop. The life expectancies of most experimental animals are under three years.

We are very much indebted to the outstanding investigators in diverse disciplines who have generously agreed to review their respective areas. The authors have attempted to provide succinct reviews with detailed bibliographies for readers who wish to explore specific areas in greater depth.

We hope this work will provide a background for those who wish to "attack" cancer in humans.

References

Boone, C. W. (1975). Malignant hemangioendothelioma produced by subcutaneous inoculation of Balb/3T3 cells attached to glass beads. *Science* **183**, 68–70.

Cowdry, E. V. (1955). "Cancer Cells." W. B. Saunders, Philadelphia.

Fridman, R., Kibbey, M. C., Royce, L. S., Zain, M., Sweeney, T. M., Jicha, D. L., Yannelli, J. R., Martin, G. R., and Kleinman, H. K. (1991). Enhanced tumor growth of both primary and established human and murine tumor cells in athymic mice after coinjection with Matrigel. *J. Natl. Cancer Inst.* **83**, 769–774.

Greenstein, J. P. (1954). "Biochemistry of Cancer." Academic Press, New York.

Chapter 1

Tumor-Suppressor Genes and Human Neoplasia

GARY R. SKUSE AND PETER T. ROWLEY

*Department of Medicine and Division of Genetics, University of Rochester
School of Medicine and Dentistry, Rochester, New York 14642*

I. Introduction

A. GENETIC HYPOTHESES ABOUT CANCER

Widely held hypotheses in cancer research today are (1) that the neoplastic cell differs from its normal counterpart at the DNA level, (2) that DNA differences between a neoplastic cell and its normal counterpart generally involve multiple loci, (3) that mutations responsible for the neoplastic phenotype may be

1

BIOCHEMICAL AND MOLECULAR ASPECTS
OF SELECTED CANCERS, VOL. 1

either inherited (present in the germline) or acquired (present only in somatic cells), and (4) that environmental agents (e.g., radiation, tumor viruses, and carcinogenic chemicals) produce their carcinogenic effect by causing mutations in DNA.

B. TYPES OF CANCER GENES

1. Two Types of Cancer Genes

Genes responsible for the neoplastic phenotype are commonly divided into two categories. In the first category are oncogenes, most commonly identified by their pathogenic role in animal tumor virsues. Their neoplasia-inducing properties are due to the production of an abnormal protein that deregulates cell division. In the second category are tumor-suppressor genes. Genes in this class encode proteins that normally inhibit cell division and contribute to neoplasia through their loss or mutational inactivation.

2. Tumor-Suppressor Genes

Tumor-suppressor genes are also called growth-suppressor genes, recessive oncogenes, antioncogenes, and emerogenes. The term *tumor-suppressor* gene derives from the method of their identification, in which an ability to suppress the tumor phenotype is the identifying characteristic. However, the term *growth-suppressor* gene may be more appropriate since the conservation of such genes throughout the course of evolution strongly suggests that they have an important function in the control of normal growth. The term *recessive* is used because mutation in both alleles is often assumed to be required for their contribution to tumorigenesis (Fig. 1); however, the possibility that one deficient allele has a subtle phenotypic effect is a matter of current investigation. The term *antioncogene* is attractive in those cases in which the product of the tumor-suppressor locus can be shown to complex with a protein required for cell division. However, at present this has been demonstrated for only a few tumor suppressors (e.g., retinoblastoma and p53). The term *emerogene* is derived from *emero:* to tame (Todaro, 1988).

This chapter is confined to tumor-suppressor genes in man, even though they have been identified in organisms as evolutionarily distant as *Drosophila melanogaster* (Mechler *et al.*, 1985). Recessive conditions that predispose to neoplasia via deficient DNA repair (e.g., xeroderma pigmentosum) are not included. Useful reviews of human tumor-suppressor genes have recently appeared by Green (1988), Klein (1988), Sager (1989), and Weinberg (1989). A list of human neoplasms for which there is evidence of tumor-suppressor gene involvement is given in Table I.

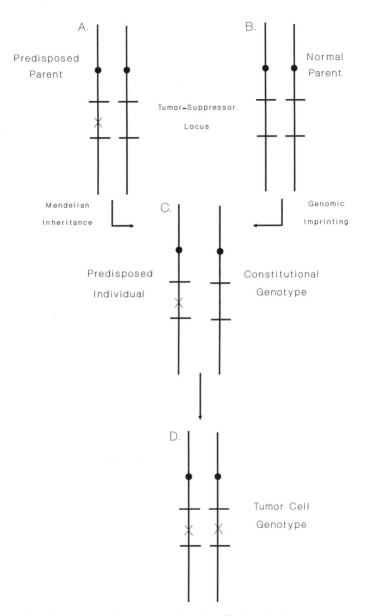

FIG. 1. Hereditary predisposition to tumor formation. The inactivated tumor-suppressor gene may be inherited *either* from a heterozygous parent (A) or from a normal parent as the result of genomic imprinting during gametogenesis (B). The predisposed individual (C) thus has one inactive allele and one active allele at the tumor-suppressor locus in all cells. A tumor forms when a post-conceptional mutation inactivates the remaining normal allele in a susceptible cell (D).

TABLE I

TUMOR SUPPRESSOR LOCI IMPLICATED IN SPORADIC AND FAMILIAL TUMORS

Chromo-somal location	Tumor or syndrome	Reference
1	Multiple endocrine neoplasia type 2	Mathew et al., 1987
1p	Neuroblastoma	Fong et al., 1989
2,6	Melanoma	Mukai and Dryja 1986; Trent et al., 1990
3p	Renal cell carcinoma	Zbar et al., 1987; Kovacs et al., 1988
3p	von Hippel–Lindau disease	King et al., 1987; Seizinger et al., 1988; Decker et al., 1988; Tory et al., 1989
3p,13q	Small cell carcinoma of the lung	Naylor et al., 1987; Brauch et al., 1987; Kok et al., 1987; Yokota et al., 1987; Harbour et al., 1988
3,11,13,17	Non–small-cell carcinoma of the lung	Weston et al., 1989
4,16	Hepatocellular carcinoma	Zhang et al., 1990
5	Familial polyposis coli	Solomon et al., 1987; Okamoto et al., 1988
5,17p,18q	Colon carcinoma	Solomon et al., 1987; Wildrick and Boman 1988; Vogelstein et al., 1988; Fearon et al., 1990
6q,11,17	Ovarian carcinoma	Lee et al., 1990
11p	Wilms' tumor	Fearon et al., 1984; Koufos et al., 1984; Orkin et al., 1984; Reeve et al., 1984
11p	Beckwith–Wiedemann syndrome	Koufos et al., 1985; Scrabie et al., 1987; Hayward et al., 1987; Little et al., 1988
11p	Bladder carcinoma	Fearon et al., 1985
11p,13q	Breast carcinoma	Lundberg et al., 1987; Theillet et al., 1986; Varley et al., 1989
13q	Retinoblastoma and osteosarcoma	Cavenee et al., 1983; Hansen et al., 1985; Friend et al., 1986
17p	Astrocytoma and glioblastoma	James et al., 1989; El-Azouzi et al., 1989
17q	Neurofibromatosis type 1 (malignancies only)	Skuse et al., 1989
22q	Neurofibromatosis type 2	Seizinger et al., 1987a
22q	Meningioma	Seizinger et al., 1987b

II. Methods for Identifying Tumor-Suppressor Genes

At least five methods have been employed to identify tumor-suppressor genes in man. First, Mendelian syndromes having as a feature a predisposition to a specific type of neoplasia have been analyzed (reviewed by Mulvihill, 1977). Second, nonrandom chromosome abnormalities have been identified in malignant disease, e.g., in retinoblastoma (Rb) (Francke, 1976). Third, nonrandom losses of heterozygosity have been found in tumors (reviewed by Hansen and Cavenee, 1987). Fourth, the tumorigenic phenotype has been suppressed either by fusion with cells of normal phenotype or by insertion of chromosomal material from a normal cell (Harris *et al.*, 1969; Huang *et al.*, 1988; Weissman *et al.*, 1987). Fifth, phenotypic reversion of transformed cells *in vitro* has been characterized (Noda *et al.*, 1983).

The methods just listed represent only the first step in identification of tumor-suppressor genes. Their isolation has required intensive effort and ingenuity. Some methods used have been those useful for isolating genes of other types, such as chromosome walking from linked markers, as in the retinoblastoma case (Friend *et al.*, 1986) or subtractive hybridization, as in the case of putative suppressors of breast epithelial cell growth (Trask *et al.*, 1989). In other cases, functional assays have been utilized to take advantage of the tumor suppressor properties of the gene sought. For example, DNA from normal cells has been transfected into malignant cells, and those cells subsequently reverting to a normal phenotype have been isolated. This method incurs the difficulty of isolating normal cells from a population of rapidly growing transformed cells; however using ouabain to select against transformed cells has permitted isolation of a putative tumor-suppressor gene by this method (Schaefer *et al.*, 1988). Human tumor-suppressor genes isolated to date include the retinoblastoma susceptibility gene (Friend *et al.*, 1986), *erbA* (Weinberger *et al.*, 1986; Benbrooke and Pfahl, 1987), p53 (Matlashewski *et al.*, 1984; Zakut-Houri *et al.*, 1985; Harlow *et al.*, 1985; Wolf *et al.*, 1985), the Wilms' tumor gene (Call *et al.*, 1990; Gessler *et al.*, 1990), and the DCC (deleted in colorectal carcinoma) gene (Fearon *et al.*, 1990).

III. Mechanisms of Tumor-Suppressor Gene Action

The mechanisms of action of tumor-suppressor genes are at present poorly understood. However, four general types of mechanisms can be delineated (Van Amsterdam *et al.*, 1989; Fearon and Vogelstein, 1990). In the first type, homozygous inactivation is associated with the development of specific tumors owing to the deficiency of a growth regulator. The Rb gene is an example. In the second type, the gene product interferes in a positive way with the activity of some oncogene by either inhibiting its expression or interfering with its product's action. An example may be the Kirsten-*ras* revertant-1 (Krev-1) gene, isolated by Kitayama *et al.*, (1989). In the third type, a single mutant allele is able to interfere with the function of the normal allele and thereby contribute to cell transformation. An example is p53 (Hicks and Mowat, 1988). In the fourth type, deficiency of an extracellular adhesion molecule may contribute to the metastatic character of the cell. An example is the DCC gene.

A. Tissue Specificity

Some tumor-suppressor genes may have activity limited to one or a few specific tissues, such as the DCC gene for colonic epithelium and the NF2 gene for the Schwann cell derivatives of the vestibular branch of the eighth cranial nerve. Other tumor-suppressor genes appear to have an important function in many tissues, whether or not their deficiency gives rise to neoplasms. Examples are the Rb gene and the p53 gene.

B. Multiple Loci Involved in Tumor Initiation

There is a growing body of evidence to suggest that many tumors arise by a tumor-suppressor mechanism, yet involve mutations at multiple loci. Wilms' tumor can occur sporadically or in a familial form. It has been established that the locus responsible for tumorigenesis in sporadic cases is located on chromosome 11p13 (Koufos *et al.*, 1984). Recently two laboratories investigated whether the locus for the familial predisposition to Wilms' tumor was linked to the 11p13 locus. Grundy and co-workers (1988) studied one family using seven polymorphic DNA markers from the short arm of chromosome 11. They failed to find linkage between the Wilms' tumor locus and the familial predisposition. Huff and co-workers (1988) performed similar studies and also failed to find linkage. These findings suggest that another gene, distinct from the Wilms' tumor locus on chromosome 11p, is involved with the familial predisposition to this disease.

There appears to be heterogeneity in the genetic mechanism responsible for tumor formation also in von Recklinghausen's neurofibromatosis (NF1). Skuse and co-workers (1989) reported finding a loss of heterozygosity for polymorphic DNA markers closely linked to the NF1 gene on chromosome 17q in malignant tumors occurring in NF1. They failed to see similar losses in benign neurofibromas occurring in NF1. Subsequent analyses (Skuse *et al.*, in press) revealed that neurofibromas are monoclonal in origin and hence must result from a mutation in a single cell. Apparently that somatic mutation occurs at a site different from the NF1 locus or is not detectable as a loss of heterozygosity.

C. MULTIPLE LOCI INVOLVED IN TUMOR PROGRESSION

1. *Colorectal Carcinoma*

In 1986 Herrera *et al.* reported the case of a retarded male with multiple developmental abnormalities, multiple adenomatous polyps of the colon, and carcinomas of the rectum and colon that had an interstitial deletion of chromosome 5q. Stimulated by this report, Bodmer *et al.* (1987) localized the gene for familial adenomatous polyposis to chromosome 5q21-q22, using DNA markers and linkage analysis. Leppert *et al.* (1987) confirmed this localization. Solomon *et al.* (1987) claimed that 20 to 40% of sporadic colorectal adenocarcinomas manifest a loss of heterozygosity for markers in this region. Later Okamoto *et al.* (1988) reported that this figure was 23%, and Ashton-Rickardt *et al.* reported 48% (1989). However, Law *et al.* (1988) found that the percentage of colorectal carcinomas showing a loss of heterozygosity for chromosome 5 was only 19%.

a. Mutations at Multiple Loci. In 1987 Fearon and co-workers reported studies of DNA markers in 50 colorectal tumors including 20 carcinomas and 30 adenomas; all tumors analyzed showed a monoclonal cellular origin as judged by the pattern of X-chromosome inactivation. Loss of 17p sequences was found in many carcinomas (75%) but in few adenomas. Law *et al.* (1988) reported that many carcinomas had lost heterozygosity for chromosome 17 markers (56%) and for chromosome 18 markers (52%), and proposed that multiple tumor-suppressor loci are involved in the development of colorectal carcinoma. On the basis of studies of *ras* gene activation (Bos *et al.*, 1987; Forrester *et al.*, 1987) and chromosome loss in both colorectal adenomas and carcinomas, Vogelstein *et al.* (1988) proposed a commonly occurring sequence of mutational events. In this common sequence, the first mutation occurs at the familial adenomatous polyposis locus on chromosome 5q. The loss or inactivation of one allele, not only in familial polyposis subjects, but also in normal individuals, may result in hyperproliferation of colonic epithelial cells. The second step is the activation of a *ras* gene, frequently K-*ras*. The third step is the loss of a tumor-suppressor allele on chromosome 18. The final step is the loss of a tumor-suppressor allele on chromosome 17p. Others also reported allele loss for markers on chromosomes 17 and 18 (Monpezat *et al.*, 1988; Boman *et al.*, 1988). Loci on other chromosomes may also be involved (Okamoto *et al.*, 1988; Vogelstein *et al.*, 1989; Sasaki *et al.*, 1989). Patients with more than the median percentage of allelic deletions have a worse prognosis than other patients (Vogelstein *et al.*, 1989).

b. Involvement of p53. In 1989 Baker *et al.* reported mutations in the p53 gene in colorectal carcinomas and suggested that p53 was the location of the previously noted 17p loss in this tumor type. Although p53 had previously been considered an oncogene, it now appears that the normal p53 gene product has suppressor activity (Finlay *et al.*, 1989). The normal p53 gene appears to interact with other macromolecules to suppress the neoplastic growth of colorectal epithelial cells.

c. Identification of a Tissue-Specific Tumor Suppressor. Fearon *et al.* (1990) reported identification of a chromosome 18q gene frequently deleted in colorectal cancers and named DCC (deleted in colorectal carcinoma), utilizing ingenious methods including a novel *exon-connection* strategy. This gene is expressed in most normal tissues, including colonic mucosa, but expression is greatly reduced or absent in most colorectal carcinomas. The amino acid sequence specifies a protein with sequence homology to neural cell adhesion molecules and related cell surface glycoproteins. They proposed that the DCC gene may play a role in the pathogenesis of human colorectal neoplasia through alteration of the normal cell–cell interactions controlling growth.

d. Sequence of Genetic Events. Fearon and Vogelstein (1990) have recently summarized their current view of the pathogenesis of colorectal tumors (Fig. 2). Most malignant colorectal tumors arise from preexisting adenomas. The development of a carcinoma involves mutations of at least four to five genes, whereas fewer mutations may suffice for an adenoma. A typical colorectal carcinoma

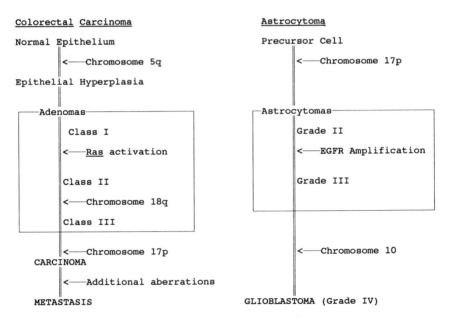

FIG. 2. Multiple loci involved in tumor progression. Models for colorectal carcinoma adapted from Fearon and Vogelstein (1990) and astrocytoma adapted from James *et al.* (1988).

would have activation of one *ras* gene and allelic losses at three or more loci, namely presumptive tumor-suppressor loci. *Ras* gene mutations are found in about 50% of colorectal carcinomas and larger adenomas and in fewer than 10% of adenomas less than 1 cm in size. A *ras* gene mutation is commonly associated with an increase in size of a preexisting adenoma. In patients without familial polyposis, losses involving chromosome 5q are observed in 20 to 50% of colon carcinomas and about 30% of colorectal adenomas.

The same group proposes that loss of a single copy of the p53 gene may provide the affected cells with a growth advantage. This may be due to a dominant negative effect, e.g., a mutant p53 gene product may inactivate the wild-type gene product by binding to it and preventing its normal association with other cellular constituents (Eliyahu *et al.*, 1988). Subsequent loss of the residual normal p53 allele may be associated with progression from adenoma to carcinoma and may augment this growth advantage. However, in adenomas from patients with familial adenomatous polyposis, allelic losses at this locus are rare. Allelic loss on chromosome 18q appears to involve the DCC gene, occurring in 70% of carcinomas and in almost 50% of adenomas (Fearon and Vogelstein, 1990). Loss of a large portion of chromosome 17p, including the p53 locus, is seen in more than 75% of colorectal carcinomas and infrequently in adenomas of any stage (Fearon and Vogelstein, 1990). A common sequence of mutations in colorectal carcinoma is presented in Fig. 2.

It may seem unlikely that 4 to 5 mutations would occur in the same cell. Vogelstein and colleagues suggest this may be explained by mutations early in the process of tumor progression that increase the rate of cell division, thus increasing the pool size of cells in which a subsequent mutation can productively occur. They emphasize that the phenotype of the fully developed carcinoma may not be dependent on the sequence of changes, but merely on their aggregation.

e. Clinical Implications.   A practical application of the identification of a mutational progression is the possibility of clinical screening for the early mutations. This might permit individuals identified as being at higher risk to change their life-styles with the hope of reducing the risk of subsequent mutations or, at least, of early detection of cancer by having frequent examinations. A Mendelian predisposition to colorectal carcinoma is found in families without polyposis. Such families are said to have hereditary nonpolyposis colorectal cancer (HNPCC), and their members may have no or few polyps (Lynch *et al.*, 1988; Cannon-Albright *et al.*, 1988; Leppert *et al.*, 1990). An important question to resolve is the locus of the germline mutation in these families.

2. *Astrocytoma and Glioma*

It has long been established that malignant tumors arise as the result of multiple genetic changes in their constituent cells. Only recently has the involvement of tumor-suppressor genes been implicated in this progression. Early studies of glial tumors revealed the overexpression of *erb*B, the gene for the epidermal growth factor receptor, located on chromosome 7 (Liberman *et al.*, 1985; Henn *et al.*, 1986). Amplification of c-*myc* on chromosome 8 was also observed (Trent *et al.*, 1986).

a. Cytogenetics.   Cytogenetic analyses confirmed the involvement of several chromosomes. Studies of chromosomal evolution in malignant human gliomas by Bigner and co-workers (1986) revealed additional copies of chromosome 7, consistent with increaseed *erb*B expression, losses of chromosome 10 and 22, and deletions and translocations of chromosome 9p. Kinzler and co-workers (1987) identified a novel gene, named *gli*, on chromosome 12q, which was amplified fiftyfold in gliomas.

b. Loss of Heterozygosity.   More recent studies employing DNA probes that detect restriction fragment–length polymorphisms have revealed consistent losses on chromosome 10 in more aggressive tumors and losses on chromosomes 13, 17, and 22 in lower-grade tumors (James *et al.*, 1988). Mitotic recombination was the mechanism leading to the reduction to homozygosity for the chromosome 17 markers studied in astrocytomas (James *et al.*, 1989). El-Azouzi and coworkers (1989) reported similar findings. The observed loss of heterozygosity suggests that both alleles at the relevant loci must be inactivated before a tumor can arise. The events in astrocytoma tumor progression are shown in Fig. 2.

IV. Dominant Effect of Mutant Alleles

According to the original formulation (Knudson, 1971), a tumor-suppressor gene contributes to the malignant phenotype only if both copies of the gene are lost or mutationally inactivated. More recently a phenotypic effect has been ascribed to mutation of only one allele. The p53 gene is a case in point.

The p53 gene was originally considered an oncogene because of its high level in transformed cells (Crawford *et al.*, 1981; Dippold *et al.*, 1981). However, the wild-type sequence of the protooncogene does not encode a transforming protein. The confusion arose because cells presumed to contain only the wild-type allele actually contained mutant forms (Finlay *et al.*, 1988; Eliyahu *et al.*, 1988; Hinds *et al.*, 1989). When overexpressed, such mutants may act in a transdominant fashion to inactivate the endogenous wild-type p53, perhaps by the formation of nonfunctional multimeric protein complexes (Herskowitz, 1987). Inactivation of p53 appears to play a role in the development of Friend virus–induced erythroleukemia (Mowat *et al.*, 1985) and in osteogenic sarcomas (Masuda *et al.*, 1987). Further, expression of high levels of the wild-type p53 can suppress transformation (Finlay *et al.*, 1989). The phenotype of the cell containing both normal and inactive alleles may depend on the relative amounts of the normal and mutant gene products.

V. Genomic Imprinting

Genomic imprinting is the modification of particular chromosomal regions during gametogenesis that affects gene expression (Allen *et al.*, 1990; Reik 1989; Surani *et al.*, 1984). Those modifications involve DNA methylation and repress the expression of genes in the affected regions (Swain *et al.*, 1987; Reik *et al.*, 1987). Genomic imprinting can occur in both males and females and leads to functional differences between the maternal and paternal genetic contribution, even though they are quantitatively equivalent (McGrath and Solter, 1984; Cattanach and Kirk, 1985).

A. Evidence from Transgenic Mice

Genomic imprinting has been observed to affect the expression of foreign genes in transgenic mice (Hadchouel *et al.*, 1987). The foreign gene introduced into the embryo, called the transgene, is differently expressed depending on whether it was received from the mother or the father. Inactivation by genomic imprinting is reversed when passed through a parent of the opposite gender. These effects can have important implications for disease genes; for example, imprinting of the wild-type allele in a heterozygote can lead to the phenotypic expression of the recessive phenotype. Can genomic imprinting of tumor suppressor genes contribute to tumorigenesis?

B. Role in Retinoblastoma (Rb)

The role of genomic imprinting in the expression of the Rb gene was investigated by Toguchida and his colleagues (1989). They employed probes from the Rb locus that detect restriction fragment–length polymorphisms in order to detect loss of heterozygosity in tumors in Rb patients. Analysis of sporadic osteosarcomas revealed that the allele remaining in the tumor, which was not detectably altered in 12 of 13 cases, was the paternal allele, suggesting that genomic imprinting may have inactivated that allele during spermatogenesis.

Parental effects on the Rb gene were also investigated in sporadic retinoblastomas (Dryja *et al.*, 1989). In that study, tumors were classified as arising by somatic mutation if they were unilateral, or as arising by a new germline mutation if they were bilateral. Seven of 15 tumors were determined to be due to postconceptional somatic mutations. The allele remaining in the tumor was paternal in three cases and maternal in four cases. Eight tumors were studied that arose by a new germline mutation. In all eight, the allele remaining in the tumor was paternal, suggesting that it was inactivated during spermatogenesis. Taken together, the studies of the Rb gene suggest that genomic imprinting may lead to its inactivation during spermatogenesis.

C. ROLE IN WILMS' TUMOR

Genomic imprinting also plays a role in the expression of several other tumor-suppressor genes. Schroeder and colleagues (1987) determined that the maternal allele was lost during tumorigenesis in all of five Wilms' tumors studied. Additional studies of the familial form of Wilms' tumor have revealed the involvement of another unlinked locus in those cases (Huff *et al.*, 1988; Grundy *et al.*, 1988), as described in Section IV, B. This unlinked locus may have a regulatory effect on the Wilms' locus and, in view of its involvement in only familial cases, may be itself regulated by an epigenetic event such as genomic imprinting.

D. ROLE IN NEUROFIBROMATOSIS TYPE I

Von Recklinghausen's neurofibromatosis (NF1) has the highest known spontaneous mutation rate of any human disorder (Huson *et al.*, 1989). Jadayel and co-workers (1990) studied 14 individuals with NF1 due to a new mutation and found that in 12, the new mutation had occurred on the paternally derived chromosome 17. Since they did not observe a paternal age effect, they concluded that genomic imprinting during spermatogenesis was probably responsible for these new mutations.

E. ROLE IN RHABDOMYOSARCOMA

Scrable and her co-workers (1989) looked at both sporadic and familial cases of embryonal rhabdomyosarcoma. This tumor has been shown to arise from cells that are isodisomic for chromosome 11p. In every case studied, the isodisomic chromosome was derived from the father. Based on these observations, the authors proposed a modification of the model originally proposed by Knudson (1971). Their modification proposes that individuals predisposed to develop tumors carry one inherited inactivating mutation that can be not only an altered DNA sequence but alternatively, the result of genomic imprinting. A tumor arises when the allele in a susceptible cell undergoes a subsequent mutation. This new model (reflected in Fig. 1) may account for nonfamilial cases of bilateral or multifocal tumors.

VI. Interactions of Tumor-Suppressor Genes with Oncogenes

A. RETINOBLASTOMA AND ADENOVIRUS E1a

Revelation of the specific role of tumor-suppressor genes in normal and tumor cells has only recently begun. The Rb gene product has been the most thoroughly characterized. In 1985 Yee and Branton reported that antisera prepared against the adenovirus E1a gene product coprecipitated certain cellular proteins from infected cells. One of these proteins was a 105-kDa phosphoprotein. This protein complexed with E1a proteins *in vitro* and was not immunoprecipitated from lysates of mock-infected cells.

Harlow and his co-workers (1986) immunoprecipitated proteins from adenovirus-transformed human 293 cells using monoclonal antibodies prepared against adenovirus E1a. One of the most abundant cellular proteins that coprecipitated with E1a had an apparent molecular mass of 110 kDa.

1. *Identification of the Rb–E1a Complex*

The protein that formed a complex with the adenovirus E1a gene product was later identified as the product of the Rb gene (Whyte *et al.*, 1988). Monoclonal antibodies were prepared against the 105-kDa protein and against synthetic peptides whose sequence was predicted by the Rb cDNA sequence. All of the monoclonal antibodies precipitated a 105-kDa protein. The identity of the polypeptides precipitated with either the monoclonal antibody prepared against the 105-kDa protein or the synthetic peptides was demonstrated by partial proteolysis mapping and Western blotting. Peptides synthesized *in vitro* from mRNAs transcribed *in vitro* from Rb cDNA also reacted with these monoclonal antibodies, further confirming that the 105-kDa protein was the Rb gene product.

2. *Delineation of the Regions Necessary for Binding*

The regions of the E1a gene product necessary for Rb binding were found to be the same regions needed for the transformation ability of E1a (Whyte *et al.*, 1989). The regions of the Rb protein that bind E1a and the SV40 large tumor (T) antigen were similarly mapped (Hu *et al.*, 1990). Those regions necessary for binding to these oncoproteins correspond to the regions commonly found to be mutated in tumors. These findings further suggest that the Rb gene product may normally regulate cell division, and its interaction with the E1a gene product may play an important role in cellular transformation by adenovirus.

B. Rb AND SV40 LARGE T ANTIGEN

The retinoblastoma gene product also interacts with the transforming proteins of several other DNA tumor viruses. DeCaprio and his co-workers (1988) determined that the SV40 large T antigen forms a complex with the Rb protein in SV40-transformed cells. Experiments demonstrated that induced mutations of the large T antigen within the transformation-controlling domain restrict complex formation with the Rb protein, while mutations outside that domain do not.

C. Role of Rb Binding in Transformation

Characterization of the Rb gene product during the cell cycle has revealed that it is underphosphorylated during G_1 and becomes phosphorylated before the cell can enter S phase (DeCaprio *et al.*, 1989). The SV40 large T antigen preferentially binds to the underphosphorylated form of the Rb protein (Ludlow *et al.*, 1989). Together these results suggest that the Rb gene product may block the transition from G_1 to S until it is either phosphorylated or bound to a viral oncogene product, a mechanism that may be important in tumor suppression, or, when defective, leads to tumor formation. The findings that the large tumor (T) antigen of several polyoma viruses (monkey, mouse, baboon, and human) also form complexes with the Rb protein (Dyson *et al.*, 1990), thus demonstrating the evolutionary conservation of this interaction.

D. Rb and Human Papilloma Virus E7

None of the viral gene products mentioned so far has been implicated in human cancers. That observation led Dyson and his co-workers (1989) to look for an interaction between the E7 oncoprotein of human papilloma virus-16 and the Rb gene product. *In vitro* mixing experiments demonstrated that the E7 protein does indeed form a complex with the Rb gene product, suggesting that the human papilloma virus may induce tumors by inactivating a normal inhibitor of cell division.

E. p53 and SV40 Large T Antigen

Interactions between viral oncogene products and the p53 tumor suppressor have also been studied (for review, see Levine, 1990). Lane and Crawford (1979) first demonstrated that monoclonal antibodies directed against the SV40 large T antigen coprecipitate a cellular protein with the same approximate molecular mass as the p53 gene product. Linzer and Levine (1979) observed similar results with antisera prepared against the SV40 large T antigen. They observed the p53 protein in both infected and uninfected cells and demonstrated that the p53 proteins from the two cell types were identical by peptide mapping.

F. p53 and Adenovirus E1a and E1b

The adenovirus E1a gene products transcriptionally activate p53 and result in increased levels of p53 protein (Braithwaite *et al.*, 1990). The adenovirus E1b gene product binds to p53 (Sarnow *et al.*, 1982). Partial peptide maps demonstrated that the cellular p53 bound to the E1b gene product and the p53 bound to the SV40 large T antigen were the same.

G. p53 AND *Ras*

Interaction of p53 with dominant oncogene products was demonstrated by Finlay *et al.* (1989). Cells transfected with an activated *ras* oncogene and either a mutant p53 gene or an adenovirus E1a gene formed foci of transformed cells. In either case, cotransfection with a wild-type copy of the p53 gene suppressed focus formation.

H. ONCOGENE ACTIVATION LEADING TO LOSS OF A TUMOR SUPPRESSOR

A final example of the interaction between an oncogene and a potential tumor suppressor comes from the laboratory of Bremner and Balmain (1990). Using a mouse model, they induced skin tumors by the topical application of chemical carcinogens. Analysis of the resulting tumors revealed that *ras* was activated and that DNA sequences from chromosome 7 had been lost. Tumors without *ras* mutations also lacked losses on chromosome 7. The specificity of chromosome losses was confirmed by analysis with probes from other chromosomes. These experiments suggest that there may be a relationship between the activation of a cellular oncogene and the loss of tumor-suppressor sequences during tumor progression.

VII. Significance

Recent advances have revealed the involvement of a tumor-suppressor gene in many types of human neoplasia. The same tumor-suppressor gene appears to be involved in both the familial and sporadic forms of several types of tumors studied. Although the role of each tumor-suppressor gene product in the normal cell is as yet unclear, the evidence to date has provided some insights. The Rb gene product is a nuclear phosphoprotein that appears to play a cell-cycle–regulatory role. Its inactivation may lead to unregulated cell proliferation. Regarding the DCC gene involved in colorectal carcinoma, its product shares some sequence homology with the neuronal cell adhesion molecule. Its inactivation may lead to greater metastatic potential. The product of the NF1 gene may play a role in growth signal transduction (Xu *et al.*, 1990). Its inactivation may result in inappropriate cell growth. Apparently tumor suppressors act at various levels of cellular growth regulation.

It is conceivable that tumor-suppressor genes play a role in an individual's susceptibility to environmentally induced cancers. Perhaps a partially dysfunctional tumor-suppressor gene product or a variant DNA sequence may render an individual atypically susceptible to environmental mutagens.

More information is needed before we can fully understand the role of tumor suppressors in both the normal and malignant cell cycle. Nevertheless it is abundantly clear that tumor-suppressor genes will continue to be a productive area of research.

Acknowledgments

G.R.S. was supported by a Research Grant from the G. Harold and Leila Y. Mathers Charitable Foundation. This work was also supported by American Cancer Society Grant CH-474, National Institutes of Health Grant CA-38685, and a grant from the American Medical Association Education and Research Fund.

References

Allen, N. D., Norris, M. L., and Surani, M. A. (1990). Epigenetic control of transgene expression and imprinting by genotype-specific modifiers. *Cell* **61**, 853–861.
Ashton-Rickardt, P. G., Dunlop, M. G., Nakamura, Y., Morris, R. G., Purdie, C. A., Steel, C. M., Evans, H. J., Bird, C. C., and Wyllie, A. H. (1989). High frequency of APC loss in sporadic colorectal carcinoma due to breaks clustered in 5q21-22. *Oncogene* **4**, 1169–1174.
Baker, S. J., Fearon, E. R., Nigro, J. M., Hamilton, S. R., Preisinger, A. C., Jessup, J. M., vanTuinen, P., Ledbetter, D. H., Barker, D. F., Nakamura, Y., White, R., and Vogelstein, B. (1989). Chromosome 17 deletions and p53 gene mutations in colorectal carcinomas. *Science* **244**, 217–221.
Benbrook, D., and Pfahl, M. (1987). A novel thyroid hormone receptor encoded by a cDNA clone from a human testis library. *Science* **238**, 788–791.
Bigner, S. H., Mark, J., Bullard, D. E., Mahaley, M. S., Jr., and Bigner, D. D. (1986). Chromosomal evolution in malignant human gliomas starts with specific and usually numerical deviations. *Cancer Genet. Cytogenet.* **22**, 121–135.
Bodmer, W. F., Bailey, C. J., Bodmer, J., Bussey, H. J. R., Ellis, A., Gorman, P., Lucibello, F. C., Murday, V. A., Rider, S. H., Scambler, P., Sheer, D., Solomon, E., and Spurr, N. K. (1987). Localization of the gene for familial adenomatous polyposis on chromosome 5. *Nature* **328**, 614–616.
Boman, B. M., Wildrick, D. M., and Alfaro, S. R. (1988). Chromosome 18 allele loss at the D18S6 locus in human colorectal carcinomas. *Biochem. Biophys. Res. Commun.* **155**, 463–469.
Bos, J. L., Fearon E. R., Hamilton, S. R., Verlaan-de Kries, M., van Boom, J. H., van der Eb, A. J., Vogelstein, B. (1987). Prevalence of *ras* gene mutation in human colorectal cancers. *Nature (London)* **327**, 293–297.
Braithwaite, A., Nelson, C., Skulimowski, A., McGovern, J., Pigott, D., and Jenkins, J. (1990). Transactivation of the p53 oncogene by E1a gene products. *Virology* **177**, 595–605.
Brauch, H., Johnson, B., Hovis, J., Yano, T., Gazdar, A., Pettengill, O. S., Graziano, S., Sorenson, G. D., Poiesz, B. J., Minna, J., Linehan, M., and Zbar, B. (1987). Molecular analysis of the short arm of chromosome 3 in small-cell and non–small-cell carcinoma of the lung. *N. Engl. J. Med.* **317**, 1109–1113.
Bremner, R., and Balmain, A. (1990). Genetic changes in skin tumor progression: Correlation between presence of a mutant *ras* gene and loss of heterozygosity on mouse chromosome 7. *Cell* **61**, 407–417.

Call, K. M., Glaser, T., Ito, C. Y., Buckler, A. J., Pelletier, J., Haber, D. A., Rose, E. A., Kral, A., Yeger, H., Lewis, W. H., Jones, C., and Housman, D. E. (1990). Isolation and characterization of a zinc finger polypeptide gene at the human chromosome 11 Wilms' tumor locus. *Cell* **60**, 509–520.

Cannon-Albright, L. A., Skolnick, M. H., Bishop, D. T., Lee, R. G., and Burt, R. W. (1988). Common inheritance of susceptibility to colonic adenomatous polyps and associated colorectal cancers. *N. Engl. J. Med.* **319**, 533–537.

Cattanach, B. M., and Kirk, M. (1985). Differential activity of maternally and paternally derived chromosome regions in mice. *Nature (London)* **315**, 496–498.

Cavenee, W. K., Dryja, T. P., Phillips, R. A., Benedict. W. F., Godbout, R., Gallie, B. L., Murphree, A. L., Strong, L. C., and White, R. L. (1983). Expression of recessive alleles by chromosomal mechanisms in retinoblastoma. *Nature (London)* **305**, 779–784.

Crawford, L. V., Pim, D. C., Gurney, E. G., Goodfellow, P., and Taylor-Papadimitriou, J. (1981). Detection of a common feature in several human tumor cell lines—a 53,000-dalton protein. *Proc. Natl. Acad. Sci. U.S.A.* **78**, 41–45.

DeCaprio, J. A., Ludlow, J. W., Figge, J., Shew, J.-Y., Huang, C.-M., Lee, W.-H., Marsilio, E., Paucha, E., and Livingston, D. M. (1988). SV40 large tumor antigen forms a specific complex with the product of the retinoblastoma susceptibility gene. *Cell* **54**, 275–283.

DeCaprio, J. A., Ludlow, J. W., Lynch, D., Furukawa, Y., Griffin, J., Piwnica-Worms, H., Huang, C.-M., and Livingston, D. M. (1989). The product of the retinoblastoma susceptibility gene has properties of a cell-cycle regulatory element. *Cell* **58**, 1085–1095.

Decker, H.-J., Neumann, H. P. H., Walter, T. A., and Sandberg, A. A. (1988). 3p involvement in a renal cell carcinoma in von Hippel–Lindau syndrome. *Cancer Genet. Cytogenet.* **33**, 59–65.

Dippold, W. G., Jay, G., DeLeo, A. B., Khoury, G., and Old, L. J. (1981). p53 transformation–related protein: Detection by monoclonal antibody in mouse and human cells. *Proc. Natl. Acad. Sci. U.S.A.* **78**, 1695–1699.

Dryja, T. P., Mukai, S., Peterson, R., Rapaport, J. M., Walton, D., and Yandell, D. W. (1989). Parental origin of mutations of the retinoblastoma gene. *Nature (London)* **339**, 556–558.

Dyson, N., Bernards, R., Friend, S. H., Gooding, L. R., Hassell, J. A., Major, E. O., Pipas, J. M., VanDyke, T., and Harlow, E. (1990). Large T antigens of many polyomaviruses are able to form complexes with the retinoblastoma protein. *J. Virol.* **64**, 1353–1356.

Dyson, N., Howley, P. M., Munger, K., and Harlow, E. (1989). The human papilloma virus-16 E7 oncoprotein is able to bind to the retinoblastoma gene product. *Science* **243**, 934–937.

El-Azouzi, M., Chung, R. Y., Farmer, G. E., Martuza, R. L., Black, P. McL., Rouleau, G. A., Hettlich, C., Hedley-Whyte, E. T., Zervas, N. T., Panagopoulos, K., Nakamura, Y., Gusella, J. F., and Seizinger, B. R. (1989). Loss of distinct regions on the short arm of chromosome 17 associated with tumorigenesis of human astrocytomas. *Proc. Natl. Acad. Sci. U.S.A.* **86**, 7186–7190.

Eliyahu, D., Goldfinger, N., Pinhasi-Kimhi, O., Shaulsky, G., Skurnik, Y., Arai, N., Rotter, V., and Oren, M. (1988). Meth A fibrosarcoma cells express two transforming mutant p53 species. *Oncogene* **3**, 313–321.

Fearon, E. R., Cho, K. R., Nigro, J. M., Kern, S. E., Simons, J. W., Ruppert, J. M., Hamilton, S. R., Preisinger, A. C., Thomas, G., Kinzler, K. W., and Vogelstein, B. (1990). Identification of a chromosome 18q gene that is altered in colorectal cancers. *Science* **247**, 49–56.

Fearon, E. R., Feinberg, A. P., Hamilton, S. H., and Vogelstein, B. (1985). Loss of genes on the short arm of chromosome 11 in bladder cancer. *Nature (London)* **318**, 377–380.

Fearon, E. R., Hamilton, S. R., and Vogelstein, B. (1987). Clonal analysis of human colorectal tumors. *Science* **238**, 193–197.

Fearon, E. R., Vogelstein, B., and Feinberg, A. P. (1984). Somatic deletion and duplication of genes on chromosome 11 in Wilms' tumors. *Nature (London)* **309**, 176–178.

Fearon, E. R., and Vogelstein, B. (1990). A genetic model for colorectal tumorigenesis. *Cell* **61**, 759–767.

Finlay, C. A., Hinds, P. W., and Levine, A. J. (1989). The p53 protooncogene can act as a suppressor of transformation. *Cell* **57**, 1083–1093.

Finlay, C. A., Hinds, P. W., Tan, T.-H., Eliyahu, D., Oren, M., and Levine, A. J. (1988). Activating mutations for transformation by p53 produce a gene product that forms an hsc70-p53 complex with an altered half-life. *Mol. Cell. Biol.* **8**, 531–539.

Fong, C.-T., Dracopoli, N. C., White, P. S., Merrill, P. T., Griffith, R. C., Housman, D. E., and Brodeur, G. M. (1989). Loss of heterozygosity for chromosome 1p in human neuroblastoma: Correlation with N-*myc* amplification. *Proc. Natl. Acad. Sci. U.S.A.* **86**, 3753–3757.

Forrester K., Almoguera C., Han K., Grizzle W. E., and Perucho M. (1987). Detection of high incidence of K-*ras* oncogenes during human colon tumorigenesis. *Nature (London)* **327**, 298–303.

Francke, U. (1976). Retinoblastoma and chromosome 13. *Birth Defects* **12**, 131–137.

Friend, S. H., Bernards, R., Rogelj, S., Weinberg, R. A., Rapaport, J.M., Albert, D. M., and Dryja, T. P. (1986). A human DNA segment with properties of the gene that predisposes to retinoblastoma and osteosarcoma. *Nature (London)* **323**, 643–646.

Gessler, M., Poustka, A., Cavenee, W., Neve, R. L., Orkin, S. H., and Bruns, G. A. P. (1990). Homozygous deletion in Wilms' tumours of a zinc-finger gene identified by chromosome jumping. *Nature (London)* **343**, 774–778.

Green, A. R. (1988). Recessive mechanisms of malignancy. *Br. J. Cancer* **58**, 115–121.

Grundy, P., Koufos, A., Morgan, K., Li, F. P., Meadows, A. T., and Cavenee, W. K. (1988). Familial predisposition to Wilms' tumour does not map to the short arm of chromosome 11. *Nature (London)* **336**, 374–376.

Hadchouel, M., Farza, H., Simon, S., Tiollais, P., and Pourcel, C. (1987). Maternal inhibition of hepatitis B surface antigen gene expression in transgenic mice correlates with. *de novo* methylation. *Nature (London)* **329**, 454–456.

Hansen, M. F., and Cavenee, W. K. (1987). Genetics of cancer predisposition. *Cancer Res.* **47**, 5518–5527.

Hansen, M. F., Koufos, A., Gallie, B. L., Phillips, R. A., Fodstad, O., Brogger, A., Gedde-Dahl, T., and Cavenee, W. K. (1985). Osteosarcoma and retinoblastoma: A shared mechanism revealing recessive predisposition. *Proc. Natl. Acad. Sci. U.S.A.* **82**, 6216–6220.

Harbour, J. W., Lai, S.-L., Whang-Peng, J., Gazdar, A. F., Minna, J. D., and Kaye, F. J. (1988). Abnormalities in structure and expression of the human retinoblastoma gene in SCLC. *Science* **241**, 353–357.

Harlow, E., Whyte, P., Franza, B. R., and Schley, C. (1986). Association of adenovirus early-region 1A proteins with cellular polypeptides. *Mol. Cell. Biol.* **6**, 1579–1589.

Harlow, E., Williamson, N. M., Ralston, R., Helfman, R. M., and Adams, T. E. (1985). Molecular cloning and *in vitro* expression of a cDNA clone for human cellular tumor antigen p53. *Mol. Cell. Biol.* **5**, 1601–1610.

Harris, H., Miller, O. J., Klein, G., Worst, P. L., and Tachibana, T. (1969). Suppression of malignancy by cell fusion. *Nature (London)* **223**, 363–368.

Hayward, N. K., Little, M. H., Mortimer, R. H., Clouston, W. M., and Smith, P. J. (1987). Generation of homozygosity at the c-Ha-*ras*-1 locus of chromosome 11p in an adrenal adenoma from an adult with Wiedemann-Beckwith syndrome. *Cancer Genet. Cytogenet.* **30**, 127–132.

Henn, W., Blin, N., and Zang, K. D. (1986). Polysomy of chromosome 7 is correlated with overexpression of the *erb*B oncogene in human glioblastoma cell lines. *Hum. Genet.* **74**, 104–106.

Herrera, L., Kakati, S., Gibas, L., Pietrzak, E., and Sandberg, A. A. (1986). Gardner syndrome in a man with an interstitial deletion of 5q. *Am. J. Med. Genet.* **25**, 473–476.

Herskowitz, I. (1987). Functional inactivation of genes by dominant negative mutations. *Nature (London)* **329**, 219–222.

Hicks, G. G., and Mowat, M. (1988). Integration of Friend leukemia virus into both alleles of the p53 oncogene in an erythroleukemia cell line. *J. Virol.* **62,** 4752–4755.

Hinds, P., Finlay, C., and Levine, A. J. (1989). Mutation is required to activate the p53 gene for cooperation with the *ras* oncogene and transformation. *J. Virol.* **63,** 739–746.

Hu, Q., Dyson, N., and Harlow, E. (1990). The regions of the retinoblastoma protein needed for binding to adenovirus E1A or SV40 large T antigen are common sites for mutations. *EMBO J.* **9,** 1147–1155.

Huang, H.-J.S., Yee, J.-K., Shew, J.-Y., Chen, P.-L., Bookstein, R., Friedmann, T., Lee, E. Y.-H. P., and Lee, W.-H. (1988). Suppression of the neoplastic phenotype by replacement of the RB gene in human cancer cells. *Science* **242,** 1563–1566.

Huff, V., Compton, D. A., Chai, L.-Y., Strong, L. C., Geiser, C. F., and Saunders, G. F. (1988). Lack of linkage of familial Wilms' tumour to chromosomal band 11p13. *Nature (London)* **336,** 377–378.

Huson, S. M., Compston, D. A. S., Clark, P., and Harper, P. S. (1989). A genetic study of von Recklinghausen neurofibromatosis in south east Wales. I. Prevalence, fitness, mutation rate, and effect of parental transmission on severity. *J. Med. Genet.* **26,** 704–711.

Jadayel, D., Fain, P., Upadhyaya, M., Ponder, M. A., Huson, S. M., Carey, J., Fryer, A., Mathew, C. G. P., Barker, D. F., and Ponder, B. A. J. (1990). Paternal origin of new mutations in von Recklinghausen neurofibromatosis. *Nature (London)* **343,** 558–559.

James, C. D., Carlbom, E., Dumanski, J. P., Hansen, M., Nordenskjold, M., Collins, V. P., and Cavenee, W. K. (1988). Clonal genomic alterations in glioma malignancy stages. *Cancer Res.* **48,** 5546–5551.

James, C. D., Carlbom, E., Nordenskjold, M., Collins, V. P., and Cavenee, W. K. (1989). Mitotic recombination of chromosome 17 in astrocytomas. *Proc. Natl. Acad. Sci. U.S.A.* **86,** 2858–2862.

King, C. R., Schimke, R. N., Arthur, T., Davoren, B., and Collins, D. (1987). Proximal 3p deletion in renal cell carcinoma cells from a patient with von Hippel–Lindau disease. *Cancer Genet. Cytogenet.* **27,** 345–348.

Kinzler, K. W., Bigner, S. H., Bigner, D. D., Trent, J. M., Law, M. L., O'Brien, S. J., Wong, A. J., and Vogelstein, B. (1987). Identification of an amplified, highly expressed gene in a human glioma. *Science* **236,** 70–73.

Kitayama, H., Sugimoto, Y., Matsuzaki, T., Ikawa, Y., and Noda, M. (1989). A *ras*-related gene with transformation-suppressor activity. *Cell* **56,** 77–84.

Klein, G. (1988). Tumour suppressor genes. *J. Cell Sci. Suppl.* **10,** 171–180.

Knudson, A. G. (1971). Mutation and cancer: Statistical study of retinoblastoma. *Proc. Natl. Acad. Sci. U.S.A.* **68,** 820–823.

Kok, K., Osinga, J., Carritt, B., Davis, M. B., van der Hout, A. H., van derVeen, A. Y., Landsvater, R. M., de Leij, L. F., Berendsen, H. H., Postmus, P. E., Poppema, S., and Buys, C. H. (1987). Deletion of a DNA sequence at the chromosomal region 3p21 in all major types of lung cancer. *Nature (London)* **330,** 578–581.

Koufos, A., Hansen, M. F., Copeland, N. G., Jenkins, N. A., Lampkin, B. C., and Cavenee, W. K. (1985). Loss of heterozygosity in three embryonal tumours suggests a common pathogenetic mechanism. *Nature (London)* **316,** 330–334.

Koufos, A., Hansen, M. F., Lampkin, B. C., Workman, M. L., Copeland, N. G., Jenkins, N. A., and Cavenee, W. K. (1984). Loss of alleles at loci on human chromosome 11 during genesis of Wilms' tumour. *Nature (London)* **309,** 170–172.

Kovacs, G., Erlandsson, R., Goldog, F., Ingvarsson, S., Muller-Brechlin, R., Klein, G., and Sumegi, J. (1988). Consistent chromosome 3p deletion and loss of heterozygosity in renal cell carcinoma. *Proc. Nat. Acad. Sci. U.S.A.* **85,** 1571–1575.

Lane, D. P., and Crawford, L. V. (1979). T antigen is bound to a host protein in SV40-transformed cells. *Nature (London)* **278,** 261–263.

Law, D. J., Olschwang, S., Monpezat, J.-P., Lefrancois, D., Jagelman, D., Petrelli, N. J., Thomas, G., and Feinberg, A. P. (1988). Concerted nonsyntenic allelic loss in human colorectal carcinoma. *Science* **241**, 961–964.

Lee, J. H., Kavanagh, J. J., Wildrick, D. M., Wharton, J. T., and Blick, M. (1990). Frequent loss of heterozygosity on chromosomes 6q, 11, 17 in human ovarian carcinomas. *Cancer Res.* **50**, 2724–2728.

Leppert, M., Dobbs, M., Scambler, P., O'Connell, P., Nakamura, Y., Stauffer, D., Woodward, S., Burt, R., Hughes, J., Gardner, E., Lathrop, M., Wasmuth, J., Lalouel, J.-M., and White, R. (1987). The gene for familial polyposis coli maps to the long arm of chromosome 5. *Science* **238**, 1411–1413.

Leppert, M., Burt, R., Hughes, J. P., Samowitz, W., Nakamura, Y., Woodward, S., Gardner, E., Lalouel, J.-M., and White, R. (1990). Genetic analysis of an inherited predisposition to colon cancer in a family with a variable number of adenomatous polyps. *N. Engl. J. Med.* **322**, 904–908.

Levine, A. J. (1990). The p53 protein and its interactions with the oncogene products of the small DNA tumor viruses. *Virology* **177**, 419–426.

Libermann, T. A., Nusbaum, H. R., Razon, N., Kris, R., Lax, I., Soreq, H., Whittle, M., Waterfield, M. D., Ullrich, A., and Schlessinger, J. (1985). Amplification and overexpression of the EGF receptor gene in primary human glioblastomas. *J. Cell Sci. Suppl.* **3**, 161–172.

Linzer, D. I. H., and Levine, A. J. (1979). Characterization of a 54 kDa cellular SV40 tumor antigen present in SV40-transformed cells and uninfected embryonal carcinoma cells. *Cell* **17**, 43–52.

Little, M. H., Thomsen, D. B., Hayward, N. K., and Smith, P. J. (1988). Loss of alleles on the short arm of chromosome 11 in a hepatoblastoma from a child with Beckwith-Wiedemann syndrome. *Hum. Genet.* **79**, 186–189.

Ludlow, J. W., DeCaprio, J. A., Huang, C.-H., Lee, W.-H., Paucha, E., and Livingston, D. M. (1989). SV40 large T antigen binds preferentially to an underphosphorylated member of the retinoblastoma susceptibility gene product family. *Cell* **56**, 57–65.

Lundberg, C., Skoog, L., Cavenee, W. K., Nordenskjold, M. (1987). Loss of heterozygosity in human ductal breast tumors indicates a recessive mutation on chromosome 13. *Proc. Nat. Acad. Sci. U.S.A.* **84**, 2372–2376.

Lynch, H. T., Lanspa, S. J., Boman, B. M., Smyrk, T., Watson, P., Lynch, J. F., Lynch, P. M., Cristofaro, G., Bufo, P., Tauro, A. V., Mingazzini, P., and DiGiulio, E. (1988). Hereditary nonpolyposis colorectal cancer—Lynch syndromes I and II. *Gastroenterol. Clin. North Am.* **17**, 679–712.

Masuda, H., Miller, C., Koeffler, H. P., Battifora, H., and Cline, M. J. (1987). Rearrangement of the p53 gene in human osteogenic sarcomas. *Proc. Natl. Acad. Sci. U.S.A.* **84**, 7716–7719.

Mathew, C. G. P., Smith, B. A., Thorpe, K., Wong, Z., Royle, N. J., Jeffreys, A. J., and Ponder, B. A. J. (1987). Deletion of genes on chromosome 1 in endocrine neoplasia. *Nature (London)* **328**, 524–526.

Matlashewski, G., Lamb, P., Pim, D., Peacock, J., Crawford, L., and Benchimol, S. (1984). Isolation and characterization of a human p53 cDNA clone: Expression of the human p53 gene. *EMBO J.* **3**, 3257–3262.

McGrath, J., and Solter, D. (1984). Completion of mouse embryogenesis requires both maternal and paternal genomes. *Cell* **37**, 179–183.

Mechler, B. M., McGinnis, W., and Gehring, W. J. (1985). Molecular cloning of lethal (2) giant larvae, a recessive oncogene of *Drosophila melanogaster*. *EMBO J.* **4**, 1551–1557.

Monpezat, J.-P, Delattre, O., Bernard, A., Grunwald, D., Remvikos, Y., Muleris, M., Salmon, R. J., Frelat, G., Dutrillaux, B., and Thomas, G. (1988). Loss of alleles on chromosome 18 and on the short arm of chromosome 17 in polyploid colorectal carcinomas. *Int. J. Cancer* **41**, 404–408.

Mowat, M., Cheng, A., Kimura, N., Bernstein, A., and Benchimol, S. (1985). Rearrangements of the cellular p53 gene in erythroleukemic cells transformed by Friend virus. *Nature (London)* **314**, 633–636.

Mukai, S., and Dryja, T. P. (1986). Loss of alleles at polymorphic loci on chromosome 2 in uveal melanoma. *Cancer Genet. Cytogenet.* **82**, 45–53.

Mulvihill, J. J. (1977). Genetic repertory of human neoplasia. *Prog. Cancer Res. Ther.* **3**, 137–143.

Naylor, S. L., Johnson, B. E., Minna, J. D., and Sakaguchi, A. Y. (1987). Loss of heterozygosity of chromosome 3p markers in small-cell lung cancer. *Nature (London)* **329**, 451–454.

Noda, M., Selinger, Z., Scolnick, E. M., and Bassin, R. H. (1983). Flat revertants isolated from Kirsten sarcoma virus–transformed cells are resistant to the action of specific oncogenes. *Proc. Natl. Acad. Sci. U.S.A.* **80**, 5602–5606.

Okamoto, M., Sasaki, M., Sugio, K., Sato, C., Iwama, T., Ikeuchi, T., Tonomura, A., Sasazuki, T., and Miyaki, M. (1988). Loss of constitutional heterozygosity from patients with familial polyposis coli. *Nature (London)* **331**, 273–277.

Orkin, S. H., Goldman, D. S., and Sallan, S. E. (1984). Development of homozygosity for chromosome 11p markers in Wilms' tumour. *Nature (London)* **309**, 172–174.

Reeve, A. E., Housiaux, P. J., Gardner, R. J. M., Chewings, W. E., Grindley, R. M., and Millow, L. J. (1984). Loss of a Harvey *ras* allele in sporadic Wilms' tumour. *Nature (London)* **309**, 174–176.

Reik, W. (1989). Genomic imprinting and genetic disorders in man. *Trends Genet.* **5**, 331–336.

Reik, W., Collick, A., Norris, M. L., Barton, S. C., and Surani, M. A. (1987). Genomic imprinting determines methylation of parental alleles in transgenic mice. *Nature (London)* **328**, 248–254.

Sager, R. (1989). Tumor-suppressor genes: The puzzle and the promise. *Science* **246**, 1406–1412.

Sarnow, P., Ho, Y. S., Williams, J., and Levine, A. J. (1982). Adenovirus Elb-58 kDa tumor antigen and SV40 large tumor antigen are physically associated with the same 54 kDa cellular protein in transformed cells. *Cell* **28**, 387–394.

Sasaki, M., Okamoto, M., Sato, C., Sugio, K., Soejima, J., Iwama, T., Ikeuchi, T., Tonomura, A., Miyaki, M., and Sasazuki, T. (1989). Loss of constitutional heterozygosity in colorectal tumors from patients with familial polyposis coli and those with nonpolyposis colorectal carcinoma. *Cancer Res.* **49**, 4402–4406.

Schaefer, R., Iyer, J., Iten, E., and Nirkko, A. C. (1988). Partial reversion of the transformed phenotype in H-ras–transfected tumorigenic cells by transfer of a human gene. *Proc. Natl. Acad. Sci. U.S.A.* **85**, 1590–1594.

Schroeder, W. T., Chao, L.-Y., Dao, D. D., Strong, L. C., Pathak, S., Riccardi, V., Lewis, W. H., and Saunders, G. F. (1987). Nonrandom loss of maternal chromosome 11 alleles in Wilms' tumors. *Am. J. Hum. Genet.* **40**, 413–420.

Scrable, H., Cavenee, W., Ghavimi, F., Lovell, M., Morgan, K., and Sapienza, C. (1989). A model for embryonal rhabdomyosarcoma tumorigenesis that involves genome imprinting. *Proc. Natl. Acad. Sci. U.S.A.* **86**, 7480–7484.

Scrable, H. J., Witte, D. P., Lampkin, B. C., and Cavenee, W. K. (1987). Chromosomal localization of the human rhabdomyosarcoma locus by mitotic recombination mapping. *Nature (London)* **329**, 645–647.

Seizinger, B. R., de la Monte, S., Atkins, L., Gusella, J. F., and Martuza, R. L. (1987). Molecular genetic approach to human meningioma: Loss of genes on chromosome 22. *Proc. Natl. Acad. Sci. U.S.A.* **84**, 5419–5423.

Seizinger, B. R., Rouleau, G. A., Ozelius, L. J., Lane, A. H., Farmer, G. E., Lamiell, J. M., Haines, J., Yuen, J. W. M., Collins, D., Majoor-Krakauer, D., Bonner, T., Mathew, C., Rubenstein, A., Halperin, J., McConkie-Rosell, A., Green, J. S., Trofatter, J. A., Ponder, B. A., Eierman, L., Bowmner, M. I., Schimke, R., Oostra, B., Aronin, N., Smith, D. I., Drabkin, H., Waziri, M. H., Hobbs, W. J., Martuza, R. L., Conneally, P. M., Hsia, Y. E., and Gusella, J. F.

(1988). Von Hippel–Lindau disease maps to the region of chromosome 3 associated with renal cell carcinoma. *Nature (London)* **332**, 268–269.

Seizinger, B. R., Rouleau, G., Ozelius, L. J., Lane, A. H., St. George-Hyslop, P., Huson, S., Gusella, J. F., and Martuza, R. L. (1987). Common pathogenetic mechanisms for three tumor types in bilateral acoustic neurofibromatosis. *Science* **236**, 317–319.

Skuse, G. R., Kosciolek, B. A., and Rowley, P. T. (1989). Molecular genetic analysis of tumors in von Recklinghausen neurofibromatosis: Loss of heterozygosity for chromosome 17. *Genes Chromosomes Cancer* **1**, 36–41.

Skuse, G. R., Kosciolek, B. A., and Rowley, P. T. (1991). The neurofibroma in von Recklinghausen neurofibromatosis has a unicellular origin. *Am. J. Hum. Genet.* (in press).

Solomon, E., Voss, R., Hall, V., Bodmer, W. F., Jass, J. R., Jeffreys, A. J., Lucibello, F. C., Patel, I., and Rider, S. H. (1987). Chromosome 5 allele loss in human colorectal carcinomas. *Nature (London)* **328**, 616–619.

Surani, M. A. H., Barton, S. C., and Norris, M. L. (1984). Development of reconstituted mouse eggs suggests imprinting of the genome during gametogenesis. *Nature (London)* **308**, 548–551.

Swain, J. L., Stewart, T. A., and Leder, P. (1987). Parental legacy determines methylation and expression of an autosomal transgene: A molecular mechanism for parental imprinting. *Cell* **50**, 719–727.

Theillet, C., Lidereau, R., Escot, C., Hutzell, P., Brunet, M., Gest, J., Schlom, J., and Callahan, R. (1986). Loss of a H-*ras*-1 allele in aggressive primary breast carcinomas. *Cancer Res.* **46**, 4776–4781.

Todaro, G. N. (1988). "Theories of Carcinogenesis" (O. H. Iversen, ed.), p. 61. Hemisphere, Washington, D.C.

Toguchida, J., Ishizaki, K., Sasaki, M.S., Nakamura, Y., Ikenaga, M., Kato, M., Sugimoto, M., Kotoura, Y., and Yamamuro, T. (1989). Preferential mutation of paternally derived RB gene as the initial event in sporadic osteosarcoma. *Nature (London)* **338**, 156–158.

Tory, K., Brauch, H., Linehan, M., Barba, D., Oldfield, E., Filling-Katz, M., Seizinger, B., Nakamura, Y., White, R., Marshall, F. F., Lerman, M. I., and Zbar, B. (1989). Specific genetic change in tumors associated with von Hippel–Lindau disease. *J. Natl. Cancer Inst.* **81**, 1097–1101.

Trask, D. K., Yaswen, P., Kroepelin, M., Stampfer, M., and Sager, R. (1989). Normal breast cell–specific clone NB-2 and keratin 5 obtained by subtractive hybridization. *Proc. Am. Assoc. Cancer Res.* **30**, 444.

Trent, J., Meltzer, P., Rosenblum, M., Harsh, G., Kinzler, K., Marshall, R., Feinberg, A., and Vogelstein, B. (1986). Evidence for rearrangement, amplification, and expression of c-*myc* in human glioblastoma. *Proc. Natl. Acad. Sci. U.S.A.* **83**, 470–473.

Trent, J. M., Stanbridge, E. J., McBride, H. L., Meese, E. U., Casey, G., Araujo, D. E., Witkowski, C. M., and Nagle, R. B. (1990). Tumorigenicity in human melanoma cell lines controlled by introduction of human chromosome 6. *Science* **247**, 568–571.

Van Amsterdam, J. R., Kho, C.-J., Boylan, M. O., Hoemann, C. D., Sullivan, R. C., and Zarbl, H. (1989). Molecular cloning of transformation effector and suppressor genes. *In* "Recessive Oncogenes and Tumor Suppression" (W. Cavenee, N. Hastie, and E. Stanbridge, eds.), pp. 163–168. Cold Spring Harbor Laboratory Press, Cold Spring Harbor, New York.

Varley, J. M., Armour, J., Swallow, J. E., Jeffreys, A. J., Ponder, B. A. J. T'ang, A. T., Fung, Y.-K. T., Brammar, W. J., and Walker, R. A. (1989). The retinoblastoma gene is frequently altered leading to loss of expression in primary breast tumours. *Oncogene* **4**, 725–729.

Vogelstein, B., Fearon, E. R., Hamilton, S. R., Kern, S. E., Preisinger, A. C., Leppert, M., Nakamura, Y., White, R., Smits, A. M. M., and Bos, J. L. (1988). Genetic alterations during colorectal tumor development. *N. Engl. J. Med.* **319**, 525–532.

Vogelstein, B., Fearon, E. R., Kern, S. E., Hamilton, S. R., Preisinger, A. C., Nakamura, Y., and White, R. (1989). Allelotype of colorectal carcinomas. *Science* **244,** 207–211.

Weinberg, R. A. (1989). Positive and negative controls on cell growth. *Biochemistry* **28,** 8263–8269.

Weinberger, C., Thompson, C. C., Ong, E. S., Lebo, R., Gruol, D. J., and Evans, R. M. (1986). The c-*erb*-A gene encodes a thyroid hormone receptor. *Nature (London)* **324,** 641–646.

Weissman, B. E., Saxon, P. J., Pasquale, S. R., Jones, G. R., Geiser, A. G., and Stanbridge, E. J. (1987). Introduction of a normal human chromosome 11 into a Wilms' tumour cell line controls its tumorigenic expression. *Science* **236,** 175–180.

Weston, A., Willey, J. C., Modali, R., Sugimura, H., McDowell, E. M., Resau, J., Light, B., Haugen, A., Mann, D. L., Trump, B. F., and Harris, C. C. (1989). Differential DNA sequence deletions from chromosomes 3, 11, 13, and 17 in squamous-cell carcinoma, large-cell carcinoma, and adenocarcinoma of the human lung. *Proc. Natl. Acad. Sci. U.S.A.* **86,** 5099–5103.

Whyte, P., Buchkovich, K. J., Horowitz, J. M., Friend, S. H., Raybuck, M., Weinberg, R. A., and Harlow, E. (1988). Association between an oncogene and an antioncogene: The adenovirus E1A proteins bind to the retinoblastoma gene product. *Nature (London)* **334,** 124–129.

Whyte, P., Williamson, N. M., and Harlow, E. (1989). Cellular targets for transformation by adenovirus E1A proteins. *Cell* **56,** 67–75.

Wildrick, D. M., and Boman, B. M. (1988). Chromosome 5 allele loss at the glucocorticoid receptor locus in human colorectal carcinoma. *Biochem. Biophys. Res. Commun.* **150,** 591–598.

Wolf, D., Laver-Rudich, Z., and Rotter, V. (1985). *In vitro* expression of human p53 cDNA clones and characterization of the cloned human p53 gene. *Mol. Cell. Biol.* **5,** 1887–1893.

Xu, G., O'Connell, P., Viskochil, D., Cawthon, R., Robertson, M., Culver, M., Dunn, D., Stevens, J., Gesteland, R., White, R., and Weiss, R. (1990). The neurofibromatosis type 1 gene encodes a protein related to GAP. *Cell* **62,** 599–608.

Yee, S.-P., and Branton, P. E. (1985). Detection of cellular proteins associated with human adenovirus type 5 early region 1A polypeptides. *Virology* **147,** 142–153.

Yokota, J., Wada, M., Shimosato, Y., Terada, M., and Sugimura, T. (1987). Loss of heterozygosity on chromosomes 3, 13, 17 in small-cell carcinoma and on chromosome 3 in adenocarcinoma of the lung. *Proc. Nat. Acad. Sci. U.S.A.* **84,** 9252–9256.

Zakut-Houri, R., Oren, M., Bienz, B., Lavie, V., Hazum, S., and Givol, D. (1983). A single gene and a pseudogene for the cellular tumour antigen p53. *Nature (London)* **306,** 594–597.

Zakut-Houri, R., Bienz-Tadmor, B., Givol, D., and Oren, M. (1985). Human p53 cellular tumor antigen: cDNA sequence and expression in COS cells. *EMBO J.* **4,** 1251–1255.

Zbar, B., Brauch, H., Talmadge, C., and Linehan, M. (1987). Loss of alleles or loci on the short arm of chromosome 3 in renal cell carcinoma. *Nature (London)* **327,** 721–724.

Zhang, W., Hirohashi, S., Tsuda, H., Shimosato, Y., Yokota, J., Terada, M., and Sugimura, T. (1990). Frequent loss of heterozygosity on chromosomes 16 and 4 in human hepatocellular carcinoma. *Jpn. J. Cancer Res.* **81,** 108–111.

Chapter 2

Protein Kinase C in Neoplastic Cells

Susan A. Rotenberg* and I. Bernard Weinstein[†]

*Department of Chemistry and Biochemistry, Queens College,
City University of New York, Flushing, New York 11367 and
[†]Institute of Cancer Research, Columbia University, New York, New York, 10032

I. Introduction

A. Protein Kinase C and Signal Transduction

Regulated cell growth is a consequence of successful communication by a physiological growth signal with cellular metabolism. It is initiated by an interaction between an extracellular growth factor and its membrane-bound receptor, conveyed via discrete biochemical reactions of finite duration, and ultimately implemented by altered gene expression. Over the last 10 years, research efforts have focused on elucidating the initiating events occurring at the plasma membrane whereby the extracellular signal is transduced into an intracellular message. Our current understanding of this process envisions a complex network of as yet ill-defined growth factor–activated pathways, many of which share a series of early enzymatic reactions, including protein phosphorylation. One vital component of these early events is protein kinase C (PKC).

PKC is a Ca^{2+}- and phospholipid-dependent protein kinase that phosphorylates

BIOCHEMICAL AND MOLECULAR ASPECTS
OF SELECTED CANCERS, VOL. 1

intracellular substrates on serine and threonine residues (Kikkawa *et al.*, 1982). The enzyme is a monomer consisting of a regulatory domain in the N-terminal region, notable for its two cysteine-rich segments and pseudosubstrate segment, and a catalytic domain in the C-terminal region that resembles catalytic domains of other protein kinases by the presence of a characteristic ATP-binding site. PKC has notable hydrophobic character (Coussens *et al.*, 1986) and is believed to be reversibly associated with cellular membranes during quiescence (Kikkawa *et al.*, 1982). Current models of PKC structure (see Fig. 1) depict inactive PKC as having its N-terminal pseudosubstrate segment tucked into the protein structure and in contact with the substrate binding site; this folded, inactive form undergoes a conformational change upon addition of PKC activators (Ca^{2+}, diacylglycerol plus phospholipid, or phorbol ester tumor promoter plus phospholipid), such that the enzyme autophosphorylates and physiological substrates are admitted to the binding site (House and Kemp, 1987; Weinstein, 1988a).

In the context of signal transduction, intracellular activation of PKC is generally believed to occur via growth factor receptor–mediated activation of phospholipase C (reviewed in Nishizuka, 1986a and Huang, 1989). Phospholipase C can be directly activated *in vitro* and *in vivo* by phosphorylation on tyrosine residues by either the platelet-derived growth factor receptor kinase (Meisenhelder *et al.*, 1989) or the epidermal growth factor receptor kinase (Margolis *et al.*, 1989). Upon being activated, phospholipase C in turn causes the hydrolysis of phosphatidylinositol- 4,5-bisphosphate into (1) diacylglycerol (DAG), which is a direct activator of PKC and (2) inositol 1,4,5-trisphosphate (IP_3), which triggers mobilization of Ca^{2+} from endoplasmic reticulum stores. Recent evidence indicates that phospholipase C can also use phosphatidylcholine (reviewed in Exton, 1990) or inositol-containing glycolipid (Chan *et al.*, 1989) as a source of DAG. Other studies indicate that DAG levels can also be elevated by phospholipase D activation (Pai *et al.*, 1991) and by *de novo* synthesis (Chiarugi *et al.*, 1989). Acting together, the elevation in DAG and Ca^{2+} levels activates PKC which in turn, participates in numerous growth factor–mediated signaling pathways, as shown in Fig. 2.

Coincident with the transitory rise in intracellular Ca^{2+} and DAG required to cause activation of PKC, a tighter association of PKC with the membrane occurs (Kikkawa *et al.*, 1982). The evidence for this phenomenon is much stronger for the phorbol ester tumor promoters, which act similar to DAG (Sharkey *et al.*, 1984) but are much more potent activators of PKC and are metabolized much more slowly, (Nishizuka, 1986b), thus accounting for what is thought to be an exaggerated DAG-like effect. (Some apparent differences between phorbol esters and DAG exist, however, as discussed in Section I, B.) The phorbol ester–driven irreversible complexing of PKC with cellular membranes is customarily referred to as *translocation*. This is an operational term since in lysates of unstimulated

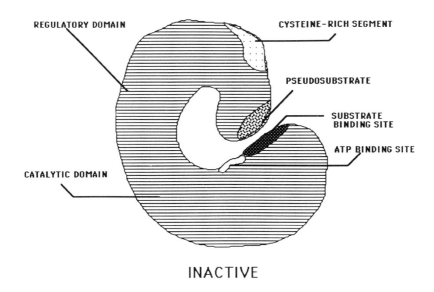

REGULATORY DOMAIN

CYSTEINE-RICH SEGMENT

PSEUDOSUBSTRATE

SUBSTRATE BINDING SITE

ATP BINDING SITE

CATALYTIC DOMAIN

INACTIVE

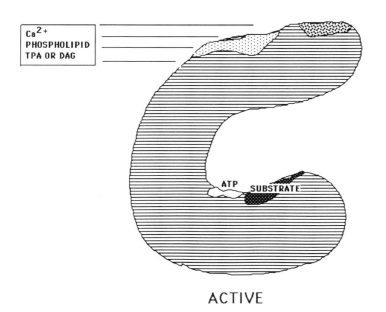

Ca^{2+}
PHOSPHOLIPID
TPA OR DAG

ATP SUBSTRATE

ACTIVE

FIG. 1. Hypothetical scheme depicting the inactive (top) and active (bottom) conformations of PKC.

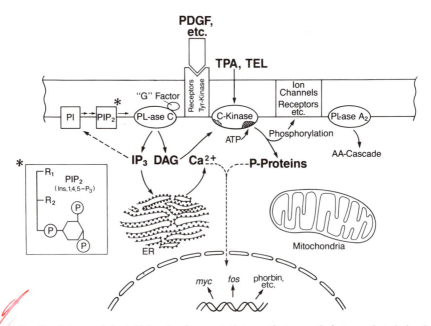

FIG. 2. Scheme of the initial molecular events that constitute growth factor–activated signal transduction. PDGF, platelet-derived growth factor; PI, phosphatidylinositol; PIP$_2$, phosphatidylinositol 4,5-bisphosphate; IP$_3$, inositol 1,4,5-trisphosphate; PL-ase C, phospholipase C; C-kinase, protein kinase C; DAG, diacylglycerol; TPA, 12-O-tetradecanoyl phorbol-13-acetate; TEL, teleocidin; PL-ase A$_2$, phospholipase A$_2$; AA, arachidonic acid; P-proteins, phosphoproteins; ER, endoplasmic reticulum.

cells, the association of PKC with the particulate fraction is dependent on the presence of Ca^{2+}; when Ca^{2+} chelators are added to the lysis buffer, PKC activity is associated primarily with the soluble fraction. When the effect of phorbol esters on PKC distribution is studied using Ca^{2+} chelators in the subcellular fractionation procedure, PKC activity becomes tightly associated with the particulate fraction (Kikkawa *et al.*, 1982). The transition from a state in which the association of PKC with the membrane is reversible and Ca^{2+}-dependent (abrogated with Ca^{2+} chelators), to a state in which the enzyme is Ca^{2+}-independent (Bazzi and Nelsestuen, 1988b) and dissociable only by detergents (Kraft and Anderson, 1983) is a phenomenon for which the physical basis and physiological significance are not well understood.

In *in vitro* assay systems, PKC activity is monitored by the phosphorylation of some exogenous substrate, such as histone IIIS or an octapeptide that represents a site of the epidermal growth factor (EGF) receptor phosphorylated by PKC *in vivo* (see below). PKC-mediated phosphorylation of an artificial substrate is measured in the presence and absence of 0.5 mmol/liter Ca^{2+} plus phospholipid micelles, typically phosphatidylserine; the difference in substrate phosphorylation occurring under these conditions is taken as the phospholipid- and Ca^{2+}-dependent kinase activity that defines PKC. The inclusion of DAG or 12-*O*-tetradecanoylphorbol-13-acetate (TPA) in this assay system dramatically lowers to low micromolar levels the Ca^{2+} required for maximal activity (Nishizuka, 1984).

Numerous studies have described both soluble and membrane-associated PKC substrates. Most prominent among them is the 80- to 87-kDa protein substrate, which was initially identified by its apparent molecular mass on SDS-PAGE (polyacrylamide gel electrophoresis). This protein has been detected in both the soluble and particulate fractions of a wide variety of tissues (Albert *et al.*, 1986). The membrane-bound form is extractable with nonionic detergents but not with high salt concentrations; this tight association has been attributed to the covalent attachment of a myristoyl moiety (Aderem *et al.*, 1988), a modification apparently not essential to its substrate function *in vivo* (Graff *et al.*, 1989a). Recent cloning of the 87-kDa protein (Stumpo *et al.*, 1989) predicts a protein having 335 amino acids (MW = 31,949), which is highly enriched in alanine residues. Based on the known characteristics of the protein, it has been named the MARCKS protein (myristoylated alanine-rich C-kinase substrate). No enzymatic function has yet been assigned to this PKC substrate. There is evidence, however, suggesting that the MARCKS protein participates in both calmodulin and PKC-related pathways. This possibility was implied by the observation that calmodulin can bind the MARCKS protein with nanomolar specificity. Upon phosphorylation of the MARCKS protein by PKC, calmodulin is released from the complex (Graff *et al.*, 1989b).

Because one of the initial events elicited by several extracellular agonists is the activation of ion-transport processes, the observation that PKC phosphorylates proteins that regulate ion channels has identified a class of PKC substrates having physiological significance (reviewed in Shearman *et al.*, 1989b). In addition, the EGF receptor–kinase is phosphorylated at threonine-654 by PKC both *in vitro* and *in vivo* (Hunter *et al.*, 1984), an event that has been associated with a lower affinity–binding interaction of EGF with its receptor and, consequently, a decrease in the intrinsic tyrosine protein kinase activity of the receptor (Cochet *et al.*, 1984), and other EGF receptor–mediated responses (Decker *et al.*, 1990). Other proteins that are substrates of PKC in various cell systems include a 40-kDa protein that is the major PKC substrate in platelets (Castagna *et al.*, 1982), pp60[src] (Gould *et al.*, 1985), the insulin receptor (Bollag *et al.*, 1986), p21 *ras* (Jeng *et al.*, 1987), the cytoskeletal proteins vinculin (Werth *et al.*, 1983) and talin (Beckerle, 1990), the nuclear envelope protein lamin B (Hornbeck *et al.*, 1988; Fields *et al.*, 1988), topoisomerase I (Samuels *et al.*,

1989), RNA polymerase II (Chuang *et al.*, 1989), and many others (Nishizuka, 1986a). The precise physiological significance of these substrates in signal transduction pathways that involve PKC is presently unknown.

B. Protein Kinase C and Tumor Promoters

In addition to serving an intricately orchestrated role in regulated signal transduction, PKC is recognized as instrumental to carcinogenesis (Nishizuka, 1984; Weinstein, 1988a). This recognition stems from the landmark work of Castagna and Nishizuka (Castagna *et al.*, 1982), which demonstrated that phorbol ester tumor promoters like TPA are potent and selective activators of PKC. Corroborative evidence was also obtained by others, including evidence that the phorbol ester receptor copurifies with protein kinase C (Niedel *et al.*, 1983). Recent evidence has shown that phorbol ester binding to the enzyme requires the presence of at least one of the cysteine-rich sequences in the regulatory domains (Ono *et al.*, 1989b). In causing PKC activation, phorbol esters are generally regarded as a substitute for DAG (Sharkey *et al.*, 1984; Jaken, 1985), thereby circumventing the stimulus by growth factors and the programmed sequence of events normally preceding PKC activation. Compared with the transitory presence of DAG during signal transduction, it is possible that the slow rate of metabolism of phorbol esters, coupled with its very high affinity for PKC, enables persistent activation of PKC, thereby producing their sustained mitogenic and tumor-promoting effects (Nishizuka, 1986b). It is of interest to note that two other classes of potent tumor promoters on mouse skin, teleocidin and aplysiatoxin, are also potent activators of PKC (Arcoleo and Weinstein, 1985).

A striking difference in the intracellular behavior of tumor promoters, when compared with DAG, is that phorbol esters can cause the down-regulation of PKC. The phenomenon of down-regulation has been attributed to proteolytic degradation by calpain, a Ca^{2+}-dependent protease (Nishizuka, 1986a), rather than to decreased expression at the level of mRNA (Young *et al.*, 1987). Although the extent and consequences of PKC proteolysis have yet to be elucidated, it is thought that either this event terminates the signal by complete proteolysis of PKC, or that owing to incomplete proteolysis, the catalytic fragment is released from the membrane and thus the constraints of the regulatory subunit that exist in the holoenzyme. It has been speculated that the catalytic fragment could then assume a distinct physiological function in the cytosol (Murray *et al.*, 1987; see also Melloni *et al.*, 1987). It should be stressed, however, that thus far there is no direct evidence for this idea.

That phorbol esters, but not DAG, have been found to cause the down-regulation of the enzyme could be attributed to the short-lived action of DAG during signal transduction (Nishizuka, 1986b). Thus, it is possible that DAG can cause down-regulation of PKC under conditions that sustain its presence in the cell.

Studies with compound R 59 022, which inhibits DAG kinase and thus leads to a sustained elevation of DAG (de Chaffoy de Courcelles *et al.*, 1985) and a pronounced activation of PKC *in vivo* (Nunn and Watson, 1987; Morris *et al.*, 1988), have not, however, yielded any evidence of PKC down-regulation. Similarly, the use of 1,2-dioctanoylglycerol (DiC$_8$), a cell-permeant analog of DAG, has not been shown to down-regulate PKC, although DiC$_8$ can produce a transient translocation of PKC (Issandou and Darbon, 1988). Evidence correlating elevated diacylglycerol levels with PKC down-regulation has been obtained, however, with cells transfected with the *ras* oncogene (see Section II,B).

The ability of phorbol esters to cause irreversible redistribution of PKC from the cytosol to the membrane fraction has been known since 1982 (Kraft *et al.*, 1982; Kikkawa *et al.*, 1982). Thus, phorbol esters can cause pronounced redistribution of PKC into membranes under conditions where growth factors, which operate through DAG, produce virtually undetectable membrane association of PKC. This was observed in 3T3-L1 fibroblasts, for example, in which phorbol ester treatment produced massive translocation of PKC, but no redistribution could be detected with platelet-derived growth factor, fibroblast growth factor, or bombesin (Halsey *et al.*, 1987). It is of interest to note that in the same study, DiC$_8$, a DAG analog, produced a small and transient association of PKC with the membrane fraction. Hence, if PKC redistribution occurs at all with growth factors, the absence of any detectable translocation may be attributable to a very short-lived association that is lost during fractionation procedures. This difference in effect by phorbol esters and DAG was also demonstrated in the *in vitro* phospholipid micelle system of Bazzi and Nelsestuen (1988a, 1988b, 1989). In their two-stage model of the Ca^{2+}-dependent association of PKC with phospholipid micelles, phorbol esters, like DAG, fostered the formation of a reversible complex that could be terminated by Ca^{2+} chelators. In the second stage of this model system, phorbol esters and, to a very small degree, DAG, could promote the formation of an irreversible complex *in vitro* (Bazzi and Nelsestuen, 1989) whereby the enzyme is physically inserted into the bilayer and becomes constitutively active. This mechanism has been invoked as a basis for long-term cell potentiation in the central nervous system (Bazzi and Nelsestuen, 1988b; Burgoyne, 1989). The precise molecular mechanism, however, is not known.

In several cell systems the activation of PKC by tumor promoters leads to increased phosphorylation of the previously mentioned 80-kDa protein (Chida *et al.*, 1986; Aderem *et al.*, 1988). In an effort to characterize the phosphorylation of this PKC substrate in the progression from the preneoplastic-to-neoplastic phenotype, Colburn and her colleagues utilized JB6 mouse epidermal cell variants, which have provided a model for studying late-stage tumor promotion. This model includes two tumorigenic JB6 cell lines, which were established by clonal selection of cells treated with TPA and exhibit anchorage-independent growth in the absence of tumor promoters. The P$^+$ cells are irreversibly transformed by addition of phorbol esters (i.e., anchorage independence and tumorigenicity) while the P^- cells are resistant to induction by promoters.

In their comparison of the phosphorylation of the PKC substrate p80 in pre-neoplastic (P^- or phorbol ester resistant) and neoplastic (P^+ or phorbol ester–sensitive) variants, the amount of ^{32}P incorporated into p80 by the treatment correlated inversely with the degree of transformation. Thus, p80 in P^- cells had a higher incorporation than in P^+ cells (Smith and Colburn, 1988). This effect was later attributed to reduced synthesis (pre- or posttranscriptional) of the p80 protein, and led the authors to suggest a tumor-suppressor role for this PKC substrate. In conjunction with this observation, it was noted that PKC levels (protein and activity) remained constant in both cell lines (Simek et al., 1989).

There is evidence that phorbol ester tumor promoters can stimulate PKC in the absence of Ca^{2+} (Arcoleo and Weinstein, 1985), and can even activate PKC, albeit submaximally, in the absence of phosphatidylserine (Da Silva et al., 1990; Rotenberg and Weinstein, unpublished studies). Such exceptions to existing conceptual models imply that phorbol esters can activate cytosolic PKC, dispensing with the requirement for membranes and even resting levels of Ca^{2+}. Observations such as these may, in part, stem from the existence of specific PKC isozymes that exhibit different cofactor requirements for activation, as will be discussed in Section I,C.

The activation of PKC by tumor promoters in the absence of the normal biochemical signals produced during the transition from quiescence to active growth metabolism suggests that the phorbol ester tumor promoters may act by releasing the enzyme from inhibitory constraints operating during cellular quiescence. In this regard, endogenous protein inhibitors of PKC have been identified (Pearson et al., 1990; Aitken et al., 1990). The mechanism of action of these proteins has not been clarified, nor is it known if these inhibitory factors are affected by growth-factor signaling or by tumor promoters. Another biomolecule receiving considerable attention as an endogenous PKC inhibitor is sphingosine (reviewed in Hannun and Bell, 1989). In view of the fundamental role portrayed by PKC in the mitogenic pathway, it is possible that, by overriding inhibitory controls, phorbol ester tumor promoters cause constitutive activation of PKC per se, producing a persistent growth signal and consequently, a state of unregulated growth. This could explain why phorbol esters and related compounds are potent tumor promoters on mouse skin and also potent modulators of cell differentiation (reviewed in Weinstein, 1988a, and Diamond, 1987), while DAG is not (Smart et al., 1988).

In an attempt to dissect the role of PKC in mitogenic pathways of normal and transformed cells, investigators have continued to search for potent and specific inhibitors of PKC. Use of the PKC inhibitors identified to date has been hampered by the low specificity and/or cytotoxicity of the available inhibitors. Intriguing, however, is the finding that several known anticancer agents such as tamoxifen

(O'Brian *et al.*, 1985), dequalinium (Rotenberg *et al.*, 1990b), adriamycin (Wise and Kuo, 1983), trifluoperazine (Schatzman *et al.*, 1981), the antineoplastic lipoidal amine CP-46,665-1 (Shojii *et al.*, 1985), and suramin (Hensey *et al.*, 1989; Mahoney *et al.*, 1990) are all potent inhibitors of PKC *in vitro* (Weinstein, 1988b). With the exception of suramin, which is anionic, the observation that these compounds are lipophilic cations is also consistent with the structures of several other PKC inhibitors so far identified such as sphingosine (Hannun and Bell, 1989), the aminoacridines (Hannun and Bell, 1988), the isoquinoline sulfonamides (Hidaka *et al.*, 1984), staurosporine (Tamaoki *et al.*, 1986) and its more highly PKC-specific derivatives (Davis *et al.*, 1989). Studies indicate that two compounds, CGP 41 251, a derivative of staurosporine (Meyer *et al.*, 1989), and dequalinium (Weiss *et al.*, 1987) also inhibit the growth of transplantable rodent tumors. Because of its purported role in regulating proliferation in many cell types, PKC continues to be a candidate target enzyme for the design of highly specific inhibitors that could have pharmacological significance (Weinstein, 1988a; Weinstein, 1988b; Gescher and Dale, 1989).

C. Protein Kinase C as a Family of Related Isozymes

Over the past five years it has become apparent that PKC exists as a family of at least seven structurally and functionally related isoenzymes whose distribution varies widely among somatic and neural tissues (Kosaka *et al.*, 1988; Nishizuka, 1988; K.-P. Huang *et al.*, 1989). The individual isoforms were originally identified by cloning methods and sequencing techniques using PKC-specific oligonucleotide probes with cDNA libraries from rat brain (Makowske *et al.*, 1986; Knopf *et al.*, 1986; Ono *et al.*, 1986; Housey *et al.*, 1987; Ohno *et al.*, 1987), bovine and human brain (Coussens *et al.*, 1986). These methods revealed that the mammalian genome contains at least six distinct genes that encode a family of PKC enzymes. The first isoforms to be characterized by these methods were the α, β_1/β_2, and γ isoforms (Parker *et al.*, 1986; Kikkawa *et al.*, 1987a) where the two β forms were determined to be splicing variants of the same gene (Ono *et al.*, 1987a; Coussens *et al.*, 1987). Based on their predicted amino acid sequences, all four isotypes share certain attributes described in Fig. 3, including the hinge region that connects the regulatory and catalytic domains and has been identified as one possible site of Ca^{2+} binding (reviewed in Kikkawa *et al.*, 1989 and Huang, 1989). Preparation and identification of the protein products encoded by these cDNAs from homogenates of brain and other tissues has been facilitated by the use of hydroxylapatite chromatography (Huang *et al.*, 1986; Pelosin *et al.*, 1987). The elution pattern of PKC isoenzymes from rat brain typically describes three major peaks designated in order of their elution, types I, II, and III, which by immunochemical analysis correspond to the γ, β_1/β_2 (generally as one peak), and α isoforms, respectively (Kikkawa *et al.*, 1987b).

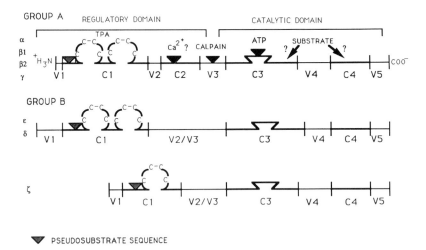

FIG. 3.   Comparison of the structural models of PKC isoforms.

Before the use of cell systems genetically engineered to overproduce a single isoform (Patel and Stabel, 1989; Rotenberg et al., 1990a; Schaap and Parker, 1990; Burns et al., 1990; also see Section II, A), hydroxylapatite chromatography offered the only means to resolve the individual isoforms to determine their biochemical properties. Although helpful in identifying which of the isoforms α, β, γ were present in a given tissue, the method has its implicit limitations for the biochemical characterization of an isoform. This is so because the three peaks often overlap, and the positions of the other isoforms in the elution profile are not known. Hence, there exists the possibility that each PKC type is contaminated by other isoforms.

Three additional members of the PKC family, δ, ε, and ζ, were discovered in mammalian cDNA libraries, by using oligonucleotide probes with less stringent screening conditions (Housey et al., 1987; Ono et al., 1987b). The primary structures of these isoforms contain the same regions of homology found for the four conventional PKC isoforms discussed above, but lack the C_2 region, which is believed to be a possible site of Ca^{2+} binding (Ono et al., 1987b; Ohno et al., 1988; Ono et al., 1989a). Consistent with this structural variation, the δ, ε, and ζ isoforms do not require Ca^{2+} for enzymatic activity. The three isoforms have been expressed individually in COS monkey cells (a commonly used transient expression system), isolated, and characterized as enzymes. This approach demonstrated that the δ and ε isoforms resemble the α, β, and γ forms in that they exhibit dependence on DAG and phospholipid with respect to kinase activity, phorbol ester binding, and translocation to the membrane fraction (Ono et al., 1988; Schaap and Parker, 1990). Interestingly, the δ and ε isoforms exhibit a threefold lower sensitivity to activation by phorbol ester tumor promoters than the α, β, γ isoforms (Akita *et al.*, 1990). Another difference that exists is the apparent *in vitro* substrate specificity of these isoforms. The ε isoform, for example, shows greatest activity with a peptide substrate modeled after its own pseudosubstrate segment (Schaap *et al.*, 1989). Compared to all isoforms studied, the ζ isoform has the lowest homology, is apparently independent of DAG, and does not bind phorbol esters, suggesting that this form is a distinct subspecies (Ono *et al.*, 1989a).

It has been suggested that the δ, ε, and ζ PKC isoforms might participate in signaling pathways distinct from those of the α, β, γ subspecies (Ono *et al.*, 1989a; Akita *et al.*, 1990; Schaap and Parker, 1990). The question as to whether the diversity of PKC isoforms is an indication of multiple PKC-dependent transduction pathways (Dreher and Hanley, 1987; Ono and Kikkawa, 1987) is still unresolved. Studies of the biochemical characteristics of types I, II, and III isolated chromatographically using hydroxylapatite from rat brain (K.-P. Huang *et al.*, 1988), bovine brain (Marais and Parker, 1989), or HL-60 cells (Beh *et al.*, 1989) demonstrated differences in the sensitivities of these conventional isoforms to activation by phorbol esters and DAG, as well as differences in substrate specificities *in vitro*. Similarly, in an *in vitro* study by K.-P. Huang *et al.*, (1988), differences in PKC activation by phorbol ester or DAG were unmasked when cardiolipin was used in place of phosphatidylserine. There have been reports claiming that arachidonic acid activates PKC type II moderately, and type III strongly, in a Ca^{2+}-dependent manner, and type I only slightly, irrespective of the Ca^{2+} concentration (Sekiguchi *et al.*, 1987). In order to detect stimulation of PKC by arachidonic acid, however, it was necessary to use high lipid concentrations (10^{-4} mol/liter). In our work with overproduced PKC-β_1 (see Section II,A), and in contrast with earlier essays of type II PKC (Nishizuka, 1988; Shearman *et al.*, 1989a), we have shown that this isoform is markedly activated by arachidonic acid in a Ca^{2+}-dependent manner. Furthermore, the maximal stimulation was achieved with 70 μmol/liter lipid and represented 55% of the activation produced when we used Ca^{2+} and phosphatidylserine in a parallel assay (Rotenberg *et al.*, 1990a). These studies demonstrated that low micromolar levels of arachidonic acid can indeed activate PKC-β_1 *in vitro*. Whether or not physiological concentrations of arachidonic acid play a role in activating PKC isoforms *in vivo* remains to be determined.

Other *in vitro* studies have indicated that the α, β, γ isoforms display differential sensitivities to the Ca^{2+}-dependent neutral protease calpain, (Kishimoto *et al.*, 1989), and to trypsin (F.L. Huang *et al.*, 1989). In the latter study, γ was the most and α, the least sensitive to proteolysis, suggesting that the isoforms may undergo different rates of *in vivo* degradation. The relevance of the *in vitro* findings was demonstrated in the same study by F.L. Huang *et al.*, (1989) with rat basophilic leukemia RBL-2H3 cells, which contain PKC types II and III (i.e.,

β and α, respectively). It was seen by immunoblot analysis using isozyme-specific antisera that, following treatment of cells with TPA, type II enzyme was degraded faster than type III, consistent with the *in vitro* studies.

Other evidence for behavioral differences of PKC isoforms was found in HL-60 cells with two isoforms that were not identified immunochemically but could be resolved by hydroxylapatite. *In vitro*, the two isoforms exhibited sensitivities to TPA-mediated activation that differed by two orders of magnitude (3 nmol/liter versus 100 nmol/liter). *In vivo*, however, both isoforms were observed to translocate similar to the particulate fraction as a function of TPA concentration (Beh *et al.*, 1989). In a related study, Fournier *et al.*, (1989), working with platelets, found that phorbol esters induced a differential association with the membrane of PKC subspecies α and β, which were identified immunochemically; the α subspecies rapidly accumulated in the particulate fraction in the presence of 150 nmol/liter TPA, while the β subspecies remained entirely in the soluble fraction. A similar pattern of isozyme behavior with TPA was observed in BC3H-1 myocytes (Cooper *et al.*, 1989) and leukemic T cells (Isakov *et al.*, 1990). In KM3 cells, a pre-B, pre-T cell line, however, the response to TPA was reversed: type II PKC was translocated and depleted more quickly than type III PKC (Ase *et al.*, 1988a).

The above examples of selective degradation, different patterns of activation and translocation by phorbol esters, differential cellular expression of PKC isoforms under different conditions (to be discussed in Section II, C), and the regiospecificity of isoform distribution in the central nervous system and other tissues (Nishizuka, 1988), suggest the possibility that PKC isoforms exhibit independent activities *in vivo* (Huang *et al.*, 1989; Kosaka *et al.*, 1988). This possibility has yet to be demonstrated by more direct evidence, such as the identification of isoform-specific *in vivo* substrates. As discussed below, the question of isoform-specific pathways is also directly relevant to the biology of specific tumors.

II. Cellular Models: Evidence for a Role of Protein Kinase C in Growth Regulation

A. CELL SYSTEMS GENETICALLY ENGINEERED TO OVERPRODUCE A SINGLE ISOFORM OF PROTEIN KINASE C

With an intention to elucidate the role(s) of specific isoforms of PKC in growth control and tumor promotion, our laboratory and other laboratories have constructed cell lines that stably produce elevated levels of a single isoform (Housey *et al.*, 1988; Persons *et al.*, 1988; Krauss *et al.*, 1989; Hsieh *et al.*, 1989; Cuadrado *et al.*, 1990). Such systems have led to the general conclusion that, although overexpression of PKC causes disturbances to growth control, it is not sufficient to cause complete cellular transformation. Moreover, the particular cell type selected for study determines the extent and nature of the growth disorder. For example, the overproduction of the rat brain β_1-isoform by 50-fold in rat 6 fibroblasts (Housey *et al.*, 1988) produced a higher saturation density in monolayer cultures and, at postconfluence, small, dense foci. These cells could also form colonies in soft agar in contrast to control cells, which were completely anchorage-dependent. Compared with control cells, treatment of the PKC-over-producing cells with TPA caused a dramatic enhancement of morphological changes. Similarly, when the β_1-isoform was overproduced by 11-fold in the mouse embryo fibroblast cell line C3H 10T1/2 (Krauss *et al.*, 1989), there was observed a pronounced morphological response to TPA, cell growth to a higher saturation density, decreased adhesiveness, and, when treated with TPA for 2 to 3 weeks postconfluence, large, dense foci occurred. Although somewhat altered morphologically in the absence of TPA, these cells did not exhibit a transformed morphology, nor were they capable of growing in soft agar or tumorigenic in nude mice. In rat liver epithelial cells, the third cell line constructed to overpro-duce PKC-β_1 (Hsieh *et al.*, 1989), there were again, despite a 10-fold higher expression of the enzyme in this cell type, no gross morphological changes char-acteristic of the transformed phenotype with regard to anchorage independence or tumorigenicity.

Other laboratories have employed similar methods to study the effects of stable overexpression of the PKC γ-isoform. In two independent studies with NIH 3T3 cells, stable overproduction of PKC-γ at a level twofold (Persons *et al.*, 1988) or threefold (Cuadrado *et al.*, 1990) higher than the PKC activity found in con-trol cells (namely, endogenous PKC-α) did not yield morphological characteris-tics of transformation (i.e., focus formation). Like the β_1-overproducing sys-tems, PKC-γ transfected cells grew to higher saturation densities. The authors observed enhanced growth in semisolid medium in the presence of TPA and a pronounced proliferative response to either TPA or cardiolipin, both mitogens of this cell line (Cuadrado *et al.*, 1990). Furthermore, following the inoculation of nude mice with these cells, their tumorigenicity could be demonstrated (Persons *et al.*, 1988). Although the role of PKC in growth regulation is complex and only poorly understood, these studies provide direct evidence for its role in growth control and in events relevant to tumor promotion and carcinogenesis.

In an effort to elucidate the significance of various structural domains of the PKC protein with respect to signal transduction or tumor promotion, recent stud-ies have developed site-specific mutants. In a study by Muramatsu *et al.*, (1989), a truncated construct of PKC-α was prepared that lacked the DNA sequence corresponding to the amino acids #6–159 of the regulatory domain. Transfec-tion of this truncated cDNA into cells produced a protein product that could no longer bind phorbol ester. As this protein primarily represented the catalytic subunit of PKC, its activity would be expressed constitutively. The authors used two *in vivo* assay methods by which to detect the constitutive PKC activity, that is, activation of the c-*fos* gene enhancer in Jurkat cells, and activation of IL-2 expression in T cells. Because the activation of IL-2 production required the presence of a Ca^{2+}-dependent ionophore, the authors further suggested that this could mean the cooperation of Ca^{2+}- and PKC-dependent pathways. It should be pointed out that this truncated version of PKC was not characterized biochemically, and thus actually proved to be Ca^{2+}-independent. However, it may well have represented the functional equivalent of the catalytic fragment of PKC. If such was the case, the expression of constitutively active PKC in the presence of Ca^{2+} led to the release of an autocrine factor that promotes proliferation in T cells. In this light, constitutively active mutants of PKC could potentially act as oncogenes.

In another study, Megidish and Mazurak (1989) sequenced PKC-α from fibrosarcoma cells derived from tumors that had been induced by UV-irradiation of mice. The results showed that these cells possessed a mutant form of PKC-α. Furthermore, the sequencing data revealed four point mutations of which three were in a highly conserved region of the regulatory domain (Ile[106] $\rightarrow$ Val; Ser[111] $\rightarrow$ Gly; Leu[240] $\rightarrow$ Gln), and one was in a conserved region of the catalytic domain (Phe[339]$\rightarrow$ Leu). By contrast with normal PKC-α cDNA, transfection of the mutant PKC-α cDNA into untransformed Balb/c 3T3 cells resulted in a large distribution of the PKC mutant protein into the membrane (also observed in the fibrosarcoma cells). Most importantly, these cells formed dense foci, exhibited anchorage-independent growth and induced solid tumors in nude mice. The significance of these point mutations to the enzymatic function of the mutant PKC was not explored in detail, leaving unresolved whether one or more of the reported mutations was (were) responsible for the transforming activity of this PKC mutant.

In a recent study by Ohno and his colleagues (1990), site-directed mutagenesis at the putative ATP-binding site of PKC eliminated kinase activity and rendered the enzyme insensitive to down-regulation, implying a functional link between autophosphorylation and down-regulation. In a related report, Flint *et al.*, (1990) demonstrated that PKC activated *in vitro* exhibits six phosphorylation sites, two of which occur at the hinge region, the target site of calpain. One interpretation emerging from these findings depicts the following scenario: phorbol ester tumor promoter binds to PKC, which is activated coincident with its autophosphorylation; this reaction causes a major conformational change in PKC such that calpain-specific cleavage sites in the hinge region are made accessible by phosphorylation, and the protein is degraded to completion and/or the catalytic fragment, as discussed in Section I,B. Future studies carried out similarly with PKC mutants, in which changes have been made in various regions of the molecule, offer a rigorous approach by which the mechanism of PKC activation and regulation can be dissected.

B. Transformed Cell Systems: Synergy between Protein Kinase C and *Ras*

Over the last five years, studies have examined the role of PKC in cell transformation, induced by specific oncogenes. The initial observation by Hsiao *et al.*, (1984) that tumor promoters markedly enhanced the formation of foci of mouse embryo fibroblasts transfected with an activated c-H-*ras* oncogene, stimulated further investigation into the complementary functions contributed to multistage carcinogenesis by tumor promoters (via PKC) and a carcinogen-activated oncogene (Balmain *et al.*, 1984; Dotto *et al.*, 1985).

Since these initial experiments were carried out, more recent studies have sought to establish a mechanistic basis for the synergy between phorbol ester tumor promoters and *ras* in cellular transformation and carcinogenesis (Hsiao *et al.*, 1989). There has been a particular emphasis to include principles emerging from studies of mitogenic signal transduction pathways (reviewed in Haliotis *et al.*, 1988). In this regard, the H-*ras* oncogene product was shown to have a direct effect on the mitogenic response of Swiss 3T3 fibroblasts to phorbol esters. This was demonstrated by the mitogenic activity evoked by microinjection of the H-*ras* p21 protein into quiescent cells. Furthermore, it was found that down-regulation of PKC by chronic treatment with TPA followed by microinjection of H-*ras* p21 resulted in a marked decrease in this mitogenic response (Lacal *et al.*, 1987). The *ras*-transformed fibroblasts displayed increased phosphatidylinositol (M. Huang *et al.*, 1988), and increased phosphatidylcholine metabolism (Teegarden *et al.*, 1990; Lopez-Barahona *et al.*, 1990), with concomitant elevation in DAG levels (Kato *et al.*, 1988; M. Huang *et al.*, 1988). The sustained higher levels of DAG were also partially accounted for by a defect in DAG kinase translocation in *ras*-transformed NIH/3T3 cells (Kato *et al.*, 1988; Wolfman *et al.*, 1987) and in H-*ras*–transformed 208F rat fibroblasts (M. Huang *et al.*, 1988). The effects of activated *ras* expression on PKC in these cell systems appear to have been at least partly mediated by the persistent elevation of DAG levels and inositol phosphates which, in turn led to continuous PKC activation and constitutive signaling to the nucleus.

The intracellular expression of an activated *ras* oncogene has been associated with partial down-regulation of PKC in C3H 10T1/2 cells (Weyman *et al.*, 1988), in NIH 3T3 cells (Wolfman *et al.*, 1987), and in 208F rat fibroblasts (M. Huang *et al.*, 1988). In view of other evidence (Section I,B and Borner *et al.*, 1990), this phenomenon of PKC down-regulation by an activated *ras* protein cannot simply be ascribed to elevated DAG levels. In fact, other metabolic pathways are activated by the *ras* protein (see below, this section). Nevertheless, because PKC was only partially down-regulated in these cell systems, it was suggested (Wolfman *et al.*, 1987) that the endogenous PKC isoforms that are expressed in these cell systems may be differentially modulated. Recent studies indicate that transfection of *ras* into rat 6 fibroblasts is associated with selective down-regulation of endogenous PKC isoforms. In these cells it was observed at both the levels of protein and mRNA that PKC-α was increased while PKC-ε was decreased in abundance (Borner *et al.*, 1990).

Coincident with down-regulation of PKC in *ras*-transfectants of NIH 3T3 cells was a corresponding decrease in the levels of the 80-kDa substrate (Wolfman *et al.*, 1987). It is not known whether this represents a *ras*-induced loss of a protein serving a tumor-suppressor function, as has been suggested for JB6 cells (see Section I,B), or if the loss of the 80-kDa substrate implicates a cellular mechanism to modulate the signal(s) produced by the *ras* oncogene protein.

That the synergy between *ras* and PKC is necessary for transformation was supported by a study by Hsiao *et al.* (1989). When normal rat 6 fibroblasts were transfected with an activated human H-*ras* oncogene, they showed a low frequency of transformation. However, rat 6 fibroblasts genetically engineered to overproduce PKC-β₁ (Housey *et al.*, 1988; see Section II,A) were extremely sensitive to transformation by this oncogene. The resulting cells formed large colonies in agar, they had a highly transformed morphology, and they were tumorigenic when introduced into nude mice. It is of interest that the rat 6 fibroblasts that overproduce PKC were also more sensitive to transformation by the v-*myc* and v-*fos* oncogenes (W.-L.W. Hsiao, H. Pei, and I.B. Weinstein, unpublished results).

The use of *ras*-transformed cell systems has provided an approach for dissecting the mechanisms of cell transformation. It is becoming clear that, in addition to stimulating phospholipase C and phosphatidylinositol hydrolysis, the *ras*-encoded protein activates other metabolic pathways, including the cyclooxygenase pathway (Hsiao *et al.*, 1990) and phosphatidylcholine hydrolysis (Lopez-Barahona *et al.*, 1990; Teegarden *et al.*, 1990). Despite the pleiotropic effects introduced by transfection of activated *ras* into cell systems (Haliotis *et al.*, 1988), PKC activation via elevated DAG levels appears to be a prominent outcome. The observation that the tyrosine protein kinase products of the oncogenes v-*src* and v-*fms* also cause an increase in steady-state levels of DAG and produce a similar effect on PKC down-regulation (Wolfman *et al.*, 1987) points to the possibility that these oncogene proteins and the *ras* protein employ a common PKC-mediated pathway in bringing about transformation.

Further evidence supporting this suggestion was found with chicken embryo fibroblasts expressing temperature-sensitive derivatives of v-*src* and v-*fps*. It was observed that induction of a transformation-related gene 9E3 by the gene products of v-*src* and v-*fps* was blocked in cells depleted of PKC, enhanced by PKC agonists, inhibited by PKC inhibitors, and was also associated with the phosphorylation of a 67-kDa PKC substrate (Spangler *et al.*, 1989). Although the precise site(s) of phosphorylation necessary for transformation by these oncogenic tyrosine protein kinases are not known, these studies indicate that PKC probably functions downstream of these sites.

An assessment of PKC-α localization in subcellular compartments of transformed cells was recently reported by Hyatt *et al.*, (1990). Using monoclonal antibodies of PKC-α, these authors addressed the distribution of this PKC isoform by immunocytofluorescence in normal and SV40-transformed REF52 cells. The results demonstrated in normal cells that PKC-α is concentrated in focal contacts, since it colocalizes with talin, also known to be an *in vivo* substrate (Beckerle, 1990). By contrast, the distribution of PKC-α in the transformed cells was much more diffuse and not strictly associated with the cytoskeleton. Furthermore, this phenotypic property of transformed cells correlated with the loss of two PKC-α binding proteins of unknown identity. The authors speculated that the alternative pattern of PKC-α subcellular localization may contribute to the transformed phenotype.

C. SELECTIVE REGULATION OF PROTEIN KINASE C ISOFORMS DURING DIFFERENTIATION

With the development of PKC isoform–specific antibodies, tools have become available for probing the relative levels of individual PKC isoforms during cellular programs of growth and differentiation. Of the small number of studies that have been completed to date, all have reported that total PKC activity (Zylber-Katz and Glazer, 1985; Wu *et al.*, 1989; Hashimoto *et al.*, 1990) or levels of specific PKC isoforms fluctuate during differentiation of cells in culture. A correlation of PKC activation–translocation and HL-60 cell maturation, for example, has been drawn (Tran *et al.*, 1989), although PKC activity alone was not sufficient to induce differentiation. Studies of PKC isoforms have included the induction of HL-60 cells by 1,25-dihydroxyvitamin D_3, TPA, retinoic acid, or dimethyl sulfoxide (Makowske *et al.*, 1988; Hashimoto *et al.*, 1990; Obeid *et al.*, 1990), the induction of mouse melanoma cells by retinoic acid (Niles and Loewy, 1989), and the induction of erythroleukemia cells by hexamethylene bisacetamide (HMBA) (Melloni *et al.*, 1989).

In their investigation of the retinoic acid–induced differentiation of the human promyelocytic cell line HL-60 to the mature granulocytic phenotype, Makowske *et al.*, (1988) were the first to profile the relative abundances of the individual PKC isoforms. In this system, the α, β, and γ isoforms, probed by Western blotting analysis with isoform-specific polyclonal antibodies, all increased in abundance following treatment with retinoic acid. Interestingly, they did not all follow the same time course and were not increased to the same extent when the effects induced by retinoic acid were compared with those induced by dimethyl sulfoxide, another inducer of these cells. Conflicting results of the effects of retinoic acid on HL-60 cells were obtained by Hashimoto *et al.* (1990). These authors monitored the abundances of PKC-α and PKC-β and a novel form of PKC identified in these cells and designated peak b; these authors claim that PKC-γ was absent in these cells. The peak b enzyme was distinct from the other isoforms, both with regard to its immunoreactivity with isoform-specific antisera and chromatography on hydroxylapatite. Following treatment with retinoic acid, the peak b enzyme was decreased dramatically within 24 hr, while within 48 hr, PKC-α was reduced twofold, and PKC-β was increased twofold. Overall, the total PKC activity in these cells was decreased 25%.

While treatment of promyelocytic HL-60 cells with retinoic acid or dimethyl sulfoxide cause HL-60 cells to differentiate into granulocytes, the use of 1,25-dihydroxyvitamin D_3 or TPA leads to their conversion into monocytes (Zylber-Katz and Glazer, 1985), implicating a mediating role for PKC in this process as well. Studies examining the effects of 1,25-dihydroxyvitamin D_3 in HL-60 cells have demonstrated an increase in PKC activity and in the number of phorbol ester–binding sites within 24 hr. This effect was inhibited by cycloheximide and thus, was dependent on protein synthesis (Martell *et al.*, 1987). It is of interest to note that steady-state levels of c-*myc* mRNA were observed to decrease in HL-60 cells treated with this inducing agent (Simpson *et al.*, 1987). Other studies have reported inducer-specific endogenous phosphorylation patterns that reflect both PKC-dependent and PKC-independent effects (Zylber-Katz and Glazer, 1985).

Studies of isoform-specific transcriptional regulation during differentiation have employed Northern blotting analysis, i.e., hybridization of isoform-specific cDNA probes to mRNA preparations from cells during progressive stages of differentiation. In this regard, Obeid *et al.* (1990) have examined levels of expression of specific isoforms of PKC in HL-60 cells, followed by the addition of 1,25-dihydroxyvitamin D_3, an inducer of macrophage differentiation in this cell system. It was found that the β-isoform showed a fourfold increase with respect to phorbol ester binding, isoform-specific mRNA levels, and rate of transcription, as determined by nuclear run-on measurements. This was associated with a twofold increase in the phosphorylation of PKC substrates, an event that occurred without the endogenous formation of DAG. Conflicting evidence was reported by Solomon *et al.* (1990) who, also working with HL-60 cells, found that 1,25-dihydroxyvitamin D_3–induced elevations in steady-state levels of PKC-α and PKC-β proteins apparently occurred by a mechanism involving posttranscriptional stabilization of PKC mRNA.

Consistent with the effects of retinoic acid on PKC in HL-60 cells, retinoic acid–mediated induction of mouse melanoma cell differentiation was attended by a large increase in PKC activity (Niles and Loewy, 1989). This effect was documented by measurement of a higher number of phorbol ester–binding sites and an increased amount of immunoreactive PKC protein. When cells were depleted of PKC by prolonged treatment with phorbol ester, melanin production, a property of the differentiated phenotype, was inhibited, and cell growth was accelerated. Although the levels of specific PKC isoforms were not monitored in this study, the elevated level of total PKC during retinoic acid–induced differentiation was consistent with the earlier studies of HL-60 cells (Makowske *et al.*, 1988; Obeid *et al.*, 1990).

In mouse erythroleukemia cells (MELC), Melloni *et al.* (1989) studied the levels of the two principal PKC isoforms α and β using PKC-specific antibodies and found that PKC activity, which is known to be required for induction by HMBA (Melloni *et al.*, 1987), is decreased within 3 hr following HMBA addition, and that this loss was largely attributable to an 80% reduction in the activity of the β-isoform; levels of PKC-α were relatively unchanged by HMBA treatment. Although the precise function of PKC-β was not addressed by these studies, this particular isoform evidently has a direct role at an early stage in the differentiation response, and is subsequently degraded. Interestingly, additional studies demonstrated that when the individual PKC isoforms were introduced into permeablized cells, β but not α could accelerate differentiation induced by HMBA (Melloni *et al.*, 1990).

A mouse neuroblastoma cell line, neuro 2a, which undergoes differentiation *in vitro* in response to various agents was studied with regard to the transcriptional regulation of specific PKC isoforms. Using cDNA probes corresponding to the α, β_1, β_2, γ, ε, and ζ, Wada *et al.* (1989) demonstrated that neuro 2a cells expressed only α, ε, and ζ. During differentiation, decreases in PKC-α and ε mRNA were observed. Furthermore, a recent report demonstrated that H-7 and suramin, both PKC inhibitors (see Section I,A), can induce morphological and functional differentiation of neuro 2a cells (Felipo *et al.*, 1990) and neuroblastoma cell clone NB2A (Hensey *et al.*, 1989), respectively.

Thus, these findings suggest that the expression of PKC isoforms is altered during differentiation. It is possible that this reflects different functions of these isoforms.

D. Effects of Protein Kinase C Activation on Gene Expression

In view of the role of PKC as the intracellular receptor for phorbol esters, the biochemical basis for tumor promotion by TPA apparently originates at the plasma membrane with the activation of PKC. Current thinking on the events that follow envisions a series of events, both cytosolic and nuclear, that produces an altered activity or steady-state level of transcriptional regulator proteins. Consequently, these DNA-binding proteins induce or repress the transcription of genes related to growth control. The participation of cytosolic PKC in this pathway, beyond the phosphorylation event initiated by its activation by TPA, is not presently known to occur, although PKC activity has been detected in nuclei of certain cell types (see Section II,E).

Using differential hybridization techniques, investigators have described the effects of TPA at the genetic level, producing a lengthy list of specific genes whose cellular expression is responsive to treatment by TPA (reviewed in Karin and Herrlich, 1989). One subset of this list contains the early response genes, which include c-*fos*, c-*jun*, and c-*myc*, all of which are likely to be under direct control by TPA via pre-existing transcriptional regulator proteins, since their expression is insensitive to cycloheximide. Other groups of TPA-inducible genes include those that encode protooncogene products, e.g., c-*sis* (Colamonici *et al.*, 1986) and c-*fms* (Rettenmier *et al.*, 1986), various extracellular matrix proteins and proteases, protease inhibitors, viral proteins, and proteins involved in DNA synthesis. Transiently activated genes, as detected in fibroblasts following TPA treatment, include actin, JUN B, EGR$_1$, TIS 8, nur/77 (=TIS 1) (reviewed in Hershman, 1989). Expression of other genes reported to be induced by TPA are those encoding collagenase (Angel *et al.*, 1986), metallothionein IIA (MT IIA) (Angel *et al.*, 1986), stromelysin (Matrisian *et al.*, 1986), ornithine decarboxylase (Rose-John *et al.*, 1987), the glucose transporter (Flier *et al.*, 1987), and the gene encoding the murine tissue inhibitor of metalloprotease (TIMP) (Edwards *et al.*, 1986); this latter inducible gene is also known as TPA-S1 or phorbin (Johnson *et al.*, 1987), and in human tissues, as erythroid-potentiating activity (Gasson *et al.*, 1985). Conversely, TPA treatment has been shown to repress the expression of some géne products such as the major surface LETS protein (Blumberg *et al.*, 1976), collagen (Finer *et al.*, 1985), phosphoenolpyruvate carboxykinase (Chu and Granner, 1986), and TPA-R1 (Johnson *et al.*, 1987).

The altered expression of many of these genes has been traced to the presence of autonomous enhancer elements acting cis to the promoter for the TPA-responsive gene. The existence of these TPA-responsive elements, or TREs, was initially described in association with genes encoding stromelysin (Matrisian *et al.*, 1986), human collagenase (Angel *et al.*, 1987a, 1987b), MT IIA (Karin and Richards, 1982; Imbra and Karin, 1987), c-*jun* (Angel *et al.*, 1988), along with many others. DNAse protection experiments and deletion analysis have shown with the collagenase TRE that there is a minimal TRE, or recognition motif, defined by a seven base–pair palindromic unit, 5′-TGAGTCA-3′. Furthermore, this sequence was found to confer TPA inducibility to various heterologous promoters (Chiu *et al.*, 1987; Angel *et al.*, 1987a; Angel *et al.*, 1987b), whereby constructs carrying multimers of TRE were more efficient than a construct containing a single TRE sequence. Consistent with its proposed function, point mutations in the TRE sequence caused loss of TPA-inducibility (Angel *et al.*, 1987b; Risse *et al.*, 1989). Although the precise mechanism has not been demonstrated, the occupation of TRE sequences by specific DNA-binding proteins is thought to influence gene expression via protein–protein interactions with transcriptional enzymes.

Identification of proteins that bind to TRE sequences was accomplished with either nuclear or whole-cell extracts from cells treated with TPA. Methods of isolation and detection included sequence-specific DNA affinity chromatography over a matrix containing the TRE sequence (Lee *et al.*, 1987), protection of DNA fragments from DNAse digestion (*in vitro* footrpinting), or retarding the electrophoretic migration of a DNA fragment (band-shift assays). TPA treatment of cells was seen to induce the synthesis or posttranslational activation of DNA-binding activity. One of the first mammalian DNA-binding proteins to be identified by these methods was a transcription factor for the SV40 promoter known as AP-1 (Lee *et al.*, 1987; Angel *et al.*, 1987a; Angel *et al.*, 1987b). Now known to be a heterodimer of various species of the *jun* and *fos* proteins (reviewed in Vogt and Bos, 1990), AP-1 is highly specific for a nine base–pair consensus TRE sequence; when this sequence was subjected to point mutations that abolished TPA-inducibility, there was a corresponding loss of AP-1 binding (Lee *et al.*, 1987). Comparison of TRE-binding activities contained in cell extracts from TPA-treated cells and control cells indicated that the abundance or activity of AP-1 increased three- to fourfold within 1 hr of TPA treatment and was unaffected by cycloheximide, suggesting a posttranslational mechanism (Angel *et al.*, 1987b). These studies also demonstrated the specificity of the effect, since levels of several other DNA-binding proteins were not increased by TPA treatment. Furthermore, band-shift experiments indicated that the complex formed between the TRE probe and the TPA-induced factor had the same electrophoretic mobility as a complex of the same probe and purified AP-1 (Angel *et al.*, 1987b). These experiments implied that AP-1 is a component of the TPA-activated signaling pathway. Efforts to identify AP-1 as a possible substrate of PKC have been unsuccessful, however. Thus the precise mechanism by which PKC activation leads to enhanced activity of AP-1 is not known.

In the context of neoplastic transformation, other studies have shown that in JB6 epithelial cells that are genetically susceptible (P^+) or resistant (P^-) to transformation by TPA (see Section I,B), the transformation-sensitive cells had an associated AP-1 activity, whereas the resistant cells did not (Bernstein and Colburn, 1989).

Studies with NF-κB, a transcriptional regulator of the immunoglobulin κ light chain enhancer (reviewed in Lenardo and Baltimore, 1989; Nigg, 1990), have implicated a more direct role for PKC. The NF-κB protein exists in the cytoplasm in an active noncovalent complex with its inhibitor protein IκB. *In vitro* experiments with cytoplasmic extracts of noninduced cells have shown that treatment of IκB with PKC causes its dissociation from the complex. In intact cells, this event would liberate NF-κB such that it can shuttle from the cytoplasm to the nucleus and activate NF-κB–dependent genes. Analogous studies with intact cells have shown that TPA triggers the dissociation of IκB and NF-κB whereby IκB is modified by the presence of TPA (Shirakawa and Mizel, 1989; Baeuerle and Baltimore, 1988). These studies have led to the formulation of a simple model of how transcriptional regulation of the NF-κB gene by TPA may be mediated by PKC.

The participation of PKC in mediating alterations in gene expression was evident with rat liver epithelial cells overexpressing PKC-β_1 (Hsieh *et al.*, 1989; see Section II,A). Northern blotting analysis of RNA using radiolabeled oligonucleotide probes for *fos*, *myc*, and the genes encoding ornithine decarboxylase, and phorbin, indicated that, relative to control cells, expression of *myc* only was enhanced in serum-fed PKC-overproducing cells, and that the expression of all four genes was markedly enhanced in PKC-overproducing cells relative to control cells, when treated with TPA. Furthermore, one gene, TPA-R1, which is constitutively high in untreated parental C3H 10T1/2 cells and repressed by TPA treatment (Johnson *et al.*, 1987), was found to have a much lower level of constitutive expression in untreated C3H 10T1/2 cells overexpressing PKC-β_1 (Krauss *et al.*, 1989). Thus, although the transcriptional effects exerted by the overproduction of PKC-β_1 were not sufficient to cause transformation in the absence of TPA, it was noted that PKC overexpression led to certain constitutive and exaggerated TPA-inducible transcriptional effects.

The study of transcriptional regulators as mediators of TPA-induced gene expression continues to provide important biochemical markers for cellular transformation. The extent to which posttranslational mechanisms, such as phosphorylation–dephosphorylation, play a general role in regulating transcription of TPA-inducible genes remains to be elucidated. Furthermore, it is possible that PKC might also influence the expression of specific genes at the levels of mRNA turnover, translation, or posttranslational modification.

E. PROTEIN KINASE C IN THE NUCLEUS

Using immunocytochemical methods, Kiss *et al.*, (1988) studied the distribution of PKC in HL-60 cells during TPA-induced differentiation. The results of this investigation revealed a time course during which PKC became transiently associated with nuclear membranes. The relocalization of PKC to the nuclear envelope has also been observed in NIH 3T3 cells following treatment with TPA (Thomas *et al.*, 1988; Leach *et al.*, 1989; Fields *et al.*, 1990). In one study with NIH 3T3 cells, it was shown that the nuclear envelope lamins A, B, and C were phosphorylated in response to TPA, while lamins A and C were preferentially phosphorylated in response to platelet-derived growth factor (Fields *et al.*, 1990). Although the consequences and precise site(s) of this nuclear localization are not known, it has been postulated that the changes in PKC distribution could have physiological significance (Kiss *et al.*, 1988). Published studies have thus far not discerned whether PKC activity is confined to peripheral nuclear structures (perinuclear) or is translocated to the intranuclear space (Nigg, 1990). Because the PKC regulatory domain contains two cysteine rich *zinc-finger*–like structures, akin to transcriptional regulatory proteins, other investigators have studied whether PKC binds directly to DNA. Only limited evidence exists, however, to support this possibility (Testori *et al.*, 1988), although the existence of PKC in isolated nuclei has been reported.

Studies of PKC in isolated nuclei are subject to the fundamental criticism of possible contamination by extranuclear PKC. The subcellular fractionation procedures employed to isolate intact nuclei generally do not include a rigorous examination of purity. Perhaps the strongest evidence regarding the existence of, and a physiological role for, a nuclear PKC activity has been obtained by D.H. Russell from studies of isolated rat liver nuclei (Buckley *et al.*, 1988; Russell, 1989). The nuclei used for these studies were pure with respect to their appearance by electron microscopy and with regard to the absence of detectable $5'$-nucleotidase activity. When isolated rat liver nuclei were treated with TPA or prolactin (10^{-12} mol/liter), an established hepatic mitogen, activation by several hundredfold of a protein kinase that exhibited dependency on both phospholipid and Ca^{2+} could be demonstrated in a time- and dose-dependent manner. Furthermore, this nuclear PKC activity was inhibited by H-7, cyclosporine, and sphingosine, all known inhibitors of PKC (Buckley *et al.*, 1988). Purification and biochemical characterization of nuclear PKC (Masmoudi *et al.*, 1989) has since shown it to exhibit an apparent MW of 80 kDa, a higher concentration of Ca^{2+} required for optimal activity, and immunoreactivity with anti-PKC antibodies specific for type II PKC (Rogue *et al.*, 1990).

Of related interest was the finding that erythropoietin was also demonstrated to activate PKC in nuclei isolated from erythroid progenitor cells (Mason-Garcia *et al.*, 1990).

Other isozymes of PKC have been identified with nuclei from other types of cells. Immunochemical assays have detected PKC-α in nuclei from NIH/3T3 cells. This enzyme was activated by TPA, DiC_8, or arachidonic acid (Leach *et al.*, 1989). When nuclei of nerve cells were examined for PKC isoforms, a ζ-related isoform was identified using immunochemical techniques (Hagiwara *et al.*, 1990).

In light of the observation that TPA treatment of nuclei causes activation of nuclear PKC in several independent studies (Buckley *et al.*, 1988; Leach *et al.*, 1989; Rogue *et al.*, 1990), it is possible that there exists an intranuclear phorbol ester signaling pathway. One possible mechanism is that nuclear PKC, activated by TPA, activates (or inhibits) by phosphorylation an enzyme or protein factor that controls DNA transcription. Indeed, TPA treatment of intact HL-60 cells is associated with the phosphorylation of nuclear matrix proteins (Macfarlane, 1986), although the nuclear kinase(s) in these studies was (were) not identified. *In vitro* assays have shown that PKC can phosphorylate RNA polymerase II (Chuang *et al.*, 1989; Lee and Greenleaf, 1989), DNA topoisomerase I (Samuels *et al.*, 1989), and DNA topoisomerase II (Sahyoun *et al.*, 1986); the latter enzyme was also shown in the same study to be activated by PKC. Recent evidence by Pommier *et al.* (1990) demonstrated that DNA topoisomerase I can be activated *in vitro* following phosphorylation by purified PKC from bovine brain. When the native topoisomerase was first dephosphorylated with calf intestine alkaline phosphatase, the activity of DNA topoisomerase I (reflected in DNA relaxation) as well as its sensitivity to camptothecin, a specific inhibitor of the topoisomerase, were abolished; rephosphorylation with purified PKC was found to restore these functions. Data supporting the possibility that PKC may also activate the enzyme in intact cells was obtained by Gorsky *et al.* (1989), who found that TPA treatment of HL-60 cells increased the activity of DNA topoisomerase I.

Thus, further studies are required to clarify the role of PKC in control of gene expression and the precise roles of cytoplasmic versus nuclear PKC in this process.

III. Role of Protein Kinase C in Tumors and Tumor Cell Lines of Specific Tissues

A. COLON TUMORS

The role of PKC in the biology of cancer has been studied in the context of its function as the high-affinity receptor for the phorbol ester tumor promoters (Nishizuka, 1986), and as an enzyme that mediates the action of certain growth factors and oncogenes (Weinstein, 1988a). Early studies of the effects of TPA on various mammalian cell lines indicated that TPA stimulates proliferation of certain cell types while inhibiting the growth of others, the latter effect sometimes being associated with the induction of differentiation (reviewed in Gesher, 1985, Weinstein, 1988a, Diamond, 1987, and Vandenbark and Niedel, 1984). The conceptual framework emerging from these findings emphasizes that the effects of PKC (or specific isoforms) on growth and differentiation is a correlate of the particular cell type in which the PKC activity is being expressed.

The etiology of human colon cancer is not known, although dietary factors have been implicated. Genetic analysis have demonstrated point mutations in c-K-*ras* and in the p53 gene, as well as deletions in loci on chromosomes 5 and 18 in many, but not all, colon tumors (Forrester *et al.*, 1987; Bos *et al.*, 1987; Vogelstein *et al.*, 1988; Fearon *et al.*, 1990). Examination of protein kinase activities in human colon tumors has revealed that, while there are elevated levels of casein kinase II (Munstermann *et al.*, 1990), there is often a decrease of PKC activity, when compared to normal colonic mucosa (Guillem and Weinstein, 1990; Guillem *et al.*, 1987a; Kopp *et al.*, 1990; Baum *et al.*, 1990).

In an effort to further elucidate the role of PKC in colon cancer, our laboratory explored the effect of stably overproducing PKC-β_1 in HT29 cells, a human colon cancer cell line that has been extensively studied with regard to its growth and differentiation properties (reviewed in Rousset, 1986). The results of these studies (Choi *et al.*, 1990) were markedly different when compared to earlier studies of PKC-β_1 overproduction in rodent fibroblasts (Housey *et al.*, 1988; Krauss *et al.*, 1989; see Section II,A). It was found that overproduction of PKC-β_1 by HT29 cells caused a dramatic suppression of growth in cell culture and a reduction in tumorigenicity in nude mice (Choi *et al.*, 1990). These results contrast with those obtained with rodent fibroblasts in which overexpression of the same isoform of PKC stimulated growth (Housey *et al.*, 1988; Krauss *et al.*, 1989). One interpretation is that in colonic epithelial cells, PKC acts to suppress growth.

If indeed PKC acts as a growth suppressor in colonic cells, then one might predict that PKC inhibitors would promote the occurrence of tumors, while PKC activators might slow proliferative growth and/or induce differentiation. There is evidence that supports this hypothetical model. First, stimulation of PKC by TPA has been associated with the appearance of differentiation-related antigens in a human colon carcinoma cell line (Baron *et al.*, 1990). Second, elevated Ca^{2+} levels, thought to play a protective role in colon cancer (Lipkin and Newmark, 1985) have also been shown to transform intestinal bile acids into PKC activators, presumably via the formation of Ca^{2+} soaps (Fitzer *et al.*, 1987).

A third piece of evidence strengthening the correlation between decreased levels of PKC and colon tumor occurrence, regards the potential for down-regulation of PKC in cells possessing an activated *ras* oncogene (see Section II,B). Although not yet well defined, this phenomenon may originate at the level of transcriptional control of PKC expression (Borner *et al.*, 1990). Our hypothetical model predicts that PKC down-regulation would release growth constraints and thus enhance proliferation. Recent studies have indicated that 40% of human colon tumors have mutations in codon 12 of the c-K-*ras* oncogene (Forrester *et al.*, 1987; Bos *et al.*, 1987). Synergy between pathways operated by the activated form of *ras* and by PKC could produce down-regulation of PKC and therefore at least partially account for diminished levels of PKC in colon carcinoma. The remaining 60% of colon tumors that do not have an activated *ras* but exhibit reduced PKC activities may be attributed to the activation of some other oncogene, such as c-*myc*. Although c-*myc* expression can be induced by certain growth factors as well as TPA, c-*myc* mRNA is also elevated in human (Guillem *et al.*, 1990) and rat (Guillem *et al.*, 1988) colon cancers. Thus, it is possible that c-*myc* expression, in addition to other derangements in growth control, might cause persistent down-regulation of PKC in colon tumors.

Deoxycholic acid, a bile acid derived from high fat diets, acts as a promoter of colon tumor formation in rats (reviewed in Guillem and Weinstein, 1990). Its effects on PKC include induction of translocation to cellular membranes (Guillem *et al.*, 1988), where down-regulation by proteolysis might occur, and stimulation of PKC activity and related pathways of signal transduction (Craven *et al.*, 1987). Regarding PKC stimulation, recent studies using normal human feces indicated that the production of DAG and monoacylglycerol was strictly dependent on the addition of bile acids, especially deoxycholic acid (Morotomi *et al.*, 1990). In a related study with Swiss 3T3 cells stimulated with fibroblast growth factor, the presence of deoxycholic acid was observed to cause an enhancement of DAG formation and PKC activation (Takeyama *et al.*, 1986). In an *in vitro* study it was also demonstrated that the bile acid fusidic acid can replace phosphatidylserine in the activation of PKC by TPA (Ward and O'Brian, 1988).

If the stimulatory effect on PKC by bile acids is indeed critical to malignant transformation, it is useful to ask whether transformation occurs by continuous activation of PKC (via elevated DAG levels) or during a subsequent refractory phase (sustained by high levels of bile acids) during which PKC is down-regulated. The latter possibility would be consistent with the observed decreases in PKC activity in human colon tumors and would support the proposed tumor suppressor role of PKC.

In view of these considerations, it has been speculated that the bile acids produced by the intestinal microflora as a consequence of high fat consumption could cause continuous activation (with concomitant down-regulation) of PKC. This condition might then foster abnormal proliferation of colonic epithelial cells and thus contribute to an elevated risk of colon cancer development in humans. Clearly, more in-depth studies are required to characterize the role of PKC activity in this process.

B. Breast Tumors

Although there have been limited studies of PKC in breast tumors (see below), several studies have been conducted with immortalized human mammary carcinoma cell lines. Comparing cell lines that exhibit estrogen dependency with those that do not, Costa *et al.* (1985) established an inverse correlation with the level of phorbol ester–binding receptors. This relationship was later corroborated by quantitating the level of total PKC using PKC-specific antisera (Borner *et al.*, 1987). Similarly, the same group confirmed this correlation and also found a positive correlation between levels of PKC and the EGF receptor in mammary carcinoma cell lines, using a direct assay of PKC kinase activity (Fabbro *et al.*, 1986b).

The above cell lines have also served as an interesting model to probe the role of PKC in the proliferation of breast carcinoma cells in culture. The basic conclusion from these studies is that prolonged TPA treatment inhibits the growth of the mammary carcinoma cells. This inhibition was coincident with the complete loss of cellular PKC activity, and was reversed upon removal of TPA, whereupon PKC enzyme activity reappeared in the cells (Fabbro *et al.*, 1986a). Furthermore, the inhibitory effect on cell growth correlated with the tumor-promoting ability of the phorbol ester, since less potent compounds induced only partial translocation, and inactive esters had no effect on PKC (Regazzi *et al.*,

1986; Darbon *et al.*, 1986). A separate study (Issandou *et al.*, 1986) examined the short-term effects of TPA on PKC in MCF-7 cells. Redistribution of PKC to the particulate fraction and down-regulation of the enzyme occurred rapidly and consumed 70% of the initial PKC activity. During this short-term exposure to TPA, PKC became activated and this was associated with the phosphorylation of a 28-kDa protein. Non–tumor promoting phorbol esters were ineffective in causing both down-regulation and the phosphorylation of this cellular protein. The same group later showed that phosphorylation of the 28-kDa protein reached a maximum at 30 min. It was phosphorylated in a dose- and time-dependent manner on serine residues, in response to treatment of the cells with either TPA or DiC_8, a permeant analog of DAG. Two-dimensional electrophoresis further demonstrated that TPA and DiC_8 treatment produced distinct patterns of phosphorylated cellular proteins, since TPA apparently induced additional phosphorylations not observed with DiC_8 treatment. Curiously, DiC_8 mimicked the effects of TPA on MCF-7 in terms of changes in morphology and inhibition of cell growth, and yet DiC_8 induced only partial and temporary translocation of PKC and did not induce PKC down-regulation (Issandou *et al.*, 1988). These results imply that down-regulation itself is not critical to the growth inhibition by DiC_8. Presumably, this same conclusion applies to the growth-inhibitory effects of TPA.

Stimulation of phosphorylation of steroid receptors has been cited as one mechanism by which phorbol esters might influence the behavior of human breast cancer cells. In particular, TPA treatment has been associated with phosphorylation of the progesterone receptor, leading to a twofold increase in progesterone-binding sites (Boyle and van der Walt, 1988).

A more detailed biochemical analysis of PKC following prolonged treatment of MCF-7 cells with TPA was carried out by Borner *et al.* (1988). Using ^{35}S-methionine labeling, these investigators demonstrated that after down-regulation of enzymatically active PKC, the cells continued to synthesize PKC-related proteins (74 and 80 kDa) that lack kinase activity and phorbol ester binding but are immunoprecipitable by anti-PKC antibodies. In addition, these proteins exhibited a V8 protease digestion pattern identical to that given by an enzymatically active PKC species (77 and 80 kDa) obtained from untreated cells. Interestingly, the amounts of inactive PKC-related protein synthesized during prolonged TPA treatment correlated inversely with the extent of TPA-mediated growth inhibition of this human breast cancer cell line. In a subsequent report, Borner *et al.* (1989) provided evidence that these PKC-related proteins are precursors of PKC that differ in their state of phosphorylation. The 74-kDa form is the primary translation product and is unphosphorylated, and the 77- and 80-kDa forms represent increasing levels of phosphorylation. The prolonged treatment of breast cancer cells with TPA apparently leads to the accumulation of the 74-kDa PKC due to an impaired conversion of the 74-kDa to the phosphorylated 77-kDa and 80-kDa forms. Tumor promoters somehow interfere, therefore, with the posttranslational processes that convert the inactive forms to the mature phosphorylated species.

Further studies are required to determine the relevance of the above findings to the previously mentioned TPA-induced phosphorylation of a 28-kDa protein, the altered levels of estrogen receptors and EGF receptors in cell lines that have high levels of PKC, and the ability of TPA and DiC_8 to induce growth inhibition. It would also be of interest to compare breast carcinoma cells to normal mammary epithelial cells with respect to these properties, and to determine whether or not PKC activation serves as a positive or negative effector of growth or differentiation in both cell types.

Preliminary studies have indicated that in contrast to colon cancer, primary breast tumors often express elevated levels of PKC (Lim *et al.*, 1987; O'Brian *et al.*, 1989a). This observation is consistent with studies on the levels of phorbol ester receptors for primary human breast tumors (Wyss *et al.*, 1987). The latter authors found an inverse relationship in levels of PKC, quantitiated by ^{3}H-phorbol ester binding, and the estrogen and progesterone receptors. Thus, tumors that are hormone-independent, and tend to be associated with a poorer prognosis, have higher phorbol ester–binding receptors than normal breast tissue or breast tumors that have retained steroid hormone dependency (Wyss *et al.*, 1987). In the same study, EGF receptors were similar to PKC in that their levels also correlated inversely with the steroid hormone receptors.

Although the results obtained with breast tumors agree with the observations made with immortalized cell lines, there are two important limitations. The first points to the difficulty in obtaining epithelial cells that are uncontaminated with adipocytes and fibroblasts from normal breast tissue for comparison of PKC levels and activities (O'Brian *et al.*, 1989a). Responding to this problem, Regenass *et al.* (1989) reported the development of short-term *in vitro* cultures of epithelial cells from normal breast tissues and epithelial cells from breast carcinoma. Examination of PKC activities and levels of estrogen and progesterone receptors in these culture systems showed that their levels were variable. Additional studies will be required, however, to establish by use of these short-term culture systems, the correlations observed for steroid receptors and PKC in cell lines and biopsies.

A second point of debate regards the possibility that normal and malignant breast cells are in different stages of mitotic activity, thereby casting elevated PKC activity as a marker of the proliferative state, rather than of malignancy per se. This possibility has not been addressed experimentally.

C. OTHER TUMORS

In view of the high abundance of PKC in the central nervous system, it is possible that changes in PKC might be associated with specific brain tumors. Immunocytochemical analysis of PKC isoforms using isoform-specific antibodies has established that in the normal brain the distribution of PKC (Wood *et al.*, 1986; Mochly-Rosen *et al.*, 1987), and of PKC isoforms (Ohno *et al.*, 1987; Ase *et al.*, 1988b; Hidaka *et al.* 1988; Yoshida *et al.*, 1988; K.-P. Huang, 1989) is regiospecific and varies according to the stage of development (Yoshida *et al.*, 1988). It is possible, therefore, that the PKC isoform expression profile in specific tumors of the central nervous system might be altered relative to the corresponding normal tissue. Evidence pertaining to this was reported in a comparative study of PKC isoform expression in human glioblastomas and neuroblastomas (Shimosawa *et al.*, 1990). It was found that cultured glioblastoma cells expressed type III PKC (PKC-α) whereas type II (PKC-β) was detected in neuroblastoma cells. This result was in marked contrast to similar studies carried out with normal rat brain (Ito *et al.*, 1990), which demonstrated that PKC-α is poorly represented in glial cells of normal tissue but was predominantly detected in neurons. Whether this was attributable to the species difference or to the development of malignancy requires additional study. Nevertheless, the results suggest that, relative to normal tissue, an altered pattern of isoform expression may occur in malignant cells. If such is the case, it might be possible to use the expression profile of PKC isoforms as a means of diagnosing malignancy.

Studies with primary melanoma cell lines have demonstrated a tumor-specific deletion within the gene encoding PKC-α as well as polymorphic alleles for this isoform of PKC (Linnenbach *et al.*, 1988). The deletion in the PKC-α gene was not detectable cytogenetically and was apparently homozygous since corresponding restriction fragments were lost completely; normal cells from the same individual, however, did not exhibit this deletion, indicating that the effect was tumor-specific. Other structural aberrations in these melanoma cell lines were observed, particularly with the MYB and EGF receptor genes, suggesting that alterations to multiple genetic loci had occurred.

The observation that PKC levels were elevated in human gastric cancers (Lim *et al.*, 1987), lung cancer cells (Hirai *et al.*, 1989), and in neoplastic squamous epithelia from the upper aero-digestive tract (Rydell *et al.*, 1988) deserves further attention.

IV. Protein Kinase C and Multidrug Resistance

The resistance of malignant cells to multiple cytotoxic drugs represents a major obstacle to effective chemotherapy. This phenomenon has been observed with cells in culture, which become increasingly insensitive to multiple cytotoxic drugs during a period of continuous exposure to a single agent (reviewed in Gottesman and Pastan, 1988). Similarly, some human tumors such as leukemias and neuroblastoma are initially responsive but acquire resistance to the drugs used to treat them, as well as to other drugs (cross-resistance). Many other types of tumors, such as adenocarcinomas of the colon and kidney, are refractory to cytotoxic drugs from the beginning, due to an intrinsic drug resistance of the malignant tissue. In some cases, the phenotype of drug resistance in cultured cells (Shen *et al.*, 1986a) and in tumors (Fojo *et al.*, 1987) has been correlated with the amplified expression of a gene designated *mdr 1*. A direct demonstration of the function of the *mdr 1* gene product was shown by Gros *et al.* (1986) and by Ueda *et al.* (1987) when a full length cDNA clone of *mdr 1*, introduced into and overexpressed in drug-sensitive cells, conferred multidrug resistance. Similarly, RNA encoding the *mdr 1b* gene (one member of the *mdr* gene family), was injected into *Xenopus laevis* oocytes and consequently produced resistance to vinblastine accumulation by this system (Castillo *et al.*, 1990).

The *mdr 1* gene, a member of a growing family of related genes (Gros *et al.*, 1988), encodes a plasma membrane–associated glycoprotein of M_r 170,000–180,000 daltons termed P-glycoprotein (or P170) where P connotes *permeability*. Upon cloning and sequencing of the *mdr 1* gene, it was found that the predicted structure of P-glycoprotein showed strongest homology with a bacterial hemolysin transport protein (Gerlach *et al.*, 1986). This observation prompted the formulation of a mechanism for drug resistance whereby P-glycoprotein functions as an energy-dependent efflux pump which, by actively exporting intracellular anticancer agents, reduces their cytotoxicity. Although other mechanisms of drug resistance are also being explored, the P-glycoprotein efflux pump has become a focus of recent investigations.

Further characterization of the P-glycoprotein has shown it to possess an associated ATPase activity (Hamada and Tsuruo, 1988). In addition, when multidrug-resistant tumor cells are treated with various substances, including phorbol esters, the protein undergoes phosphorylation (Hamada *et al.*, 1987). These observations suggested that the function of the P-glycoprotein can be activated by phosphorylation. Indeed, the coincidence of phosphorylation of membrane surface glycoproteins and drug resistance had been observed in earlier studies by V. Ling (Carlsen *et al.*, 1977) and by M. Center (1985). Analyses of tryptic phosphopeptide maps obtained for P-glycoprotein purified from cells that had been treated with different stimuli, suggested that several protein kinases are involved in this phenomenon (Hamada *et al.*, 1987). There is also evidence that a membrane-associated cAMP-dependent protein kinase can phosphorylate P-glycoprotein *in vitro* (Mellado and Horwitz, 1987) and in cells (Abraham *et al.*, 1987). Furthermore, in membranes isolated from drug-resistant HL-60 cells, a novel membrane-associated protein kinase (PK-1), that is neither PKC nor cAMP-dependent protein kinase, was observed to phosphorylate P-glycoprotein (Staats *et al.*, 1990).

Several studies have focused on the phosphorylation of P-glycoprotein by PKC, and its role in the mechanism of drug resistance (see Fig. 4). In this regard, correlation between elevated levels of PKC activity and drug resistance has been

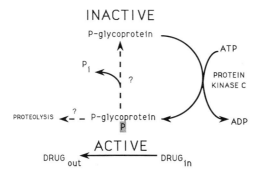

FIG. 4. Mechanistic model of PKC-mediated activation of P-glycoprotein and its role in multi-drug resistance.

observed. This correlation was reported in studies of drug-resistant human breast cancer cells (MCF-7), in which there was a sevenfold elevation in PKC (Fine *et al.*, 1988). Other studies have shown twofold increases of PKC in adriamycin-resistant murine fibrosarcoma cells (O'Brian *et al.*, 1989b) and HL-60 leukemia cells (Aquino *et al.*, 1988), and a fourfold elevation of PKC in human KB carcinoma cells (Chambers *et al.*, 1990a). The latter change is apparently due to increased expression of the α-isoform, although the presence of other isoforms was not examined (Posada *et al.*, 1989a). Additional evidence has shown that inhibitors of PKC, such as H-7, staurosporine and several antineoplastic agents, can transiently confer drug sensitivity to resistant cells (Center, 1985; Palayoor *et al.*, 1987; O'Brian *et al.*, 1989b; Posada *et al.*, 1989a; Chambers *et al.*, 1990b; Sachs *et al.*, 1990). Conversely, activators of PKC, such as tumor promoting phorbol esters, engender transient resistance and are associated with reduced intracellular levels of anticancer drugs (Chambers *et al.*, 1990b; Fine *et al.*, 1988). There is also evidence of a transient conferral of adriamycin resistance by the bile acid deoxycholate, which is known to activate PKC (C.A. O'Brian, personal communication; see Section III,A).

A direct correlation of drug resistance with PKC-mediated phosphorylation of the P-glycoprotein and decreased drug accumulation has been demonstrated in MCF-7 cells breast carcinoma cells (Yu *et al.*, 1990) and in KB carcinoma cells (Chambers *et al.*, 1990b). In the breast carcinoma model, MCF-7 cells were transfected with the *mdr 1* gene, producing a cell line, BC19, that displayed resistance to adriamycin. This resistance, however, was 30- to 50-fold less than that seen in cells that had acquired adriamycin resistance through drug selection. Transfection of BC19 cells with PKC-α led to a further several-fold increase in drug resistance, which was associated with increased PKC activity and phosphorylation of P-glycoprotein, and reduced retention of drug. Treatment of the

PKC-α–expressing BC19 cells with phorbol dibutyrate, a tumor-promoting phorbol ester, further enhanced drug resistance and P-glycoprotein phosphorylation (Yu et al., 1990). Studies with the multidrug–resistant KB human carcinoma cells showed that when the P-glycoprotein was immunoprecipitated from cells incubated with [γ-^{32}P]ATP in the absence and presence of TPA, the phosphopeptide map was the same as that produced in vitro by purified PKC-mediated phosphorylation of P-glycoprotein. In the same study, TPA was shown to increase by twofold the level of P-glycoprotein phosphorylation in ^{32}P-labeled cells; the basal and TPA-stimulated levels of ^{32}P-labeled P-glycoprotein were both reduced with H-7, an inhibitor of PKC (Chambers et al., 1990b). These experiments demonstrated that the phosphorylation of P-glycoprotein is mediated by phorbol ester–activated PKC and can modulate the transport activity that is believed to define multidrug resistance in these cell models.

It is of interest to note that the calcium channel blocker, verapamil, can reverse the multidrug-resistance phenotype (Gottesman and Pastan, 1988). Current thinking of how verapamil might act envisions a direct competitive interaction with sites on the P-glycoprotein occupied by drugs that are normally transported out of the cell. This mode of action would be expected to enhance sensitivity dramatically by rendering the P-glycoprotein efflux pump ineffective, and thus increasing the intracellular retention of antineoplastic drugs. Since several antineoplastic agents are potent PKC inhibitors (see Section I,B), this could also block phosphorylation of the P-glycoprotein, thus further augmenting drug sensitivity. Direct proof of the competitive action of verapamil with other drugs for sites on P-glycoprotein will require the reconstitution of the efflux pump into artificial membranes.

Although the mechanistic model of multidrug resistance has been strengthened by much of the biochemical evidence obtained thus far, there exist other observations that are not included in the model. The complexity of multidrug resistance is implied a priori by the existence of multiple forms of P-glycoprotein (Greenberger et al., 1988), the expression of which is a function of the specific drug used for selection (Peterson et al., 1983; Roy and Horwitz, 1985; Shen et al., 1986). Two types of P-glycoprotein, expressed by mdr-1a and mdr-1b, have also been shown to exhibit functional differences with regard to drug binding and efficiencies of transport (Yang et al., 1990). Moreover, a novel resistance-related membrane protein, P-95, was overexpressed in cells selected for adriamycin resistance in the presence of verapamil (Chen et al., 1990).

One striking counterexample of the function of PKC in P-glycoprotein activation and consequent drug resistance, was a study reported by Posada et al. (1989b). In that report, treatment of adriamycin-resistant murine sarcoma 180 cells with TPA actually enhanced cytotoxicity by adriamycin, and prolonged treatment with TPA led to protection from adriamycin-induced toxicity. The authors speculated that a different mechanism of resistance may be responsible in their cell system (Posada *et al.*, 1989a). In another study carried out by D. Kessel (1988), it was shown that drug-responsive murine leukemia cells, when treated with TPA for 2 hr, displayed an impaired ability to take up anthracycline. The observation that the entry of drug into cells was blocked by TPA treatment and was not reversed by verapamil pointed to a different TPA-related mechanism operating in these cells, possibly PKC-mediated inhibition of a different route of drug entry.

There is evidence for numerous other molecular mechanisms of drug resistance, such as the glutathione redox cycle, that do not involve the P-glycoprotein system (Deffie *et al.*, 1988; Harker *et al.*, 1989). Nevertheless, the strongest evidence implicates P-glycoprotein and related efflux proteins as a key mechanism for cellular detoxification of not only antineoplastic reagents but also chemical carcinogens (Gottesman, 1988). The functional modulation of drug efflux by PKC has generated new possibilities for circumventing the clinical difficulties posed by multidrug resistance. Furthermore, the expulsion of antineoplastic drugs that occurs as a consequence of PKC activation in certain drug-resistant cells, creates new imperatives for the development of novel and specific PKC inhibitors, which might be useful in counteracting drug resistance.

V. Future Directions

In light of the evidence that PKC may play a role in certain types of multidrug resistance in cancer cells, the development of highly specific PKC inhibitors could provide a new approach to overcoming this drug resistance. Recent studies, being carried out in our laboratory in collaboration with D. Rideout (Scripps Institute) have focused on the characterization of a phosphonium salt that is a novel PKC inhibitor; this compound assembles from noninhibitory precursors that are selectively concentrated by carcinoma cells relative to normal cells, resulting in synergistic and selective inhibition of cell growth (Rideout *et al.*, 1990; Rotenberg *et al.*, 1991). The development of compounds that are potent and selective inhibitors of PKC is essential for the development of chemical tools with which to dissect the role of PKC in various signal transduction pathways and as a possible basis for developing novel pharmacological agents. Furthermore, because our knowledge of the enzymology of the various PKC isoforms is limited, the possible use of inhibitors to discriminate between the two classes of PKC, namely the Ca^{2+}-dependent and Ca^{2+}-independent forms, has not been explored in detail. Last, the observation of an endogenous PKC inhibitor(s) (see Section I,B), implies a potential cellular strategy by which PKC may be regulated physiologically, and suggests a line of inquiry for further study.

It is clear that protein kinase C is a critical component in signal-transduction pathways that regulate growth, and in the development of tumors. The identification of specific PKC isoforms in pathways of signal transduction, tumor promotion, and programs of differentiation, predicts the possibility that these isoforms have distinct functions. Furthermore, it is possible that changes in isoform expression profiles in a specific tissue may precede or accompany the development of neoplasia, thus providing an early diagnostic marker of malignancy. Documentation of PKC isoform–expression profiles in normal and malignant cells will require more extensive study.

Preliminary studies demonstrate that human colon, breast, and brain tumors display altered levels of PKC when compared to their normal counterparts. Much more extensive studies are required in various human tumors to determine the significance of these findings. Furthermore, it will be essential to examine specific isoforms of PKC, rather than total PKC activity, and to determine whether mutations, which inactivate or activate specific PKC genes, occur in specific human tumors.

Because no isoform-specific substrates have yet been identified *in vivo*, it is not known whether the structural diversity of PKC implies diversity of function. The future use of isoform-specific overexpression systems, as well as direct reconstitution of signal pathway components, will afford important insights into the putative functional differences of PKC isoforms and their relationship to the generation of aberrant growth signals.

Acknowledgments

The authors wish to thank Doctors Christoph M. B. Borner, Susan Jaken, Robert S. Krauss, Catherine A. O'Brian, and Kevin O'Driscoll for critically reading the manuscript. During the preparation of this work, S.A.R. was supported by NIH PO1 ES05294–01.

NOTE ADDED IN PROOF: Since the preparation of this article, a new member of the protein kinase C family, designated PKCη, was discovered to be the predominant PKC isoform of lung tissue [Osada *et al.*, (1990) *J. Biol. Chem.* **265**, 22434–22440; Bacher *et al.*, (1991) *Mol. Cell. Biol.* **11**, 126–133]. As another Ca^{2+}-independent protein kinase which binds phorbol ester, PKCη shows the highest sequence similarity to PKC-ε (59.4% homology).

References

Abraham, I., Hunter, R. J., Sampson, K. E., Smith, S., Gottesman, M. M., and Mayo, J. K. (1987). Cyclic AMP–dependent protein kinase regulates sensitivity of cells to multiple drugs. *Mol. Cell. Biol.* **7**, 3098–3106.
Aderem, A. A., Albert, K. A., Keum, M. M., Wang, J. K. T., Greengard, P., and Cohn, Z. A. (1988). Stimulus-dependent myristoylation of a major substrate for protein kinase C. *Nature (London)* **332**, 362–364.
Aitken, A., Ellis, C. A., Harris, A., Sellers, L. A., and Toker, A. (1990). Kinase and neurotransmitters. *Nature (London)* **344**, 594.
Akita, Y., Ohno, S., Konno, Y., Yano, A., and Suzuki, K. (1990). Expression and properties of

two distinct classes of the phorbol ester receptor family, four conventional protein kinase C types, and a novel protein kinase C. *J. Biol. Chem.* **265,** 354–362.

Albert, K. A., Walass, S. I., Wang, J. K.-T., and Greengard, P. (1986). Widespread occurence of "87 kDa," a major specific substrate for protein kinase C. *Proc. Natl. Acad. Sci. U.S.A.* **83,** 2822–2826.

Angel, P., Poting, A., Mallick, U., Rahmsdorf, H. J., Schorpp, M., and Herrlich, P. (1986). Induction of metallothionein and other mRNA species by carcinogens and tumor promoters in primary human skin fibroblasts. *Mol. Cell. Biol.* **6,** 1760–1766.

Angel, P., Baumann, I., Stein, B., Delius, H., Rahmsdorf, H. J., and Herrlich, P. (1987a). 12-*O*-Tetradecanoylphorbol-13-acetate induction of the human collagenase gene is mediated by an inducible enhancer element located in the 5'-flanking region. *Mol. Cell. Biol.* **7,** 2256–2266.

Angel, P., Imagawa, M., Chiu, R., Stein, B., Imbra, R. J., Rahmsdorf, H. J., Jonat, C., Herrlich, P., and Karin, M. (1987b). Phorbol ester-inducible genes contain a common *cis* element recognized by a TPA-modulated *trans*-acting factor. *Cell* **49,** 729–739.

Angel, P., Hattori, K., Smeal, T., and Karin, M. (1988). The *jun* protooncogene is positively autoregulated by its product, Jun/AP-1. *Cell* **55,** 875–885.

Aquino, A., Hartman, K. D., Knode, M. C., Grant, S., Huang, K.-P., Niu, C.-H., and Glazer, R. I. (1988). Role of protein kinase C in phosphorylation of vinculin in adriamycin-resistant HL-60 leukemia cells. *Cancer Res.* **48,** 3324–3329.

Arcoleo, J. P., and Weinstein, I. B. (1985). Activation of protein kinase C by tumor-promoting phorbol esters, teleocidin and aplysiatoxin in the absence of added calcium. *Carcinogenesis* **6,** 213–217.

Ase, K., Berry, N., Kikkawa, U., Kishimoto, A., and Nishizuka, Y. (1988a). Differential downregulation of protein kinase C subspecies in KM3 cells. *FEBS Lett.* **236,** 396–400.

Ase, K., Saito, N., Shearman, M. S., Kikkawa, U., Ono, Y., Igarashi, K., Tanaka, C., and Nishizuka, Y. (1988b). Distinct cellular expression of βI- and βII-subspecies of protein kinase C in rat cerebellum. *J. Neurosci.* **8,** 3850–3856.

Baeuerle, P. A., and Baltimore, D. (1988). IκB: A specific inhibitor of the NF-κB transcription factor. *Science* **242,** 540–546.

Balmain, A., Ramsden, M., Bowden, G. T., and Smith, J. (1984). Activation of the mouse cellular Harvey-*ras* gene in chemically induced benign skin papillomas. *Nature (London)* **307,** 658–660.

Baron, P. L., Koretz, M. J., Carchman, R. A., Collins, J. M., Tokarz, A. S., Parker, G. A. (1990). Induction of the expression of differentiation-related antigens on human colon carcinoma cells by stimulating protein kinase C. *Arch. Surg.* **125,** 344–350.

Baum, C. L., Wali, R., Sitrin, M. D., Bolt, M. J. G., Brasitus, T. A. (1990). 1,2-Dimethylhydrazine–induced alterations in protein kinase C activity in the rat preneoplastic and neoplastic colon. *Gastroenterology (Suppl.)* **98**(2), A272.

Bazzi, M. D., and Nelsestuen, G. L. (1988a). Constitutive activity of membrane-inserted protein kinase C. *Biochem. Biophys. Res. Commun.* **152,** 336–343.

Bazzi, M. D., and Nelsestuen, G. L. (1988b). Properties of membrane-inserted protein kinase C. *Biochemistry* **27,** 7589–7593.

Bazzi, M. D., and Nelsestuen, G. L. (1989). Differences in the effects of phorbol esters and diacylglycerols on protein kinase C. *Biochemistry* **28,** 9317–9323.

Beckerle, M. C. (1990). The adhesion plaque, talin, is phosphorylated *in vivo* in chicken embryo fibroblasts exposed to a tumor-promoting phorbol ester. *Cell Regul.* **1,** 227–236.

Beh, I., Schmidt, R., and Hecker, E. (1989). Two isozymes of PKC found in HL-60 cells show a difference in activation by the phorbol ester TPA. *FEBS Lett.* **249,** 264–266.

Bernstein, L. R., and Colburn, N. H. (1989). AP1/*jun* function is differentially induced in promoter-sensitive and -resistant JB6 cells. *Science* **244,** 566–569.

Blumberg, P. M., Driedger, P. E., and Rossow, P. W. (1976). Effect of a phorbol ester on a transformation-sensitive surface protein of chick fibroblasts. *Nature* **264,** 446–447.

Bollag, G. E., Roth, R. A., Beaudoin, J., Mochly-Rosen, D., and Koshland, D. E. (1986). Protein kinase C directly phosphorylates the insulin receptor *in vitro* and reduces its protein–tyrosine kinase activity. *Proc. Natl. Acad. Sci. U.S.A.* **83**, 5822–5824.

Borner, C., Wyss, R., Regazzi, R., Eppenberger, U., and Fabbro, D. (1987). Immunological quantitation of phospholipid/Ca^{2+}-dependent protein kinase of human mammary carcinoma cells: Inverse relationship to estrogen receptors. *Int. J. Cancer* **40**, 344–348.

Borner, C., Eppenberger, U., Wyss, R., and Fabbro, D. (1988). Continuous synthesis of two protein kinase C–related proteins after down-regulation by phorbol esters. *Proc. Natl. Acad. Sci. U.S.A.* **85**, 2110–2114.

Borner, C., Filipuzzi, I., Wartmann, M., Eppenberger, U., Fabbro, D. (1989). Biosynthesis and posttranslational modifications of protein kinase C in human breast cancer cells. *J. Biol. Chem.* **264**, 13902–13909.

Borner, C., Guadagno, S. N., Hsieh, L.-L., Hsiao, W.-L. W., and Weinstein, I. B. (1990). Transformation by a *ras* oncogene causes increased expression of protein kinase C-α and decreased expression of protein kinase C-ε. *Cell Growth Differ.* **1**, 653–660.

Bos, J. L., Fearon, E. R., Hamilton, S. R., Verlaan-de Vries, M., van Boom, J. H., van der Eb, A. J., and Vogelstein, B. (1987). Prevalence of *ras* gene mutations in human colorectal cancers. *Nature (London)* **327**, 293–297.

Boyle, D. M., and van der Walt, A. L. (1988). Enhanced phosphorylation of progesterone receptor by protein kinase C in human breast cancer cells. *J. Steroid Biochem.* **30**, 239–244.

Buckley, A. R., Crowe, P. D., and Russell, D. H. (1988). Rapid activation of protein kinase C in isolated rat liver nuclei by prolactin, a known hepatic mitogen. *Proc. Natl. Acad. Sci. U.S.A.* **85**, 8649–8653.

Burgoyne, R. D. (1989). A role for membrane-inserted protein kinase C in cellular memory? *Trends Biochem. Sci.* **14**, 87–88.

Burns, D. J., Bloomenthal, J., Lee, M.-H., Bell, R. M. (1990). Expression of the α, βII, and γ-protein kinase C isozymes in the baculovirus-insect cell expression system. *J. Biol. Chem.* **265**, 12044–12051.

Carlsen, S. A., Till, J. E., and Ling, V. (1977). Modulation of drug permeability in Chinese hamster ovary cells. *Biochim. Biophys. Acta* **467**, 238–250.

Castagna, M., Takai, Y., Kaibuchi, K., Sano, K., Kikkawa, U., and Nishizuka, Y. (1982). Direct activation of calcium-activated, phospholipid-dependent protein kinase by tumor-promoting phorbol esters. *J. Biol. Chem.* **257**, 7847–7851.

Castillo, G., Vera, J. C., Yang, C.-P. H., Horwitz, S. B., and Rosen, O. M. (1990). Functional expression of murine multidrug resistance in *Xenopus laevis* oocytes. *Proc. Natl. Acad. Sci. U.S.A.* **87**, 4737–4741.

Center, M. S. (1985). Mechanisms regulating cell resistance to adriamycin. *Biochem. Pharmacol.* **34**, 1471–1476.

Chambers, T. C., Chalikonda, I., and Eilon, G. (1990a). Correlation of protein kinase C translocation, P-glycoprotein phosphorylation, and reduced drug accumulation in multidrug-resistant human KB cells. *Biochem. Biophys. Res. Commun.* **169**, 253–259.

Chambers, T. C., McAvoy, E. M., Jacobs, J. W., and Eilon, G. (1990b). Protein kinase C phosphorylates P-glycoprotein in multidrug-resistant human KB carcinoma cells. *J. Biol. Chem.* **265**, 7679–7686.

Chan, B. L., Chao, M. V., and Saltiel, A. R. (1989). Nerve growth factor stimulates the hydrolysis of glycosylphosphatidylinositol in PC-12 cells: A mechanism of protein kinase C regulation. *Proc. Natl. Acad. Sci. U.S.A.* **86**, 1756–1760.

Chen, Y.-N., Mickley, L. A., Schwartz, A. M., Acton, E. M., Hwang, J., and Fojo, A. T. (1990). Characterization of adriamycin-resistant human breast cancer cells which display overexpression of a novel resistance-related membrane protein. *J. Biol. Chem.* **265**, 10073–10080.

Chiarugi, V., Bruni, P., Pasquali, F., Magnelli, L., Basi, G., Ruggiero, M., and Farnararo, M. (1989). Synthesis of diacylglycerol *de novo* is responsible for permanent activation and down-regulation of protein kinase C in transformed cells. *Biochem. Biophys. Res. Commun.* **164**, 816–823.

Chida, K., Hahiba, H., Sasaki, K., and Kuroki, T. (1986). Activation of protein kinase C and specific phosphorylation of a M_r 90,000 membrane protein of promotable BALB/3T3 and C3H 10T1/2 cells by tumor promoters. *Cancer Res.* **46**, 1055–1062.

Chiu, R., Imagawa, M., Imbra, R. J., Bockoven, J. R., and Karin, M. (1987). Multiple *cis*- and *trans*-acting elements mediate the transcriptional response to phorbol esters. *Nature* **329**, 648–651.

Choi, P. M., Tchou-Wong, K.-M., and Weinstein, I. B. (1990). Overexpression of protein kinase C in HT29 colon cancer cells causes growth inhibition and tumor suppression. *Mol. Cell. Biol.* **10**, 4650–4657.

Chu, D. T. W., and Granner, D. K. (1986). The effect of phorbol esters and diacylglycerol on expression of the phosphoenolpyruvate carboxykinase (GTP) gene in rat hepatoma H4IIE cells. *J. Biol. Chem.* **261**, 16848–16853.

Chuang, L. F., Zhao, F.-K., and Chuang, R. Y. (1989). Isolation and purification of protein kinase C from human leukemia ML-1 cells: Phosphorylation of human leukemia RNA polymerase II *in vitro. Biochim. Biophys. Acta* **992**, 87–95.

Cochet, C., Gill, G. N., Meisenhelder, J., Cooper, J. A., and Hunter, T. (1984). C-kinase phosphorylates the epidermal growth factor receptor and reduces its epidermal growth factor–stimulated tyrosine protein kinase activity. *J. Biol. Chem.* **259**, 2553–2558.

Colamonici, O. R., Trepel, J. B., Vidal, C. A., and Neckers, L. M. (1986). Phorbol ester induces c-*sis* gene transcription in stem cell line K-562. *Mol. Cell. Biol.* **6**, 1847–1850.

Cooper, D. R., Watson, J. E., Acevedo-Duncan, M., Pollet, R. J., Standaert, M. L., and Farese, R. V. (1989). Retention of specific protein kinase C isozymes following chronic phorbol ester treatment in BC3H-1 myocytes. *Biochem. Biophys. Res. Commun.* **161**, 327–334.

Costa, S. D., Fabbro, D., Regazzi, R., Kung, W., and Eppenberger, U. (1985). The cytosolic phorboid receptor correlates with hormone dependency in six mammary carcinoma cell lines. *Biochem. Biophys. Res. Commun.* **133**, 814–822.

Coussens, L., Parker, P. J., Rhee, L., Yang-Feng, T. L., Chen, E., Waterfield, M. D., Francke, U., and Ullrich, A. (1986). Multiple, distinct forms of bovine and human protein kinase C suggest diversity in cellular signaling pathways. *Science* **233**, 859–866.

Coussens, L., Rhee, L., Parker, P. J., and Ullrich, A. (1987). Alternative splicing increases the diversity of the human protein kinase C family. *DNA* **6**, 389–394.

Craven, P. A., Pfanstiel, J., and DeRubertis, F. R. (1987). Role of activation of protein kinase C in the stimulation of colonic epithelial proliferation and reactive oxygen formation by bile acids. *J. Clin. Invest.* **79**, 532–541.

Cuadrado, A., Molloy, C. J., and Pech, M. (1990). Expression of protein kinase C in NIH 3T3 cells increases its growth response to specific activators. *FEBS Lett.* **260**, 281–284.

Darbón, J.-M., Valette, A., and Bayard, F. (1986). Phorbol esters inhibit the proliferation of MCF-7 cells. *Biochem. Pharmacol.* **35**, 2683–2686.

Da Silva, C., Fan, X., Martelly, I., and Castagna, M. (1990). Phorbol esters mediate phospholipid-free activation of rat brain protein kinase C. *Cancer Res.* **50**, 2081–2087.

Davis, P. D., Hill, C. H., Keech, E., Lawton, G., Nixon, J. S., Sedgwick, A. D., Wadsworth, J., Westmacott, D., and Wilkinson, S. E. (1989). Potent selective inhibitors of protein kinase C. *FEBS Lett.* **259**, 61–63.

de Chaffoy de Courcelles, D., Roevens, P., and Van Belle, H. (1985). R 59 022, a diacylglycerol kinase inhibitor. *J. Biol. Chem.* **260**, 15762–15770.

Decker, S. J., Ellis, C., Pawson, T., and Velu, T. (1990). Effects of substitution of threonine 654 of the epidermal growth factor receptor on epidermal growth factor–mediated activation of phospholipase C. *J. Biol. Chem.* **265**, 7009–7015.

Deffie, A. M., Alam, T., Seneviratne, C., Beenken, S. W., Batra, J. K., Shea, T. C., Henner, W. D., and Goldenberg, G. J. (1988). Multifactorial resistance to adriamycin: Relationship of DNA repair, glutathione transferase activity, drug efflux, and P-glycoprotein in cloned cell lines of adriamycin-sensitive and -resistant P388 leukemia. *Cancer Res.* **48**, 3595–3602.

Diamond, L. (1987). Tumor promoters and cell transformation. *In* "Mechanisms of cellular transformation by carcinogenic agents" (D. Grunberger, and S. Goff, eds.), pp. 73–134. Pergamon Press, Elmsford, NY.

Dotto, G. P., Parada, L. F., and Weinberg, R. A. (1985). Specific growth response of *ras*-transformed embryo fibroblasts to tumor promoters. *Nature (London)* **318**, 472–475.

Dreher, M. L., and Hanley, M. R. (1987). Multiple modes of protein kinase C regulation and their significance in signaling. *Trends Pharmacol. Sci.* **9**, 114–115.

Edwards, D. R., Waterhouse, P., Holman, M. L., and Denhardt, D. T. (1986). A growth-responsive gene (16C8) in normal mouse fibroblasts homologous to a human collagenase inhibitor with erythroid-potentiating activity: Evidence for inducible and constitutive transcripts. *Nucleic Acids Res.* **14**, 8863–8878.

Exton, J. H. (1990). Signaling through phosphatidylcholine breakdown. *J. Biol. Chem.* **265**, 1–4.

Fabbro, D., Regazzi, R., Costa, S. D., Borner, C., and Eppenberger, U. (1986a). Protein kinase C desensitization by phorbol esters and its impact on growth of human breast cancer cells. *Biochem. Biophys. Res. Commun.* **135**, 65–73.

Fabbro, D., Kung, W., Roos, W., Regazzi, R., and Eppenberger, U. (1986b). Epidermal growth factor binding and protein kinase C activities in human breast cancer cell lines: Possible quantitative relationship. *Cancer Res.* **46**, 2720–2725.

Fearon, E. R., Cho, K. R., Nigro, J. M., Kern, S. E., Simons, J. W., Ruppert, J. M., Hamilton, S. R., Preisinger, A. C., Thomas, G., Kinzler, K. W., and Vogelstein, B. (1990). Identification of a chromosome 18q gene that is altered in colorectal cancers. *Science* **247**, 49–56.

Felipo, V., Minana, M.-D., and Grisolia, S. (1990). A specific inhibitor of protein kinase C induces differentiation of neuroblastoma cells. *J. Biol. Chem.* **265**, 9599–9601.

Fields, A. P., Pettit, G. R., and May, W. S. (1988). Phosphorylation of lamin B at the nuclear membrane by activated protein kinase C. *J. Biol. Chem.* **263**, 8253–8260.

Fields, A. P., Tyler, G., Kraft, A. S., and May, W. S. (1990). Role of nuclear protein kinase C in the mitogenic response to platelet-derived growth factor. *J. Cell Sci.* **96**, 107–114.

Fine, R. L., Patel, J., and Chabner, B. A. (1988). Phorbol esters induce multidrug resistance in human breast cancer cells. *Proc. Natl. Acad. Sci. U.S.A.* **85**, 582–586.

Finer, M. H., Gerstenfeld, L. C., Young, D., Doty, P., and Boedtker, H. (1985). Collagen expression in embryonic chicken chondrocytes treated with phorbol myristate acetate. *Mol. Cell. Biol.* **5**, 1415–1424.

Fitzer, C. J., O'Brian, C. A., Guillem, J. G., and Weinstein, I. B. (1987). The regulation of protein kinase C by chenodeoxycholate, deoxycholate, and several structurally related bile acids. *Carcinogenesis* **8**, 217–220.

Flier, J. S., Mueckler, M. M., Usher, P., and Lodish, H. F. (1987). Elevated levels of glucose transport and transporter messenger RNA are induced by *ras* or *src* oncogenes. *Science* **235**, 1492–1495.

Flint, A. J., Paladin, R. D., and Koshland, D. E., Jr. (1990). Autophosphorylation of protein kinase C at three separated regions of its primary sequence. *Science* **249**, 408–411.

Fojo, A. T., Ueda, K., Slamon, D. J., Poplack, D. G., Gottesman, M. M., and Pastan, I. (1987). Expression of a multidrug-resistance gene in human tumors and tissues. *Proc. Natl. Acad. Sci. U.S.A.* **84**, 265–269.

Forrester, K., Almoguera, C., Han, K., Grizzle, W. E., and Perucho, M. (1987). Detection of high incidence of K-*ras* oncogenes during human colon tumorigenesis. *Nature (London)* **327**, 298–303.

Fournier, A., Hardy, S. J., Clark, K. J., and Murray, A. W. (1989). Phorbol ester induces differential membrane-association of protein kinase C subspecies in human platelets. *Biochem. Biophys. Res. Commun.* **161,** 556–561.

Gasson, J. C., Golde, D. W., Kaufman, S. E., Westbrook, C. A., Hewick, R. M., Kaufman, R. J., Wong, G. G., Temple, P. A., Leary, A. C., Brown, E. L., Orr, E. C., and Clark, S. C. (1985). Molecular characterization and expression of the gene encoding human erythroid–potentiating activity. *Nature (London)* **315,** 768–771.

Gerlach, J. H., Endicott, J. A., Juranka, P. F., Henderson, G., Sarangi, F., Deuchars, K. L., and Ling, V. (1986). Homology between P-glycoprotein and a bacterial haemolysin transport protein suggests a model for multidrug resistance. *Nature (London)* **324,** 485–489.

Gesher, A. (1985). Antiproliferative properties of phorbol ester tumor promoters. *Biochem. Pharmacol.* **34,** 2587–2592.

Gesher, A., and Dale, I. L. (1989). Protein kinase C—a novel target for rational anti-cancer drug design? (Mini-review). *Anticancer Drug Des.* **4,** 93–105.

Gorsky, L. D., Cross, S. M., and Morin, M. J. (1989). Rapid increase in the activity of DNA topoisomerase I but not topoisomerase II, in HL-60 promyelocytic leukemia cells treated with a phorbol diester. *Cancer Commun.* **1,** 83–92.

Gottesman, M. M. (1988). Multidrug resistance during chemical carcinogenesis: A mechanism revealed? *J. Natl. Cancer Inst.* **80,** 1352–1353.

Gottesman, M. M., and Pastan, I. (1988). The multidrug transporter, a double-edged sword. *J. Biol. Chem.* **263,** 12163–12166.

Gould, K. L., Woodgett, J. R., Cooper, J. A., Buss, J. E., Shalloway, D., and Hunter, T. (1985). Protein kinase C phosphorylates pp60^{src} at a novel site. *Cell* **42,** 849–857.

Graff, J. M., Gordon, J. I., and Blackshear, P. J. (1989a). Myristoylated and nonmyristoylated forms of a protein are phosphorylated by protein kinase C. *Science* **246,** 503–506.

Graff, J. M., Young, T. N., Johnson, J. D., and Blackshear, P. J. (1989b). Phosphorylation-regulated calmodulin binding to a prominent cellular substrate for protein kinase C. *J. Biol. Chem.* **264,** 21818–21823.

Greenberger, L. M., Lothstein, L., Williams, S. S., and Horwitz, S. B. (1988). Distinct P-glycoprotein precursors are overproduced in independently isolated drug-resistant cell lines. *Proc. Natl. Acad. Sci. U.S.A.* **85,** 3762–3766.

Gros, P., Ben-Neriah, Y., Croop, J., and Housman, D. E. (1986). Isolation and expression of a cDNA that confers multidrug resistance. *Nature (London)* **323,** 728–731.

Gros, P., Raymond, M., Bell, J., and Housman, D. (1988). Cloning and characterization of a second member of the mouse *mdr* gene family. *Mol. Cell. Biol.* **8,** 2770–2778.

Guillem, J. G., O'Brian, C. A., Fitzer, C. J., Forde, K. A., LoGerfo, P., Treat, M., and Weinstein, I. B. (1987a). Altered levels of protein kinase C and Ca^{2+}-dependent protein kinases in human colon carcinomas. *Cancer Res.* **47,** 2036–2039.

Guillem, J. G., O'Brian, C. A., Fitzer, C. J., Johnson, M. D., Forde, K. A., LoGerfo, P., and Weinstein, I. B. (1987b). Studies on protein kinase C and colon carcinogenesis. *Arch. Surg.* **122,** 1475–1478.

Guillem, J. G., Hsieh, L.-L. O'Toole, K. M., Forde, K. A., LoGerfo, P., and Weinstein, I. B. (1988). Changes in expression of oncogenes and endogenous retroviral-like sequences during colon carcinogenesis. *Cancer Res.* **48,** 3964–3971.

Guillem, J. G., Levy, M. F., Hsieh, L. L., Johnson, M. D., LoGerfo, P., Forde, K. A., and Weinstein, I. B. (1990). Increased levels of phorbin, c-*myc*, and ornithine decarboxylase RNAs in human colon cancer. *Mol. Carcinogenesis* **3,** 68–74.

Guillem, J. G., and Weinstein, I. B. (1990). The role of protein kinase C in colon neoplasia. *In* "Familial Adenomatous Polyposis," pp. 325–332. Alan R. Liss, Inc, New York.

Hagiwara, M., Uchida, C., Usuda, N., Nagata, T., and Hidaka, H. (1990). ζ-Related protein kinase C in nuclei of nerve cells. *Biochim. Biophys. Res. Commun.* **168,** 161–168.

Haliotis, T., Trimble, W., Chow, S., Mills, G., Girard, P., Kuo, J. F., Govindji, N., and Hozumi, N. (1988). The cell biology of ras-induced transformation: Insights from studies utilizing an inducible hybrid oncogene system. Anticancer Res. 8, 935–946.

Halsey, D. L., Girard, P. R., Kuo, J. F., and Blackshear, P. J. (1987). Protein kinase C in fibroblasts. J. Biol. Chem. 262, 2234–2241.

Hamada, H., Hagiwara, K.-I., Nakajima, T., and Tsuruo, T. (1987). Phosphorylation of the M_r 170,000 to 180,000 glycoprotein specific to multidrug-resistant tumor cells: Effects of verapamil, trifluoperazine, and phorbol esters. Cancer Res. 47, 2860–2865.

Hamada, H., and Tsuruo, T. (1988). Characterization of the ATPase activity of the M_r 170,000 to 180,000 membrane glycoprotein (P-glycoprotein) associated with multidrug resistance in K562/ADM cells. Cancer Res. 48, 4926–4932.

Hannun, Y. A., and Bell, R. M. (1988). Aminoacridines, potent inhibitors of protein kinase C. J. Biol. Chem. 263, 5124–5131.

Hannun, Y. A., and Bell, R. M. (1989). Functions of sphingolipids and sphingolipid breakdown products in cellular regulation. Science 243, 500–507.

Harker, W. G., Slade, D. L., Dalton, W. S., Meltzer, P. S., and Trent, J. M. (1989). Multidrug resistance in mitoxantrone-selected HL-60 leukemia cells in the absence of P-glycoprotein overexpression. Cancer Res. 49, 4542–4549.

Hashimoto, K., Kishimoto, A., Aihara, H., Yasuda, I., Mikawa, K., and Nishizuka, Y. (1990). Protein kinase C during differentiation of human promyelocytic leukemia cell line, HL-60. FEBS Lett. 263, 31–34.

Hensey, C. E., Boscoboinik, D., and Azzi, A. (1989). Suramin, an anticancer drug, inhibits protein kinase C and induces differentiation in neuroblastoma cell clone NB2A. FEBS Lett. 258, 156–158.

Herschman, H. R. (1989). Extracellular signals, transcriptional responses, and cellular specificity. Trends Biochem. Sci. 14, 455–458.

Hidaka, H., Inagaki, M., Kawamoto, S., and Sasaki, Y. (1984). Isoquinolinesulfonamides, novel and potent inhibitors of cyclic nucleotide–dependent protein kinase and protein kinase C. Biochemistry 23, 5036–5041.

Hidaka, H., Tanaka, T., Onoda, K., Hagiwara, M., Watanabe, M., Ohta, H., Itoh, Y., Tsurudome, M., and Yoshida, T. (1988). Cell type–specific expression of protein kinase C isozymes in the rabbit cerebellum. J. Biol. Chem. 263, 4523–4526.

Hirai, M., Gamou, S., Kobayashi, M., and Shimizu, N. (1989). Lung cancer cells often express high levels of protein kinase C activity. Jpn. J. Cancer Res. 80, 204–208.

Hornbeck, P., Huang, K.-P., and Paul, W. E. (1988). Lamin B is rapidly phosphorylated in lymphocytes after activation of protein kinase C. Proc. Natl. Acad. Sci. U.S.A. 85, 2279–2283.

House, C., and Kemp, B. E. (1987). Protein kinase C contains a pseudosubstrate prototype in its regulatory domain. Science 238, 1726–1728.

Housey, G. M., O'Brian, C. A., Johnson, M. D., Kirschmeier, P., and Weinstein I. B. (1987). Isolation of cDNA clones encoding protein kinase C: Evidence for a protein kinase C–related gene family. Proc. Natl. Acad. Sci. U.S.A. 84, 1065–1069.

Housey, G. M., Johnson, M. D., Hsiao, W.-L. W., O'Brian, C. A., Murphy, J. P., Kirschmeier, P., and Weinstein, I. B. (1988). Overproduction of protein kinase C causes disordered growth control in rat fibroblasts. Cell 52, 343–354.

Hsiao, W.-L. W., Gattoni-Celli, S., and Weinstein, I. B. (1984). Oncogene-induced transformation of C3H 10T1/2 cells is enhanced by tumor promoters. Science 226, 552–555.

Hsiao, W.-L. W., Housey, G. M., Johnson, M. D., and Weinstein, I. B. (1989). Cells that overproduce protein kinase C are more susceptible to transformation by an activated H-ras oncogene. Mol. Cell. Biol. 9, 2641–2647.

Hsiao, W.-L. W., Pai, H.-L. H., Matsui, M. S., and Weinstein, I. B. (1990). Effects of specific fatty acids on cell transformation induced by an activated c-H-*ras* oncogene. *Oncogene* **5,** 417–421.

Hsieh, L. L., Hoshina, S., and Weinstein, I. B. (1989). Phenotypic effects of overexpression of PKCβ$_1$ in rat liver epithelial cells. *J. Cell. Biochem.* **41,** 179–188.

Huang, F. L., Yoshida, Y., Cunha-Melo, J. R., Beaven, M. A., and Huang, K.-P. (1989). Differential down-regulation of protein kinase C isozymes. *J. Biol. Chem.* **264,** 4238–4243.

Huang, K.-P., Nakabayashi, H., and Huang, F. L. (1986). Isozymic forms of rat brain Ca^{2+}-activated and phospholipid-dependent protein kinase. *Proc. Natl. Acad. Sci. U.S.A.* **83,** 8535–8539.

Huang, K.-P., Huang, F. L., Nakabayashi, H., and Yoshida, Y. (1988). Biochemical characterization of rat brain protein kinase C isozymes. *J. Biol. Chem.* **263,** 14839–14845.

Huang, K.-P., Huang, F. L., Nakabayashi, H., and Yoshida, Y. (1989). Expression and function of protein kinase C isozymes. *Acta Endocrinol.* **121,** 307–316.

Huang, K.-P. (1989). The mechanism of protein kinase C activation. *Trends Neurosci.* **11,** 425–432.

Huang, M., Chida, K., Kamata, N., Nose, K., Kato, M., Homma, Y., Takenawa, T., and Kuroki, T. (1988). Enhancement of inositol phospholipid metabolism and activation of protein kinase C in *ras*-transformed rat fibroblasts. *J. Biol. Chem.* **263,** 17975–17980.

Hunter, T., Ling, N., and Cooper, J. A. (1984). Protein kinase C phosphorylation of the EGF receptor at a threonine residue close to the cytoplasmic face of the plasma membrane. *Nature (London)* **311,** 480–483.

Hyatt, S. L., Klauck, T., and Jaken, S. (1990). Protein kinase C is localized in focal contacts of normal but not transformed fibroblasts. *Mol. Carcinogenesis* **3,** 45–53.

Imbra, J. R., and Karin, M. (1987). Metallothionein gene expression is regulated by serum factors and activators of protein kinase C. *Mol. Cell. Biol.* **7,** 1358–1363.

Isakov, N., McMahon, P., and Altman, A. (1990). Selective post-transcriptional down-regulation of protein kinase C isozymes in leukemic T cells chronically treated with phorbol ester. *J. Biol. Chem.* **265,** 2091–2097.

Issandou, M., Bayard, F., and Darbon, J.-M. (1986). Activation by phorbol esters of protein kinase C in MCF-7 human breast cancer cells. *FEBS Lett.* **200,** 337–342.

Issandou, M., and Darbon, J. M. (1988). 1,2-Dioctanoyl-glycerol induces a discrete but transient translocation of protein kinase C as well as the inhibition of MCF-7 cell proliferation. *Biochem. Biophys. Res. Commun.* **151,** 458–465.

Issandou, M., Bayard, F., and Darbon, J.-M. (1988). Inhibition of MCF-7 cell growth by 12-*O*-tetradecanoyl-13-acetate and 1,2-dioctanoyl-*sn*-glycerol: Distinct effect on protein kinase C activity. *Cancer Res.* **48,** 6943–6950.

Ito, A., Saito, N., Hirata, M., Kose, A., Tsujino, T., Yoshihara, C., Ogita, K., Kishimoto, A., Nishizuka, Y., and Tanaka, C. (1990). Immunocytochemical localization of the α-subspecies of protein kinase C in rat brain. *Proc. Natl. Acad. Sci. U.S.A.* **87,** 3195–3199.

Jaken, S. (1985). Increased diacylglycerol content with phospholipase C or hormone treatment: Inhibition of phorbol ester binding and induction of phorbol ester–like biological responses. *Endocrinology* **117,** 2301–2306.

Jeng, A. Y., Srivastava, S. K., Lacal, J. C., and Blumberg, P. M. (1987). Phosphorylation of *ras* oncogene product by protein kinase C. *Biochem. Biophys. Res. Commun.* **145,** 782–788.

Johnson, M. D., Housey, G. M., Kirschmeier, P. T., and Weinstein, I. B. (1987). Molecular cloning of gene sequences regulated by tumor promoters and mitogens through protein kinase C. *Mol. Cell. Biol.* **7,** 2821–2829.

Karin, M., and Richards, R. I. (1982). Human metallothionein genes—primary structure of the metallothionein-II gene and a related processed gene. *Nature* **299,** 797–802.

Karin, M., and Herrlich, P. (1989). Cis- and trans-acting genetic elements responsible for induction of specific genes by tumor promoters, serum factors, and stress. *In* "Genes and signal transduction in multistage carcinogenesis" (N. H. Colburn, ed.), pp. 415–440. Marcel Dekker, New York-Basel.

Kato, H., Kawai, S., Takenawa, T. (1988). Disappearance of diacylglycerol kinase translocation in *ras*-transformed cells. *Biochem. Biophys. Res. Commun.* **154**, 959–966.

Kessel, D. (1988). Effects of phorbol esters on doxorubicin transport systems. *Biochem. Pharmacol.* **37**, 2297–2299.

Kikkawa, U., Takai, Y., Minakuchi, R., Inohara, S., and Nishizuka, Y. (1982). Calcium-activated, phospholipid-dependent protein kinase from rat brain. *J. Biol. Chem.* **257**, 13341–13348.

Kikkawa, U., Ogita, K., Ono, Y., Asaoka, Y., Shearman, M. S., Fujii, T., Ase, K., Sekiguchi, K., Igarashi, K., and Nishizuka, Y. (1987a). The common structure and activities of four subspecies of rat brain protein kinase C family. *FEBS Lett.* **223**, 212–216.

Kikkawa, U., Ono, Y., Ogita, K., Fujii, T., Asaoka, Y., Sekiguchi, K., Kosaka, Y., Igarashi, K., and Nishizuka, Y. (1987b). Identification of the structures of multiple subspecies of protein kinase C expressed in rat brain. *FEBS Lett.* **217**, 227–231.

Kikkawa, U., Kishimoto, A., and Nishizuka, Y. (1989). The protein kinase C family: Heterogeneity and its implications. *Ann. Rev. Biochem.* **58**, 31–44.

Kishimoto, A., Mikawa, K., Hashimoto, K., Yasuda, I., Tanaka, S., Tominaga, M., Kuroda, T., and Nishizuka, Y. (1989). Limited proteolysis of protein kinase C subspecies by calcium-dependent neutral protease (calpain). *J. Biol. Chem.* **264**, 4088–4092.

Kiss, Z., Deli, E., and Kuo, J. F. (1988). Temporal changes in intracellular distribution of protein kinase C during differentiation of human leukemia HL-60 cells induced by phorbol ester. *FEBS Lett.* **231**, 41–46.

Knopf, J. L., Lee, M.-H., Sultzman, L. A., Kriz, R. W., Loomis, C. R., Hewick, R. M., and Bell, R. M. (1986). Cloning and expression of multiple protein kinase C cDNAs. *Cell* **46**, 491–502.

Kopp, R., Noelke, B., Sauter, G., and Pfeiffer, A. (1990). Early alterations of protein kinase-C activity in the colonic adenoma-carcinoma sequence in humans. *Gastroenterology (Suppl.)* **98**(2), A290.

Kosaka, Y., Ogita, K., Ase, K., Nomura, H., Kikkawa, U., and Nishizuka, Y. (1988). The heterogeneity of protein kinase C in various rat tissues. *Biochem. Biophys. Res. Commun.* **151**, 973–981.

Kraft, A. S., Anderson, W. B., Cooper, H. L., and Sando J J. (1982). Decrease in cytosolic calcium phospholipid-dependent protein kinase activity following phorbol ester treatment of EL4 thymoma cells. *J. Biol. Chem.* **257**, 13193–13196.

Kraft, A. S., and Anderson, W. B. (1983). Phorbol esters increase the amount of Ca^{2+} phospholipid-dependent protein kinase with plasma membrane. *Nature (London)* **301**, 621–623.

Krauss, R. S., Housey, G. M., Johnson, M. D., and Weinstein, I. B. (1989). Disturbances in growth control and gene expression in a C3H 10T1/2 cell line that stably overproduces protein kinase C. *Oncogene* **4**, 991–998.

Lacal, J. C., Fleming, T. P., Warren, B. S., Blumberg, P. M., and Aaronson, S. A. (1987). Involvement of functional protein kinase C in the mitogenic response to the H-*ras* oncogene product *Mol. Cell. Biol.* **7**, 4146–4149.

Leach, K. L., Powers, E. A., Ruff, V. A., Jaken, S., and Kaufmann, S. (1989). Type 3 protein kinase localization to the nuclear envelope of phorbol ester-treated NIH 3T3 cells. *J. Cell. Biol.* **109**, 685–695.

Lee, J. M., and Greenleaf, A. L. (1989). A protein kinase that phosphorylates the C-terminal repeat domain of the largest subunit of RNA polymerase II. *Proc. Natl. Acad. Sci. U.S.A.* **86**, 3624–3628.

Lee, W., Mitchell, P., and Tjian, R. (1987). Purified transcription factor AP-1 interacts with TPA-inducible enhancer elements. *Cell* **49**, 741–752.

Lenardo, M. J., and Baltimore, D. (1989). NF-κB: A pleiotropic mediator of inducible and tissue-specific gene control. *Cell* **58**, 227–229.

Lim, I. K., Lee, D. J., Lee, K. H., and Yun, T. K. (1987). High activities of protein kinases C and M in fresh human stomach and breast tumors. *Yonsei Med. J.* **28**, 255–260.

Linnenbach, A. J., Huebner, K., Reddy, E. P., Herlyn, M., Parmiter, A. H., Nowell, P. C., and Koprowski, H. (1988). Structural alteration in the MYB protooncogene and deletion within the genes encoding α-type protein kinase C in human melanoma cell lines. *Proc. Natl. Acad. Sci. U.S.A.* **85,** 74–78.

Lipkin, M., and Newmark, H. (1985). Effect of added dietary calcium on colonic epithelial-cell proliferation in subjects at high risk for familial colonic cancer. *N. Engl. J. Med.* **313,** 1381–1384.

Lopez-Barahona, M., Kaplan, P. L., Cornet, M. E., Diaz-Meco, M. T., Larrodera, P., Diaz-Laviada, I., Municio, A. M., and Moscat, J. (1990). Kinetic evidence of a rapid activation of phosphatidylcholine hydrolysis by Ki-*ras* oncogene. *J. Biol. Chem.* **265,** 9022–9026.

Macfarlane, D. E. (1986). Phorbol diester-induced phosphorylation of nuclear matrix proteins in HL60 promyelocytes. *J. Biol. Chem.* **261,** 6947–6953.

Mahoney, C. W., Azzi, A., Huang, K.-P. (1990). Effects of suramin, an anti-human immunodeficiency virus reverse transcriptase agent, on protein kinase C. *J. Biol. Chem.* **265,** 5424–5428.

Makowske, M., Birnbaum, M. J., Ballester, R., and Rosen, O. M. (1986). A cDNA encoding PKC identifies two species of mRNA in brain and GH3 cells. *J. Biol. Chem.* **261,** 13389–13392.

Makowske, M., Ballester, R., Cayre, Y., and Rosen, O. M. (1988). Immunochemical evidence that three protein kinase C isozymes increase in abundance during HL-60 differentiation induced by dimethylsulfoxide and retinoic acid. *J. Biol. Chem.* **263,** 3402–3410.

Marais, R. M., and Parker, P. J. (1989). Purification and characterisation of bovine brain protein kinase C isotypes α, β, and γ. *Eur. J. Biochem.* **182,** 129–137.

Margolis, B., Rhee, S. G., Felder, S., Mervic, M., Lyall, R., Levitzki, A., Ullrich, A., Zilberstein, A., and Schlessinger, J. (1989). EGF induces tyrosine phosphorylation of phospholipase C-II: A potential mechanism for EGF signaling. *Cell* **57,** 1101–1107.

Martell, R. E., Simpson, R. U., and Taylor, J. M. (1987). 1,25-Dihydroxyvitamin D₃ regulation of phorbol ester receptors in HL-60 leukemia cells. *J. Biol. Chem.* **262,** 5570–5575.

Masmoudi, A., Labourdette, G., Mersel, M., Huang, F. L., Huang, K.-P., Vincendon, G., and Malviya, A. N. (1989). Protein kinase C located in rat liver nuclei. *J. Biol. Chem.* **264,** 1172–1179.

Mason-Garcia, M., Weill, C. L., and Beckman, B. S. (1990). Rapid activation by erythropoietin of protein kinase C in nuclei of erythroid progenitor cells. *Biochem. Biophys. Res. Commun.* **168,** 490–497.

Matrisian, L. M., Leroy, P., Ruhlmann, C., Gesnel, M.-C., and Breathnach, R. (1986). Isolation of the oncogene and epidermal growth factor–induced transin gene: Complex control in rat fibroblasts. *Mol. Cell. Biol.* **6,** 1679–1686.

Megidish, T., and Mazurek, N. (1989). A mutant protein kinase C that can transform fibroblasts. *Nature (London)* **342,** 807–811.

Meisenhelder, J., Suh, P.-G., Rhee, S. G., and Hunter, T. (1989). Phospholipase C-γ is a substrate for the PDGF and EGF protein–tyrosine kinases *in vivo* and *in vitro. Cell* **57,** 1109–1122.

Mellado, W., and Horwitz, S. B. (1987). Phosphorylation of the multidrug resistance–associated glycoprotein. *Biochemistry* **26,** 6900–6904.

Melloni, E., Pontremoli, S., Michetti, M., Sacco, O., Cakiroglu, A. G., Jackson, J. F., Rifkind, R. A., and Marks, P. A. (1987). Protein kinase C activity and hexamethylene bisacetamide–induced erythroleukemia cell differentiation. *Proc. Natl. Acad. Sci. U.S.A.* **84,** 5282–5286.

Melloni, E., Pontremoli, S., Viotti, P. L., Patrone, M., Marks, P. A., and Rifkind, R. A. (1989). Differential expression of protein kinase C isozymes and erythroleukemia cell differentiation. *J. Biol. Chem.* **264,** 18414–18418.

Melloni, E., Pontremoli, S., Sparatore, B., Patrone, M., Grossi, F., Marks, P. A., Rifkind, R. A. (1990). Introduction of the β isozyme of protein kinase C accelerates induced differentiation of murine erythroleukemia cells. *Proc. Natl. Acad. Sci. U.S.A.* **87,** 4417–4420.

Meyer, T., Regenass, U., Fabbro, D., Alteri, E., Rosel, J., Muller, M., Caravatti, G., and Matter,

A. (1989). A derivative of staurosporine (CGP 41 251) shows selectivity for protein kinase C inhibition and *in vitro* antiproliferative as well as *in vivo* antitumor activity. *Int. J. Cancer* **43**, 851–856.

Mochly-Rosen, D., Basbaum, A. I., and Koshland, D. E., Jr. (1987). Distinct cellular and regional localization of immunoreactive protein kinase C in rat brain. *Proc. Natl. Acad. Sci. U.S.A.* **84**, 4660–4664.

Morotomi, M., Guillem, J. G., LoGerfo, P., and Weinstein, I. B. (1990). Production of diacylglycerol, an activator of protein kinase C, by human intestinal microflora. *Cancer Res.* **50**, 3595–3599.

Morris, C., Rice, P., and Rozengurt, E. (1988). The diacylglycerol kinase inhibitor R 59 022 potentiates bombesin stimulation of protein kinase C activity and DNA synthesis in Swiss 3T3 cells. *Biochem. Biophys. Res. Commun.* **155**, 561–568.

Munstermann, U., Fritz, G., Seitz, G., Yiping, L., Schneider, H. R., and Issinger, O.-G. (1990). Casein kinase II is elevated in solid human tumours and rapidly proliferating non-neoplastic tissue. *Eur. J. Biochem.* **189**, 251–257.

Muramatsu, M., Kaibuchi, K., and Arai, K.-I. (1989). A protein kinase C cDNA without the regulatory domain is active after transfection *in vivo* in the absence of phorbol ester. *Mol. Cell. Biol.* **9**, 831–836.

Murray, A. W., Fournier, A., and Hardy, S. J. (1987). Proteolytic activation of protein kinase C: A physiological reaction? *Trends Biochem. Sci.* **12**, 53–54.

Niedel, J. E., Kuhn, L. J., and Vandenbark, G. R. (1983). Phorbol diester receptor copurifies with protein kinase C. *Proc. Natl. Acad. Sci. U.S.A.* **80**, 36–40.

Niles, R. M., and Loewy, B. P. (1989). Induction of protein kinase C in mouse melanoma cells by retinoic acid. *Cancer Res.* **49**, 4483–4487.

Nigg, E. A. (1990). Mechanisms of signal transduction to the cell nucleus. *Adv. Cancer Res.* **55**, 271–310.

Nishizuka, Y. (1984). The role of protein kinase C in cell surface signal transduction and tumour production. *Nature (London)* **308**, 693–698.

Nishizuka, Y. (1986a). Studies and perspectives of protein kinase C. *Science* **233**, 305–312.

Nishizuka, Y. (1986b). Perspectives on the role of protein kinase C in stimulus–response coupling. *J. Natl. Cancer Inst.* **76**, 363–370.

Nishizuka, Y. (1988). The molecular heterogeneity of protein kinase C and its implications for cellular regulation. *Nature (London)* **334**, 661–665.

Nunn, D. L., and Watson, S. P. (1987). A diacylglycerol kinase inhibitor, R 59 022, potentiates secretion by and aggregation of thrombin-stimulated human platelets. *Biochem. J.* **243**, 809–813.

Obeid, L. M., Okazaki, T., Karolak, L. A., and Hannun, Y. A. (1990). Transcriptional regulation of protein kinase C by 1,25-dihydroxyvitamin D_3 in HL-60 cells. *J. Biol. Chem.* **265**, 2370–2374.

O'Brian, C. A., Liskamp, R. M., Solomon, D. H., and Weinstein, I. B. (1985). Inhibition of protein kinase C by tamoxifen. *Cancer Res.* **45**, 2462–2465.

O'Brian, C. A., Vogel, V. G., Singletary, S. E., and Ward, N. E. (1989a). Elevated protein kinase C expression in human breast tumor biopsies relative to normal breast tissue. *Cancer Res.* **49**, 3215–3217.

O'Brian, C. A., Fan, D., Ward, N. E., Seid, C., and Fidler, I. J. (1989b). Level of protein kinase C activity correlates directly with resistance to adriamycin in murine fibrosarcoma cells. *FEBS Lett.* **246**, 78–82.

Ohno, S., Kawasaki, H., Imajoh, S., Suzuki, K., Inagaki, M., Yokohura, H., Sakoh, T., and Hidaka, H. (1987). Tissue-specific expression of three distinct types of rabbit protein kinase C. *Nature (London)* **325**, 161–166.

Ohno, S., Akita, Y., Konno, Y., Imajoh, S., and Suzuki, K. (1988). A novel phorbol ester receptor/protein kinase, nPKC, distantly related to the protein kinase C family. *Cell* **53**, 731–741.

Ohno, S., Konno, Y., Akita, Y., Yano, A., and Suzuki, K. (1990). A point mutation at the putative ATP-binding site of protein kinase C α abolishes the kinase activity and renders it down-regulation–insensitive. *J. Biol. Chem.* **265,** 6296–6300.

Ono, Y., Kurokawa, T., Fujii, T., Kawahara, K., Igarashi, K., Kikkawa, U., Ogita, K., and Nishizuka, Y. (1986). Two types of complementary DNAs of rat brain protein kinase C. *FEBS Lett.* **206,** 347–352.

Ono, Y., Kikkawa, U., Ogita, K., Tomoko, F., Kurokawa, T., Asaoka, Y., Sekiguchi, K., Ase, K., Igarashi, K., and Nishizuka, Y. (1987a). Expression and properties of two types of protein kinase C: Alternative splicing from a single gene. *Science* **236,** 1116–1120.

Ono, Y., Fujii, T., Ogita, K., Kikkawa, U., Igarashi, K., and Nishizuka, Y. (1987b). Identification of three additional members of rat protein kinase C family: δ-, ε- and ζ-subspecies. *FEBS Lett.* **226,** 125–128.

Ono, Y., and Kikkawa, U. (1987). Do multiple species of protein kinase C transduce different signals? *Trends Biochem. Sci.* **12,** 421–423.

Ono, Y., Fujii, T., Ogita, K., Kikkawa, U., Igarashi, K., and Nishizuka, Y. (1988). The structure, expression, and properties of additional members of the protein kinase C family. *J. Biol. Chem.* **263,** 6927–6932.

Ono, Y., Fujii, T., Ogita, K., Kikkawa, U., Igarashi, K., and Nishizuka, Y. (1989a). Protein kinase C ζ subspecies from rat brain: Its structure, expression, and properties. *Proc. Natl. Acad. Sci. U.S.A.* **86,** 3099–3103.

Ono, Y., Fujii, T., Igarashi, K., Kuno, T., Tanaka, C., Kikkawa, U., and Nishizuka, Y. (1989b). Phorbol ester binding to protein kinase C requires a cysteine-rich zinc-finger–like sequence. *Proc. Natl. Acad. Sci. U.S.A.* **86,** 4868–4871.

Pai, J.-K., Pachter, J. A., Weinstein, I. B., and Bishop, W. R. (1991). Overexpression of protein kinase C-β1 enhances phospholipase D activity and diacylglycerol formation in phorbol ester-stimulated rat fibroblasts. *Proc. Natl. Acad. Sci. U.S.A.* **88,** 598–602.

Palayoor, S. T., Stein, J. M., and Hait, W. N. (1987). Inhibition of protein kinase C by antineoplastic agents: Implications for drug resistance. *Biochem. Biophys. Res. Commun.* **148,** 718–725.

Parker, P. J., Coussens, L., Totty, N., Rhee, L., Young, S., Chen, E., Stabel, S., Waterfield, M. D., and Ullrich, A. (1986). The complete primary structure of protein kinase C—the major phorbol ester receptor. *Science* **233,** 853–859.

Patel, G., and Stabel, S. (1989). Expression of a functional protein kinase-γ using a baculovirus vector: Purification and characterisation of a single protein kinase C iso-enzyme. *Cell. Signalling* **1,** 227–240.

Pearson, J. D., DeWald, D. B., Mathews, W. R., Mozier, N. M., Zurcher-Neely, H. A., Heinrickson, R. L., Morris, M. A., McCubbin, W. D., McDonald, J. R., Fraser, E. D., Vogel, H. J., Kay, C. M., and Walsh, M. P. (1990). Amino acid sequence and characterization of a protein inhibitor of protein kinase C. *J. Biol. Chem.* **265,** 4583–4591.

Pelosin, J. M., Vilgrain, I., and Chambaz, E. M. (1987). A single form of protein kinase C is expressed in bovine adrenocortical tissue, as compared to four chromatographically resolved isozymes in rat brain. *Biochem. Biophys. Res. Commun.* **147,** 382–391.

Persons, D. A., Wilkison, W. O., Bell, R. M., and Finn, O. J. (1988). Altered growth regulation and enhanced tumorigenicity of NIH 3T3 fibroblasts transfected with protein kinase C-1 cDNA. *Cell* **52,** 447–458.

Peterson, R. H. F., Meyers, M. B., Spengler, B. A., and Biedler, J. L. (1983). Alteration of plasma membrane glycopeptides and gangliosides of Chinese hamster cells accompanying development of resistance to daunorubicin and vincristine. *Cancer Res.* **43,** 222–228.

Pommier, Y., Kerrigan, D., Hartman, K. D., Glazer, R. I. (1990). Phosphorylation of mammalian DNA topoisomerase I and activation by protein kinase C. *J. Biol. Chem.* **265,** 9418–9422.

Posada, J. A., McKeegan, E. M., Worthington, K. F., Morin, M. J., Jaken, S., and Tritton, T. R.

(1989a). Human multidrug-resistant KB cells overexpress protein kinase C: Involvement in drug resistance. *Cancer Commun.* **1**, 285–292.

Posada, J., Vichi, P., and Tritton, T. R. (1989b). Protein kinase C in adriamycin action and resistance in mouse sarcoma 180 cells. *Cancer Res.* **49**, 6634–6639.

Regazzi, R., Fabbro, D., Costa, S. D., Borner, C., and Eppenberger, U. (1986). Effects of tumor promoters on growth and on cellular redistribution of phospholipid/Ca^{2+}–dependent protein kinase in human breast cancer cells. *Int. J. Cancer* **37**, 731–737.

Regenass, U., Geleick, D., Curschellas, E., Meyer, T., and Fabbro, D. (1989). *In vitro* cultures of epithelial cells from healthy breast tissues and cells from breast carcinomas. *Recent Results Cancer Res.* **113**, 5–15.

Rettenmier, C. W., Sacca, R., Furman, W. L., Roussel, M. F., Holt, J. T., Nienhuis, A. W., Stanley, E. R., and Sherr, C. J. (1986). Expression of the human c-*fms* protooncogene product colony-stimulating factor-1 receptor on peripheral blood mononuclear cells and choriocarcinoma cell lines. *J. Clin. Invest.* **77**, 1740–1746.

Rideout, D. C., Calogeropoulou, T., Jaworski, J. S., and McCarthy, M. R. (1990). Synergism through direct covalent bonding between agents: A strategy for rational design of chemotherapeutic combinations. *Biopolymers* **29**, 247–262.

Risse, G., Jooss, K., Neuberg, M., Bruller, H.-J., and Muller, R. (1989). Asymmetrical recognition of the palindromic AP1 binding site (TRE) by Fos protein complexes. *EMBO J.* **8**, 3825–3832.

Rogue, P., Labourdette, G., Masmoudi, A., Yoshida, Y., Huang, F. L., Huang, K.-P., Zwiller, J., Vincendon, G., and Malviya, A. N. (1990). Rat liver nuclei protein kinase C is the isozyme type II. *J. Biol. Chem.* **265**, 4161–4165.

Rose-John, S., Rincke, G., and Marks, F. (1987). The induction of ornithine decarboxylase by the tumor promoter TPA is controlled at the post-transcriptional level in murine Swiss 3T3 fibroblasts. *Biochem. Biophys. Res. Commun.* **147**, 219–225.

Rotenberg, S. A., Krauss, R. S., Borner, C. M. B., and Weinstein, I. B. (1990a). Characterization of a specific form of protein kinase C overproduced by a C3H 10T1/2 cell line. *Biochem. J.* **266**, 173–178.

Rotenberg, S. A., Smiley, S., Ueffing, M., Krauss, R. S., Chen, L. B., and Weinstein, I. B. (1990b). Inhibition of rodent protein kinase C by the anticarcinoma agent dequalinium. *Cancer Res.* **50**, 677–685.

Rotenberg, S. A., Calogeropoulou, T., Jaworski, J. S., Weinstein, I. B., and Rideout, D. (1991). A self-assembling protein kinase C inhibitor. *Proc. Natl. Acad. Sci. U.S.A.* **88**, 2490–2494.

Rousset, M. (1986). The human colon carcinoma cell lines HT29 and Caco-2: Two *in vitro* models for the study of intestinal differentiation. *Biochimie* **68**, 1035–1040.

Roy, S. N., and Horwitz, S. B. (1985). A phosphoglycoprotein associated with taxol resistance in J774.2 cells. *Cancer Res.* **45**, 3856–3863.

Russell, D. H. (1989). New aspects of prolactin and immunity: A lymphocyte-derived prolactin-like product and nuclear protein kinase C activation. *Trends Pharmacol. Sci.* **10**, 40–44.

Rydell, E. L., Axelsson, K. L., and Olofsson, J. (1988). Protein kinase C activity in normal and neoplastic squamous epithelia from the upper aero-digestive tract. *Second Messengers Phosphoproteins* **12**, 155–162.

Sachs, C., Schnur, D., Balla, L., Hannun, Y., Loomis, C., Carroll, I., Bell, R., and Fine, R. L. (1990). Protein kinase C (PKC) inhibitors increase drug accumulation and are cytotoxic to a human multidrug resistant (mdr) breast cancer line. *Proc. Amer. Assoc. Cancer Res.* **31**, Abst. #2128.

Sahyoun, N., Wolf, M., Besterman, J., Hsieh, T.-s., Sander, M., LeVine, H., III, Chang, K.-J., and Cuatrecasas, P. (1986). Protein kinase C phosphorylates topoisomerase II: Topoisomerase activation and its possible role in phorbol ester–induced differentiation of HL-60 cells. *Proc. Natl. Acad. Sci. U.S.A.* **83**, 1603–1607.

Samuels, D. S., Shimizu, Y., and Shimizu, N. (1989). Protein kinase C phosphorylates DNA topoisomerase I. *FEBS Lett.* **259**, 57–60.

Schaap, D., Parker, P. J., Bristol, A., Kriz, R., and Knopf, J. (1989). Unique substrate specificity and regulatory properties of PKC-ε: A rationale for diversity. *FEBS Lett.* **243,** 351–357.

Schaap, D., and Parker, P. J. (1990). Expression, purification, and characterization of protein kinase C-ε. *J. Biol. Chem.* **265,** 7301–7307.

Schatzman, R. C., Wise, B. C., and Kuo, J. F. (1981). Phospholipid-sensitive calcium-dependent protein kinase: Inhibition by antipsychotic drugs. *Biochem. Biophys. Res. Commun.* **98,** 669–676.

Sekiguchi, K., Tsukuda, M., Ogita, K., Kikkawa, U., and Nishizuka, Y. (1987). Three distinct forms of rat brain protein kinase C: Differential response to unsaturated fatty acids. *Biochem. Biophys. Res. Commun.* **145,** 797–802.

Sharkey, N. A., Leach, K. L., and Blumberg, P. M. (1984). Competitive inhibition by diacylglycerol of specific phorbol ester binding. *Proc. Natl. Acad. Sci. U.S.A.* **81,** 607–610.

Shearman, M. S., Naor, Z., Sekiguchi, K., Kishimoto, A., and Nishizuka, P. (1989a). Selective activation of the γ-subspecies of protein kinase C from bovine cerebellum by arachidonic acid and its lipoxygenase metabolites. *FEBS Lett.* **243,** 177–182.

Shearman, M. S., Sekiguchi, K., and Nishizuka, Y. (1989b). Modulation of ion channel activity: A key function of the protein kinase C enzyme family. *Pharmacol. Rev.* **41,** 211–237.

Shen, D.-W., Fojo, A., Roninson, I. B., Chin, J. E., Soffir, R., Pastan, I., and Gottesman, M. M. (1986a). Multidrug resistance of DNA-mediated transformants is linked to transfer of the human *mdr* 1 gene. *Mol. Cell. Biol.* **6,** 4039–4044.

Shen, D.-W., Cardarelli, C., Hwang, J., Cornwell, M., Richert, N., Ishii, S., Pastan, I., and Gottesman, M. M. (1986b). Multiple drug–resistant human KB carcinoma cells independently selected for high-level resistance to colchicine, adriamycin, or vinblastine show changes in expression of specific proteins. *J. Biol. Chem.* **261,** 7762–7770.

Shimosawa, S., Hachiya, T., Hagiwara, M., Usuda, N., Sugita, K., and Hidaka, H. (1990). Type-specific expression of protein kinase C isozymes in CNS tumor cells. *Neurosci. Lett.* **108,** 11–16.

Shirakawa, F., and Mizel, S. B. (1989). *In vitro* activation and nuclear translocation of NF-κB catalyzed by cyclic AMP–dependent protein kinase and protein kinase C. *Mol. Cell. Biol.* **9,** 2424–2430.

Shoji, M., Vogler, W. R., and Kuo, J. F. (1985). Inhibition of phospholipid/Ca^{2+}–dependent protein kinase and phosphorylation of leukemic cell proteins by CP-46,665-1, a novel antineoplastic lipoidal amine. *Biochem. Biophys. Res. Commun.* **127,** 590–595.

Simek, S. L., Kligman, D., Patel, J., and Colburn, N. H. (1989). Differential expression of an 80-kDa protein kinase C substrate in preneoplastic and neoplastic mouse JB6 cells. *Proc. Natl. Acad. Sci. U.S.A.* **86,** 7410–7414.

Simpson, R. U., Hsu, T., Begley, D. A., Mitchell, B. S., and Alizadeh, B. N. (1987). Transcriptional regulation of the c-*myc* protooncogene by 1,25-dihydroxyvitamin D$_3$ in HL-60 promyelocytic leukemia cells. *J. Biol. Chem.* **262,** 4104–4108.

Smart, R. C., Huang, M.-T., Monteiro-Riviere, N. A., Wong, C.-Q., Mills, K. J., and Conney, A. H. (1988). Comparison of the effect of sn-1,2-didecanoyl-glycerol and 12-*O*-tetradecanoyl-phorbol-13-acetate on cutaneous morphology, inflammation, and tumor promotion in CD-1 mice. *Carcinogenesis* **9,** 2221–2226.

Smith, B. M., and Colburn, N. H. (1988). Protein kinase C and its substrates in promoter-sensitive and -resistant cells. *J. Biol. Chem.* **263,** 6424–6431.

Solomon, D. H., O'Driscoll, K., Sosne, G., Weinstein, I. B., and Cayre, Y. E. (1991). 1α,25-Dihydroxyvitamin D3–induced regulation of protein kinase C gene expression during HL60 cell differentiation. *Cell. Growth Diff.* **2,** 187–194.

Spangler, R., Joseph, C., Qureshi, S. A., Berg, K. L., and Foster, D. A. (1989). Evidence that v-*src* and v-*fps* gene products use a protein kinase C–mediated pathway to induce expression of a transformation-related gene. *Proc. Natl. Acad. Sci. U.S.A.* **86,** 7017–7021.

Staats, J., Marquardt, D., and Center, M. S. (1990). Characterization of a membrane-associated protein kinase of multidrug-resistant HL 60 cells which phosphorylates P-glycoprotein. *J. Biol. Chem.* **265**, 4084–4090.

Stumpo, D. J., Graff, J. M., Albert, K. A., Greengard, P., and Blackshear, P. J. (1989). Molecular cloning, characterization, and expression of a cDNA encoding the "80-87–kDa" myristoylated alanine-rich C kinase substrate: A major cellular substrate for protein kinase C. *Proc. Natl. Acad. Sci. U.S.A.* **86**, 4012–4016.

Takeyama, Y., Tanimoto, T., Hoshijima, M., Kaibuchi, K., Ohyanagi, H., Saitoh, Y., and Takai, Y. (1986). Enhancement of fibroblast growth factor–induced diacylglycerol formation and protein kinase C activation by colon tumor–promoting bile acid in Swiss 3T3 cells. *FEBS Lett.* **197**, 339–343.

Tamaoki, T., Nomoto, H., Takahashi, I., Kato, Y., Morimoto, M., and Tomita, F. (1986). Staurosporine, a potent inhibitor of phospholipid/Ca^{2+}–dependent protein kinase. *Biochem. Biophys. Res. Commun.* **135**, 397–402.

Teegarden, D., Taparowsky, E. J., and Kent, C. (1990). Altered phosphatidylcholine metabolism in C3H 10T1/2 cells transfected with the Harvey-*ras* oncogene. *J. Biol. Chem.* **265**, 6042–6047.

Testori, A., Hii, C. S. T., Fournier, A., Burgoyne, L. A., and Murray, A. W. (1988). DNA-binding proteins in protein kinase C preparations. *Biochem. Biophys. Res. Commun.* **156**, 222–227.

Thomas, T. P., Talwar, H. S., and Anderson, W. B. (1988). Phorbol ester-mediated association of protein kinase C to the nuclear fraction of NIH 3T3 cells. *Cancer Res.* **48**, 1910–1919.

Tran, P. L., Le Peuch, C., and Basset, M. (1989). Effects of fluorescent derivatives of TPA on HL-60 cells: Dissociation between the differentiation-induced and protein kinase C activity. *J. Cell. Physiol.* **139**, 313–319.

Ueda, K., Cardarelli, C., Gottesman, M. M., and Pastan, I. (1987). Expression of a full-length cDNA for the human "MDR 1" gene confers resistance to colchicine, doxorubicin, and vinblastine. *Proc. Natl. Acad. Sci. U.S.A.* **84**, 3004–3008.

Vandenbark, G., and Niedel, J. (1984). Phorbol diesters and cellular differentiation. *J. Natl. Cancer Inst.* **73**, 1013–1019.

Vogelstein, B., Fearon, E. R., Hamilton, S. R., Kern, S. E., Preisinger, A. C., Leppert, M., Nakamura, Y., White, R., Smits, A. M. M., and Bos, J. L. (1988). Genetic alterations during colorectal-tumor development. *N. Engl. J. Med.* **319**, 525–532.

Vogt, P. K., and Bos, T. J. (1990). *Jun:* oncogene and transcription factor. *Adv. Cancer Res.* **55**, 1–35.

Wada, H., Ohno, S., Kubo, K., Taya, C., Tsuji, S., Yonehara, S., and Suzuki, K. (1989). Cell type–specific expression of the genes for the protein kinase C family: Down-regulation of mRNAs for PKCα and nPKCε upon *in vitro* differentiation of a mouse neuroblastoma cell line neuro 2a. *Biochem. Biophys. Res. Commun.* **165**, 533–538.

Ward, N. E., and O'Brian, C. A. (1988). The bile acid analog fusidic acid can replace phosphatidylserine in the activation of protein kinase C by 12-O-tetradecanoylphorbol-13-acetate *in vitro*. *Carcinogenesis* **9**, 1451–1454.

Weinstein, I. B. (1988a). The origins of human cancer: Molecular mechanisms of carcinogenesis and their implications for cancer prevention and treatment. 27th G. H. A. Clowes Memorial Award Lecture. *Cancer Res.* **48**, 4135–4143.

Weinstein, I. B. (1988b). Strategies for inhibiting multistage carcinogenesis based on signal transduction pathways. *Mutation Res.* **202**, 413–420.

Weiss, M. J., Wong, J. R., Ha, C. S., Bleday, R., Salem, R. R., Steele, G. D., Jr., and Chen, L. B. (1987). Dequalinium, a tropical antimicrobial agent, displays anticarcinoma activity based on selective mitochondrial accumulation. *Proc. Natl. Acad. Sci. U.S.A.* **84**, 5444–5448.

Werth, D. K., Niedel, J. E., and Pastan, I. (1983). Vinculin, a cytoskeletal substrate of protein kinase C. *J. Biol. Chem.* **258**, 11423–11426.

Weyman, C. M., Taparowsky, E. J., Wolfson, M., and Ashendel, C. L. (1988). Partial down-regulation of protein kinase C in C3H 10T1/2 mouse fibroblasts transfected with the human Ha-*ras* oncogene. *Cancer Res.* **48,** 6535–6541.

Wise, B. C., and Kuo, J. F. (1983). Modes of inhibition by acylcarnitines, adriamycin, and trifluo-perazine of cardiac phospholipid-sensitive calcium-dependent protein kinase. *Biochem. Pharmacol.* **32,** 1259–1265.

Wolfman, A., Wingrove, T. G., Blackshear, P. J., and Macara, I. G. (1987). Down-regulation of protein kinase C and of an endogenous 80-kDa substrate in transformed fibroblasts. *J. Biol. Chem.* **262,** 16546–16552.

Wood, J. G., Girard, P. R., Mazzei, G. J., and Kuo, J. F. (1986). Immunocytochemical location of protein kinase C in identified neuronal compartments of rat brain. *J. Neurosci.* **6,** 2571–2577.

Wu, X., Shao, G., Chen, S., Wang, X., Wang, Z.-Y. (1989). Studies on the relationship between protein kinase C and differentiation of human promyelocytic leukemia cells induced by retinoic acid. *Leuk. Res.* **13,** 869–874.

Wyss, R., Fabbro, D., Regazzi, R., Borner, C., Takahashi, A., and Eppenberger, U. (1987). Phorbol ester and epidermal growth factor receptor in human breast cancer. *Anticancer Res.* **7,** 721–728.

Yang, C.-P. H., Cohen, D., Greenberger, L. M., Hsu, S. I.-H., and Horwitz, S. B. (1990). Differential transport properties of two *mdr* gene products are distinguished by progesterone. *J. Biol. Chem.* **265,** 10282–10288.

Yoshida, Y., Huang, F. L., Nakabayashi, H., and Huang, K.-P. (1988). Tissue distribution and developmental expression of protein kinase C isozymes. *J. Biol. Chem.* **263,** 9868–9873.

Young, S., Parker, P. J., Ullrich, A., and Stabel, S. (1987). Down-regulation of protein kinase C is due to an increased rate of degradation. *Biochem. J.* **244,** 775–779.

Yu, G., Aquino, A., Fairchild, C. R., Cowan, K. H., Ohno, S., and Glazer, R. I. (1990). Adriamycin resistance in MCF-7 cells expressing P-glycoprotein following transfection with protein kinase Cα. *Proc. Amer. Assoc. Cancer. Res.* **31,** Abst. #2168.

Zylber-Katz, E., and Glazer, R. I. (1985). Phospholipid- and Ca^{2+}–dependent protein kinase activity and protein phosphorylation patterns in the differentiation of human promyelocytic leukemia cell line HL-60. *Cancer Res.* **45,** 5159–5164.

Chapter 3

HER-2/*neu* Oncogene Amplification and Expression in Human Mammary Carcinoma

D. Craig Allred*, Atul K. Tandon†, Gary M. Clark†,
and William L. McGuire†

*University of Texas Health Science Center,
Department of Pathology, and Department of Medicine/Oncology,
San Antonio, Texas 78284*

I. Introduction

The treatment of patients with breast cancer has evolved from a historical reliance on surgery alone to include many other potentially beneficial options such as radiation, endocrine therapy, and chemotherapy. Ideally, the decision to use any of these additional (*adjuvant*) therapies should be based on a comparison of the anticipated clinical outcomes (prognosis) with and without adjuvant therapy. If the expected outcome without treatment is very promising, additional therapy may do more harm than good. If the prognosis is poor, adjuvant therapy offers at least the chance for improvement.

About half of all breast cancer patients have metastatic disease in axillary lymph nodes when they are first seen by a physician. The untreated prognosis for these patients is very poor, and the decision to use adjuvant therapy has become almost routine. The other half of patients first present without clinical–pathological evidence of nodal disease, and appear to be cured by initial surgery. Unfortunately, the disease will eventually recur in and kill 20–30% of these patients. The choice for adjuvant therapy in this setting is difficult and controversial. On the one hand, there is unequivocal evidence from recent studies that adjuvant endocrine and/or chemotherapy can significantly improve disease-free survival (DFS) in some patients with apparently localized breast cancer (i.e., axillary node–negative tumors) (Fisher *et al.*, 1989a, Fisher *et al.*, 1989b,

BIOCHEMICAL AND MOLECULAR ASPECTS
OF SELECTED CANCERS, VOL. 1

Mansour *et al.*, 1989). This has lead to an official recommendation by the National Cancer Institute in 1988 that all such patients be considered as candidates for adjuvant therapy. On the other hand, the majority of node-negative tumors do not recur, supporting the alternative point of view that not all of these patients should receive potentially harmful adjuvant therapy (McGuire, 1989). Proponents of both views would probably agree that patients at high risk for recurrence should receive adjuvant therapy if there were reliable means to identify them.

The prospective recognition of high-risk, node-negative breast cancers has traditionally been based on the size, hormone receptor status, histological grade, and nuclear grade of the primary tumor (McGuire *et al.*, 1990). Recently, flow cytometric determinations of tumor DNA content and growth fraction have been used to predict the course of disease (Clark *et al.*, 1989). However, consideration of all these factors combined has still been unable to accurately predict the clinical outcome of all patients, and there is a need for more powerful markers to identify specific patients with poor prognosis who might benefit from adjuvant therapy.

Among the candidates in the search for more powerful prognostic factors are activated (amplified and/or overexpressed) protooncogenes. One of the most intensely studied of these is HER-2/*neu*. Several recent studies have demonstrated that HER-2/*neu* is amplified or overexpressed in a significant percentage of breast carcinomas, and that these manifestations of oncogene activation are associated with poor prognosis. This chapter will briefly review some of the molecular biology of HER-2/*neu*, followed by a more detailed discussion of the clinical biology of this oncogene in breast cancer.

II. Molecular Biology of HER-2/*neu*

In 1981, Shih and co-workers described a novel transforming gene, which they identified in the DNA of chemically induced rat neuroblastomas using the NIH-3T3 transfection assay. This gene, called *neu*, was shown to be highly homologous to the epidermal growth factor–receptor (EGFR) gene and coded for a 185-kDa membrane protein (p185) (Padhy *et al.*, 1982; Schecter *et al.*, 1984). The human equivalent of *neu* was soon independently cloned from a human cDNA library (and referred to as HER-2) (Coussens *et al.*, 1985), from human genomic DNA (and referred to as c-*erb*B-2) (Semba *et al.*, 1985), and from the DNA of a human breast carcinoma cell line in which it was highly amplified (and referred to as *erb*B-related gene) (King *et al.*, 1985). Additional studies involving nucleotide sequencing and chromosomal mapping confirmed that the human gene was also very homologous to the EGFR gene, and resided on chromosome 17 (Coussens *et al.*, 1985, Semba *et al.*, 1985, Schecter *et al.*, 1985). Human p185 was shown to be similar to EGFR with respect to amino acid sequence and intracellular tyrosine-kinase activity (Coussens *et al.*, 1985; Semba *et al.*, 1985; Schecter *et al.*, 1985). The structural and functional activities shared with EGFR, and results from animal experiments in which antibodies to p185 inhibited the growth of xenografts containing activated *neu* (Drebin *et al.*, 1986), suggested that the HER-2/*neu* oncoprotein was a growth factor receptor. However, results obtained from clinical studies attempting to correlate HER-2/*neu* activation with various measures of tumor proliferation rate have been conflicting, with some finding (Heintz *et al.*, 1990; Tsuda *et al.*, 1990; Bacus *et al.*, 1990) and others not finding (Kommoss *et al.*, 1990; Allred *et al.*, 1991a) a significant relationship between the two.

Additional studies have shown that transfection of HER-2/*neu* is not transforming in the NIH-3T3 assay when the gene is normal, and that to be transforming, the gene must be overexpressed, which can occur by at least two mechanisms including amplification and mutation (DiFiore *et al.*, 1987; Bargmann *et al.*, 1988; DiMarco *et al.*, 1990). In fact, the originally described rat *neu* gene was mutationally activated. Related investigations have shown that overexpression of HER-2/*neu* also occurs in short-term cultures of normal breast epithelial cells (Benz *et al.*, 1989), suggesting that overexpression per se is not sufficient to induce malignant transformation. Of great interest was the recent development of transgenic mice that carry an activated *neu* gene, and overexpress p185 in several tissues (Muller *et al.*, 1988). These animals rapidly developed diffuse polyclonal adenocarcinomas only in breast tissue, suggesting the *neu*-induced malignant transformation is a tissue-restricted, single-step transforming event in mice. Slightly different results have come from more recent studies involving similarly constructed transgenic mice, in which transgene expression was detected in histologically normal mammary glands before and during the asynchronous development of tumors, suggesting that activated *neu* is necessary but not sufficient to induce malignant transformation in mouse mammary tissue (Bouchard *et al.*, 1989).

Clearly, the molecular biology of HER-2/*neu* in the context of both its normal and oncogenic functions is complex and incompletely understood at this time. Studies of early human fetuses showing prominent HER-2/*neu* expression in all 3 germ layers provide convincing evidence that the normal gene plays a central role in embryogenesis, which may involve regulation of cell proliferation and/or differentiation (Mori *et al.*, 1989; Quirke *et al.*, 1989). Other studies showing a high incidence of HER-2/*neu* amplification and expression in a variety of malignant tumors provide equally convincing evidence that the gene plays an important role in oncogenesis (Yokota *et al.*, 1986; Tal *et al.*, 1988; Gutman *et al.*, 1989; McCann *et al.*, 1990). With the recent report of a ligand being identified for HER-2/*neu* (Lupur *et al.*, in press), perhaps the issue of its biological function will begin to be resolved.

III. Clinical Biology of HER-2/*neu*

A. HER-2/*NEU* AMPLIFICATION AND EXPRESSION IN HUMAN BREAST CANCER

Amplification and/or overexpression of protooncogenes are often thought of as manifestations of their *oncogenic* potential when associated with malignant tumors. The first report of the involvement of the HER-2/*neu* oncogene in clinical breast cancer was by Slamon *et al.*, (1987), showing that HER-2/*neu* was amplified from 2 to 20 times in 30% of 189 samples of human breast carcinomas. Soon thereafter, Venter *et al.*, (1987) provided the first evidence of HER-2/*neu* overexpression in clinical breast tumors. These initial studies have motivated many others within the past 3 years, which have shown evidence of Her-2/*neu* activation in 10 to 40% of human breast cancers (reviewed in Table I). This wide range of values is most likely a reflection of technical and biological variability, and has been a serious impediment to our understanding of the clinical biology of this oncogene.

In our review of the literature, Southern blotting was the most sensitive method for measuring HER-2/*neu* amplification. The average incidence of amplification from 19 published studies involving over 2000 patients was about 22%. The range between values was large (10–34%), emphasizing several potential pitfalls of using this technique, including an absolute necessity for uniformly and properly handled fresh-frozen specimens, a requirement for considerable technical expertise in conducting the test, and the nearly unavoidable dilutional effect of nontumor cells contaminating the samples.

Several methods have been used to measure HER-2/*neu* expression. At least four studies using Western blotting have been published. The combined results from these efforts showed an average of 18.9% overexpression in 1135 breast tumors. Like Southern blotting, this method requires pampered fresh-frozen specimens, considerable technical expertise, and is subject to inaccuracies resulting from the presence of nontumor cells in the specimens. When performed properly, however, Western blots provide a reliable, semiquantitative assessment of HER-2/*neu* expression, which can be routinely performed in clinical laboratories on a large scale (Fig. 1).

Permanent section immunohistochemistry is by far the easiest method to measure HER-2/*neu* expression, relying on routinely prepared (i.e., formalin-fixed, paraffin-embedded) histopathological specimens. It also appears to have about the same sensitivity as Western blotting. A review of 16 studies showed an average incidence of about 19% positive staining in over 3600 patients. Fig. 2 shows a typical example of a HER-2/*neu*–positive breast carcinoma detected by this technique. Staining is primarily localized to the surface membranes of tumor cells, and most positive tumors are diffusely positive. Interestingly, it has also recently been shown that positive staining appears to be restricted to the more

TABLE I

SUMMARY OF LITERATURE REVIEW REGARDING THE RESULTS OF
DIFFERENT METHODS OF MEASURING AMPLIFICATION AND EXPRESSION OF
THE HER-2/neu ONCOGENE IN HUMAN BREAST CANCERS

Reference[a]	Amplification by Southern blot	
	Number of cases[b]	% Positive
Slamon et al. (1987)	189	30
van de Vijver et al. (1987)	95	17
Cline et al. (1987)	53	16
Varley et al. (1987)	41	19
Venter et al. (1987)	36	33
Zhou et al. (1987)	86	17
Berger et al. (1988)	51	25
Tal et al. (1988)	21	10
Ali et al. (1988)	122	10
Tavassoli et al. (1989)	52	28
Slamon et al. (1989)	345[c]	27
	181[d]	25
Zeilinger et al. (1989)	291	18
Lacroix et al. (1989)	57	19
Ro et al. (1989)	66	20
Adane et al. (1989)	219	20
Garcia et al. (1989)	125	22
Yamada et al. (1989)	50	20
Heintz et al. (1990)	50	34
Hanna et al. (1990)	66	25
	total = 2196	average[e] = 22.2

Reference	Amplification by slot blot	
	Number of cases[f]	% Positive
Paterson et al. (1988)	157	13
Tsuda et al. (1988)	176	16
Zhou et al. (1989)	157	11
Tsuda et al. (1990)	176	18
Borg et al. (1990)	300	17
	total = 966	average = 15.3

Reference	Expression by Western blot or immunoblot	
	Number of cases[b]	% Positive
Tandon et al. (1989)	728	17
Lacroix et al. (1989)	57	26
Yamada et al. (1989)	50	38
Borg et al. (1990)	300	19
	total = 1135	average = 18.9

(continued)

TABLE I
CONTINUED

Reference	Expression by permanent-section immunohistochemistry Number of cases[f]	% Positive
Gusterson *et al.* (1988a)	34	35
van de Vijver *et al.* (1988)	189	14
	45[g]	42
Barnes *et al.* (1988)	195	10
Gusterson *et al.* (1988b)	103	14
Gusterson *et al.* (1988c)	180	16
	93[g]	44
Wright *et al.* (1989)	189	17
de Potter *et al.* (1989a)	67	29
Thor *et al.* (1989)	47[h]	15
Walker *et al.* (1989)	85	17
Paik *et al.* (1990)	292	21
McCann *et al.* (1990)	405	17
Kommoss *et al.* (1990)	50	10
Hanna *et al.* (1990)	66	33
Lovekin *et al.* (in press)	229[c]	20
	250[d]	15
Gullick *et al.* (in press)	437	21
Allred *et al.* (1991a)	736	17
	total = 3692	average = 18.7

Reference	Expression by frozen-section immunohistochemistry Number of cases[f]	% Positive
Venter *et al.* (1987)	36	33
Kommoss *et al.* (1990)	50	22
Bacus *et al.* (1990)	45	47
Marx *et al.* (1990)	163	33
	total = 294	average = 33.3

[a] References are listed by first author in chronological order.
[b] Cases represented by fresh-frozen tumor specimens.
[c] Axillary node-positive cases.
[d] Axillary node-negative cases.
[e] Averages are weighted with respect to the number of cases from each study.
[f] Cases represented by formalin-fixed, paraffin-embedded tumor specimens.
[g] *In situ* carcinomas of the breast.
[h] Cases showing "strong" staining in over 40% of tumor cells.

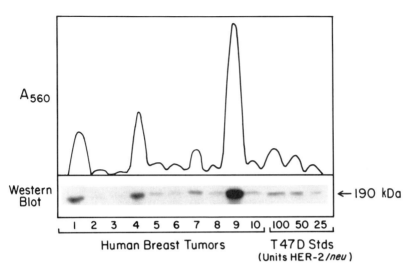

FIG. 1.   Semiquantitation of HER-2/*neu* protein in tumor specimens by Western blot analysis. An SDS extract of human breast cancer cells (T47D) was used as our laboratory standard. The HER-2/*neu* bands at 190 kDa along with densitometric scan are shown. From Tandon *et al.* (1989).

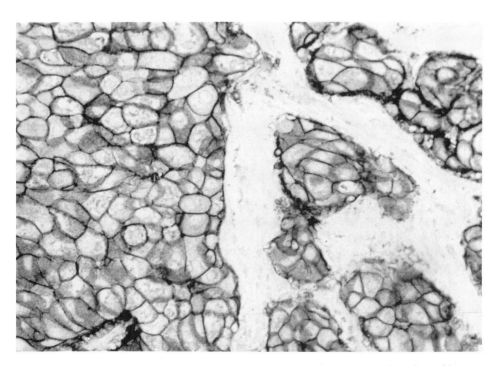

FIG. 2.   Example of breast carcinoma overexpressing the HER-2/*neu* oncoprotein as detected by permanent-section immunohistochemistry. Positive staining is localized to the surface membranes of malignant cells. (154× magnification)

common subtypes of ductal carcinomas of the breast (Gusterson *et al.*, 1988b; Allred *et al.*, 1991a). Because high concentrations of anti-Her-2/*neu* antibody can result in membrane (and occasionally cytoplasmic) staining of both benign and malignant cells, the reagents must be titered to react only with the latter, or the test will not discriminate between overexpression and baseline expression. The cellular localization of the signal is also probably biologically important, as suggested by recent *in vitro* studies showing that development of the malignant phenotype in *neu*-transfected cells is strictly dependent on the presence of the oncoprotein at the cell surface (Drebin *et al.*, 1985; Drebin *et al.*, 1986). In addition, De Potter *et al.*, (1988a) have shown that the molecular weight of the protein associated with cytoplasmic staining (155 kDa) is less than that of the protein associated with membrane staining (185 kDa). More recent work by De Potter *et al.*, (1989b) suggests that the cytoplasmic signal represents crossreactivity with an uncharacterized mitochondrial protein. Despite its problems, permanent-section immunostaining will very likely become the method of choice for measuring HER-2/*neu* expression because it is easy to interpret, and the samples are easy to obtain.

Frozen-section immunohistochemistry is more sensitive than its permanent-section counterpart. Results from 4 frozen-section studies involving nearly 300 breast cancers showed an average of 33% cases positive for HER-2/*neu* expression. A few studies have directly compared permanent and frozen-section techniques in the same series of patients and found frozen-section immunostaining to be more sensitive (Slamon *et al.*, 1989; Kommoss *et al.*, 1990). The reason for this increased sensitivity is most likely better preservation of the oncoprotein in frozen sections.

At least two potential problems may arise when tumor specimens are fixed. First, it takes considerable time for fixatives to permeate tissue, allowing degradation of the antigen before fixation. Second, most fixatives progressively crosslink or precipitate proteins, which alters their configuration and ability to bind antibodies. Our results using a polyclonal antibody prepared in our laboratory against a synthetic peptide of HER-2/*neu* (21N-SAT) suggest that the first type of insult is more critical than the second. In our experience, small biopsy specimens can remain for up to 48 hr in 10% buffered fromalin without appreciable loss of staining reactivity, presumably owing to rapid fixation. In contrast, larger specimens often show poor staining reactivity, regardless of fixation time, presumably because penetration of formalin is too slow for adequate fixation. The latter problem often arises when dealing with large biopsy or mastectomy specimens, which were not thoroughly sectioned before submerging in fixative.

Despite the increased sensitivity of frozen-section compared to permanent-section immunohistochemistry, the logistical problems involved in obtaining fresh-frozen specimens will probably prohibit the former from becoming the routine method for measuring HER-2/*neu* expression.

As illustrated in Table I, the rate of HER-2/*neu* amplification and expression in many clinical breast cancers appears to be nearly the same, suggesting that there is biological concordance of these phenomena. Consistent with this, several studies have directly examined the relationship between amplification and expression of HER-2/*neu* in the same series of tumors, and found a high correlation between the two (Venter *et al.*, 1987; Gusterson *et al.*, 1988a; Berger *et al.*, 1988; Tandon *et al.*, 1989). Other studies, however, have shown that while expression and amplification are similar in late-clinical-stage tumors, expression is much more common than amplification in early-stage tumors (Yamada *et al.*, 1989). Similarly, the incidence of expression has been shown to be very high in *in situ* carcinomas (van de Vijver *et al.*, 1988; Gusterson *et al.*, 1988b; Allred *et al.*, 1991a), while the only study measuring amplification in these early noninvasive lesions found none (Tsuda *et al.*, 1990). Our studies (Allred *et al.*, 1991a) have extended these findings by showing significant differences in HER-2/*neu* expression in tumors stratified on the basis of histological composition (Fig. 3). In a study involving over 700 tumors, we found a very high rate of expression in pure *in situ* carcinomas (56%), an intermediate incidence of expression in invasive carcinomas with an *in situ* component (22%), and very low levels in pure invasive carcinomas (11%). These histologically distinct categories arguably represent progressive stages in tumor development. The decrease in oncogene expression observed during this evolutionary sequence, combined with results from the studies above, suggest that HER-2/*neu* expression is a very early event in malignant transformation, and precedes oncogene amplification. Furthermore, to explain the relatively low incidence of expression in pure invasive carcinomas, one must hypothesize that individual tumors lose expression over time and/or that many invasive carcinomas arise *de novo* by mechanisms not

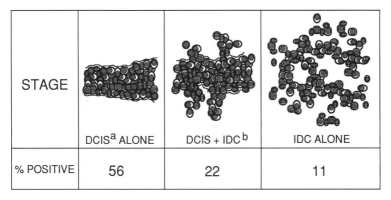

Fig. 3. HER-2/*neu* expression in tumors stratified on the basis of histological composition and evolutionary stage of development: (a) Duct carcinoma *in situ*. (b) Infiltrating ductal carcinoma.

involving HER-2/*neu*. We have observed rare tumors in which the *in situ* component was HER-2/*neu* positive, while the invasive component was negative, providing circumstantial evidence that some tumors lose expression. The observation that very small, pure invasive carcinomas are common favors the hypothesis that these lesions may also arise *de novo,* independent of HER-2/*neu* activation.

To be meaningful, the interpretation and comparison of results between different studies must take into account both the techniques being utilized to measure HER-2/*neu* activation, and the evolutionary or histological composition of the tumors being studied. It is probably reasonable to assume that amplification and expression are concordant in the average infiltrating carcinoma encountered in clinical practice, and that the true incidence of HER-2/*neu* activation in these lesions is somewhere between 20 and 30%. This assumption is consistent with recent results by Naber *et al.,* (1990), in which amplification and expression were measured by several methods in the same series of fresh specimens, and found to occur at a concordant rate of about 30%.

B. CORRELATION OF HER-2/*NEU* WITH CLINICAL–PATHOLOGICAL FEATURES

One approach to studying the possible function of a potential prognostic marker is to evaluate the strength of its relationships with other established indicators of clinical outcome. Many studies have evaluated the relationship of HER-2/*neu* amplification and/or expression with other prognostically important clinical–pathological variables in human breast carcinoma. The most consistent findings that have emerged from these studies (summarized in Table II) are that HER-2/*neu* activation is significantly associated with negative estrogen receptors, negative progesterone receptors, high histological grade, high nuclear grade, and positive axillary lymph nodes, all of which are indicators of poor prognosis.

Results from our studies (Allred *et al.,* 1991a) suggest that the relationships between HER-2/*neu* expression and other prognostic features are dependent on the histological composition and evolutionary stage of the tumors (Table III). In 221 tumors composed of both *in situ* and invasive carcinoma, oncogene expression showed significant correlations with younger patient age, premenopause, negative estrogen receptors, negative progesterone receptors, and high nuclear grade. In contrast, only negative estrogen receptors correlated significantly with expression in 408 pure invasive carcinomas. There are currently no data available to explain the apparent independence that emerges between HER-2/*neu* expression and other prognostic features as lesions progress from *early* invasive carcinomas with a significant *in situ* component, to *late* pure invasive lesions where, presumably, the *in situ* component has been completely overgrown.

While it is generally believed that HER-2/*neu* codes for a growth factor

TABLE II

SUMMARY OF LITERATURE REVIEW REGARDING PROGNOSTICALLY IMPORTANT
CLINICAL–PATHOLOGICAL FEATURES THAT ARE SIGNIFICANTLY ASSOCIATED WITH AMPLIFICATION
AND/OR EXPRESSION OF HER-2/neu IN HUMAN BREAST CANCERS

Reference[a]	Association with negative estrogen receptors Number of patients	Significance[b]
Slamon et al. (1987)	189	0.05[c]
Berger et al. (1988)	51	0.01[c]
Wright et al. (1989)	189	0.03[d]
Tandon et al. (1989)	350	0.02[d]
Zeillinger et al. (1989)	291	0.02[c]
de Potter et al. (1989a)	67	0.01[d]
Adnane et al. (1989)	292	0.003[c]
Garcia et al. (1989)	125	0.04[c]
Marx et al. (1990)	163	0.001[d]
Kommoss et al. (1990)	50	0.005[d]
Borg et al. (1990)	300	0.001[c,d]
Allred et al. (1991a)	629	0.002[d]

Reference[a]	Association with negative progesterone receptors Number of patients	Significance[b]
Tandon et al. (1989)	350	0.0003[d]
Zeillinger et al. (1989)	291	0.01[c]
Adnane et al. (1989)	292	0.004[c]
Garcia et al. (1989)	125	0.04[c]
Marx et al. (1990)	163	0.05[d]
Kommoss et al. (1990)	50	0.01[d]
Borg et al. (1990)	300	0.001[c,d]
Allred et al. (1991a)	629	0.003[d]

Reference[a]	Association with poor histological grade Number of patients	Significance[b]
Wright et al. (1989)	189	0.04[d]
Walker et al. (1989)	85	0.02[d]
Garcia et al. (1989)	125	0.005[c]
Marx et al. (1990)	163	0.05[d]
Tsuda et al. (1990)	176	0.001[c]

Reference[a]	Association with poor nuclear grade Number of patients	Significance[b]
Berger et al. (1988)	51	0.0002[c]
Barnes et al. (1988)	195	0.04[d]
Tsuda et al. (1990)	176	0.001[c]
Allred et al. (1991a)	629	0.005[d]

(continued)

TABLE II
CONTINUED

Reference[a]	Association with positive axillary lymph nodes Number of patients	Significance[b]
Cline et al. (1987)	53	0.05[c]
Berger et al. (1988)	51	0.02[d]
Tavassoli et al. (1989)	52	0.03[c]
Tandon et al. (1989)	350	0.04[d]
Borg et al. (1990)	300	0.04[c,d]

[a] References are listed by first author in chronological order.
[b] Level of significance is indicated by p-value rounded to one significant figure.
[c] Significance relative to HER-2/neu amplification.
[d] Significance relative to HER-2/neu expression.

receptor, the few studies that have directly addressed this relationship have found conflicting results. Heintz et al. (1990) and Tsuda et al. (1990) have reported a significant association between HER-2/neu amplification and growth fraction as measured by mitotic rate. Similarly, Bacus et al. (1990) recently described a strong relationship between HER-2/neu expression and proliferation rate in non-

TABLE III
ASSOCIATION OF HER-2/neu EXPRESSION WITH CLINICAL–PATHOLOGICAL
FEATURES KNOWN TO HAVE PROGNOSTIC SIGNIFICANCE
IN HUMAN BREAST CANCER

Characteristic	"Early" IDC[a] + DCIS[b]	"Late" pure IDC
Number of patients	221	408
Age	$p = 0.03$ (young)	ns
Menopause	$p = 0.02$ (pre)	ns
Tumor size	ns[c]	ns
Estrogen receptors	$p = 0.002$ (neg)	$p = 0.01$ (neg)
Progesterone receptors	$p = 0.003$ (neg)	ns
Nuclear grade	$p = 0.005$ (high)	ns
Histologic grade	ns	ns
Ploidy	ns	ns
S phase	ns	ns

[a] Infiltrating ductal carcinoma.
[b] Duct carcinoma in situ.
[c] Not significant.

invasive carcinomas of the breast. In contrast, Kommoss *et al.* (1990) found no correlation between HER-2/*neu* expression and tumor growth fraction using Ki-67 immunostaining as a measure of cell-cycle activity. We also found no significant relationship between expression and S phase as determined by flow cytometry (Allred *et al.*, 1991a). These findings may not be contradictory in the sense that, while HER-2/*neu* may be expressed, its ligand may not be present in the same quantities in all tumors. The recent identification of a ligand for the HER-2/*neu* protein may help resolve some of these issues (Lupur *et al.*, 1991).

C. Prognostic Significance of HER-2/*neu*

The first study regarding the prognostic significance of HER-2/*neu* activation was by Slamon *et al.* (1987), showing that amplification of the oncogene was associated with significantly decreased DFS and overall survival (OS) in 86 node-positive breast cancer patients. Since this initial report, there have been many others looking at the prognostic significance of HER-2/*neu* activation (summarized in Table IV). At least 17 studies have been published that evaluated the prognostic ability of HER-2/*neu* activity in breast cancer patients irrespective of clinical stage, with 9 finding and 8 not finding a relationship between HER-2/*neu* and clinical outcome. The issue is much clearer in studies analyzing only axillary node-positive patients, where 8 of 9 published reports have shown a strong relationship between HER-2/*neu* activation and poor clinical outcome. These include results from our laboratory involving 350 node-positive patients in which HER-2/*neu* expression, as measured by Western blotting, was strongly correlated with early recurrence and decreased survival (Fig. 4) (Tandon *et al.*, 1989).

In contrast, the relationship between prognosis and HER-2/*neu* activation is not clear in node-negative patients, which is unfortunate considering the controversy regarding which of these patients should receive adjuvant chemotherapy. Results from seven published studies have shown no significant relationship between HER-2/*neu* activation and clinical outcome, while four other studies have reported positive correlations between activation of this gene and poor prognosis. In three of the positive studies involving node-negative disease, significant relationships were observed between HER-2/*neu* activation and OS, but not with DFS (Wright *et al.*, 1989; Ro *et al.*, 1989; Paik *et al.*, 1990). In the positive study by Paik *et al.* (1990), the correlation between oncogene activation and decreased OS was restricted to a subset of node-negative patients with low-risk tumors defined on the basis of having *good* nuclear grade tumors.

Results from our studies (Allred *et al.*, 1991b) failed to show a significant influence of HER-2/*neu* expression on clinical outcome in 453 untreated patients with axillary node-negative tumors (Fig. 5A). We also found no relationship

TABLE IV

SUMMARY OF LITERATURE REVIEW REGARDING THE PROGNOSTIC SIGNIFICANCE
OF HER-2/neu AMPLIFICATION AND/OR EXPRESSION IN BREAST CANCER PATIENTS
STRATIFIED ON THE BASIS OF CLINICAL STAGE

| Reference[a] | Prognosis in mixed clinical stages | | |
	Number of patients	Recurrence[b]	Survival[c]
Negative studies			
Cline et al. (1987)	53	ns[d]	na[e]
Ali et al. (1988)	122	ns	ns
Barnes et al. (1988)	195	ns	ns
Gusterson et al. (1988c)	103	ns	ns
Thor et al. (1989)	290	ns	ns
Zhou et al. (1989)	157	ns	na
Tandon et al. (1989)	728	ns	ns
Heintz et al. (1990)	50	ns	ns
Positive studies			
Varley et al. (1987)	41	0.0002	na
Zhou et al. (1987)	86	0.06	na
van de Vijver et al. (1988)	189	ns	0.04
Wright et al. (1989)	185	0.005	0.001
Tsuda et al. (1989)	176	0.001	0.001
Walker et al. (1989)	85	0.0002	0.009
Paik et al. (1990)	292	ns	0.001
Gullick et al. (in press)	483	0.001	0.0007
Lovekin et al. (in press)	497	na	0.0003

| Reference[a] | Prognosis in node-positive patients | | |
	Number of patients	Recurrence[b]	Survival[c]
Negative studies			
Thor et al. (1989)	120	ns	ns
Positive studies			
Slamon et al. (1987)	86	0.0001	0.001
Wright et al. (1989)	62	0.03	0.05
Slamon et al. (1989)	345	0.01	0.04
Tsuda et al. (1989)	91	0.01	0.001
Tandon et al. (1989)	350	0.001	0.0001
Thor et al. (1989)	49[f]	0.002	0.0002
Borg et al. (1990)	120	0.04	na
Lovekin et al. (in press)	229	na	0.003

TABLE IV
CONTINUED

Reference[a]	Prognosis in node-negative patients		
	Number of patients	Recurrence[b]	Survival[c]
Negative studies			
Slamon et al. (1989)	181	ns	ns
Tsuda et al. (1989)	73	ns	ns
Tandon et al. (1989)	378	ns	ns
Thor et al. (1989)	141	ns	ns
Borg et al. (1990)	192	ns	ns
Lovekin et al. (in press)	250	ns	ns
Allred et al. (1991b)	453	ns	ns
Positive studies			
Wright et al. (1989)	44	ns	0.05
Ro et al. (1989)	66	ns	0.02
Paik et al. (1990)	94[g]	ns	0.0004
Allred et al. (1991b)	179[h]	0.0001	0.0001

[a]References are listed by first author in chronological order.

[b]Significance of HER-2/neu activation with respect to association with early recurrence of disease. Level of significance indicated by univariate p-value rounded to one significant figure.

[c]Significance of HER-2/neu activation with respect to association with decreased survival. Level of significance indicated by univariate p-value rounded to one significant figure.

[d]Not significant.

[e]Not available.

[f]Patients with advanced clinical stage tumors (T3 and T4).

[g]Low-risk patients defined as having tumors with "good" nuclear grade.

[h]Low-risk patients defined as having small (< 3 cm), estrogen receptor–positive tumors composed of pure invasive ductal carcinoma.

between HER-2/neu expression and poor clinical outcome in a subset of these untreated patients defined as having low-risk tumors on the basis of small size (< 3 cm) and ER positivity. When we evaluated the subset of low-risk untreated patients with tumors composed of both in situ and invasive carcinoma, again, no relationship between HER-2/neu expression and clinical outcome was observed. In contrast, expression strongly correlated with early recurrence and death in the subset of low-risk untreated patients with pure invasive carcinomas (Figs. 5B and 5C). The latter findings are consistent with the results of Paik et al. (1990) in the sense that both studies identified small subsets of node-negative, otherwise low-risk patients who have very poor prognosis on the basis of HER-2/neu expression.

The reason for our observation of a difference in prognosis between invasive carcinomas with and without an in situ component is unkown. This difference

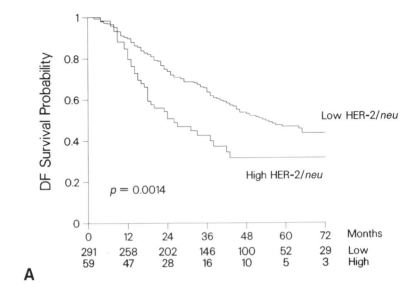

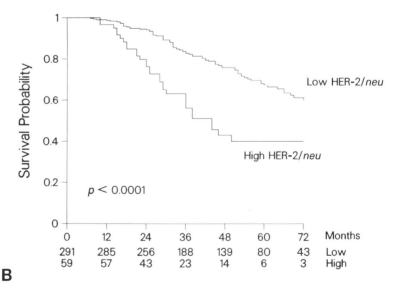

FIG. 4.   Disease-free (A) and overall (B) survival curves in node-positive breast cancer patients as a function of HER-2/*neu* expression measured by Western blotting. High HER-2/*neu* protein was defined as equal to or greater than 100 U as determined by densitometry. Median follow-up was 50 months. Values below the x-axis indicate the number of patients at risk at the interval shown. From Tandon *et al.* (1989).

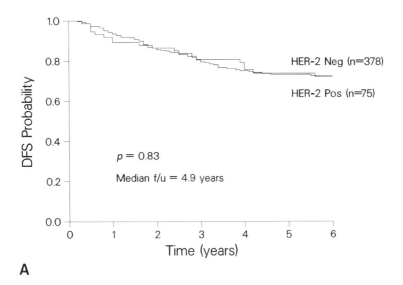

A

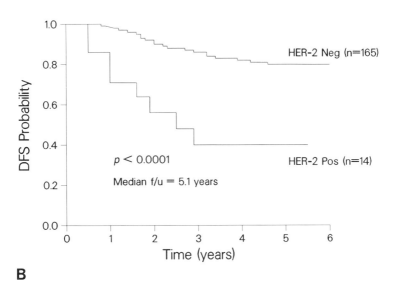

B

FIG. 5. (A) Disease-free survival curve in all untreated node-negative breast cancer patients stratified on the basis of HER-2/*neu* expression. (B) Disease-free survival curve for a subset of untreated node-negative patients with low-risk, pure invasive carcinomas. Low risk was defined as small (< 3 cm), estrogen receptor–positive tumors. (C) Overall survival curve for untreated, low-risk patients with tumors composed of pure invasive carcinoma. Modified from Allred *et al.* (1991b).

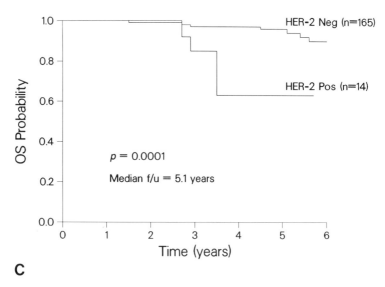

C

Fig. 5. Continued

may reflect associations between HER-2/*neu* and other prognostic factors that assume importance only in pure invasive lesions. For example, Bacus *et al.* (1990) have recently shown a positive correlation between the growth rate of tumors and HER-2/*neu* expression in *in situ* carcinomas of the breast. They further demonstrated that invasive HER-2/*neu* positive tumors were not associated with rapid proliferation unless they coexpressed EGFR and, in this sense, perhaps invasive carcinomas have accumulated multiple activated oncogenes, or lost tumor-suppressor genes, which cumulatively contribute to poor clinical outcome. Consistent with this idea, several recent studies have described simultaneous activation of multiple oncogenes in human breast tumors (Cline *et al.*, 1987; Varley *et al.*, 1987; Garcia *et al.*, 1989). Other possible explanations for the emergence of prognostic significance associated with HER-2/*neu* expression in pure invasive carcinomas may involve the ligand for HER-2/*neu*. For example, an autocrine loop may exist between the ligand and oncoprotein in the small subset of *late* pure invasive tumors that have retained HER-2/*neu* expression, and this interaction may result in uncontrolled growth leading to poor prognosis.

IV. Summary

HER-2/*neu* is a protooncogene highly homologous to the EGFR gene that resides on human chromosome 17. It codes for a 185-kDa membrane protein with intracellular tyrosine-kinase activity, and is thought to function as a growth-factor receptor. Amplification and/or overexpression of the HER-2/*neu* oncogene is present in up to 30% of invasive human breast cancers. The incidence of expression is nearly twice as high in pure *in situ* carcinomas of the breast, suggesting that HER-2/*neu* plays an important role in the early stages of tumor development. The observation that expression dramatically declines, as tumors progress from noninvasive to pure invasive lesions, suggests that individual tumors lose expression over time, and/or that many invasive carcinomas arise *de novo* by mechanisms not involving HER-2/*neu*. Amplification and expression of HER-2/*neu* are strongly associated with poor prognosis in breast cancer patients with positive axillary lymph nodes. In contrast, the prognostic significance of HER-2/*neu* in patients with node-negative disease appears to be restricted to small subsets of these patients.

Acknowledgments

This work was supported by NIH Grant CA 30195. William L. McGuire is a Clinical Research Professor of the American Cancer Society.

References

Adnane, J., Gaudray, P., Simon, M. P., Simony-Lafontaine, J., Jeanteur, P., and Theillet, C. (1989). Protooncogene amplification and human breast tumor phenotype. *Oncogene* **4**, 1389–1395.

Ali, I. U., Campbell, G., Lidereau, R., and Callahan, R. (1988). Amplification of c-*erb*B-2 and aggressive human breast tumors. *Science* **240**, 1795–1796.

Allred, D. C., Clark, G. M., Tandon, A. K., Molina, R., Tormey, D. C., Osborne, C. K., Schnitt, S. J., Gilchrist, K. W., and McGuire, W. L. (1991a). HER-2/*neu* oncogene expression during the evolutionary progression of human breast carcinoma (submitted).

Allred, D. C., Clark, G. M., Tandon, A. K., Molina, R., Tormey, D. C., Osborne, C. K., Gilchrist, K. W., Gray, R., Mansour, E. G., Abeloff, M., Eudey, L., and McGuire, W. L. (1991b). HER-2/*neu* expression identifies a restricted subset of axillary node-negative breast cancer patients with poor prognosis (submitted).

Bacus, S. S., Ruby, S. G., Weinberg, D. S., Chin, D., Ortiz, R., and Bacus, J. W. (1990). HER-2/ *neu* oncogene expression and proliferation in breast cancers. *Am. J. Pathol.* **137**, 103–111.

Bargmann, C. I., and Weinberg, R. A. (1988). Oncogenic activation of the *neu*-encoded receptor protein by point mutation and deletion. *EMBO J.* **7**, 2043–2052.

Barnes, D. M., Lammie, G. A., Millis, R. R., Gullick, W. L., Allen, D. S., and Altman, D. G. (1988). An immunohistochemical evaluation of c-*erb*B-2 expression in human breast carcinoma. *Br. J. Cancer* **58**, 448–452.

Benz, C. C., Scott, G. K., Santos, G. F., and Smith, H. S. (1989). Expression of c-*myc*, c-Ha-*ras*1, and c-*erb*B-2 protooncogenes in normal and malignant human breast epithelial cells. *J. Natl. Cancer Inst.* **81**, 1704–1709.

Berger, M. S., Locher, G. W., Saurer, S., Gullick, W. J., Waterfield, M. D., Groner, B., and Hynes, N. E. (1988). Correlation of c-*erb*B-2 gene amplification and protein expression in human breast carcinoma with nodal status and nuclear grading. *Cancer Res.* **48**, 1238–1243.

Borg, A., Tandon, A. K., Sigurdsson, H., Clark, G. M., Ferno, F., Fuqua, S. A. W., Killander, D., and McGuire, W. L. (1990). HER-2/*neu* amplification predicts poor survival in node-positive breast cancer. *Cancer Res.* **50,** 4332–4337.

Bouchard, L., Lamarre, L., Tremblay, P. J., and Jolicoeur, P. (1989). Stochastic appearance of mammary tumors in transgenic mice carrying the MMTV/c-*neu* oncogene. *Cell* **57,** 931–936.

Clark, G. M., Dressler, L. G., Owens, M. A., Pounds, G., Oldaker, T., and McGuire, W. L. (1989). Prediction of relapse or survival in patients with node-negative breast cancer by DNA flow cytometry. *N. Engl. J. Med.* **320,** 627–633.

Cline, M. J., Battifora, H., and Yokota, J. (1987). Protooncogene abnormalities in human breast cancer: Correlations with anatomic features and clinical course of disease. *J. Clin. Oncol.* **5,** 999–1006.

Coussens, L., Yang-Fen, T. L., Liao, Y. C., Chen, E., Gray, A., McGrath, J., Seeburg, P. H., Libermann, T. A., Schlessinger, J., Francke, U., Levinson, A., and Ullrich A. (1985). Tyrosine kinase receptor with extensive homology to EGF receptor shares chromosomal location with *neu* oncogene. *Science* **230,** 11321–11339.

De Potter, C. R., Van Dalle, S., van de Vijver, M. J., Pauwels, C., Maertens, G., de Boever, J., Vandekerckhove, D., and Roels, H. (1989a). The expression of the *neu* oncogene product in breast lesions and in normal fetal and adult human tissues. *Histopathology* **15,** 351–362.

De Potter, C. R., Quatacker, J., Maertens, G., Van Daele, S., Pauwels, C., Verhofstede, C., Eechaute, W., and Roels, H. (1989b). The subcellular localization of the *neu* protein in human normal and neoplastic cells. *Int. J. Cancer* **44,** 969–974.

Di Fiore, P. P., Pierce, J. H., Kraus, O. S., King, C. R., and Aaronson, S. A. (1987). *Erb*B-2 is a potent oncogene when overexpressed in NIH/3T3 cells. *Science* **237,** 178–182.

Di Marco, E., Pierce, J. H., Knicley, C. L., and Di Fiore, P. P. (1990). Transformation of NIH/3T3 cells by overexpression of the normal coding sequence of the rat *neu* gene. *Mol. Cell. Biol.* **10,** 3247–3252.

Drebin, J. A., Link, V. C., Stern, D. F., Weinberg, R. A., and Greene, M. I. (1985). Downmodulation of an oncogene protein product and reversion of the transformed phenotype of monoclonal antibodies. *Cell* **41,** 695–706.

Drebin, J. A., Link, V. C., Weinberg, R. A., and Greene, M. I. (1986). Inhibition of tumor growth by a monoclonal antibody reactive with an oncogene-encoded tumor antigen. *Proc. Natl. Acad. Sci. U.S.A.* **83,** 9129–9133.

Fisher, B., Constantino, J., Redmond, C., Poisson, R., Bowman, D., Couture, J., Dimitrov, N. V., Wolmark, N., Wickerham, D. L., Fisher, E. R., Margolese, R., Robidoux, A., Shibata, H., Terz, J., Paterson, A. H. G., Feldman, M. I., Farrar, W., Evans, J., Lickley, H. L., Ketner, M., and Others. (1989a). A randomized clinical trial evaluating tamoxifen in the treatment of patients with node-negative breast cancer who have estrogen-receptor–positive tumors. *N. Engl. J. Med.* **320,** 479–484.

Fisher, B., Redmond, C., Nikolay, V., Dimitro, V., Bowman, D., Legault-Poisson, S., Wickerham, D. L., Wolmark, N., Fisher, E. R., Margolese, R., Sutherland, C., Glass, A., Foster, R., Caplan, R., and Others. (1989b). A randomized clinical trial evaluating sequential methotrexate and fluorouracil in the treatment of patients with node-negative breast cancer who have estrogenreceptor–negative tumors. *N. Engl. J. Med.* **320,** 473–478.

Garcia, I., Dietrich, P. Y., Aapro, M., Vauthier, G., Vadas, L., and Engel, E. (1989). Genetic alterations of c-*myc*, c-*erb*B-2, and c-Ha-*ras* protooncogenes and clinical associations in human breast carcinomas. *Cancer Res.* **49,** 6675–6679.

Gullick, W. J., Love, S. B., Wright, C., Barnes, D. M., Gusterson, B., Harris, A. L., and Altman, D. G. (1991). C-*erb*B-2 protein overexpression in breast cancer is a risk factor in patients with involved and uninvolved lymph nodes. *Br. J. Cancer* (in press).

Gusterson, B. A., Gullick, W. J., Venter, D. J., Powles, T. J., Elliott, C., Ashley, S., Tidy, A., and

Harrison, S. (1988a). Immunohistochemical localization of c-*erb*B-2 in human breast carcinomas. *Mol. Cell. Probes* **2,** 383–391.

Gusterson, B. A., Machin, L. G., Gullick, W. J., Gibbs, N. M., Powles, T. J., McKinna, A., and Harrison, S. (1988b). Immunohistochemical distribution of c-*erb*/b-2 in infiltrating and *in situ* breast cancer. *Int. J. Cancer* **42,** 842–845.

Gusterson, B. A., Machin, L, G., Gullick, W. J., Gibbs, N. M., Powles, T. J., Elliot, C., Ashley, S., Monaghan, P., and Harrison, S. (1988c). C-*erb*B-2 expression in benign and malignant breast disease. *Br. J. Cancer* **58,** 453–457.

Gutman, M., Ravia, Y., Assaf, D., Yamamoto, Y., Rozin, R., and Shiloh, Y. (1989). Amplification of c-*myc* and c-*erb*B-2 protooncogenes in human solid tumors: Frequency and clinical significance. *Int. J. Cancer* **44,** 802–805.

Hanna, W., Kahn, H. J., Andrulis, I., and Pawson, T. (1990). Distribution and patterns of staining of *neu* oncogene product in benign and malignant breast diseases. *Mod. Pathol.* **3,** 455–461.

Heintz, N. H., Leslie, K. O., Rogers, L. A., and Howard, P. L. (1990). Amplification of the c-*erb*B-2 oncogene and prognosis of breast adenocarcinoma. *Arch. Pathol. Lab. Med.* **114,** 160–163.

King, C. R., Kraus, M. H., and Aaronson, S. A. (1985). Amplification of a novel v-*erb*B–related gene in human mammary carcinoma. *Science* **229,** 974–976.

Kommoss, F., Colley, M., Hart, C. E., and Franklin, W. A. (1990). *In situ* distribution of oncogene products and growth factor receptors in breast carcinoma: C-*erb*B-2 oncoprotein, EGFR and PDGFR-b-subunit. *Mol. Cell. Probes* **4,** 11–23.

Lacroix, H., Iglehart, J. D., Skinner, M. A., and Kraus, M. H. (1989). Overexpression of *erb*-2 or EGF receptor proteins present in early stage mammary carcinoma is detected simultaneously in matched primary tumors and regional metastases. *Oncogene* **4,** 145–151.

Lovekin, C., Ellis, I. O., Locker, A., Robertson, J. F. R., Bell, J., Elston, C. W., and Blamey, R. W. (1991). C-*erb*B-2 oncoprotein expression in primary and advanced breast cancer. *Br. J. Cancer* (in press).

Lupur, R., Colomer, R., Zugmaier, G., Shepard, M., Slamon, D. J., and Lippman, M. E. (1991). Direct interaction of a ligand for the *erb*B-2 oncogene product with the EGF receptor and p185 c-*erb*B-2. *Science* **249,** 1552–1555.

Mansour, E. G., Gray, R., Shatila, A. H., Osborne, C. K., Tormey, D. C., Gilchrist, K. W., Cooper, M. R., and Falkson, G. (1989). Efficacy of adjuvant chemotherapy in high-risk node-negative breast cancer. *N. Engl. J. Med.* **320,** 485–490.

Marx, D., Schauer, A., Reiche, C., May, A., Ummenhofer, L., Reles, A., Rauschecker, H., Sauer, R., and Schumacher, M. (1990). C-*erb*B-2 expression in correlation to other biological parameters of breast cancer. *J. Cancer Res. Clin. Oncol.* **116,** 15–20.

McCann, A., Dervan, P. A., Johnston, P. A., Gullick, W. J., and Carney, D. N. (1990). C-*erb*B-2 oncoprotein expression in primary human tumors. *Cancer* **65,** 88–92.

McGuire, W. L. (1989). Adjuvant therapy of node-negative breast cancer (Editorial). *N. Engl. J. Med.* **320,** 525–527.

McGuire, W. L., Tandon, A. K., Allred, D. C., Chamness, G. C., and Clark, G. M. (1990). How to use prognostic factors in axillary node–negative breast cancer patients. *J. Natl. Cancer Inst.* **82,** 1006–1015.

Mori, S., Akiyama, T., Yamada, Y., Morishita, Y., Sagawaras, I., Toyoshima, K., and Yamamoto, T. (1989). C-*erb*B-2 gene product, a membrane protein commonly expressed on human fetal epithelial cells. *Lab. Invest.* **61,** 93–97.

Muller, W. J., Sinn, E., Pattengale, P. K., Wallace, R., and Leder, P. (1988). Single-step induction of mammary adenocarcinoma in transgenic mice bearing the activated c-*neu* oncogene. *Cell* **54,** 105–115.

Naber, S. P., Tsutsumi, Y., Yin, S., Zolnay, S. A., Mobtaker, H., Marks, P. J., McKenzie, S. J.,

DeLellis, R. A., and Wolfe, H. J. (1990). Strategies for the analysis of oncogene overexpression. Studies of the *neu* oncogene in breast carcinoma. *Am. J. Clin. Pathol.* **94**, 125–136.

Padhy, L. C., Shih, C., Cowing, D., Finkelstien, R., and Weinberg, R. A. (1982). Identification of a phosphoprotein specifically induced by the transforming DNA of rat neuroblastomas. *Cell* **28**, 865–871.

Paik, S., Hazan, R., Fisher, E. R., Sass, R. E., Fisher, B., Redmond, C., Schlessinger, J., Lippman, M. E., and King, C. R. (1990). Pathological findings from the National Surgical Adjuvant Breast Project (protocol B-06): Prognostic significance of *erb*-2 protein overexpression in primary breast cancer. *J. Clin. Oncol.* **8**, 103–112.

Paterson, A. H. B., Fourney, R. M., Dietrich, K. D., Danyluk, J., Jamil, N., Lees, A. W., Krause, B., McEwan, A., Lukka, H., Hanson, J., McBlain, W. H., Willin, B., Slamon, D. J., and Paterson, M. C. (1988). HER-2/*neu* oncogene is a prognostic factor in node-negative breast cancer. *Breast Cancer Res. Treat.* **12**, 109.

Quirke, P., Pickles, A., Tuzi, N. L., Mohamdee, O., and Gullick, W. J. (1989). Pattern of expression of c-*erb*B-2 oncoprotein in human fetuses. *Br. J. Cancer* **60**, 64–69.

Ro, J., El-Naggar, A., Ro, J. Y., Blick, M., Frye, D., Fraschini, G., Fritsche, H., and Gortobagyi, G. (1989). C-*erb*B-2 amplification in node-negative human breast cancer. *Cancer Res.* **49**, 6931–6944.

Schecter, A. L., Stern, D. F., Vaidyanathan, L., Decker, S., Drebin, J. A., Greene, M. I., and Weinberg, R. A. (1984). The c-*neu* oncogene: An *erb*B-related gene encoding a 185,000 MW tumour antigen. *Nature* **312**, 513–516.

Schecter, A. L., Hung, M. C., Vaidyanathan, L., Weinberg, R. A., Yang-Feng, T. L., Francke, U., Ullrich, A., Coussens, L. (1985). The c-*neu* gene: An *erb*B-homologous gene distinct from and unlinked to genes encoding the EFG receptor. *Science* **229**, 976–978.

Semba, K., Kamata, N., Toyoshima, K., and Yamamoto, T. (1985). A v-*erb*–related protooncogene, c-*erb*B-2, is distinct from c-*erb*B-1/epidermal growth factor receptor gene and is amplified in a human salivary gland adenocarcinoma. *Proc. Natl. Acad. Sci. U.S.A.* **82**, 6497–6501.

Shih, C., Padhy, L. C., Murray, M., and Weinberg, R. A. (1981). Transforming genes of carcinomas and neuroblastomas introduced into mouse fibroblasts. *Nature* **290**, 261–264.

Slamon, D. J., Clark, G. M., Wong, S. G., Levin, L. J., Ullrich, A., and McGuire, W. L. (1987). Human breast cancer: Correlation of relapse and survival with amplification of the HER-2/*neu* oncogene. *Science* **235**, 177–181.

Slamon, D. J., Godolphin, W., Jones, L. A., Holt, J. A., Wong, G., Keith, D. E., Levin, W. J., Stuart, S. G., Udove, J., Ullrich, A., and Press, M. F. (1989). Studies of the HER-2/*neu* protooncogene in human breast and ovarian cancer. *Science* **244**, 707–712.

Tal, M., Wetzler, M., Josefberg, Z., Deutch, A., Gutman, M., Assag, D., Kris, R., Shiloh, Y., Givol, D., and Schlessinger, J. (1988). Sporadic amplification of the HER-2/*neu* protooncogene in adenocarcinomas of various tissues. *Cancer Res.* **48**, 1517–1520.

Tandon, A. K., Clark, G. M., Chamness, G. C., Ullrich, A., and McGuire, W. L. (1989). HER-2/*neu* oncogene protein and prognosis in breast cancer. *J. Clin. Oncol.* **7**, 1120–1128.

Tavassoli, M., Quirke, P., Farzaneh, F., Lock, N. J., Mayne, L. V., and Kirkham, N. (1989). C-*erb*B-2/c-*erb*A coamplification indicative of lymph node metastasis, and c-*myc* amplification of high tumour grade in human breast carcinoma. *Br. J. Cancer* **60**, 505–510.

Thor, A. D., Schwartz, L. H., Koerner, F. C., Edgerton, S. M., Skates, S. J., Yin, S., McKenzie, S. J., Panicali, D. L., Marks, P. J., Fingert, H. J., and Wood, W. C. (1989). Analysis of c-*erb*B-2 expression in breast carcinomas with clinical follow-up. *Cancer Res.* **49**, 7147–7152.

Tsuda, H., Hirohashi, S., Shimosato, Y., Hirota, T., Tsugane, S., Yamamoto, H., Miyajima, N., Toyoshima, K., Yamamoto, T., Yokota, J., Yoshida, T., Sakamoto, H., Terada, M., and Sugimura, T. (1989). Correlation between long-term survival in breast cancer patients and amplification of two putative oncogene-coamplification units: *Hst*-1/*int*-2 and c-*erb*B-2/ear-1. *Cancer Res.* **49**, 3104–3108.

Tsuda, H., Hirohashi, S., Shimosato, Y., Hirota, T., Tsugane, S., Watanabe, S., Terada, M., and Yamamoto, H. (1990). Correlation between histologic grade of malignancy and copy number of c-*erb*B-2 gene in breast carcinoma. *Cancer* **65**, 1794–1800.

van de Vijver, M. J., Peterse, J. L., Mooi, W. J., Wisman, P., Lomans, J., Dalesio, O., and Nusse, R. (1988). *Neu*-protein overexpression in breast cancer. Association with comedo-type ductal carcinoma *in situ* and limited prognostic value in stage II breast cancer. *N. Engl. J. Med.* **319**, 1239–1245.

Varley, J. M., Swallow, J. E., Brammar, W. J., Whittaker, J. L., and Walker, R. A. (1987). Alterations to either c-*erb*B-2 (neu) or c-*myc* protooncogenes in breast carcinomas correlate with poor short-term prognosis. *Oncogene* **1**, 423–430.

Venter, D. J., Kumar, S., Tuzi, N. L., and Gullick, W. J. (1987). Overexpression of the c-*erb*B-2 oncoprotein in human breast carcinomas: Immunohistological assessment correlates with gene amplification. *Lancet* **II**, 69–72.

Walker, R. A., Gullick, W. J., and Varley, J. M. (1989). An evaluation for immunoreactivity for c-*erb*B-2 protein as a marker for poor short-term prognosis in breast cancer. *Br. J. Cancer* **60**, 426–429.

Wright, C., Angus, B., Nicholson, S., Sainsbury, J. R. C., Cairns, J., Gullick, W. J., Kelly, P., Harris, A. L., and Wilson, C. H. (1989). Expression of c-*erb*B-2 oncoprotein: A prognostic indicator in human breast cancer. *Cancer Res.* **49**, 2087–2090.

Yamada, Y., Yoshimoto, M., Murayama, Y., Ebuchi, M., Mori, S., Yamamoto, T., Sugano, H., and Toyoshima, K. (1989). Association of elevated expression of the c-*erb*B-2 protein with spread of breast cancer. *Jpn. J. Cancer Res.* **80**, 1192–1198.

Yokota, J., Yamamoto, T., Toyoshima, K., Terada, M., Sugimaura, T., Battifora, H., and Cline, M. J. (1986). Amplification of c-*erb*B-2 oncogene in human adenocarcinomas *in vivo*. *Lancet* **1**, 765–767.

Zeillinger, R., Kury, F., Czerwenka, K., Kubista, E., Sliutz, G., Knogler, W., Huber, J., Zielinski, C., Reiner, G., Jakesz, R., Staffen, A., Reiner, A., Wrba, F., and Spona, J. (1989). HER-2 amplification, steroid receptors and epidermal growth factor receptor in primary breast cancer. *Oncogene* **34**, 109–114.

Zhou, D., Battifora, H., Yokota, J., Yamamoto, T., and Cline, M. J. (1987). Association of multiple copies of the c-*erb*B-2 oncogene with spread of breast cancer. *Cancer Res.* **47**, 6123–6125.

Zhou, D. J., Ahuja, H., and Cline, M. J. (1989). Protooncogene abnormalities in human breast cancer: C-*erb*B-2 amplification does not correlate with recurrence of disease. *Oncogene* **4**, 105–108.

Chapter 4

Extracellular Matrix Interactions with Tumor-Progressing Cells: Tumor versus Cell Type-Specific Mechanisms

LLOYD A. CULP, ROBERT RADINSKY,[1] AND WEN-CHANG LIN

*Department of Molecular Biology and Microbiology,
Case Western Reserve University School of Medicine,
Cleveland, Ohio 44106*

[1] Present address: Department of Cell Biology, University of Texas M. D. Anderson Cancer Center, Houston, Texas 77030

BIOCHEMICAL AND MOLECULAR ASPECTS
OF SELECTED CANCERS, VOL. 1

I. Introduction

A. GENERAL CONCEPTS—MATRIX ORGANIZATION AND ADHESION PROCESSES

An intricate meshwork of multiple and interacting macromolecules constitute extracellular matrices (ECM). These versatile protein and polysaccharide components are secreted by cells locally and assemble into an organized meshwork in extracellular spaces of all tissues (Fig. 1). In addition to serving as a universal "biological glue," they also form highly specialized structures such as cartilage, tendons, and basal laminae (McDonald, 1988). Until recently, the vertebrate ECM was thought to act as an inert scaffold that stabilized the physical structure of tissues. Now it is clear that the adhesion-promoting molecules of the ECM regulate cellular migration, differentiation, and growth (Juliano, 1987). They also contribute actively to the pathogenesis of disease characterized by aberrant adhesion, including cancer (Poste and Fidler, 1980; Nicolson, 1988; Humphries *et al.*, 1989). This chapter will focus on the mechanisms by which fibronectin (FN) mediates the adhesion of various tumor cell types and the significance of these mechanisms in tumor progression.

The ECM is composed of various collagens; proteoglycans containing multiple chains of the glycosaminoglycans heparan sulfate, dermatan sulfate, and/or chondroitin sulfate; adhesion-mediating proteins such as FN and/or laminin; and other proteins less well characterized (Fig. 1). To effect adhesive responses from cells, adhesion-mediating proteins recognize various classes of cell-surface receptors, which signal across the plasma membrane during various physiological responses (Fig. 1). To study FN-mediated adhesion at the molecular level, our laboratory and others have used several experimental approaches, including isolation and characterization of specific components involved in the FN responses of specific cell types (Culp *et al.*, 1986). An *in vitro* assay system consists of a tissue-culture substratum coated with FN and a specific cell type (Fig. 1).

Our laboratory has studied extensively the substratum adhesion processes of BALB/c 3T3 mouse fibroblasts and two different tumor cell systems, whose analyses will be reviewed in Section II. Two general methods were used to evaluate mechanics of cell adhesion in this tissue-culture assay system. The first approach involved analyzing adhesive responses of cells on substrata coated with intact FNs or isolated functional domains of FNs, as well as with model binding proteins that mimic particular binding activities of FNs. The second approach involved biochemical analysis of substratum-attached material (SAM), adhesion sites or *footprints* left on the substratum after ethyleneglycol-bis (β-aminoethyl ether)-N,N,N',N'-tetraacetic acid (EGTA)-mediated detachment of cells (Rollins *et al.*, 1982). Analysis of cell–matrix adhesions using interference reflection microscopy identified two types of contact regions between the cell and FN-coated substrata (Izzard and Lochner, 1980; Laterra *et al.*, 1983b). One class, a

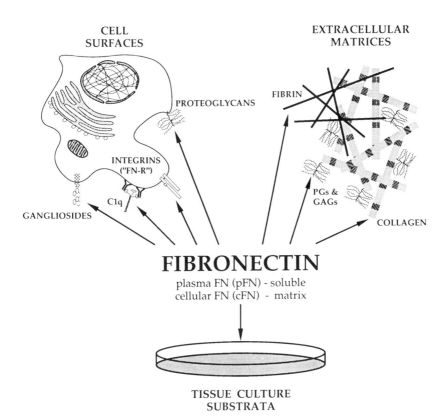

CELL
SURFACES

EXTRACELLULAR
MATRICES

PROTEOGLYCANS

FIBRIN

INTEGRINS
("FN-R")

C1q

GANGLIOSIDES

PGs &
GAGs

COLLAGEN

FIBRONECTIN

plasma FN (pFN) - soluble
cellular FN (cFN) - matrix

TISSUE CULTURE
SUBSTRATA

FIG. 1.   Tissue culture model of cell adhesion mechanisms. For analyzing matrix adhesion processes of various tumor cell populations, tissue culture substrata are coated with various fibronectins
(plasma FN,pFN; cellular FN,cFN), their proteolytic fragments harboring specified binding domains,
or heterologous proteins that mimic FN binding activities. Extracellular matrices *in situ* are composed of specific types of collagens or, in some cases such as wound sites or certain tumors (see
chapter by Dvorak *et al.* in Volume 2 of this work), fibrin. For collagen matrices, proteoglycans
(PGs) or glycosaminoglycans (GAGs), particularly for tumor cells where catabolism of PGs generate
GAGs into the environment, are bound to the collagen molecules, as well as other proteins whose
structures and functions remain to be characterized. The surfaces of various cell types can express a
wide variety of molecules that can bind to FNs in matrices and/or modulate FN receptor function.
These include glycolipids, such as certain gangliosides; the collagen-like glycoprotein, C1q; the
integrin glycoprotein complex (FN-R), and heparan sulfate proteoglycans whose core protein can
contain a hydrophobic domain, permitting intercalation into the plasma membrane. The reactions
and their consequences between defined matrices and cells expressing subsets of "receptors" can be
readily analyzed in this tissue-culture model system. This knowledge and the reagents generated
from such studies *in vitro* can be applied to processes of tumor progression *in vivo*. [Model is
courtesy of Richard Hershberger of this laboratory.]

tight-focal contact, is the site of microfilament stress-fiber condensation and participates in cell spreading–migrating activity over matrices. Tumor cells are generally incompetent for forming tight-focal contacts and stress fibers, defects that have considerable significance in the altered social behavior of tumor cells (Juliano, 1987). The second adhesion class, the close contact, is thought to be responsible for the marginal spreading during forward movement of the cell (Izzard and Lochner, 1980). Close contacts are probably the principal mechanism by which tumor cells interact with FN matrices (Culp et al., 1986, 1989).

B. Fibronectin—Structure and Binding Activities

FNs are heterodimers of two similar but nonidentical, disulfide-linked subunits, each of which has a molecular mass of ~250 kDa (Fig. 2). Two general classes of FN exist (Hynes, 1985): cellular FNs synthesized by many cell types, particularly mesenchymal cells, and plasma FN synthesized by hepatocytes and secreted into the blood. FNs form fibrillar networks at the cell surface, between cells and substrata, and between adjacent cells in some cases (Juliano, 1987; Ruoslahti, 1988a). FN functions during interaction of normal or transformed cells with substrata by cytoskeletal reorganization leading to cell spreading, normal physiological responses, and anchorage-dependent gene expression required for migration, proliferation, morphogenesis, and wound healing.

The functional diversity of FN is reflected in its structure. Many binding domains for a variety of cell-surface receptors and ECM-containing macromolecules map along the lengths of each chain (Fig. 2). Some of these domains are observed in all twenty alternatively spliced forms of human FNs, while other domains are observed only in spliced-in sequences. Some domains interact with the glycoprotein receptor complex, called integrin (see Sections I,D and II). Other domains bind to unidentified receptors on the cell surface; to cell-surface heparan sulfate proteoglycan, which acts as a receptor in some situations; to various gangliosides on the cell surface; and to various ECM macromolecules (collagen, fibrin–fibrinogen, and heparan sulfate proteoglycans) (Ruoslahti, 1988a,b) (Fig. 2).

Examination of amino acid sequences of FN subunits revealed a series of homologous, repeating polypeptide units (Fig. 2) (Hynes, 1985). Three patterns of intrachain homologies are present: type I and II repeats, which are double-disulfide-bonded structures containing 40–50 amino acids; and type III repeats, which are cysteine-free and which contain 80–100 amino acids (Hynes, 1985). There are two types of alternative splicing of FN pre-mRNA in most species (Hynes, 1985): the inclusion–exclusion of an entire type III homology repeat (ED_a and ED_b) or the differentiation of one type III repeat into five variants in the IIICS region of the human (Hershberger and Culp, 1990) (Fig. 2). Proteolysis of FNs typically cleaves the chains within the short stretches of nonhomologous

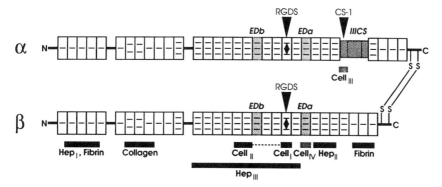

FIG. 2. Structure and binding activities of fibronectins. Displayed are the two chains of plasma FN (α and β) with addition of generic information for cellular FNs. Three types of homologous repeats of protein sequence are shown in the boxes: type I repeats (single dash), type II repeats (double dashes), and type III repeats (triple dashes). One binding domain per chain for collagen is shown; two domains for binding fibrin; and three domains for binding heparan sulfates/heparin/dermatan sulfates (Hep$_{I,II,III}$ with the last domain imprecisely mapped). Although these domains are only shown along one chain, they are found in all forms of alternatively spliced FNs. Three different cell-binding domains have been mapped along these sequences as well: Cell$_I$ containing the *RGDS* sequence responsible for binding to some select integrin receptors (Table 1) on cell surfaces and found in all FN chains; Cell$_{II}$ maps to common sequences N-terminal to the ED$_b$ sequences, operates cooperatively with Cell$_I$ (therefore, the dashed line between the two domains), is observed in all chains of FNs, and recognizes an unidentified receptor on some tumor cell populations; Cell$_{III}$ containing the CS1 peptide sequence within the alternatively spliced IIICS region which recognizes the $\alpha_4\beta_1$ integrin receptor and is therefore restricted to only FN chains containing the A subsegment of IIICS (Hershberger and Culp, 1990); and Cell$_{IV}$ which may be located in alternatively spliced ED$_a$ sequences and which recognizes an unidentified receptor molecule on some tumor cell populations. Alternative splicing of FN pre-mRNA generates 20 different variant forms of FN in the human: the splicing in or out of complete type III repeats at extra domains$_{a \, and \, b}$ (ED$_a$ and ED$_b$), as well as five different splicing permutations in the IIICS region that introduce various portions of one type III repeat (Hershberger and Culp, 1990). (Model is courtesy of Richard Hershberger of this laboratory.)

sequence, facilitating the isolation of the multiple binding domains in various permutations (Castellani *et al.*, 1986; Zardi *et al.*, 1987), providing important reagents for various *in vitro* and *in vivo* adhesion analyses (Fig. 1).

C. Other Adhesion-Mediating Proteins of Cells and Matrices

Other adhesion-regulating components of ECMs include laminin, entactin, and vitronectin (Liotta *et al.*, 1986; see Liotta chapter in Volume 2 of this work). These glycoproteins are interwoven into a highly insoluble matrix, supported by collagen and elastin fibers with a network of interlacing proteoglycans. Proteoglycans contain negatively charged glycosaminoglycan chains of one or, in some cases, two classes (Ruoslahti, 1988b; Iozzo, 1988). The exception is hyaluronic acid, which is synthesized as a free polysaccharide. Each of these proteins and polysaccharides is thought to interact and to assemble into a large variety of different three-dimensional structures, ordered in part by the cells secreting specific matrix components and two different cell types secreting complementary matrix components. Similar to FNs, laminins are large, complex molecules, each of which has a variety of functional activities, and which are not so well characterized structurally or functionally as the FNs. Laminins also share a common structural pattern of protease-resistant functional domains with binding activities for other macromolecules and for various cell-surface receptors, linked by protease-sensitive interdomain sequences (Liotta *et al.*, 1986; Ruoslahti, 1988b).

D. MATRIX RECEPTORS—INTEGRINS, PROTEOGLYCANS, GANGLIOSIDES

Integrin receptor binding to one cell-binding domain of FN (Cell$_l$ of Fig. 2) occurs at a specific tetrapeptide sequence, Arg-Gly-Asp-Ser (RGDS) (Buck and Horwitz, 1987; Ruoslahti, 1988a). Characterization of this and other integrin receptors identifies a large family of closely related genes coding for 140 to 160 kDa glycoprotein complexes (Hynes, 1987; Buck and Horwitz, 1987) (Fig. 3).

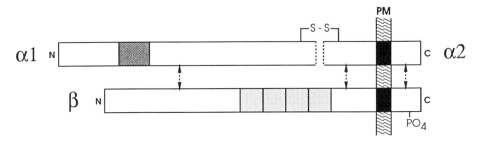

FIG. 3. Model of an integrin receptor. Each integrin receptor is composed of two glycoprotein subunits (termed the α and β subunits) which are encoded by separate genes. There are a large family of integrin genes (Table 1) whose products recognize specific extracellular matrix molecules and which are selectively expressed in differentiated cell types, conferring specificity for both the matrix and the cell type during matrix adhesion. The β chain is approximately 140 kDa with a plasma membrane (PM) spanning domain, contains four repeats with extensive intrachain disulfide bonding (stippled areas), and a cytoplasmic domain that can be phosphorylated. The α chain is synthesized as a large precursor glycoprotein of approximate molecular weight 160,000–180,000 which in some cases is cleaved into two subunits that remain disulfide-linked to each other: α_1 of 105–120 kDa and a smaller α_2 subunit of 20–30 kDa which spans the PM. The α_1 subunit also contains a Ca^{2+}-binding domain (cross-hatched area) that confers considerable conformational sensitivity of the molecule to chelation. Bonding between the α and β chains is noncovalent and has not been mapped along the two sequences. (Model is courtesy of Richard Hershberger of this laboratory.)

Each integrin is composed of a heterodimer of noncovalently associated α and β subunits (Fig. 3), some of which share binding specificity for the tetrapeptide sequence RGDS in FNs or in other matrix ligands (Table 1) (Hynes, 1987; Cassiman et al., 1989). They provide tissue integrity by allowing cells to attach to ECM components (Hynes, 1987; Cassiman et al., 1989). As classified in Table 1, three different β chains associate with a particular group of structurally related α chains, subdividing the larger integrin family into three subfamilies, each with its particular β subunit (Hynes, 1987; Cassiman et al., 1989). Based on differences in the function of each protein, six different heterodimers can be identified in the $\beta 1$ subfamily, also referred to as the very late antigens (VLA) initially described for T cells (Hemler, 1990). The $\beta 2$ subfamily, expressed on cells of lymphocyte or myeloid lineage, constitute the receptors for the intercellular adhesion molecules (ICAM). The third subfamily shares the $\beta 3$ subunit and comprises the vitronectin receptor and platelet glycoprotein IIb/IIIa receptor (Table 1). The fundamental importance of these molecules is further demonstrated by their expression in all species including *Drosophila* (Cassiman et al., 1989) and by the pathology associated with the functional inactivity of some family members (Springer et al., 1984).

Different cell types cultured on FN substrata or its individual binding domains display various adhesion responses independent of any integrin interaction (Culp

TABLE I
CLASSIFICATION OF HUMAN INTEGRIN RECEPTORS[a]

Integrin Class	Other designation	Matrix moiety for binding
$\alpha_1\beta_1$	VLA-1	LN, Collagens I and IV
$\alpha_2\beta_1$	VLA-2	Collagen I
$\alpha_3\beta_1$	VLA-3	FN (Cell$_I$ domain), LN, Collagen I
$\alpha_4\beta_1$	VLA-4	FN (Cell$_{III}$ domain)
$\alpha_5\beta_1$	VLA-5	FN (Cell$_I$ domain)
$\alpha_6\beta_1$	VLA-6	LN
$\alpha_V\beta_X$		FN (Cell$_I$ domain), VN
$\alpha_V\beta_3$	VN-R	FN (Cell$_I$ domain), VN, fibrinogen, osteopontin, von Willebrand factor
$\alpha_{IIb}\beta_3$	gp IIb/IIIa (platelet)	FN (Cell$_I$ domain), VN fibrinogen, von Willebrand factor
$\alpha_L\beta_2$	LFA-1	ICAM-1, ICAM-2
$\alpha_M\beta_2$	MAC-1	fibrinogen, C3bi complement

[a] Human integrins are composed of two subunits (α and β), as illustrated in Fig. 3, whose evidence is summarized in Juliano, 1987; Buck and Horwitz, 1987; Ruoslahti, 1988; Hemler, 1990. The following abbreviations are used to designate the target ligands for specific integrins: FN, fibronectin; LN, laminin; VN, vitronectin.

et al., 1986, 1989). These studies established that cell-surface heparan sulfate proteoglycan acts as a receptor for transmembrane signaling in some situations, either by binding to the heparin-binding domains of the substratum ligand directly (Culp *et al.*, 1989; see Section II) or by influencing the interaction of other cell-surface receptors with their recognition sites on the substratum ligand (Ruoslahti, 1988b; Iozzo, 1988). Additionally, evidence has accumulated that di- and trisialogangliosides may be involved in the interaction of cells with FN (Yamada *et al.*, 1981; Matyas *et al.*, 1986; Mugnai *et al.*, 1988b). Thus, individual cell types can establish different morphological and physiological responses based on adhesion preferences mediated by FNs binding to multiple receptors (Section II).

E. POSTTRANSCRIPTIONAL SPLICING REGULATION OF FIBRONECTIN BIOSYNTHESIS

Comparison of FNs from different sources has revealed diversity in the amino acid sequence at three sites (Hynes, 1985) as a result of alternative splicing of FN pre-mRNA at three regions (Fig. 2). One site is more complex and is termed the type III connecting segment (IIICS of Fig. 2); it comprises a region of 120 amino acids, which can be included completely or partially in the polypeptide or completely deleted, resulting in five variant mRNAs in human (Hynes, 1987; Hershberger and Culp, 1990). The biological significance of these alternative splicings is not well understood, but they may affect FN functions (Hershberger and Culp, 1990; Guan *et al.*, 1990).

Evaluation of many different cultured untransformed and tumor cell populations for their distributions of IIICS mRNA variants revealed some particularly interesting distributions (Fig. 4) (Hershberger and Culp, 1990). Liver contained the highest proportion of O variant (missing the entire IIICS sequence) (Fig. 4A). Most untransformed cells had a high proportion of O variant as well, particularly dermal fibroblasts, when compared with colon or lung fibroblasts, indicating tissue type–specificity in these mRNA distributions within one cell class. When O variant decreased, the AB variant increased (this variant contains the first two subsegments of IIICS (Hershberger and Culp, 1990), while the ABC and B variants remained reasonably constant (Fig. 4B). Finally, all tumor and transformed cell lines had uniformly low levels of O variant mRNA and very high levels of AB variant mRNA. This latter observation is particularly interesting in light of the identification of a unique cell-binding domain in the A subsegment of IIICS that some tumor cells generate for recognition of a unique integrin (Table 1) (Humphries *et al.*, 1986a, 1987). This evidence, along with that described in Section II, suggests that tumor cells have expressed unique molecular mechanisms for interacting with FN matrices.

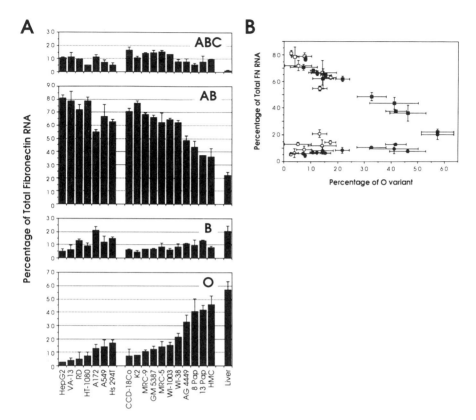

Fig. 4. (A) Quantitation of the relative abundance of the four major alternatively spliced IIICS mRNA variants. A double-primer extension assay was developed (Hershberger and Culp, 1990) to evaluate the relative amounts of the IIICS mRNA variants. Whole cell RNAs were isolated from many cell types and assayed for their distributions of these variants: O, which lacks all IIICS sequence; ABC, which contains the entire sequence of IIICS; and AB, BC (not shown), or B variants, which contain only subsegments of IIICS. Autoradiograms from the primer-extension assay were densitometrically scanned to derive values for the relative amounts of each variant. Bars represent standard errors obtained from multiple assays of each cell line. Results are grouped among tumor and transformed cell lines (left), normal cell strains (center), and liver tissue (far right). (B) AB and B variant levels in relation to O-variant expression. The percentages of AB variant (squares) and B variant (circles) levels are plotted against O-variant levels for each tumor (open symbols) and normal (filled symbols) cell type. Percentage values and errors are as described for panel (A). The following human tumor lines were analyzed: HepG2, hepatocellular carcinoma; VA-13, Simian virus 40–transformed WI-38 cells; RD, rhabdomyosarcoma; HT-1080, fibrosarcoma; A172, glioblastoma; A549, adenocarcinoma; and Hs 294T, melanoma. The following normal human cell strains were analyzed: CCD-18Co, colon fibroblasts; K2, keratinocytes; MRC-9, fetal lung fibroblasts; GM 5387, fetal lung fibroblasts; MRC-5, fetal lung fibroblasts; WI-1003, adult lung fibroblasts; WI-38, fetal lung fibroblasts; AG4449, fetal skin fibroblasts (full thickness); 8 Pap, papillary dermal fibroblasts from a 78-year-old Caucasian male; 13 Pap, papillary dermal fibroblasts from a 17-year-old Caucasian female; and HMC, human kidney mesangial cells. [Taken with permission from R. P. Hershberger and L. A. Culp. (1990). *Molecular and Cellular Biology* **10,** 662–671.]

II. Tumor Cell-Specific Adhesion Mechanisms

A. Hypotheses under Investigation in Model Culture Systems

Knowledge of the structure and binding activities of FNs, laminin, proteogly-cans, and integrins (Section I) provides opportunity for evaluating differences in the mechanisms by which various tumor cell populations interact with extracellular matrices and the significance of these differences for tumor progression. This applies not only to the static concept of attachment of tumor cells to matrices but also to the dynamics of spreading, migration, and detachment, where cell–matrix contacts must be made and broken at selected sites of the cell's undersurface and at various matrices of target organs. These latter processes become particularly significant for clonal selection during tumor progression (McCarthy et al., 1985; Partin et al., 1988; Kerbel et al., 1988; Kerbel, 1990).

The breakage of cell–matrix contacts can result from a variety of disorganiz-ing principles (Rollins et al., 1982). First, factors in specific localities of the cytosol could disrupt the cytoskeletal architecture required to stabilize adhesive contacts. For example, this occurs during experimental treatment of cells with the Ca^{2+} chelator, EGTA, whereby cytoskeletal disruption results in plasma membrane retraction from the adhesive contacts and subsequent breakage of re-traction fibers, liberating cells into suspension and leaving adhesive contacts as footprints or substratum-attached material (Rosen and Culp, 1977; Rollins et al., 1982). This occurs during natural movement of many cells in culture model systems (Rosen and Culp, 1977; Chen, 1981). Src oncogene–transformed cells have specialized adhesive contacts, called podosomes, that differ in several re-gards from the contacts of untransformed cells (Tarone et al., 1985).

Second, proteases secreted from tumor cells in autocrine-like fashion (alter-natively, secreted from host stromal cells upon stimulation by factors from tumor cells in a paracrine-like mechanism) could cleave receptors at the periphery of adhesive contacts, resulting in disruption of the cytoskeleton, retraction, and footprint evolution (Chen et al., 1984). This mechanism may operate at podo-some contacts of some transformed fibroblasts (Chen, 1989; Radinsky et al., 1990). A variant of this mechanism would be secretion of proteases that selec-tively degrade the FN or laminin molecules themselves (Chen et al., 1984; Fair-bairn et al., 1985; Grinnell, 1986).

Third, glycosaminoglycan lyases can alter adhesive processes during secretion by various tumor cells (Eldor et al., 1987; Kramer et al., 1982; Robertson et al., 1989; Radinsky et al., 1990). Since heparan sulfate proteoglycans inter-calated into the plasma membrane mediate some adhesion processes of untrans-formed cells by recognizing the heparin-binding domains of FN or laminin in matrices (Laterra et al., 1983a,b; Beyth and Culp, 1984; Izzard et al., 1986;

Culp *et al.*, 1986; Hall *et al.*, 1988; Saunders and Bernfield, 1988), cleavage of heparan sulfate chains would significantly perturb their adhesive functions.

Fourth, specific chondroitin or dermatan sulfate proteoglycans secreted from some cells interfere with attachment and spreading of some untransformed cells (Knox and Wells, 1979; Rich *et al.*, 1981; Lewandowska *et al.*, 1987; Perris and Johansson, 1987; Yamagata *et al.*, 1989) and tumor cells (Brennan *et al.*, 1983; Mugnai *et al.*, 1988b). This inhibition is effected in two different ways. Binding of medium-borne proteoglycans to the heparin-binding domains of FN on the substratum (Brennan *et al.*, 1983; Lewandowska *et al.*, 1987) or, under some conditions, core protein binding to FN (Schmidt *et al.*, 1987) results in steric interference of cell-surface integrin and/or heparan sulfate proteoglycan interactions. Alternatively, occupancy of substrata by proteoglycans interferes with FN occupancy of the same substrata (Yamagata *et al.*, 1989). Similar processes may be operating to facilitate *detachment of cells previously attached* to the matrix. Fifth, the collagenous substratum with which cells must ultimately interface could be degraded by secreted collagenases, as reviewed by Liotta and his colleagues in Volume 2 of this work.

These many possibilities for facilitating detachment of cells would require a large array of genes and their products for various classes of tumor cells to facilitate matrix interactions. It is also likely that the embryonic origin of specific tumor cell types and the biochemical nature of the matrices in target host organs dictate which of these mechanisms dominate. Matrices also provide the incredibly selective environment that results in clonal dominance of rare tumor cell types in complex tumor populations, as discussed more fully in Section IIIB below.

With regard to the concepts considered above, tumor biologists must initially describe the matrix-adhesion processes of various tumor cell classes and their significance for selection mechanisms operating during tumor progression (Poste and Fidler, 1980; Nicolson, 1988; Kerbel *et al.*, 1988; Kerbel, 1990; see review chapter by Nicolson in Volume 2 of this work). Two general possibilities for altered adhesion mechanisms may operate in tumor cell populations. First, many embryologically different tumor cells may have evolved a common mechanism for interacting with FNs; this would be described as a tumor-specific mechanism not observed in untransformed cell populations, but instigated upon activation of many different oncogenes. Second, the embryological origin of the tumor cell class may dictate the uniqueness of the FN adhesive mechanisms, as originally described for melanoma cells by Humphries *et al.* (1986a, 1987) as a cell type–specific mechanism not completely divorced from the mechanisms of its differentiated precursor cell. We will focus on the details of FN-mediated adhesion mechanisms of two different tumor cell classes being analyzed in our laboratory, compare and contrast these findings with those of other tumor cell systems, and draw some interesting parallels with studies of embryonic systems and with clonal dominance studies during tumor progression.

B. NEUROBLASTOMA—MODEL OF A NERVOUS SYSTEM–DERIVED TUMOR

Evidence has shown that neuroblastoma tumors develop by malignant conversion of a presumptive neuron from the embryonic neural crest destined for the peripheral nervous system (Tsokos et al., 1985; Imashuku et al., 1985; Reynolds et al., 1988). During metastasis of neuroblastoma into the bone marrow, selection occurs for cell variants with highly amplified copies and expression levels of the N-myc oncogene (Schwab et al., 1983; Kohl et al., 1983; Emanuel et al., 1985; see review chapter by Brodeur in this volume). Rat and mouse neuroblastoma cells were shown to attach and extend neurite processes on plasma FN-coated substrata (Culp, 1980; Culp et al., 1980; Domen and Culp, 1981), to develop growth cone structures at the ends of neurites visualized in scanning electron micrographs (Domen and Culp, 1981), and to generate a pattern of proteins and glycosaminoglycans in their substratum-attached material different from the patterns of fibroblasts (Culp et al., 1980). Since the morphologies and biochemical compositions of substratum-attached material under growth cones and cell bodies of neuroblastoma cells on FN were also different, the hypothesis was developed that differing receptor activities for FN mediated these two adhesion processes (Culp et al., 1980; Domen and Culp, 1981). This was verified by other experimental approaches.

1. Multiple Receptor Recognition

Adhesion of human or rodent neuroblastoma cells was evaluated using several proteins that mimicked the binding activities of FNs (Tobey et al., 1985). Platelet factor-4 (PF4) is a tetravalent heparan sulfate–binding protein and is used as a model of the heparan sulfate–binding activity of FNs while avoiding any recognition of integrin receptors (Laterra et al., 1983a,b). A chymotrypsin-generated fragment of plasma FN (Pierschbacher et al., 1981), referred to as the 120K CBF (cell-binding fragment) and containing the RGDS recognition site for some integrins (Pierschbacher and Ruoslahti, 1984; Yamada and Kennedy, 1984) but not heparin/heparan sulfate–binding activity, was also evaluated. PF4 substrata promoted attachment and spreading of all neuroblastoma populations tested, but would not promote neurite outgrowth (Tobey et al., 1985). Conversely, 120K CBF substrata promoted both attachment and neurite outgrowth. This suggested that cell-surface heparan sulfate proteoglycan and integrin could mediate stable attachment and spreading of cells, but that integrin is specifically required for growth cone initiation–migration. The topography of these binding relationships was established by coating two adjacent regions of substrata with CBF and PF4 and by evaluating cells interfacing with the two substrata (Tobey et al., 1985).

Only on the CBF side would cells extend neurites. Cells bridging the interface (i.e., with one portion of their surface contacting PF4 and the other, CBF) were competent for forming neurites only on the CBF side. This important experiment demonstrated that surface receptors exclusively regulated these adhesion processes and that there was no positive or negative regulatory signal transmitted within the cytosol.

Roles for neuroblastoma integrin in these responses were tested further by using a synthetic peptide containing the RGDS sequence as a medium-borne inhibitor (Waite *et al.*, 1987). Attachment and neurite outgrowth of neuroblastoma cells on 120K CBF were completely inhibited by RGDS peptide in the medium, indicating that an RGDS-recognizing integrin (Table 1) is principally responsible for responses on this FN proteolytic fragment. In contrast, attachment and neurite outgrowth on intact plasma FN were *not* inhibited by the RGDS peptide, suggesting that these neuronal tumor cells can effect an *RGDS-heparan sulfate–independent mechanism of adhesion*. An alternative hypothesis for this resistance—namely, that these tumor cells have highly elevated levels of integrin overcoming peptide inhibition—does not apply because low concentrations of the peptide were effective at inhibition on the 120K CBF harboring the $Cell_I$ domain (Fig. 2). This unique adhesion mechanism of all rodent and human neuroblastoma cells tested to date contrasts with the complete sensitivity of the adhesion responses of rat pheochromocytoma PC12 cells on FN matrices to RGDS peptide (Akeson and Warren, 1986) and later shown to utilize an RGDS-recognizing integrin receptor (Tomaselli *et al.*, 1987). Neural crest cells of the developing embryo also respond to FN matrices in an RGDS-independent manner; this required cooperativity between $Cell_I$ and $Cell_{III}$ domains, the latter mapping to the CS1 peptide sequence in alternatively spliced IIICS region of FNs (Fig. 2) (Dufour *et al.*, 1988).

A larger array of proteolytic fragments of plasma FNs was screened to map the RGDS-independent adhesion activity for neuroblastoma cells (Mugnai *et al.*, 1988a). A thermolysin-generated 110-kDa fragment (F110), containing $Cell_I$ domain, also contained RGDS-independent attachment, neurite–promoting activities. F110 adhesive activity was not inhibitable by pretreatment of cells with glycosaminoglycan lyases, thereby discounting a proteoglycan-binding domain in F110. In contrast, adhesion responses of fibroblasts on F110 are completely sensitive to RGDS peptide inhibition (Hall *et al.*, 1988), revealing the cell type–specificity of this adhesion activity. Since ganglioside binding of FNs had been localized to an N-terminal domain (Thompson *et al.*, 1986), it is also unlikely that F110 recognizes a ganglioside on the cell surface. Since F110 does not contain any sequence from the IIICS region, there must be an additional cell-binding domain (labeled $Cell_{II}$ in Fig. 2) harbored in F110, but not in chymotrypsin-generated 120K CBF (Mugnai *et al.*, 1988a).

This study made additional observations into various receptor functions of neuroblastoma cells (Mugnai *et al.*, 1988a). When larger proteolytic fragments of plasma FN, containing all of the protein sequence of F110 as well as the Hep$_{II}$ domain (e.g., F145 or F155), were tested in this paradigm, cell attachment and neurite outgrowth displayed significant sensitivity to inhibition by the RGDS peptide. This indicates one of two possibilities—either these particular fragments have an altered conformation when bound to the culture substratum, such that Cell$_I$ plays a more prominent role than Cell$_{II}$ or, alternatively, interaction between Hep$_{II}$ and cell-surface heparan sulfate proteoglycan modulates Cell$_{II}$ activity. In this regard, mixtures of F110 and Hep$_{II}$ fragments (e.g., F29 or F38 from the two different chains of plasma FN or F44 + 47 from the many chains of cellular FNs) failed to increase RGDS peptide sensitivity of responses, indicating that the intact F145 or F155 was required to shift adhesive activity from Cell$_{II}$ to Cell$_I$ domains (Mugnai *et al.*, 1988a). While cells attached reasonably well on Hep$_{II}$ fragments only, spreading was minimal and neurite outgrowth nonexistent.

These experiments raised the question of where the neuroblastoma-specific, adhesion-promoting activity maps along FN sequences, since it cannot be ascribed to Cell$_{III}$ activity. Since thermolysin-generated F110 but not chymotrypsin-generated 120K CBF contained this activity, F110 would be the logical choice for sequence analysis. However, this fragment resists further proteolytic cleavage (Mugnai *et al.*, 1988a; Lewandowska *et al.*, 1990). The identical fragment (F120) from human transformed cell FNs contains alternatively spliced ED$_b$ sequences, in addition to F110 sequences (Fig. 2); this fragment is susceptible to thermolysin cleavage into two subfragments—(1) F35 harboring the Cell$_I$ domain, and (2) F90 harboring virtually all of ED$_b$ and the remainder of F110-identical sequences. Neuroblastoma cells responded to substrata of F120 (Fig. 5) from transformed cellular FNs by attaching and extending neurites identically to their responses on F110 or intact FNs (Lewandowska *et al.*, 1990). Analyses of the F120 subfragments were even more informative. Cells attached stably on either F35 (containing RGDS-dependent Cell$_I$) or on F90 while murine fibroblasts (Balb/c 3T3) attached stably on F35 but not on F90 (Fig. 5). Therefore, the Cell$_{II}$ domain must map within F90 sequences (Lewandowska *et al.*, 1990). It should also be noted that on *either* F35 or F90 substrata, neuroblastoma cells failed to generate neurites. On substrata of F35/F90 mixtures, some neurite generation was observed, but not nearly so effectively as on intact F120 (Lewandowska *et al.*,1990). This suggests cooperativity between Cell$_I$ and Cell$_{II}$ domains for effecting maximal differentiation of neuronal tumor cells. Also, topology of receptors may be a critical element in its regulation. Obara *et al.* (1988) also reported synergy between the Cell$_I$ domain and sequences that are close to or identical with those of F90 described here, using site-directed mutagenesis of FN cDNA.

These experiments provide insight into the complexity by which one class of tumor cells responds to FN matrices by using multiple binding domains along

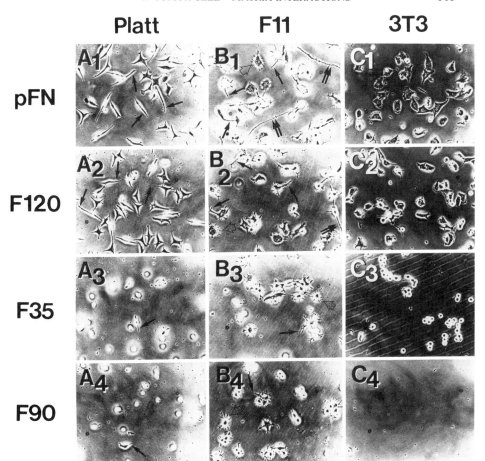

Fig. 5. Morphological responses of three cell types on FN and three proteolytic fragments. Wells of a 48-well cluster dish were adsorbed with 20 μg/ml of one of the following: plasma FN (series 1); F120 from human transformed cellular FNs and containing ED_b (series 2); F35 which is one subfragment of F120 cleavage and which contains the $Cell_1$ domain but not ED_b (series 3); or F90, which is the other subfragment of F120 cleavage and which contains the ED_b sequence and common sequences N-terminal to ED_b (series 4). Wells were then rinsed twice with phosphate-buffered saline, postadsorbed with adhesion medium, and finally inoculated with cells in adhesion medium that had been detached from stock cultures by EGTA treatment. At 16 hr for Platt human neuroblastoma cells (series A) and the F11 hybrid cells (series B), which is sufficient time for neurites to form if conditions are permissive (or at 4 hr for the Balb/c 3T3 cells [series C]), wells were rinsed twice with phosphate-buffered saline and the cells fixed with glutaraldehyde for phase-contrast microscopy. Arrows define short linear neurites that have been characterized several ways previously; double arrows define long irregular neurites characteristic of primary neurons; broad open arrows identify multiple spiky projections that emanate from some cells. Magnification, ×76. [Taken with permission from K. Lewandowska, E. Balza, L. Zardi, and L. A. Culp (1990). *J. Cell Science* **95**, 75–83.]

FN sequences and multiple receptors. These domains include $Cell_I$, $Cell_{II}$, and Hep_{II} (Fig. 2). In addition, $Cell_{III}$ in alternatively spliced IIICS may also function in neuroblastoma responses in analogous fashion to $Cell_{II}$ by complementing the functions of $Cell_I$, although this possibility remains to be explored. While Hep_{II} recognizes heparan sulfate proteoglycan as a receptor (Laterra *et al.*, 1983a,b; Saunders and Bernfield, 1988), $Cell_I$ recognizes multiple members of the integrin family ($\alpha_5\beta_1$, $\alpha_3\beta_1$, and $\alpha_v\beta_3$), and $Cell_{III}$ recognizes integrin $\alpha_4\beta_1$ associated with melanoma cells and certain lymphopoietic T- and B-cell subsets (Wayner *et al.*, 1989; Guan and Hynes, 1990; Garcia-Pardo and Ferreira, 1990). The identity of the receptor for $Cell_{II}$ must be determined, as well as its cell type– or tumor-specific identity. Other tumor cell classes fail to recognize $Cell_{II}$, consistent with its recognizing a cell type–specific receptor (see Section IIC2 below). Since F110 and F120 contain identical activities, it cannot be located in alternatively spliced ED_b sequences, which are much more common in transformed cellular FNs (Zardi *et al.*, 1987). However, this does not rule out the possibility that ED_b sequences regulate its functions in various contexts.

2. Ganglioside-Dependent Adhesion

Using the precedence of proteoglycan-binding proteins such as PF4 to evaluate the significance of FN–proteoglycan binding in adhesion (Laterra *et al.*, 1983a,b), experiments were initiated to evaluate the mediation by one specific ganglioside of neuroblastoma cells, particularly in light of the considerable enrichment of gangliosides in nervous system cells. Cholera toxin B subunit (CTB) binds specifically to ganglioside GM1 and was used to test GM1's role in responses (Mugnai and Culp, 1987). Neuroblastoma cells attached stably to CTB substrata in a GM1-dependent process that excluded the possibility of replacement of CTB on the substratum with secreted cellular FNs. Attached cells generated neurites on CTB, but much more slowly and with differing morphologies than neuritogenesis on FN substrata. Neuritogenesis, but not attachment on CTB, was inhibited by cycloheximide or trypsin pretreatments of cells, indicating that some GM1-"associated" proteins at the cell surface mediate transmembrane signaling to effect neurite formation (Mugnai and Culp, 1987).

Properties of cell-surface proteins mediating $CTB_{substratum}$–$GM1_{cell\ surface}$ responses were explored (Mugnai *et al.*, 1988b). In contrast to the resistance of responses on FN substrata upon addition of the RGDS synthetic peptide described above, this peptide completely inhibited neurite formation, but not attachment, on CTB substrata. This indicates that one of the RGDS-recognizing integrins must participate in neurite formation on GM1-binding substrata. Proteoglycan-mediated regulation was tested by two approaches (Mugnai *et al.*, 1988b). First, PF4 was mixed with CTB or plasma FN on the substratum or, alternatively, added to the medium of cells responding to homogeneous substrata of either CTB or FN. Diluting the substratum ligand with PF4 had little effect on cell attachment on either substratum but inhibited neurite formation on CTB very effectively (with a less-pronounced inhibition of neuritogenesis on FN). Similarly, PF4 addition to the medium had little effect on FN responses or of attachment on CTB; it completely inhibited neurite formation on CTB. Second, responses were tested upon addition of bovine cartilage dermatan sulfate proteoglycan or chondroitin–keratan sulfate proteoglycan to the medium. Dermatan sulfate proteoglycan, but not the chondroitin–keratan sulfate proteoglycan, completely inhibited responses on CTB and partially inhibited attachment (but not neurite formation) on FN. Therefore, cell-surface proteoglycan interactions with cell-surface GM1 and/or one of the FN receptors must modulate the responses of these cells on GM1 substrata.

These results identify a fourth extracellular matrix-recognition process—namely, to specific cell-surface gangliosides—as a potential participant in neuroblastoma cell responses. They also demonstrate the functional interrelationships among several classes of cell-surface molecules. These include one or more RGDS-recognizing integrins, the RGDS-independent receptor recognizing Cell$_{II}$, heparan sulfate proteoglycan as the predominant proteoglycan on the surface of neuroblastoma cells (Maresh *et al.*, 1984; Vallen *et al.*, 1988), and ganglioside GM1.

3. *Hybrid Neuronal Cells—An "Intermediate" Biological System*

An alternative biological system was developed recently that is proving beneficial in analyzing neuron- and tumor-specific properties of cells. Somatic cell hybridization of rat embryonic dorsal root neurons with mouse neuroblastoma cells was achieved with the prospect of "fixing" the differentiated properties of these neurons from the neural crest in immortalized hybrid cells (Platika *et al.*, 1985). Our laboratory has been studying the F11 hybrid cell, which was cloned soon after hybridization and which has one complement of rat and one complement of mouse chromosomes, verifying fusion of a single dorsal root neuron with a single neuroblastoma cell. Furthermore, this system will be particularly valuable for analyzing regulation of the amplified copies of the mouse N-*myc* oncogene upon the differentiation phenotype and upon tumor progression in this nervous system tumor model.

Mugnai *et al.* (1988c) initiated analyses of matrix adhesion of F11 cells. Attachment of these cells was excellent on both plasma FN and PF4 substrata, while attachment on CTB substrata was poor, unless the cells were supplemented with ganglioside GM1. This indicates that FN receptors and heparan sulfate proteoglycan are stably associated with the cell surface of these cells but that GM1 is present in limiting amounts or experiences rapid turnover. Two morphological classes of neurites were observed on FN, suggestive of multiple FN receptors in their responses. Only a relatively few cells formed a third morphological class of neurites on PF4. CTB-generated neurites resembled one class of FN-generated neurites. Both FN classes were sensitive to inhibition of their formation by RGDS peptide, contrasting with the resistance of neurite formation of neuroblastoma cells (Waite *et al.*, 1987). F11 neurite formation on FN or CTB was also sensitive to cytochalasin D, suggesting mediation by microfilament bundles (Mugnai *et al.*, 1988c). In contrast to neuroblastoma neuritogenesis, this process in F11 cells on CTB was highly resistant to cycloheximide treatment and indicates that different proteins mediate GM1-dependent neurite formation in the two cell types. These data argue for multiple and alternative adhesive responses in F11 hybrid cells from genetic information contributed by two neuronal derivative cells, one of which is tumorigenic and metastatic. They also suggest that these hybrid cells make several classes of neurites using several different receptors.

Many *subclones* of F11 parent cells were obtained based on the premise that hybrid cells shed some chromosomes randomly soon after hybridization and ultimately achieve stable genotypes (Barletta and Culp, 1990). This paradigm tests whether F11 differentiation utilizes only one pluripotent cell type in the population or whether differing subpopulations evolve, characterized by independent and/or overlapping mechanisms of differentiation. In the latter case, these subclones could be particularly valuable for assessing the cell and molecular biological mechanisms by which one dorsal root neuron can execute its specialized functions and the dominance or recessiveness of the tumorigenic phenotype in subclones.

Attachment of nine F11 subclones was significantly lower on CTB substrata than on FN or PF4 substrata (Barletta and Culp, 1990). However, neurite formation followed a substratum-specific pattern, with the CTB and PF4 patterns comparable to each other and quite different from the pattern on FN. This probably reflects the multiple receptors to FN that some subclones would utilize preferentially. This was verified by the demonstration that F11 cells attach to substrata coated with proteolytic fragments of FN harboring the Cell$_{II}$ domain but not the Cell$_I$ domain (Lewandowska *et al.*, 1990), supporting the concept that the Cell$_{II}$ domain is neuron-specific. Neurite morphologies of F11 subclones on CTB, PF4, or FN differed and were variably inhibited by pretreatment of cells with cycloheximide. These experiments led to two classification systems for the nine subclones—one system based on substratum selectivity and the second, on cycloheximide sensitivity (Fig. 10 of Barletta and Culp, 1990). These analyses resolved six or more different transmembrane signaling processes for generating different neurite classes, with some mechanisms segregated into individual subclones, while others overlap in other subclones.

4. *Regulation of Receptor Function*

The experiments described above reveal that there are many different cell-surface receptors that recognize different domains of FNs. They reveal the multiplicity and complexity of neuronal differentiation by analyzing processes in malignantly converted presumptive neurons. In the F11 hybrid subclones, it remains to be determined whether the highly amplified copies of mouse N-*myc* are observed in all subclones, whether amplified copies of N-*myc* are down-regulated in their expression in specific subclones, and whether expression of this oncogene correlates with specific differentiation mechanisms and/or differing tumor-progression pathways. The many receptors utilized by F11 subclones remain to be identified, including the one or more integrins that recognize the Cell$_I$ domain, the receptor that recognizes the Cell$_{II}$ domain and any differences from Cell$_{II}$-recognizing receptors of neuroblastoma cells, the heparan sulfate proteoglycan(s) that mediate neuritogenesis on PF4 substrata, and ganglioside GM1-binding proteins that would regulate adhesive responses on CTB substrata. Obviously, such a complex array of receptor functions offers considerable versatility for neuronal tumor cells to progress, to exhibit matrix plasticity, and to clonally dominate in highly selective environments.

Two approaches have been used to examine regulation of matrix adhesion functions in this laboratory. In the first approach, tissue culture glass substrata were derivatized with an alkyl chain, at the ends of which specific chemical endgroups can be inserted for interfacing with the adsorbed FN (Lewandowska *et al.*, 1989). Six different endgroups were used in comparison with underivatized glass: methyl and olefin as hydrophobic surfaces; bromo and cyano as intermediate hydrophilic surfaces; and diol and carboxy groups as highly polar surfaces. Plasma FN bound effectively, stably, and comparably to all these surfaces, and both Balb/c 3T3 fibroblasts and human neuroblastoma cells attached comparably to all surfaces. However, the patterns of cell differentiation responses varied between the two cell types and among the seven surfaces. For example, hydrophobic substrata were poor for neurite outgrowth of neuroblastoma cells but generated excellent F-actin stress fibers in fibroblasts. Bromo surfaces yielded poor neuritogenesis but excellent stress fibers that were highly resistant to inhibition of their formation by RGDS peptide. While hydrophobic surfaces were poor for neurite generation when plasma FN was adsorbed alone, neurite formation was *rescued* if a FN–bovine albumin mixture was adsorbed, demonstrating complex conformational interactions between substratum-bound FN and adhesion-inert neighboring molecules. These studies (Lewandowska *et al.*, 1989) confirmed that different chemical endgroups modulate FN functions in adhesion, principally by affecting the conformation of FN on substrata and not the amounts bound, and that multiple receptor interactions occur with FN molecules in cell type–specific adhesion patterns.

A complementary investigation explored receptor regulation in F11 subclones (Barletta *et al.*, 1991). When cycloheximide was included in the medium to inhibit protein synthesis during active neuritogenesis, neurite formation increased significantly for *all subclones on all three substrata* (FN, PF4, and CTB), virtually eliminating substratum selectivity for differentiation mediated by cell surface integrin, ganglioside GM1, or proteoglycans. Therefore, one or more labile proteins (we refer to these receptor-regulatory proteins as *disintegrins*) must modulate functions of matrix receptors (e.g., integrins) mediating neurite formation. To verify whether cycloheximide-induced neuritogenesis was also regulated by integrin interaction with cell surface GM1, two approaches were used. When the RGDS peptide was added to the medium, it completely inhibited cycloheximide-induced neuritogenesis *on all three substrata of all subclones,* indicating stringent requirement for integrin function in these mechanisms. In contrast, when CTB or a monoclonal anti-GM1 antibody was also added to the medium, cycloheximide-induced neuritogenesis was amplified further on FN, and sensitivity to RGDS peptide inhibition abolished. Therefore, in some contexts ganglioside GM1 must complex with integrin receptors at the cell surface to modulate their function. These results also indicate that (a) cycloheximide treatment leads to loss of substratum selectivity in neuritogenesis, (b) this negative regulation of neurite outgrowth is effected by integrin receptor association with labile regulatory proteins (*disintegrins*) as well as with GM1, and (c) complexing of GM1 by multivalent GM1-binding proteins shifts neuritogenesis from an RGDS-dependent integrin mechanism to an RGDS-independent receptor mechanism (Barletta *et al.*, 1991).

5. *Cell-Type Specificity*

The results described above provide conclusive evidence for the specificity by which various cell types interact with chemically defined extracellular matrices. The embryological origin of the tumor cell types plays a prominent role in determining which receptors are expressed in specific tumor cell populations and how they function in transmembrane signaling processes. That many different neuroblastoma tumor populations of rodent and human origin behave identically provides assurance of the generality of this cell-type specificity. Therefore, within one well-defined tumor cell class, there is consistency of the matrix adhesion mechanisms being utilized across species lines and among multiple independent malignant conversion processes of the same neuronal precursor class. These data can now be compared with similar analyses of other tumor model systems, described in Sections II,C and II,D, to provide insight into cell type–versus tumor-specific alterations in matrix adhesion mechanisms and their potential significance in tumor-progression mechanisms.

C. *Ras*/3T3—Model of Fibrosarcoma

The Balb/c 3T3 cell provides a relatively generic fibroblast that has been immortalized but not converted into fully malignant cells, except under unusual selection pressures over long periods *in vivo* or *in vitro* (Wells *et al.*, 1982). It offers advantages also in being susceptible to full malignant conversion upon introduction of a wide variety of oncogenes (Thorgeirsson *et al.*, 1985; Greig *et al.*, 1985; Bradley *et al.*, 1986; Egan *et al.*, 1987; Radinsky *et al.*, 1987, 1988; Lin *et al.*, 1990a,b). In addition, 3T3 FN adhesive mechanisms are being analyzed in some detail (Rollins *et al.*, 1982; Culp *et al.*, 1986, 1989), providing opportunity to apply this information to selection environments and clonal dominance processes that regulate tumor progression.

1. *3T3 Adhesion Responses*

Balb/c 3T3 cells also adhere to FN by use of multiple surface receptors (Laterra *et al.*, 1983a,b). 3T3 cells on FN demonstrate two specialized processes indicative of fibroblast–matrix interactions: (a) tight-focal contacts identified by interference reflection microscopy and (b) polymerization of F-actin into microfilament stress fibers, detectable with phalloidin staining (Fig. 6), that span distant regions of the cytoplasm and that terminate at tight-focal contacts. Laterra *et al.* (1983a,b) initially demonstrated that heparan sulfate–binding PF4 substrata facilitated stable attachment, partial cytoplasmic spreading, and F-actin bundling in the cytoplasm; however, fully mature stress fibers were never observed. This indicates that heparan sulfate–binding activity on the substratum, upon binding to membrane-intercalated proteoglycans, effects transmembrane signaling with subsequent cytoskeletal reorganization. However, this binding activity of FNs was insufficient by itself to generate tight-focal contacts at the cell's undersurface or microfilament stress-fiber formation. These studies were then extended to heparin-binding fragments of FNs (Lark *et al.*, 1985; Izzard *et al.*, 1986).

Parallel analyses of 3T3 cells on substrata coated with one proteolytic fragment of plasma FNs, the 120K CBF fragment harboring only the Cell$_1$ domain (Fig. 2), revealed responses complementary to those on PF4 or heparin-binding FN fragments. Again, cells were incompetent for forming microfilament stress fibers. F-actin was observed in condensations at select areas of the ruffling plasma membrane (Lark *et al.*, 1985). Cells were also unable to form tight-focal contacts with the 120K CBF substratum but formed only close contacts, which were inhibitable with the RGDS peptide in the medium (Izzard *et al.*, 1986).

A larger array of FN proteolytic fragments was used to determine the binding requirements of various fibroblast responses (Hall *et al.*, 1988; Flickinger and Culp, 1990). The smallest fragment that could effect physiologically normal

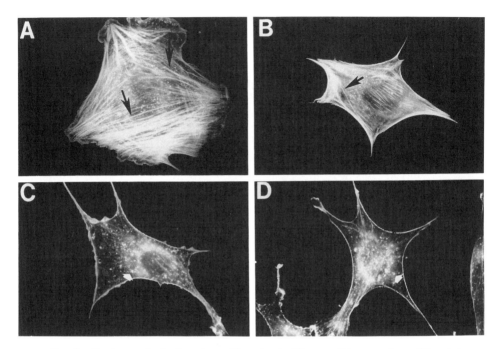

FIG. 6.   F-actin organization in various v-Ki-*ras*⁺ and v-Ki-*ras*⁻ cell types on plasma FN-coated substrata. Balb/c 3T3 cells (A), v-Ki-*ras*⁻ revertant IIIA-4 cells (B), KiMSV early-passage cells (all are v-Ki-*ras*⁺) (C), and lung metastatic tumor cells after subcutaneous injection into nude mice (all are v-Ki-*ras*⁺) (D) were detached from stock cultures by EGTA treatment and 1.5 × 10⁴ cells inoculated onto plasma FN-coated glass coverslips in cluster dishes. After 4 hr, cells were fixed with paraformaldehyde, stained with rhodamine-phalloidin, which binds to filamentous actin, and photographed under fluorescence microscopy. Excellent stress fibers are observed in untransformed 3T3 cells (arrows in A) and in v-Ki-*ras*⁻ revertant cells (arrow in B). Stress fibers are not evident in KiMSV early-passage cells, which displayed small clusters of F-actin (broad white arrow in C). Similarly, all primary tumor and lung metastatic tumor cells (e.g., D) were also defective at forming stress fibers and generated only small clusters of F-actin condensation in the cytoplasm (broad white arrow in D). All micrographs, × 194. [Taken with permission from R. Radinsky, K. S. Flickinger, M. A. Kosir, L. Zardi, and L. A. Culp. (1990). *Cancer Res.* **50,** 4388-4400.]

spreading and microfilament stress-fiber formation of human skin fibroblasts or 3T3 cells, identical to responses on intact FNs, was F155 harboring both Cell$_I$ and Hep$_{II}$ domains (Hall *et al.*, 1988). Separate fragments harboring these domains, even in various molar mixtures, were incompetent for generating complete responses, indicating the specificity and the topological requirements of both integrin and heparan sulfate proteoglycan–binding reactions in these mechanisms. Furthermore, the topology of the fragments on the substratum was critical

(Flickinger and Culp, 1990). If two adjacent regions of substrata were coated with F110 (harboring only Cell$_I$) and with F155 (or collagen, or intact FNs), cells bridging this interface generated stress fibers *only on the F155-facing side of their undersurfaces;* these stress fibers terminated abruptly at the F155–F110 interface (Flickinger and Culp, 1990). These important experiments demonstrate that (a) fibroblasts require only two binding domains of FNs (Cell$_I$ and Hep$_{II}$) in a precise topological arrangement to effect their major responses; (b) they do not require specialized receptors, such as those recognizing Cell$_{II}$ or Cell$_{III}$ and characteristic of neuroblastoma, F11, or other differentiated cell types, for these responses; and (c) cell type–specific adhesion processes are supported by these data, along with 3T3 responses on chemically derivatized substrata reviewed in Section II,B,5 above.

2. Ras/3T3 Adhesion Responses—Different but Overlapping Mechanisms

With this knowledge of 3T3 adhesion mechanisms, we have the opportunity to compare these mechanisms directly with those of various malignant derivatives of 3T3, an opportunity not afforded so easily with cells from the nervous system (Cepko, 1989). Kirsten murine sarcoma virus–transformed Balb/c 3T3 cells (KiMSV cells) were available to relate levels and expression of the v-Ki-*ras* oncogene to altered matrix adhesion (Aaronson and Wallace, 1970; Radinsky *et al.*, 1987). This transformant contains a replication-defective copy of the retrovirus genome and only one copy of the viral oncogene; it has lost ability to generate F-actin stress fibers in its cytoplasm (Fig. 6C), as have tumor cells derived from this cell type (Fig. 6D). Long-term growth of these cloned, transformed cells in culture results in deletion of the v-Ki-*ras* oncogene and selective overgrowth of v-Ki-*ras*⁻ revertant cells during culturing (Radinsky *et al.*, 1987, 1988). V-Ki-*ras*⁻ cells have also *reverted* their ability to form stress fibers in the cytoplasm (Fig. 6B). Conversely, inoculation of KiMSV cells into nude mice by many different routes selects for cells that harbor v-Ki-*ras* in all cells of all tumors; in some cases, formation of lung metastases results from selection of cells with amplified/rearranged copies of the oncogene (Radinsky *et al.*, 1988). This affords opportunity to evaluate one tumor cell system full cycle: from untransformed 3T3, to v-Ki-*ras*–transformed cells, to primary and metastatic tumor populations containing the oncogene, and back to a 3T3-like phenotype as a consequence of deleting the oncogene.

Radinsky *et al.* (1990) initiated FN adhesion analyses of this homologous cell system using approaches proved successful for neuroblastoma systems, as described in Section II,B. Of particular significance and contrasting with 3T3 analyses (Izzard *et al.*, 1986), attachment of early-passage KiMSV cells (all of which harbor v-Ki-*ras*), primary tumor, and lung metastatic tumor cells was resistant to inhibition with the RGDS peptide in the medium on FN, on proteolytic fragment F155 (harboring Cell$_I$ and Hep$_{II}$ domains), on PF4, and on heparin-binding fragments. In contrast, attachment on F110 (harboring both Cell$_I$ and Cell$_{II}$ domains) was highly sensitive to the RGDS peptide. This latter result also contrasts with the noted resistance of neuroblastoma processes on this same fragment (Mugnai *et al.*, 1988a; Lewandowska *et al.*, 1990) and indicates again cell-type specificity in adhesion, i.e., KiMSV cells do not express the receptor recognizing Cell$_{II}$ (Radinsky *et al.*, 1990). Cytoplasmic spreading of early-passage KiMSV cells and all tumor cells was very good on intact FN and on F155 (Radinsky *et al.*, 1990), paralleling similar observations with untransformed fibroblasts (Hall *et al.*, 1988; Flickinger and Culp, 1990).

On heparin-binding proteins, additional differences were noted between v-Ki-*ras*$^+$ and v-Ki-*ras*$^-$ revertant cells (Radinsky *et al.*, 1990). On F38 derived from plasma FN or on PF4, v-Ki-*ras*$^+$ cells remained rounded or detached (Fig. 7A); on F44 + 47 from cellular FNs that harbor ED$_a$ sequences (Fig. 2), cells spread more effectively, with long linear processes evident in many cells (Fig. 7B). The same differences were noted for primary tumor (Fig. 7C and D) and lung metastatic tumor (Fig. 7E and F) cells. Evidence that F44 + 47 contains a new cell-binding domain (called Cell$_{IV}$ in Fig. 2), specific for v-Ki-*ras*$^+$ cultured or tumor cells, was obtained (Radinsky *et al.*, 1990). First, attachment on F44 + 47 but not on the other heparin-binding proteins was resistant to pretreatment of cells with bacterial heparitanase, which destroys cell-surface heparan sulfate. Therefore, there must be a proteoglycan-independent binding site in F44 + 47. Second, neuroblastoma cells respond poorly to these same fragments (Mugnai *et al.*, 1988a), indicating cell-type specificity for fibrosarcoma cells. Third, v-Ki-*ras*$^-$ revertant cells have lost competence for spreading on F44 + 47 and resemble untransformed 3T3 cells in this regard. Fourth, F44 + 47 lack peptide sequences required for Cell$_{III}$ activity. Finally, biochemical evaluation of the substratum-attached material of all primary and metastatic tumor cell populations in culture established considerable catabolism of their heparan sulfate proteoglycans, consistent with their inability to mediate stable attachment of these cells on heparin-binding proteins. Therefore, all of this evidence establishes a new adhesion domain in FNs (Cell$_{IV}$) that may be located in alternatively spliced sequences of ED$_a$, since fragments containing these sequences are the only effectors of excellent responses from *ras* oncogene–expressing cells (Radinsky *et al.*, 1990).

D. Oncogene-Dependent Regulation of Adhesion Receptor Function

The studies described above reveal that multiple receptors function in the adhesion processes of tumor cell populations derived from 3T3 fibroblasts. By comparing these results with those of neuroblastoma cells (Section II,B), we can draw some interesting and important conclusions. First, these two tumor cell classes express different receptors, permitting them to interact with FN matrices

PF4   F44+47

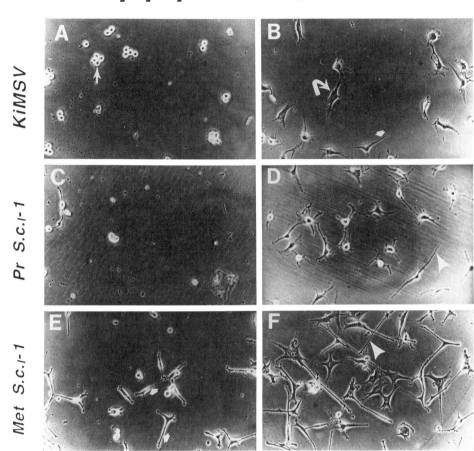

FIG. 7. Morphology of various v-Ki-*ras*$^+$ cells on substrata of PF4 or cellular FN fragments F44 + 47. KiMSV early-passage cells (A and B), primary tumor cells from a subcutaneous injection of nude mice with late-passage KiMSV cells (referred to as Pr. S.c.$_I$-1; C and D), and lung metastatic tumor cells from a subcutaneous injection of nude mice (referred to as Met. S.c.$_I$-1; E and F) were detached from stock cultures with EGTA treatment. After rinsing, 2.5×10^4 cells were inoculated into tissue culture wells coated with PF4 (A, C, and E) or cellular FN heparin-binding fragments F44 + 47 (B,D, and F). After incubation in adhesion medium for 24 hr at 37°C, samples were rinsed twice with phosphate-buffered saline plus divalent cations and fixed for 1 hr with 3% glutaraldehyde in buffered saline. A, C, and E—after 24 hr of attachment on PF4-coated substrata, KiMSV cells demonstrated a rounded morphology (white arrow in A), in contrast to Pr. S.c.$_I$-1 cells, which extended short linear processes. Met. S.c.$_I$-1 cells had increased numbers of attaching cells that displayed short extensions on PF4 (broad white arrows in E). B, D, and F—After 24 hr on F44 + 47, KiMSV cells showed increased cytoplasmic spreading (hooked arrow in B) and extension of short processes. Pr. S.c.$_I$-1 cells extended long linear processes, as similarly observed in the Met. S.c.$_I$-1 cells (white arrowheads in D and F). These processes were more pronounced at this 24-hr point as compared to the 4-hr point. Other tumor cell populations demonstrated the same differences on the two substrata (see Radinsky *et al.*, 1990). All micrographs, ×92. [Taken with permission from R. Radinsky, K. S. Flickinger, M. A. Kosir, L. Zardi, and L. A. Culp. (1990). *Cancer Res.* **50,** 4388–4400.]

in cell type–specific ways (i.e., receptors directed to $Cell_{II}$ and $Cell_{IV}$). This raises the question of how many more receptors and FN-binding domains remain to be discovered. Use of FN proteolytic fragments and molecular biologically generated *deminectins* (Schwarzbauer *et al.*, 1987) for adhesion analyses will be particularly important in this regard, with the latter approach beneficial in assessing binding site–sequence requirements and the topological alignment of binding domains. Second, some binding activities of FNs are shared in common among all untransformed and transformed cell classes examined to date (e.g., $Cell_I$ and Hep_{II}). $Cell_{III}$ receptor (integrin $\alpha_4\beta_1$) has been observed in melanoma tumor cells (Humphries *et al.*, 1986a, 1987) and some T/B cell classes (Wayner *et al.*, 1989; Guan and Hynes, 1990; Garcia-Pardo and Ferreira, 1990). It remains to be determined whether many other tumor cell classes also utilize $\alpha_4\beta_1$. Third, the differing adhesion mechanisms of neuroblastoma and fibrosarcoma cells could result from the embryological origins of these particular cell types and/or the elevated expressions of the N-*myc* or *ras* oncogenes, respectively. The results of Radinsky *et al.* (1990) are certainly consistent with *ras*-dependent regulation of the $Cell_{IV}$ receptor. Therefore, it will be important to transfect several different oncogenes into a common parent cell (e.g., N-*myc* into Balb/c 3T3; v-Ki-*ras* into human neuroblastoma cells) and determine whether distinctive FN adhesion mechanisms are observed. Fourth, two FN-binding domains, $Cell_{III}$ and $Cell_{IV}$, occur in alternatively spliced sequences of the molecule and provide potential regulation for tumor cells at the site of their nuclear splicing apparatus. Tumor cells preferentially include IIICS sequences in their mRNA populations when compared to untransformed cells (Hershberger and Culp, 1990). Similarly, transformed–tumor cells preferentially include ED_a and ED_b sequences (Zardi *et al.*, 1987). However, these studies averaged mRNA distributions over large numbers of cells; it remains to be determined what diversity in mRNA distributions occurs among single tumor cells, an important issue considering clonal dominance during tumor progression (Kerbel *et al.*, 1988; Kerbel, 1990; see review by Nicolson in this series). Finally, these analyses establish the diversity of adhesion mechanisms that tumor cells can utilize when confronting various FN matrices. Modulation of the functions of multiple tumor cell receptors by a variety of mechanisms described in Section II,A also affords cells opportunity to facilitate their interactions with organ-specific matrices.

III. Matrix Adhesion during Tumor Progression

A. THE PARADOX OF ADHESION VERSUS DETACHMENT–INVASION

As metastatic tumor cells spread to target organs, they must continuously break adhesions and form new ones (McCarthy *et al.*, 1985; Juliano, 1987; Nicolson, 1988; Humphries *et al.*, 1989). The interactions of tumor cells with several different adhesion molecules, as well as tumor cell migration within the ECM, are critical for metastasis. Liotta *et al.* (1986) have proposed a stepwise model to account for tumor cell interaction/invasion of ECMs during metastasis, including cell attachment to the ECM by surface receptor functions that recognize specific adhesion molecules, digestion of ECM with tumor- or host-associated hydrolases, migration into the newly created space, formation of new adhesions, and repetition of the cycle until the entire basement membrane is penetrated. FN plays a central role in these interactions (Humphries *et al.*, 1989). Proteolytic fragments of FNs may have physiological relevance to adhesion of tumor cells displaying proteases on their surfaces, which could cleave them (Liotta *et al.*, 1986; Chen and Chen, 1987). Thus, ECM invasion by malignant tumor cells involves both tumor cell adhesive properties and specific cell-surface components as important determinants in this process.

Alteration of FN function in cell-adhesion processes of tumor-progressing cells has not been well characterized. Transformation may lead to decreased FN biosynthesis (Humphries *et al.*, 1989), synthesis of variant forms (Hynes, 1985; Castellani *et al.*, 1986), increased turnover and degradation, posttranslational modifications (Wagner *et al.*, 1981), or changes in the distribution or quality of FN receptor(s) (Plantefar and Hynes, 1989). Additionally, overexpression of the FN receptor $\alpha_5\beta_1$ leads to suppression of the transformed phenotype, with acquisition of normal growth-control characteristics (Giancotti and Ruoslahti, 1990). These observations suggest that invading tumor cells must express adequate numbers and/or quality of receptors to interact with basement membrane components. A great deal must be learned about the metabolism of FN receptors and in selected tumor cell subpopulations at various host tissue sites.

B. Clonal Dominance during Tumor Progression— Implications for Studying Adhesion

Fidler (1973a,b) originally reported evidence for the selective nature of the metastatic phenotype based on the hypothesis that metastases are generated from highly specialized and genetically mutated subpopulations of tumor cells that emerge during the course of primary tumor growth. To date many malignant tumors from different systems have been shown to contain cell subpopulations that differ in many properties, including metastatic capability (Poste and Fidler, 1980; Heppner and Miller, 1983; Kerbel, 1990). This model predicts that authentic metastatic variants, as a result of phenotypic instability, would remain a minority subpopulation, not only in the primary tumor but also within metastases themselves (Kerbel, 1990; Weiss, 1990). The variability in metastatic and other phenotypic properties of subpopulations isolated from the same tumor is an important consideration when analyzing tumor cell–surface properties and their

relationship to metastasis (Heppner and Miller, 1983; Nicolson, 1988). If biochemical analyses are to be meaningful, they must either utilize tumor cells from
uniform cell populations with similar metastatic characteristics (see below) or
compensate for clonal variability. In tumors with cell subpopulations, as in those
in which the highly metastatic cells represent only a small proportion, random
analyses of the entire cellular repertoire may mask important characteristics.

Recently, late-stage primary tumors transfected with pSV2neo or infected with
a retroviral vector harboring the neo[R] gene showed nonrandom overgrowth
of genotypically marked metastatic subpopulations of tumor cells (using the
pSV2neo or the retroviral integration sites as genetic markers) (Kerbel et al.,
1988; Kerbel, 1990; Radinsky and Culp, 1991). These results indicate that the
metastatic-competent variant cells manifest a strong growth preference over
their nonmetastatic counterparts even within the primary tumor and, with time,
come to clonally dominate it. This model predicts that the primary tumor,
given enough time, will become increasingly indistinguishable genotypically
and phenotypically from its metastases (Kerbel, 1990; Price et al., 1990;
Staroselsky et al., 1990; Radinsky and Culp, 1991). Furthermore, it would
suggest that genotypic and phenotypic differences could be detected between
metastatic cells and the primary tumor cells at discrete growth stages of the
primary tumor itself. An example of this was reported recently where the intercellular adhesion molecule (ICAM-1) was expressed only in the late and
metastatic stages during melanoma progression (Johnson et al., 1989). It will
now be essential to evaluate FN and other matrix-receptor distributions at
various stages of primary tumor growth, at multiple metastatic sites, and for
multiple single-cell clones of various tumor populations (Radinsky et al., 1988,
1990).

C. TARGET ORGAN SPECIFICITY—ROLES FOR MATRIX RECEPTORS AND MULTIPLE CELL CLASSES

Clinical observations over a long period have revealed that certain tumors have
a marked preference for metastasis to specific organs and that these metastatic
patterns are not determined entirely by vascular anatomy, rate of blood flow, or
number of tumor cells delivered (Fidler, 1984; Nicolson, 1988). The adherence
of circulating malignant cells to specific organ microvessel endothelial cells is
one important mechanism in determining organ-specific metastasis (Nicolson,
1988). For example, B16 melanoma sublines that efficiently colonize the lung
site display increased rates of adherence to murine lung microvessel endothelial
cells, while brain-colonizing B16 cells showed increased rates of adhesion to
brain microvessel endothelial cells (Nicolson, 1988). The mechanisms of tumor
cell–endothelial cell interactions are believed to be similar to those of lymphocytes adhering to specialized high endothelial venules at sites of lymphocyte exit

from the blood into *home* lymphoid tissues (Springer *et al.*, 1984; Sher *et al.*, 1988; Hemler, 1990). VLA integrins may provide an important element in the specificity of host organ implantation of select tumor cells.

Following tumor cell–endothelial cell interactions, the malignant cells can stimulate endothelial cell retraction to expose the underlying basement membrane and thereby to permit tumor cell matrix receptors to bind (Juliano, 1987). The basement membrane, being a better adhesive substrate, would mediate net movement of tumor cells, probably because of an adhesion gradient (McCarthy *et al.*, 1985). These adhesion events must involve a variety of molecules including FN, laminin, type IV collagen, various proteoglycans, and vitronectin (see Section I). A great deal remains to be learned about the dynamics of tumor cell receptor interactions in these complex environments. Although these differential adhesion properties are important, they are probably insufficient by themselves for determining the organ specificity of metastasis, and it is likely that factors generated by specific host-cell populations must act as a paracrine-like mechanism during these events.

D. Deregulation of Matrix-Dependent Genes

Malignant transformation frequently, but not invariably, results in decreased expression of ECM components, increased capability to actively invade basement membranes, and active migration through surrounding stroma. It follows that invading tumor cells must express adequate numbers of receptors for ECM components. Humphries *et al.* (1986a, 1987) described two important regions in the alternately spliced IIICS region of human FN that promote B16-F10 melanoma adhesion and spreading but are inactive with baby hamster kidney cells. Additionally, neural crest cells and lymphocytes recognize the $Cell_{III}$ domain, suggesting its involvement in migration during development and lymphocyte trafficking (Humphries *et al.*, 1989). McCarthy *et al.* (1986, 1988) identified an RGDS-resistant attachment–spreading activity for B16-F10 mouse melanoma cells in a tryptic–catheptic 33-kDa COOH-terminal, heparin-binding fragment from the α-chain of pFN involving multiple domains, i.e., Hep_{II} plus $Cell_{III}$ domains. Recently, the human melanoma–specific receptor for the FN IIICS region was identified as $\alpha_4\beta_1$ integrin (Mould *et al.*, 1990). These results suggest that tumor cell–specific expression and/or deregulation of ECM components and receptors is an important determinant for tumor progression.

Proteoglycans can also act as modulators of tumorigenesis (Iozzo, 1988; Ruoslahti, 1988b). As reviewed in Section II,C, v-Ki-*ras*–mediated alteration of proteoglycan metabolism correlates with the tumor-progressing phenotype of KiMSV cells (Radinsky *et al.*, 1990). Some proteoglycans bind to soluble ligands and matrix proteins involved in cell growth and adhesion; their synthesis in some tumors has been shown to be altered (Iozzo, 1988; Ruoslahti, 1988b). Highly metastatic

B16 melanoma subclones degraded sulfated glycosaminoglycans at a higher rate than B16 cells of poor lung-colonizing ability (Nakajima *et al.*, 1984). This was attributed to a tumor cell–associated heparanase (Nakajima *et al.*, 1984) and confirmed in other systems (Iozzo, 1988). Furthermore, variants of Swiss 3T3 cells produced undersulfated heparan sulfate chains that correlated with defects in formation of focal contacts and cytoskeletal organization, similar to the phenotypic changes observed in many tumor cells (Keller *et al.*, 1988). Proteoglycan-deficient Chinese hamster ovary variants were less tumorigenic, suggesting the participation of cell-surface proteoglycans in immune recognition of foreign cells (Esko *et al.*, 1988). All of these observations suggest alteration of various classes of tumor cell-surface receptors as a contributing factor in the complex processes of tumor progression.

IV. Interference with Tumor Progression at the Cell–Matrix Interface

The ability of metastatic tumor cells to adhere and migrate through various extracellular matrices suggests that highly specific inhibitors of tumor cell–matrix interactions may selectively interfere with this critical step of tumor progression. Several such inhibitors have been described for reducing tumor cell colonization of host target organs: proteolytic fragments of FN or laminin with specific binding domains; synthetic peptides mimicking adhesion-recognition sites in FNs or laminin; reagents interfering with cellular oligosaccharide processing or other biochemical pathways; and inhibitors of matrix metalloproteinase and collagenase IV. These inhibition mechanisms will be reviewed separately.

A. Proteolytic Fragments of Fibronectin and/or Laminin at Metastatic Sites

FNs and laminin in matrices are essential for promoting attachment, spreading, and migration of most tumor cell types (Akiyama *et al.*, 1986; McCarthy *et al.*, 1985). Preincubation of murine melanoma cells with FN *or* laminin reduced their lung colonization following intravenous injection into animals (Terranova *et al.*, 1984). Some malignant cells display more laminin on their surfaces, bind more laminin, and attach more readily to laminin substrata (Terranova *et al.*, 1982; Terranova *et al.*, 1984). Conversely, laminin increases the invasive–metastatic activity and induces the secretion of collagenase IV of some tumor cells (Turpeenniemi-Hujanen *et al.*, 1986).

To study the specific interaction of the metastatic cells with different domains of FN, proteolytic fragments of FNs are used in adhesion experiments *in vitro* (Section II), as well as in metastasis-inhibition experiments *in vivo* (McCarthy *et al.*, 1986). A heparin-binding fragment of FNs, which promoted tumor cell adhesion by an RGD-independent mechanism, inhibited lung colonization of metastatic tumor cells upon intravenous injection and enhanced survival rates of animals (McCarthy *et al.*, 1988). It remains to be determined whether fragments of FN harboring Cell$_{I,II,III \text{ or } IV}$ domains, separately or in combination, inhibit metastasis more or less effectively than heparin-binding fragments, and whether they inhibit in cell type–specific ways.

Proteolytic fragments of laminin have also been used to inhibit experimental metastasis of melanomas (Barsky *et al.*, 1984; McCarthy *et al.*, 1988). Several laminin fragments (600-kDa thrombin fragment; 440-kDa chymotrypsin fragment; 330-kDa/110-kDa thermolysin fragments) promoted cell adhesion *in vitro* on tissue-culture substrata, but only the thrombin fragment or intact laminin promoted adhesion of tumor cells to type IV collagen substrata (McCarthy *et al.*, 1985). The 440-kDa chymotrypsin and 330-kDa/110-kDa thermolysin fragments completely inhibited metastasis formation *in vivo* (Barsky *et al.*, 1984; McCarthy *et al.*, 1985; McCarthy *et al.*, 1988). It appears that interference with the binding of laminin to high-affinity receptors on the cell surface might be the basis for this effect (Barsky *et al.*, 1984; Terranova *et al.*, 1984).

B. INHIBITION BY SYNTHETIC PEPTIDES THAT MIMIC ADHESION PROTEIN ACTIVITIES

Synthetic peptides containing the RGD sequence of the Cell$_I$ domain of FNs (Fig. 2) and that recognize specific integrins (Table 1) inhibit these receptor–ligand interactions during adhesion *in vitro* (Piershbacher and Ruoslahti, 1984; Yamada and Kennedy, 1984). *In vitro* invasion of the amniotic membrane by malignant cells is inhibited by specific RGD peptides in a dose-dependent manner. A hexapeptide, GRGDTP, which inhibits the attachment of cells to type I collagen in addition to inhibiting FN- and vitronectin-mediated attachment, was more inhibitory than those RGD peptides that inhibit only FN and vitronectin attachment (Gehlsen *et al.*, 1988). Coinjection of GRGDS peptide with B16-F10 melanoma cells resulted in a marked reduction of melanotic colonies 14 days postinjection in the lungs of mice (Humphries *et al.*, 1986b). The inhibition of experimental metastasis was also demonstrated by using several other tumor lines and RGD peptides or polymeric peptides (Bretti *et al.*, 1989; Saiki *et al.*, 1989; Ugen *et al.*, 1988). The effect of the peptides on inhibiting lung colonization seems to increase the rate of clearance of the injected cells from the lungs (Humphrics *et al.*, 1986b). *Possible* mechanisms of RGD-mediated clearance of the cells from the lungs and inhibition of colony formation include disruption of cell attachment, interference with cell migration during invasion, inhibition of platelet aggregation, and effects on host stromal cells (Humphries *et al.*, 1988). It remains to be determined whether synthetic peptides mimicking the activities of

Cell$_{II-IV}$ domains of FNs display cell type–specific inhibition of metastasis. Some B16 melanoma cells escape inhibition of metastasis (Humphries *et al.*, 1988), and it will be informative to determine whether these are tumor cell variants that rely on different FN and/or laminin adhesion mechanisms.

In the case of laminin, a synthetic nonapeptide (CDPGYIGSR) from the B1 chain was identified as a major site for melanoma cell adhesion *in vitro* (Graf *et al.*, 1987). A pentapeptide within the nonapeptide sequence (YIGSR) was later found to reduce the formation of lung colonies in mice injected with melanoma cells and to inhibit the invasiveness of the cells *in vitro* (Iwamoto *et al.*, 1987). YIGSR peptide may inhibit lung tumor formation by competing with laminin for receptor recognition of tumor cells, thus blocking the binding of the cells to basement membranes. On the other hand, the metastasis-promoting activity of laminin has been located at 19 amino acid sequences in the A chain of laminin (Kanemoto *et al.*, 1990). This peptide *increases* experimental metastasis by possibly stimulating the production of collagenase IV activity and cell motility.

Other synthetic peptides have been shown to alter tumor progression in a few systems. A synthetic nonapeptide fragment of thrombin inhibits the cell motility in culture of a human melanoma subclone that possesses a high metastatic potential in mice (Packard, 1987). The peptide SRGDTG of collagen inhibits colon carcinoma cell attachment to collagen (Pignatelli and Bodmer, 1988). The effect of these new peptide sequences on the metastasis formation must be determined. Two synthetic peptides from the Hep$_{II}$ domain of FN have been shown to have adhesion-promoting activity for melanoma cells (Skubitz *et al.*, 1988). A heparin-binding synthetic peptide from the B1 chain of laminin also exhibited adhesion-promoting activity for melanoma cells (Skubitz *et al.*, 1988). It must be determined whether mixtures of RGD peptide and heparin-binding peptides have an additive effect on inhibiting metastasis to the lung. In addition, metastasis to other target organs remains to be tested in suitable tumor model systems.

C. INTERFERENCE WITH TUMOR CELL BIOSYNTHETIC PROCESSES

Neoplastic transformation in both rodent and human tumor systems is often accompanied by alterations in the carbohydrate structures of glycoproteins and glycolipids, which are important biochemical determinants of cell–matrix recognition (Sections I and II). Increased β1-6 branching of asparagine-linked oligosaccharides is closely associated with enhanced metastatic potential in several tumor models (Dennis *et al.*, 1989a). Swainsonine, a plant alkaloid and a potent inhibitor of Golgi α-mannosidase II, inhibited organ colonization by metastatic cells and the growth of transformed fibroblasts in soft agar. When administered systemically to mice, swainsonine also inhibited pulmonary metastatis of i.v.-injected B16-F10 melanoma cells by a mechanism involving interleukin-2 production and augmentation of natural killer cell activity (Newton *et al.*, 1989). The antiproliferative activity of swainsonine was additive with that of interferon-α2 *in vitro*. Combination of swainsonine and interferon *in vivo* reduced tumor growth even more effectively (Dennis *et al.*, 1989b). In some cases however, treatment with succinylated lectins or with tunicamycin or swainsonine had no specific effects on metastatic colonization of the lung (Sargent *et al.*, 1987).

A sialyltransferase inhibitor (KI-8110) reduced experimental metastasis by inhibiting the interaction between tumor cells and host platelets, possibly because of reduction of sialic acid contents of tumor cell–surface components (Kijima-Suda *et al.*, 1988). Pertussis toxin, an agent known to inactivate certain G-protein-mediated signal transductions, inhibits entry of normal lymphocytes into tissues and affects invasion and metastasis of malignant lymphoma and T-cell hybridoma cells (Roos *et al.*, 1987). Sulfated polysaccharides heparin, dextran sulfate, and xylose sulfate can inhibit tumor metastasis as well, owing to the anticoagulant activity of these molecules (Coombe *et al.*, 1987). Warfarin, an anticoagulant, also inhibited metastasis without having any effect on growth of the primary tumor, although the mechanism of inhibition by warfarin may not necessarily be mediated by its anticoagulant activity (McCulloch and George, 1989).

D. Interference with Matrix-Degrading Enzymes

Adherence of malignant cells to specific matrices is a prerequisite for invasion of these matrices. Ultimately, tumor cells must traverse basement membranes for successful metastasis. Degradation of the type IV collagen is essential for these processes, and metastatic potential correlates well with the collagenase IV activity of tumor cells (Garbisa *et al.*, 1987; Liotta *et al.*, 1986; see chapter by Liotta in Volume 2 of this work). In this regard, both natural (tissue inhibitor of metalloproteases; TIMP) and synthetic (SC-44463) collagenase IV inhibitors greatly reduced invasion of metastatic tumor cells into model basal lamina (Reich *et al.*, 1988). Retinoic acid inhibited tumor-cell invasion through a model basal lamina by suppressing production of collagenase IV and plasminogen activator (Hendrix *et al.*, 1990; Nakajima *et al.*, 1989). The desmoplastic response inhibits both tumor cell invasion and metastasis; this response induces high levels of metalloproteinase inhibitors directed against tumor-derived type I/IV collagenases (Barsky *et al.*, 1987; Barsky *et al.*, 1988). Inhibition of collagenase IV converts melanoma cells into a dormant noninvasive state, reducing the incidence of lung lesions (Reich *et al.*, 1988; Schultz *et al.*, 1988). Inhibitors of metalloproteinases (TIMP) and chelating agents, such as 1, 10-phenanthroline, are very effective at inhibiting invasion and extracellular matrix degradation (Khokha and Denhardt, 1989). All of these studies taken together indicate a variety of potential mechanisms for interfering with tumor progression, but in no case is there complete efficiency, consistent with clonal plasticity and dominance of selected tumor subpopulations in various environments of the host animal.

V. Molecular Biological Approaches for Evaluating Tumor Progression Events

Metastasis comprises a very complex series of interrelated steps (Poste and Fidler, 1980; Nicolson, 1988), making cell and molecular biological evaluation of these processes difficult at the single-cell level. Several methods have been used to tag metastatic cells in order to study their fate *in vivo*, their interactions with host cells, and the clonal origin of metastatic subpopulations: radioisotopes for evaluating organ distribution (Fidler, 1970; Juacaba *et al.*, 1989); specific chromosome markers (Frost *et al.*, 1987; Hu *et al.*, 1987; McMorrow *et al.*, 1988); transfected foreign DNA sequences (Talmadge *et al.*, 1987; Itaya *et al.*, 1989; Kerbel *et al.*, 1988; Kerbel, 1990) for studying the clonal origin of tumor cells; monoclonal antibodies against tumor cell–specific antigens for studies *in situ* (Schlimok *et al.*,1987; Sheth *et al.*,1987); drug resistance markers for analyzing clonal interactions and dominance (Miller *et al.*, 1988); and melanin-producing melanoma cells for ease of identification of black pigments (Fidler, 1973a,b; Hisano and Hanna, 1982; Ishikawa *et al.*, 1988). Unfortunately, none of these markers can be used as both a phenotypic and genotypic marker in a wide variety of tumor systems. They also have limitations for *in vivo* studies at the single-cell level.

A. TRANSFECTION WITH A HETEROLOGOUS AND ULTRASENSITIVE MARKER GENES

A marker gene (*Escherichia coli lacZ*) has been utilized to genetically and histochemically tag tumor cells *in vitro*, facilitating their location during tumor progression (Lin *et al.*, 1990a,b). *LacZ* codes for a β-galactosidase whose activity is detectable by a chromogenic substrate (X-Gal) and which operates at a neutral pH optimum, therefore readily differentiating tumor cells from host cells with their lysosomal acidic β-galactosidase (Sanes *et al.*, 1986). Bacterial *lacZ* gene can be used not only as a stable and ultrasensitive histochemical marker for metastasis studies but also as a molecular biological marker for clonal dominance studies because of its sequence uniqueness as a prokaryotic gene (Lin *et al.*, 1990a). For example, a specific subclone with a distinct phenotype can be labeled with the *lacZ* marker and mixed with one or more subclones with different phenotypic markers. The *lacZ*-bearing cells can then be identified easily and quickly by the X-Gal staining *in vivo* or *in vitro*, facilitating studies on phenotypic expression–stabilization of tumor-progressing properties among various clones.

A human EJ Ha-*ras* oncogene–transfected BALB/c 3T3 clone was obtained by transfection and subsequently transfected with *lacZ* (Lin *et al.*, 1990a). These are referred to as LZEJ cells. The stability of *lacZ* gene expression has been reported for both *in vitro* (Sanes *et al.*, 1986) and *in vivo* (Goring *et al.*, 1987) systems. *LacZ* expression in LZEJ cells was also stable following at least one round of tumor growth in nude mice (Lin *et al.*, 1990a), a critical element considering the noted genetic instability of tumor cells. After inoculating LZEJ cells into athymic nude mice, rapidly growing primary tumors developed in all animals. These tumors stained intensely blue with the X-Gal assay (Fig. 8A), as did any large lung metastatic nodules, only observed in a few instances (Fig. 8C, large blue nodules).

The X-Gal staining assay is extremely sensitive for detecting small numbers of micrometastatic tumor cells (Lin *et al.*, 1990a), as shown during staining of whole lungs (Fig. 8B–D), where extremely small staining foci could be identified. Of particular note, micrometastases were observed in this 3T3 system for the first time in both brain (Fig. 8E and 8F) and kidney (Lin *et al.*, 1990a); other assays had failed to detect tumor cells in these target organs with the *ras* oncogene/3T3 system (Radinsky *et al.*, 1987). As shown in Figs. 8D and 8F at higher magnification, staining of the smallest micrometastases illustrates the sensitivity and utility of this *lacZ* marker gene for evaluating foci at many organ sites in the animal, foci that would otherwise be undetectable by current methodologies.

Blue-staining foci at target organs can also be readily quantitated for different cell lines injected by various routes (Lin *et al.*, 1990a). The vast majority of lung foci observed in the LZEJ cell model were micrometastases, ranging from a few sites at 28 days subsequent to subcutaneous injection to more than 60 sites at 52 days postinjection (Fig. 8D). In virtually all cases, these foci failed to thrive and enlarge with time. By the intravenous injection route, lung micrometastases were observed 1–30 days postinjection (Fig. 8B) while variably sized lung metastatic nodules and many micrometastases were observed 42 days postinjection (Fig. 8C). A few lung metastatic nodules were observed via the footpad injection route at 72 days postinjection in a milieu of many micrometastases that failed to develop. Therefore, the *lacZ* gene has broad application to metastasis and tumor-progression studies in virtually any tumor cell system, since the *lacZ* gene can be introduced into any tumor or transformed cell line.

B. EVALUATION OF EARLIEST STEPS IN INVASION AND MICROMETASTASIS DEVELOPMENT

In order to study the development of micrometastases at the earliest times, *lacZ*-tagged LZEJ cells were injected into animals, and their lungs were examined soon after injection (Lin *et al.*, 1990b). Pulmonary implantations (less than 30 μm in diameter) were easily detected by X-Gal staining 5 min after tail-vein injection (Fig. 9A). A comparable density of blue-staining sites was also observed in lungs at 15, 25, and 60 min, with the number of staining sites on the surface of the lung remaining very high (greater than 3,000 separate foci) (Lin et al., 1990b). The number of blue-staining foci decreased by 5 to 15 hr postinjection. By 24 hr (Fig. 9C), most LZEJ tumor cells had been cleared from the lung with only a small number of foci persisting (approximately 100 foci), indicating that only about 1 to 2% of tumor cells successfully attach and/or invade this organ. The mechanism(s) of clearance of tumor cells from the lung can be analyzed more readily with the *lacZ* marker in concert with histochemical and/or immunochemical markers for host stromal cells (Lin et al., 1990b).

In this experimental paradigm at 4 days postinjection, micrometastasis development was revealed by the increased size of blue-staining foci ($>100\mu m$ diameter), although the number of pulmonary micrometastases remained approximately the same as that at the 24-hr point (Lin et al., 1990b). By 8 days (Fig. 9D), development was also evidenced by the larger size of blue-staining foci. In addition, the total number of micrometastases increased somewhat, perhaps because some foci are hidden during earlier times or some micrometastases yield other micrometastases. For a 14-day lung, a relatively large, linear focus of tumor cells (approximate 400 μm length) was observed by either whole-organ

---

FIG. 8. X-Gal staining of whole organs from nude mice injected with LZEJ cells by different routes. LZEJ cells, described by Lin et al. (1990a,b), were generated by transfecting the human Harvey-*ras* oncogene (isolated from the EJ bladder carcinoma) into Balb/c 3T3 cells, along with the neomycin[R] gene and the *E. coli lacZ* gene to provide an ultrasensitive histochemical marker for tumor cells in various organs. In all cases, tumors or organs were removed intact and histochemically stained with the X-Gal staining reaction to identify tumor cells by their intense blue staining, as described (Lin et al., 1990a,b). The blue staining results from pH 7-optimal activity of bacterial β-D-galactosidase, coded for by the *lacZ* gene, in the cytoplasm of tumor/transfected cells upon cleavage of the X-Gal substrate (while the lysosomal galactosidase remains inactive at this pH, thereby preventing blue staining of host cells in various organs). (A) Primary tumor obtained from a mouse 4 wk after subcutaneous injection. $\times 23$. (B) Lung from a mouse given an injection at an intravenous (tail vein) site, 4 wk postinjection. Four micrometastases can be identified by X-Gal staining (black arrows) in this particular region of the lung ($\times 23$); other regions of this same lung also demonstrated a comparable density of X-Gal–stained tumor foci. (C) Lung from a mouse given an intravenous injection, 6 wk postinjection. Three X-Gal-staining metastatic nodules and one micrometastasis (black arrow) were identified in this region of the lung, $\times 7$. (D) Lung from a mouse given a subcutaneous injection, 7 wk postinjection. Three micrometastases (black arrows) were observed in this particular region of the lung. $\times 70$. Note that the magnification of D is higher than that of B. (E) Brain from a mouse given an injection at a subcutaneous site, 6 wk postinjection. One micrometastasis (white arrowhead) was identified. $\times 11.5$. (F) Brain from a mouse given a subcutaneous injection, 7 wk postinjection. Two micrometastatic foci (open arrows) were identified. $\times 173$. Note the higher magnification in this panel. [Taken with permission from W.-c. Lin, T. P. Pretlow, T. G. Pretlow II, and L. A. Culp. (1990a) *Cancer Res.* **50**, 2808–2817.]

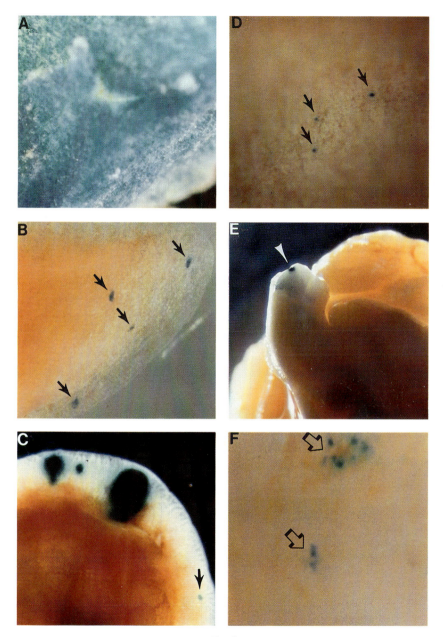

FIG. 8.

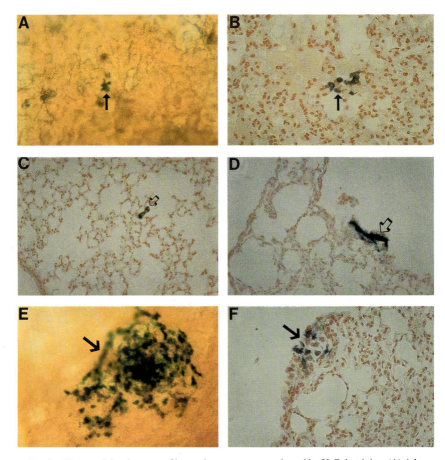

FIG. 9.   Temporal development of lung micrometastases evaluated by X-Gal staining. (A) A lung (whole-organ staining, not a section) from a mouse given an intravenous injection (1×10^5 LZEJ cells), 5 min postinjection. See Lin *et al.* (1990a,b) for description of the LZEJ cells. A small blue-staining focus of one (or only a few) tumor cell(s), less than 30 μm in diameter, is indicated by the black arrow. Note the high magnification in this panel permitting facile identification of X-Gal-staining tumor cells ($\times$ 126). (B) Methacrylate-embedded section of the lung shown in (A) from a mouse given an intravenous injection, 5 min postinjection. A small micrometastasis (or possibly two adjacent micrometastases) (black arrow) is (are) composed of several blue-staining cells ($\times$ 168). Note that this panel is approximately the same magnification as (A), thereby permitting direct comparison of tumor invasion events using either whole organs or embedded sections. (C) A section from a lung after intravenous injection (1×10^5 LZEJ cells), 24 hr postinjection. A micrometastatic focus (small open arrow) contains only one or two cells ($\times$ 84). (D) A section from a lung after intravenous injection (1×10^5 LZEJ cells), 8 days postinjection. A developing micrometastasis (large open arrow) is observed. Note the increased number of blue-staining cells within the micrometastatic focus ($\times$ 84). (E) A lung (whole-organ staining, not a section) after intravenous injection (1×10^5 LZEJ cells), 14 days postinjection. A large developing micrometastasis (large black arrow), approximately 400 μm in diameter, is observed after X-Gal staining. Note the migration of X-Gal-staining tumor cells among host lung cells ($\times$ 79). (F) A section from a lung after intravenous injection (1×10^5 LZEJ cells), 14 days postinjection. An expanding micrometastasis (large black arrow) is observed ($\times$ 168). [Taken with permission from W.-c. Lin, T. P. Pretlow, T. G. Pretlow II, and L. A. Culp. (1990b). *J. Natl. Cancer Res.* **82**, 1497–1503.]

staining (Fig. 9E) or section staining (Fig. 9F); this linear pattern suggests growth of tumor cells along a lymphatic and/or blood vessel at this lung site.

This system can be evaluated by whole-organ staining and by staining of lung sections, permitting excellent characterization of single-cell interactions in sections for correlation with data on whole organs (Lin *et al.*, 1990b). At the highest magnification of whole-organ staining (Fig. 9A), a representative blue-staining focus can be easily observed 5 min after injection. In Fig. 9B at a similar magnification of a section from the same lung, a small micrometastasis (or possibly two adjacent micrometastases) is composed of several blue-staining cells easily distinguished from unstained host lung cells. This demonstrates the sensitivity of the *lacZ* marker for detecting single tumor cells in an overwhelming background of host cells in tissues. Most early foci of tumor cells observed in sections consisted of several blue-staining cells (Fig. 9B and 9C), while foci with only a single blue-staining cell were observed in only a few cases.

This last observation has some important implications. Since precautions were taken to utilize a suspension of single cells for injection, formation of tumor emboli in the lung may result from entrapping tumor cells upon their entering the microvascular network. This result also suggests a requirement for the activity of multiple cells at any one site for tumor cell invasion. If enzymatic and other activities of several cells are used cooperatively at lung sites, as suggested by these data (Lin *et al.*, 1990b), this raises the intriguing issue of the clonal dominance observed in lung metastatic tumors in virtually all tumor systems (Poste and Fidler, 1980; Nicolson, 1988; Kerbel, 1990). Presumably, a single cell among multiple cells at the invasion site acquires growth advantages and soon overtakes the population during micrometastasis development. This important issue remains to be proven. The cooperation among the activities of multiple cells may also be important for the earliest stabilization and extravasation of tumor cells (Kawaguchi and Nakamura, 1986). For example, it has been shown in the B16 melanoma system that pulmonary metastases are more numerous when dead tumor cells or viable mouse embryo cells are coinjected with viable B16 tumor cells (Fidler, 1973b). Although arrest of tumor cell emboli is important to metastasis formation (Fidler, 1973a,b; Zeidman, 1957), the outcome and incidence of metastases may not be determined only by the presence of tumor cell emboli (Tarin and Price, 1981; Tarin *et al.*, 1984).

At 24 hr postinjection, the number of tumor foci decreased in whole-organ stains, and the average size of blue-staining foci was smaller than those foci at earlier times in tissue sections, i.e., there are fewer blue-staining cells in any one focus at 24 hr (Fig. 9C) than at earlier times (Fig. 9B). Successful micrometastases expand and proliferate by 4 to 8 days postinjection (Fig. 9D). Upon further development of micrometastases, LZEJ cells migrate and proliferate by penetration of host lung tissue, as evidenced by the scattered pattern of blue-staining cells (Fig. 9E) by whole-organ staining and when serial sections (Fig. 9F) are examined. These experiments reveal the power of this approach for analyzing the cell and molecular mechanisms of micrometastasis development, as well as the roles of selective matrix adhesion mechanisms in these processes.

C. INTERACTIONS AMONG MULTIPLE TUMOR-CELL AND WITH SPECIFIC HOST-CELL CLASSES

During the earliest stages of micrometastatic foci development, it will be essential to analyze many potential tumor cell–host cell interactions. The *lacZ* marker will be particularly effective in this regard. Blood vessel angiogenesis is crucial for tumor growth and development (Folkman *et al.*, 1987; Weiss *et al.*, 1989). In a transgenic mouse model, angiogenesis is critical for the transition from hyperplasia to neoplasia (Folkman *et al.*, 1989). During tumor invasion and metastasis, circulating tumor cells must adhere to blood vessel endothelial cells at specific organs (Auerbach *et al.*, 1987; Pauli and Lee, 1988; see chapter by Nicolson in Volume 2 of this work) and subsequently invade basement membranes underlying endothelia (Liotta *et al.*, 1986; McCarthy *et al.*, 1985). Adjacent blood vessels and their endothelial linings might serve as exit points of tumor cells for lung invasion from the circulation, as well as the nutrient and growth-factor supply for proliferation of tumor cells subsequently. Metastatic cells may also respond to growth factors secreted by endothelial cells upon tumor-cell recognition and subsequent immune responses (Gasic, 1984; Ryan, 1988). Growth of metastatic cells *in vitro* can be regulated specifically by different organ-conditioned media or growth factors purified from such conditioned media (Naito *et al.*, 1987; Cavanaugh and Nicholson, 1989). These organ-specific growth factors may be secreted by specific endothelial cells in different organs upon tissue injury. Damage induced by a monoclonal antibody against endothelial cells (Kennel *et al.*, 1988) or tumor-elicited polymorphonuclear leucocytes (Welch *et al.*, 1989) enhance the number of metastatic foci.

These studies indicate the importance of endothelial cells for organ specificity and subsequent development of micrometastases into overt metastases. The *lacZ* marker provides an effective approach for studying this microenvironment. A suitable histochemical staining method has been described to distinguish tumor cells from endothelial cells (Lin *et al.*, 1990a). Sections of lung where LZEJ cells were metastasizing were used for X-Gal staining to identify tumor cells (as blue), as described in Section V,B, and for alkaline phosphatase staining (as red) as a histochemical marker for capillary and blood vessel endothelial cells (Lin *et al.*, 1990a). Small capillaries were also observed in some sections. In most cases, blue-staining micrometastatic cells were found proximal to red-staining blood vessels.

The mechanism(s) of clearance of tumor cells from the lung can also be analyzed more readily with the *lacZ* marker in concert with histochemical or immunohistochemical markers for host stromal cells (Iskandar *et al.*, 1989; Mc-Ginnis *et al.*, 1989). Detection of host macrophages and/or monocytes in the micrometastasis foci region can be facilitated by assaying acid phosphatase and/or nonspecific esterase of macrophages and/or monocytes and β-galactosidase for tumor cells.

D. PCR AND *In Situ* HYBRIDIZATION TO EVALUATE GENE REGULATION DURING TUMOR PROGRESSION

In human colorectal carcinoma systems, multiple genetic alterations have been related to the progression of the tumor. By comparing the tumor-cell DNA and adjacent normal-tissue DNA collected from pathological sections, the malignant progression phenotype (distant metastasis and tumor recurrence) is more likely to occur in patients with multiple chromosome deletions in their tumor cells, in addition to *ras*-oncogene mutations (Bos *et al.*, 1987; Fearon *et al.*, 1987; Vogelstein *et al.*, 1989). The *lacZ* gene provides an opportunity to study the expressions of tumor cell genes *in situ* in highly specific sites of target organs in this model system. Growth factor and/or receptor gene expression in metastatic cells and their neighbor host cells can be studied by *in situ* hybridization techniques using cDNA or oligonucleotide probes. A complementary approach can be used as well with the polymerase-chain-reaction technology on extremely small numbers of cells collected from tissue sections after the blue-staining tumor cells have been identified by the X-Gal assay. In these ways, metastasis-related genes and their expression can be studied at the single-cell level at the earliest stages in micrometastatic foci development, and the genetic contributions of surrounding host cells can be evaluated more precisely. This also eliminates the potential problem of selection of tumor-cell subpopulations when tumor cells need to be grown out in tissue culture for molecular biological analyses.

VI. Summary and Future Directions

The FN adhesion mechanisms reviewed here for only two tumor-cell systems indicate the complexity by which tumor cells interact with various matrices that they would encounter during tumor progression. Even within one tumor-cell class, multiple cell-surface receptors to FNs are required, as well as multiple binding domains along FN sequences, which can be found in both common and alternately spliced sequences. Not only can tumor cells regulate adhesion processes at the level of matrix receptor gene expression, but they also can regulate the nature and degrees of splicing of FN pre-mRNAs. When consideration is given to the genetic complexity of laminins, other adhesion-promoting proteins that are not as well studied as FNs, and detachment-facilitating molecules such as certain proteoglycans, thrombospondin, and tenascin, tumor cells are afforded an incredible diversity of mechanisms for regulating their matrix interactions. These facts also suggest two things: (a) many different tumor-cell classes can use very different arrays of receptors and adhesion-modulating molecules to be successful in various target-organ environments, and (b) within one tumor-cell class there may not be a single array of these molecules that function in making and/or breaking adhesive contacts but, rather, a diversity of arrays. This latter point does not bode well for clinical intervention in cancer treatment by interfering with the specific adhesion mechanisms; tumor cells would merely alter their gene expressions and/or select for clones with mechanisms unaffected by the reagents of clinical intervention. These considerations also make it unlikely that there is a *metastasis gene*, i.e., a single dominant regulatory gene whose expression is an overriding aspect of tumor progression (Fidler and Radinsky, 1990). Rather, a very large array of genes must act together.

The results analyzed in this chapter provide insight into cell type–specific adhesion mechanisms, as differentiated from commonly shared tumor-specific mechanisms. That all neuroblastoma cells analyzed to date respond to the $Cell_{II}$ domain of FNs, while all 3T3 transformants and untransformed fibroblasts do not, reflects cell-type specificity based on the neural crest origin of these particular tumor cells. Likewise, *ras*/3T3 transformants, but not neuroblastoma, respond uniquely to the $Cell_{IV}$ domain of FNs. In addition to transformant-associated changes in the amounts or catabolism of various integrin receptors (Plantefar and Hynes, 1989), there are also cell type–specific differences in the catabolism of membrane-intercalated heparan sulfate proteoglycans in the substratum adhesion sites of these two tumors. Neuroblastoma cells display very little degradation of their substratum-interfacing proteoglycans (Maresh *et al.*, 1984; Vallen *et al.*, 1988) while *ras*/3T3 cells and their tumorigenic derivatives display considerable degradation of both protein and glycosaminoglycan chains of proteoglycans (Radinsky *et al.*, 1990). The important question now remains whether tumor cell–specific differences truly reflect the embryological origin of tumor classes or reflect the differing oncogenes activated in them.

Conversely, there are now indications for tumor-specific mechanisms in matrix adhesion that may be shared by many different tumor cell classes. Both neuroblastoma and *ras*/3T3 tumor cells utilize some degree of cooperativity between the $Cell_I$ domain of FNs and a second domain, $Cell_X$. In the case of neuroblastoma, this combination is $Cell_I$ plus $Cell_{II}$, for *ras*/3T3 it is $Cell_I$ plus $Cell_{IV}$, and for melanoma it is $Cell_I$ plus $Cell_{III}$. It remains to be seen whether this pattern will hold true for many other tumor-cell classes and how many more $Cell_X$ domains remain to be discovered.

Experimental systems in the future must address many aspects of matrix adhesion processes and their significance during metastatic spread and/or selection of tumor cell subpopulations. Many more tumor cell systems must be analyzed, both *in vitro* and *in vivo* during tumor progression, for their matrix-adhesion mechanisms. Other $Cell_x$ domains in FNs and laminins must be evaluated and their receptors identified and characterized. The possibility must also be considered that particular host organ environments lead to modulation of $Cell_x$-R gene expression and/or function, particularly by gangliosides and proteoglycans neighboring $Cell_x$-R at the cell surface or by proteases and/or factors secreted from neighboring cells. Analyses of adhesion mechanisms must consider more precisely clonal selection processes that occur, both within the primary tumor during its development as well as in single and multiple sites of tumor metastasis (Kerbel *et al.,* 1988; Kerbel, 1990). Conversely, there are indications for interclonal interactions among multiple tumor cells during metastasis that are suggestive of complementary gene products from two or more cell types acting synergistically in these processes (Lin *et al.,* 1990b; Kerbel, 1990). For analyzing gene expression and its consequences at the single-cell level during micrometastasis development, there are several molecular biological approaches that can now be exploited. The last decade of this century should see exponential growth in our understanding of the cell and molecular events that regulate tumor progression.

Acknowledgments

These studies were performed under the auspices of National Institutes of Health Research Grants CA27755 and NS17139 (to LAC). The authors are indebted to Dr. Luciano Zardi of Genoa, Italy, for contributing fibronectin proteolytic fragments; Dr. Paul Kraemer of Los Alamos National Laboratory for assistance with analyses of tumors in nude mice; Dr. Mark Fishman of the Massachusetts General Hospital, Boston, Massachusetts, for contributing the F11 neuronal hybrid cells; Dr. Joshua Sanes of Washington University, St. Louis, Missouri, for contributing the bacterial *lacZ* gene construct; and Dr. Hsing-Jien Kung of this department for assistance with oncogene probes. Case Western Reserve University is a clinical cancer center sponsored by the National Cancer Institute (P30 CA43703).

References

Aaronson, S. A., and Wallace, R. P. (1970). Nonproducer clones of murine sarcoma virus-transformed Balb/c 3T3 cells. *Virology* **42,** 9–19.

Akeson, R., and Warren, S. L. (1986). PC12 adhesion and neurite formation on selected substrates are inhibited by some glycosaminoglycans and a fibronectin-derived tetrapeptide. *Exp. Cell Res.* **162,** 347–362.

Akiyama, S. K., and Yamada, K. M. (1986). Fibronectin. *Adv. Enzymol.* **59,** 1–57.

Auerbach, R., Lu, W. C., Pardon, E., Gumkowski, F., Kaminska, G., and Kaminski, M. (1987). Specificity of adhesion between murine tumor cells and capillary endothelium: An *in vitro* correlate of preferential metastasis *in vivo. Cancer Res.* **47,** 1492–1496.

Barletta, E., Bremer, E. G., and Culp, L. A. (1991). Neurite outgrowth in dorsal root neuronal hybrid clones modulated by ganglioside GM1 and disintegrins. *Exp. Cell Res.* **193,** 101–111.

Barletta, E., and Culp, L. A. (1990). Clonal segregation of multiple and overlapping matrix adhesive responses in dorsal root neuronal derivative cells. *J. Cell. Physiol.* **143,** 263–278.

Barsky, S. H., Rao, C. N., Williams, J. E., and Liotta, L. A. (1984). Laminin molecular domains which alter metastasis in a murine model. *J. Clin. Invest.* **74**, 843–848.

Barsky, S. H., and Gopalakrishna, R. (1987). Increased invasion and spontaneous metastasis of B16 melanoma with inhibition of the desmoplastic response in C57BL/6 mice. *Cancer Res.* **47**, 1663–1667.

Barsky, S. H., and Gopalakrishna, R. (1988). High metalloproteinase inhibitor content of human cirrhosis and its possible consequence for metastasis resistance. *J. Natl. Cancer Inst.* **80**, 102–108.

Beyth, R. J., and Culp, L. A. (1984). Complementary adhesive responses of human skin fibroblasts to the cell-binding domain of fibronectin and the heparan sulfate-binding protein, platelet factor-4. *Exp. Cell Res.* **155**, 537–548.

Bos, J. L., Fearon, E. R., Hamilton, S. R., Verlaan-de Vries, M., van Boom, J. H., van der Eb, A. J., and Vogelstein, B. (1987). Prevalence of *ras* gene mutations in human colorectal cancers. *Nature* **327**, 293–297.

Bradley, M. O., Kraynak, A. R., Storer, R. D., and Gibbs, J. B. (1986). Experimental metastasis in nude mice of NIH 3T3 cells containing various *ras* genes. *Proc. Natl. Acad. Sci. U.S.A.* **83**, 5277–5281.

Brennan, M. J., Oldberg, A., Hayman, E. G., and Ruoslahti, E. (1983). Effect of a proteoglycan produced by rat tumor cells on their adhesion to fibronectin-collagen substrata. *Cancer Res.* **43**, 4302–4307.

Bretti, S., Nert, P., Lozzi, L., Rustici, M., Comoglio, P., Giancotti, F., and Tarone, G. (1989). Inhibition of experimental metastasis of murine fibrosarcoma cells by oligopeptide analogues to the fibronectin cell-binding site. *Int. J. Cancer* **43**, 102–106.

Buck, C. A., and Horwitz, A. F. (1987). Cell surface receptors for extracellular matrix molecules. *Annu. Rev. Cell Biol.* **3**, 179–205.

Cassiman, J-J. (1989). The involvement of the cell matrix receptors, or VLA integrins, in the morphogenetic behavior of normal and malignant cells is gradually being uncovered. *Cancer Genet. Cytogenet.* **41**, 19–32.

Castellani, P., Siri, A., Rosellini, C., Infusini, E., Borsi, L., and Zardi, L. (1986). Transformed human cells release different fibronectin variants than do normal cells. *J. Cell Biol.* **103**, 1671–1677.

Cavanaugh, P. G., and Nicolson, G. L. (1989). Purification and some properties of a lung-derived growth factor that differentially stimulates the growth of tumor cells metastatic to the lung. *Cancer Res.* **49**, 3928–3933.

Cepko, C. L. (1989). Immortalization of neural cells via retrovirus-mediated oncogene transduction. *Annu. Rev. Neurosci.* **12**, 47–65.

Chen, J-M., and Chen, W-T. (1987). Fibronectin-degrading proteases from the membranes of transformed cells. *Cell* **48**, 193–203.

Chen, W.-T. (1981). Mechanism of retraction of the trailing edge during fibroblast movement. *J. Cell Biol.* **90**, 187–200.

Chen, W.-T. (1989). Proteolytic activity of specialized surface protrusions formed at rosette contact sites of transformed cells. *J. Exp. Zool.* **251**, 167–185.

Chen, W.-T., Olden, K., Bernard, B. A., and Chu, F. F. (1984). Expression of transformation-associated protease(s) that degrade fibronectin at cell contact sites. *J. Cell Biol.* **98**, 1546–1555.

Coombe, D. R., Parish, C. R., Ramshaw, I. A., and Snowden, J. M. (1987). Analysis of the inhibition of tumour metastasis by sulphated polysaccharides. *Int. J. Cancer* **39**, 82–88.

Culp, L. A. (1980). Behavioural variants of rat neuroblastoma cells. *Nature (London)* **286**, 77–79.

Culp, L. A., Ansbacher, R., and Domen, C. (1980). Adhesion sites of neural tumor cells: Biochemical composition. *Biochemistry* **19**, 5899–5907.

Culp, L. A., Laterra, J., Lark, M. W., Beyth, R. J., and Tobey, S. L. (1986). Heparan sulphate proteoglycan as mediator of some adhesive responses and cytoskeletal reorganization of cells on fibronectin matrices: Independent versus cooperative functions. *In* "Functions of the Proteogly-cans" (D. Evered and J. Whelan, eds.), CIBA Symposium 124, pp. 158–183. John Wiley & Sons, London.

Culp, L. A., Mugnai, G., Lewandowska, K., Vallen, E. A., Kosir, M. A., and Houmiel, K. L. (1989). Heparan sulfate proteoglycans of *ras*-transformed 3T3 or neuroblastoma cells. Differing functions in adhesion on fibronectin. *Ann. N.Y. Acad. Sci.* **556**, 194–216.

Dennis, J., Koch, K., and Beckner, D. (1989a). Inhibition of human HT29 colon carcinoma growth *in vitro* and *in vivo* by swainsonine and human interferon-α2. *J. Natl. Cancer Inst.* **81**, 1028–1033.

Dennis, J. W., Laferte, S., Yagel, S., and Breitman, M. L. (1989b). Asparagine-linked oligosac-charides associated with metastatic cancer. *Cancer Cell* **1**, 87–92.

Domen, C., and Culp, L. A. (1981). Adhesion sites of neural tumor cells: Morphogenesis of sub-stratum-attached material. *Exp. Cell Res.* **134**, 329–338.

Dufour, S., Duband, J.-L., Humphries, M. J., Obara, J., Yamada, K. M., and Thiery, J. P. (1988). Attachment, spreading, and locomotion of avian neural crest cells are mediated by multiple adhe-sion sites on fibronectin molecules. *EMBO J.* **7**, 2661–2671.

Egan, S. E., McClarty, G. A., Jarolim, L., Wright, J. A., Spiro, I., Hager, G., and Greenberg, A. H. (1987). Expression of H-*ras* correlates with metastatic potential: Evidence for direct regu-lation of the metastatic phenotype in 10T1/2 and NIH 3T3 cells. *Mol. Cell. Biol.* **7**, 830–837.

Eldor, A., Bar-Ner, M., Yahalom, J., Fuks, Z., and Vlodavsky, I. (1987). Role of heparanase in platelet and tumor cell interactions with the subendothelial extracellular matrix. *Semin. Thromb. Hemost.* **13**, 475–488.

Emanuel, B. S., Balaban, G., Boyd, J. P., Grossman, A., Negishi, M., Parmiter, S., and Glick, M. C. (1985). N-*myc* amplification in multiple homogeneously staining regions in two human neuroblastomas. *Proc. Natl. Acad. Sci. U.S.A.* **82**, 3736–3740.

Esko, J. D., Rostand, K. S., and Weinke, J. L. (1988). Tumor formation dependent on proteoglycan biosynthesis. *Science* **241**, 1092–1096.

Fairbairn, S., Gilbert, R., Ojakian, G., Schwimmer, R., and Quigley, J. P. (1985). The extracellular matrix of normal chicken embryo fibroblasts: Its effects on transformed chicken fibroblasts and its proteolytic degradation by the transformants. *J. Cell Biol.* **101**, 1790–1798.

Fearon, E. R., Hamilton, S. R., and Vogelstein, B. (1987). Clonal analysis of human colorectal tumors. *Science* **238**, 193–197.

Fidler, I. J. (1970). Metastasis: Quantitative analysis of distribution and fate of tumor emboli labeled with ¹²⁵I-5-iodo-2'-deoxyuridine. *J. Natl. Cancer Inst.* **45**, 773–782.

Fidler, I. J. (1973a). Selection of successive tumour lines for metastasis. *Nature (New Biol.)* **242**, 148–149.

Fidler, I. J. (1973b). The relationship of embolic homogeneity, number, size, and viability to the incidence of experimental metastasis. *Eur. J. Cancer* **9**, 223–227.

Fidler, I. J. (1978). Tumor heterogeneity and the biology of cancer invasion and metastasis. *Cancer Res.* **38**, 2651–2660.

Fidler, I. J. (1984). The Ernst W. Berrtner Memorial Award Lecture: The evolution of biological heterogeneity in metastatic neoplasms. In: "*Cancer invasion and metastasis: Biologic and thera-peutic aspects*" (G. L. Nicolson and L. Milas, eds.), pp. 5–26. Raven Press, New York.

Fidler, I. J., and Radinsky, R. (1990). Editorial: Genetic control of cancer metastasis. *J. Natl. Cancer Inst.* **82**, 166–168.

Flickinger, K. S., and Culp, L. A. (1990). Aging-related changes and topology of adhesion re-sponses sensitive to cycloheximide on collagen substrata by human dermal fibroblasts. *Exp. Cell Res.* **186**, 158–168.

Folkman, J., and Klagsburn, M. (1987). Angiogenic factors. *Science* **235**, 442–447.

Folkman, J., Watson, K., Ingber, D., and Hanahan, D. (1989). Induction of angiogenesis during the transition from hyperplasia to neoplasia. *Nature* **339**, 58–61.

Frost, P., Kerbel, R. S., Hunt, B., Man, S., and Pathak, S. (1987). Selection of metastatic variants with identifiable karyotypic changes from a nonmetastatic murine tumor after treatment with 2'-deoxy-5-azacytidine or hydroxyurea: Implications for the mechanisms of tumor progression. *Cancer Res.* **47**, 2690–2695.

Garbisa, S., Pozzatti, R., Muschel, R. J., Saffiotti, U., Ballin, M., Goldfarb, R. H., Khoury, G., and Liotta, L. A. (1987). Secretion of type IV collagenolytic protease and metastatic phenotype: Induction by transfection with c-Ha-*ras* but not c-Ha-*ras* plus Ad2-E1a. *Cancer Res.* **47**, 1523–1528.

Garcia-Pardo, A., and Ferreira, O. C. (1990). Adhesion of human T-lymphoid cells to fibronectin is mediated by two different fibronectin domains. *Immunology* **69**, 121–126.

Gasic, G. J. (1984). Role of plasma, platelets, and endothelial cells in tumor metastasis. *Cancer Metastasis Rev.* **3**, 99–116.

Gehlsen, K. R., Argraves, W. S., Pierschbacher, M. D., and Ruoslahti, E. (1988). Inhibition of *in vitro* tumor cell invasion by Arg-Gly-Asp–containing synthetic peptides. *J. Cell Biol.* **106**, 925–930.

Giancotti, F. G., and Ruoslahti, E. (1990). Elevated levels of the $\alpha_5\beta_1$ fibronectin receptor suppress the transformed phenotype of Chinese hamster ovary cells. *Cell* **60**, 849–859.

Goring, D. R., Rossant, J., Clapoff, S., Breitman, M. L., and Tsui, L.-C. (1987). *In situ* detection of β-galactosidase in lenses of transgenic mice with a γ-crystallin/*lacZ* gene. *Science* **235**, 456–458.

Graf, J., Iwamota, Y., Sasaki, M., Martin, G. R., Kleinman, H. K., Robey, F. A., and Yamada, Y. (1987). Identification of an amino acid sequence in laminin mediating cell attachment, chemotaxis, and receptor binding. *Cell* **48**, 989–996.

Grieg, R. G., Koestler, T. P., Trainer, D. L., Corwin, S. P., Miles, L., Kline, T., Sweet, R., Yokoyama, S., and Poste, G. (1985). Tumorigenic and metastatic properties of "normal" and *ras*-transfected NIH/3T3 cells. *Proc. Natl. Acad. Sci. U.S.A.* **82**, 3698–3701.

Grinnell, F. (1986). Focal adhesion sites and the removal of substratum-bound fibronectin. *J. Cell Biol.* **103**, 2697–2706.

Guan, J. L., and Hynes, R. O. (1990). Lymphoid cells recognize an alternatively spliced segment of fibronectin via the integrin receptor $\alpha_4\beta_1$. *Cell* **60**, 53–61.

Guan, J-L., Trevethick, J. E., and Hynes, R. O. (1990). Retroviral expression of alternatively spliced forms of rat fibronectin. *J. Cell Biol.* **110**, 833–847.

Hall, M. D., Flickinger, K. S., Cutolo, M., Zardi, L., and Culp, L. A. (1988). Adhesion of human dermal reticular fibroblasts on complementary fragments of fibronectin: Aging *in vivo* or *in vitro*. *Exp. Cell Res.* **179**, 115–136.

Hemler, M. (1990). VLA proteins in the integrin family: Structures, functions, and their roles on leukocytes. *Annu. Rev. Immunol.* **8**, 365–400.

Hendrix, M. J. C., Wood, W. R., Seftor, E. A., Lotan, D., Nakajima, M., Misiorowski, R. L., Seftor, R. E. B., Stetler-Stevenson, W. G., Bevacqua, S. J., Liotta, L. A., Sobel, M. E., Raz, A., and Lotan, R. (1990). Retinoic acid inhibition of human melanoma cell invasion through a reconstituted basement membrane and its relation to decreases in the expression of proteolytic enzymes and motility factor receptor. *Cancer Res.* **50**, 4121–4130.

Heppner, G. J., and Miller, B. E. (1983). Tumor heterogeneity: Biological implications and therapeutic consequences. *Cancer Metastasis Rev.* **2**, 5–23.

Hershberger, R. P., and Culp, L. A. (1990). Cell type–specific expression of alternatively spliced human fibronectin IIICS mRNAs. *Mol. Cell. Biol.* **10**, 662–671.

Hisano, G., and Hanna, N. (1982). A cytochemical procedure for the *in vivo* identification of melanoma micrometastasis. *Invasion Metastasis* **2**, 299–312.

Hu, F., Wang, R.-Y., and Hsu, T. C. (1987). Clonal origin of metastasis in B16 murine melanoma: A cytogenetic study. *J. Natl. Cancer Inst.* **78,** 155–163.

Humphries, M. J., Akiyama, S. K., Komoriya, A., Olden, K., and Yamada, K. M. (1986a). Identification of an alternatively spliced site in human plasma fibronectin that mediates cell type–specific adhesion. *J. Cell Biol.* **103,** 2637–2647.

Humphries, M. J., Olden, K., and Yamada, K. (1986b). A synthetic peptide from fibronectin inhibits experimental metastasis of murine melanoma cells. *Science* **233,** 467–470.

Humphries, M. J., Komoriya, A., Akiyama, S. K., Olden, K., and Yamada, K. M. (1987). Identification of two distinct regions of the type III connecting segment of human plasma fibronectin that promote cell type–specific adhesion. *J. Biol. Chem.* **262,** 6886–6892.

Humphries, M. J., Obara, M., Olden, K., and Yamada, K. M. (1989). Role of fibronectin in adhesion, migration, and metastasis. *Cancer Invest.* **7,** 373–393.

Humphries, M. J., Yasuda, Y., Olden, K., and Yamada, K. M. (1988). The cell interaction sites of fibronectin in tumour metastasis. *In* "Metastasis" (J. Whelan, ed.), pp. 75–93. Wiley, Chichester, U.K.

Hynes, R. O. (1985). Molecular biology of fibronectin. *Annu. Rev. Cell Biol.* **1,** 67–90.

Hynes, R. O. (1987). Integrins: A family of cell surface receptors. *Cell* **48,** 549–554.

Imashuku, S., Todo, S., Esumi, N., Hashida, T., Tsunamoto, K., and Nakajima, F. (1985). Tumor differentiation—application of prostaglandins in the treatment of neuroblastoma. *In* "Advances in Neuroblastoma Research" (A. E. Evans, G. J. D'Angio, and R. C. Seeger, eds.), Vol. 1, pp. 89–98. Alan R. Liss, New York.

Iozzo, R. V. (1988). Proteoglycans and neoplasia. *Cancer Metastasis Rev.* **7,** 39–50.

Ishikawa, M., Fernandez, B., and Kerbel, R. S. (1988). Highly pigmented human melanoma variant which metastasizes widely in nude mice, including to skin and brain. *Cancer Res.* **48,** 4897–4903.

Iskandar, S. S., Emancipator, S. N., and Pretlow II, T. G. (1989). Enzyme histochemistry of monocytes/macrophages: A study in a murine model of immune complex–mediated glomerulonephritis. *J. Histochem. Cytochem.* **37,** 25–29.

Itaya, T., Judde, J.-G., Hunt, B., and Frost, P. (1989). Genotypic and phenotypic evidence of clonal interactions in murine tumor cells. *J. Natl. Cancer Inst.* **81,** 664–668.

Iwamoto, Y., Robey, F. A., Graf, J., Sasaki, M., Kleinman, H. K., Yamada, Y., and Martin, G. R. (1987). YIGSR, a synthetic laminin pentapeptide, inhibits experimental metastasis formation. *Science* **238,** 1132–1134.

Izzard, C. S., and Lochner, L. R. (1980). Formation of cell-to-substrate contacts during fibroblast motility: An interference reflexion study. *J. Cell Sci.* **42,** 81–116.

Izzard, C. S., Radinsky, R., and Culp, L. A. (1986). Substratum contacts and cytoskeletal reorganization of Balb/c 3T3 cells on a cell-binding fragment and heparin-binding fragments of plasma fibronectin. *Exp. Cell Res.* **165,** 320–336.

Johnson, J. P., Lehmann, J. M., Stade, B. G., Rothbacher, U., Sers, C., and Riethmuller, G. (1989). Functional aspects of three molecules associated with metastasis development in human malignant melanoma. *Invasion Metastasis.* **9,** 338–350.

Juacaba, S. F., Horak, E., Price, J. E., and Tarin, D. (1989). Tumor cell dissemination patterns and metastasis of murine mammary carcinoma. *Cancer Res.* **49,** 570–575.

Juliano, R. L. (1987). Membrane receptors for extracellular matrix macromolecules: Relationship to cell adhesion and tumor metastasis. *Biochim. Biophys. Acta* **907,** 261–278.

Kabat, E. A., and Furth, J. (1941). A histochemical study of the distribution of alkaline phosphatase in various normal and neoplastic tissues. *Am. J. Pathol.* **17,** 303–343.

Kanemoto, T., Reich, R., Royce, L., Greatorex, D., Adler, S. H., Shiraishi, N., Martin, G. R., Yamada, Y., and Kleinman, H. K. (1990). Identification of an amino acid sequence from the laminin A chain that stimulates metastasis and collagenase IV production. *Proc. Natl. Acad. Sci. U.S.A.* **87,** 2279–2283.

Kawaguchi, T., and Nakamura, K. (1986). Analysis of the lodgement and extravasation of tumor cells in experimental models of hematogenous metastasis. *Cancer Metastasis Rev.* **5**, 77–94.

Keller, K. M., Brauer, P. R., and Keller, J. M. (1988). Isolation of Swiss 3T3 cell variants with altered heparan sulfate. *Exp. Cell Res.* **179**, 137–158.

Kennel, S. J., Lankford, T. K., Ullrich, R. L., and Jamasbi, R. J. (1988). Enhancement of lung tumor colony formation by treatment of mice with monoclonal antibodies to pulmonary capillary endothelial cells. *Cancer Res.* **48**, 4964–4968.

Kerbel, R. S., Waghorne, C., Korczak, B., Lagarde, A., and Breitman, M. L. (1988). Clonal dominance of primary tumours by metastatic cells: Genetic analysis and biological implications. *Cancer Surv.* **7**, 597–629.

Kerbel, R. S. (1990). Growth dominance of the metastatic cancer cell: Cellular and molecular aspects. *Adv. Cancer Res.* **55**, 87–132.

Khokha, R., and Denhardt, D. T. (1989). Matrix metalloproteinases and tissue inhibitor of metalloproteinases: A review of their role in tumorigenesis and tissue invasion. *Invasion Metastasis* **9**, 391–405.

Kijima-Suda, I., Miyazawa, T., Itoh, M., Toyoshima, S., and Osawa, T. (1988). Possible mechanism of inhibition of experimental pulmonary metastasis of mouse colon adenocarcinoma 26 sublines by a sialic acid:nucleoside conjugate. *Cancer Res.* **48**, 3728–3732.

Knox, P., and Wells, P. (1979). Cell adhesion and proteoglycans. I. The effect of exogenous proteoglycans on the attachment of chick embryo fibroblasts to tissue culture plastic and collagen. *J. Cell Sci.* **40**, 77–88.

Kohl, N. E., Kanda, N., Schreck, R. R., Bruns, G., Latt, S. A., Gilbert, F., and Alt, F. W. (1983). Transposition and amplification of oncogene-related sequences in human neuroblastomas. *Cell* **35**, 359–367.

Kramer, R. H., Vogel, K. C., and Nicolson, G. (1982). Solubilization and degradation of subendothelial matrix glycoproteins and proteoglycans by metastatic tumor cells. *J. Biol. Chem.* **257**, 2678–2686.

Lark, M. W., Laterra, J., and Culp, L. A. (1985). Close and focal contact adhesions of fibroblasts to a fibronectin-containing matrix. *Fed. Proc.* **44**, 394–403.

Laterra, J., Silbert, J. E., and Culp, L. A. (1983a). Cell-surface heparan sulfate mediates some adhesive responses to glycosaminoglycan-binding matrices, including fibronectin. *J. Cell Biol.* **96**, 112–123.

Laterra, J., Norton, E. K., Izzard, C. S., and Culp, L. A. (1983b). Contact formation by fibroblasts adhering to heparan sulfate–binding substrata (fibronectin or platelet factor 4). *Exp. Cell Res.* **146**, 15–27.

Lewandowska, K., Choi, H. U., Rosenberg, L. C., Zardi, L., and Culp, L. A. (1987). Fibronectin-mediated adhesion of fibroblasts: Inhibition by dermatan sulfate proteoglycan and evidence for a cryptic glycosaminoglycan-binding domain. *J. Cell Biol.* **105**, 1443–1454.

Lewandowska, K., Balachander, N., Sukenik, C. N., and Culp, L. A. (1989). Modulation of fibronectin adhesive functions for fibroblasts and neural cells by chemically derivatized substrata. *J. Cell. Physiol.* **141**, 334–345.

Lewandowska, K., Balza, E., Zardi, L., and Culp, L. A. (1990). Requirement for two different cell-binding domains in fibronectin for neurite extension of neuronal derivative cells. *J. Cell Sci.* **95**, 75–83.

Lin, W.-c., Pretlow, T. P., Pretlow, T. G., and Culp, L. A. (1990a). Bacterial *lacZ* gene as a highly sensitive marker to detect micrometastasis formation during tumor progression. *Cancer Res.* **50**, 2808–2817.

Lin, W.-c., Pretlow, T. P., Pretlow, T. G., and Culp, L. A. (1990b). Development of micrometastases: Earliest events detected with bacterial *lacZ*-tagged tumor cells. *J. Natl. Cancer Inst.* **82**, 1497–1503.

Liotta, L. A., Rao, C. N., and Wewer, U. M. (1986). Biochemical interactions of tumor cells with the basement membrane. *Annu. Rev. Biochem.* **55,** 1037–1057.

Maresh, G. A., Chernoff, E. A. G., and Culp, L. A. (1984). Heparan sulfate proteoglycans of human neuroblastoma cells. Affinity fractionation on columns of platelet factor-4. *Arch. Biochem. Biophys.* **233,** 428–437.

Matyas, G. R., Evers, D. C., Radinsky, R., and Morre, D. J. (1986). Fibronectin binding to gangliosides and rat liver plasma membranes. *Exp. Cell Res.* **162,** 296–318.

McCarthy, J. B., Basara, M. L., Palm, S. L., Sas, D. F., and Furcht, L. T. (1985). The role of adhesion proteins—laminin and fibronectin—in the movement of malignant and metastatic cells. *Cancer Metastasis Rev.* **4,** 125–152.

McCarthy, J. B., Hagen, S. T., and Furcht, L. T. (1986). Human fibronectin contains distinct adhesion- and motility-promoting domains for metastatic melanoma cells. *J. Cell Biol.* **102,** 179–188.

McCarthy, J. B., Skubitz, A. P. N., Palm, S. L., and Furcht, L. T. (1988). Metastasis inhibition of different tumor types by purified laminin fragments and a heparin-binding fragment of fibronectin. *J. Natl. Cancer Inst.* **80,** 108–116.

McCulloch, P., and George, W. D. (1989). Warfarin inhibits metastasis of Mtln3 rat mammary carcinoma without affecting primary tumour growth. *Br. J. Cancer* **59,** 179–183.

McDonald, J. A. (1988). Extracellular matrix assembly. *Annu. Rev. Cell Biol.* **4,** 183–207.

McGinnis, M. C., Bradley, E. L., Pretlow, T. P., Ortiz-Reyes, R., Bowden, C. J., Stellato, T. A., and Pretlow, T. G. (1989). Correlation of stromal cells by morphometric analysis with metastatic behavior of human colonic carcinoma. *Cancer Res.* **49,** 5989–5993.

McMorrow, L. E., Wolman, S. R., Bornstein, S., and Talmadge, J. E. (1988). Irradiation-induced marker chromosomes in a metastasizing murine tumor. *Cancer Res.* **48,** 999–1003.

Miller, B. E., Miller, F. R., Wilburn, D., and Heppner, G. H. (1988). Dominance of a tumor subpopulation line in mixed heterogeneous mouse mammary tumors. *Cancer Res.* **48,** 5747–5753.

Mould, A. P., Wheldon, L. A., Komoriya, A., Wayner, E. A., Yamada, K. M., and Humphries, M. J. (1990). Affinity chromatography isolation of the melanoma adhesion receptor for the IIICS region of fibronectin and its identification as the integrin $\alpha_4\beta_1$. *J. Biol. Chem.* **265,** 4020–4024.

Mugnai, G., and Culp, L. A. (1987). Cooperativity of ganglioside-dependent with protein-dependent substratum adhesion and neurite extension of human neuroblastoma cells. *Exp. Cell Res.* **169,** 328–344.

Mugnai, G., Lewandowska, K., Carnemolla, B., Zardi, L., and Culp, L. A. (1988a). Modulation of matrix adhesive responses of human neuroblastoma cells by neighboring sequences in the fibronectins. *J. Cell Biol.* **106,** 931–943.

Mugnai, G., Lewandowska, K., Choi, H. U., Rosenberg, L. C., and Culp, L. A. (1988b). Ganglioside-dependent adhesion events of human neuroblastoma cells regulated by the RGDS-dependent fibronectin receptor and proteoglycans. *Exp. Cell Res.* **175,** 229–247.

Mugnai, G., Lewandowska, K., and Culp, L. A. (1988c). Multiple and alternative adhesive responses on defined substrata of an immortalized dorsal root neuron hybrid cell line. *Eur. J. Cell Biol.* **46,** 352–361.

Naito, S., Giavazzi, R., and Fidler, I. J. (1987). Correlation between the *in vitro* interaction of tumor cells with an organ environment and metastatic behavior *in vivo. Invasion Metastasis* **7,** 16–29.

Nakajima, M., Irimura, T., DiFerrante, N., and Nicolson, G. L. (1984). Metastatic melanoma cell heparanase: Characterization of heparan sulfate degradation fragments produced by B16 melanoma endoglucuronidase. *J. Biol. Chem.* **259,** 2283–2290.

Nakajima, M., Lotan, D., Baig, M. M., Carralero, R. M., Wood, W. R., Hendrix, M. J. C., and Lotan, R. (1989). Inhibition by retinoic acid of type IV collagenolysis and invasion through reconstituted basement membrane by metastatic rat mammary adenocarcinoma cells. *Cancer Res.* **49,** 1698–1706.

Newton, S. A., White, S. L., Humphries, M. J., and Olden, K. (1989). Swainsonine inhibition of spontaneous metastasis. *J. Natl. Cancer Inst.* **81,** 1024–1028.

Nicolson, G. L. (1988). Organ specificity of tumor metastasis: Role of preferential adhesion, invasion, and growth of malignant cells at specific secondary sites. *Cancer Metastasis Rev.* **7,** 143–188.

Obara, M., Kang, M. S., and Yamada, K. M. (1988). Site-directed mutagenesis of the cell-binding domain of human fibronectin: Separable, synergistic sites mediate adhesive function. *Cell* **53,** 649–657.

Packard, B. S. (1987). Identification of a synthetic nonapeptide sequence that inhibits motility in culture of a melanoma subclone that possesses a high metastatic potential. *Proc. Natl. Acad. Sci. U.S.A.* **84,** 9015–9019.

Partin, A. W., Isaacs, J. T., Treiger, B., and Coffey, D. S. (1988). Early cell motility changes associated with an increase in metastatic ability in rat prostatic cancer cells transfected with the v-Harvey-*ras* oncogene. *Cancer Res.* **48,** 6050–6053.

Pauli, B. U., and Lee, C.-L. (1988). Organ preference of metastasis: The role of organ-specifically modulated endothelial cells. *Lab. Invest.* **58,** 379–387.

Perris, R., and Johansson, S. (1987). Amphibian neural crest cell migration on purified extracellular matrix components: A chondroitin sulfate proteoglycan inhibits locomotion on fibronectin substrates. *J. Cell Biol.* **105,** 2511–2521.

Pierschbacher, M. D., and Ruoslahti, E. (1984). Cell attachment activity of fibronectin can be duplicated by small synthetic fragments of the molecule. *Nature (London)* **309,** 30–33.

Pierschbacher, M. D., Hayman, E. G., and Ruoslahti, E. (1981). Location of the cell attachment site in fibronectin with monoclonal antibodies and proteolytic fragments of the molecule. *Cell* **26,** 259–267.

Pignatelli, M., and Bodmer, W. F. (1988). Genetics and biochemistry of collagen binding–triggered glandular differentiation in a human colon carcinoma cell line. *Proc. Natl. Acad. Sci. U.S.A.* **85,** 5561–5565.

Plantefar, L. C., and Hynes, R. O. (1989). Changes in integrin receptors on oncogenically transformed cells. *Cell* **56,** 281–290.

Platika, D., Boulos, M. H., Baizer, L., and Fishman, M. C. (1985). Neuronal traits of clonal cell lines derived by fusion of dorsal root ganglia neurons with neuroblastoma cells. *Proc. Natl. Acad. Sci. U.S.A.* **82,** 3499–3503.

Poste, G., and Fidler, I. J. (1980). The pathogenesis of cancer metastasis. *Nature (London)* **283,** 139–146.

Price, J. E., Bell, C., and Frost, P. (1990). The use of a genotypic marker to demonstrate clonal dominance during the growth and metastasis of a human breast carcinoma in nude mice. *Int. J. Cancer* **45,** 968–971.

Radinsky, R. and Culp, L. A. (1991). Clonal dominance of select subsets of viral kirsten *ras*⁺-transformed 3T3 cells during tumor progression. *Int. J. Cancer* **48,** 148–159.

Radinsky, R., Kraemer, P. M., Raines, M. A., Kung, H.-J., and Culp, L. A. (1987). Amplification and rearrangement of the Kirsten *ras* oncogene in virus-transformed Balb/c 3T3 cells during malignant tumor progression. *Proc. Natl. Acad. Sci. U.S.A.* **84,** 5143–5147.

Radinsky, R., Kraemer, P. M., Proffitt, M. R., and Culp, L. A. (1988). Clonal diversity of the Kirsten-*ras* oncogene during tumor progression in athymic nude mice: Mechanisms of amplification and rearrangement. *Cancer Res.* **48,** 4941–4953.

Radinsky, R., Flickinger, K. S., Kosir, M. A., Zardi, L., and Culp, L. A. (1990). Adhesion of Kirsten-*ras*⁺ tumor-progressing and Kirsten-*ras*⁻ revertant 3T3 cells on fibronectin proteolytic fragments. *Cancer Res.* **50,** 4388–4400.

Reich, R., Stratford, B., Klein, K., Martin, G. R., Mueller, R. A., and Fuller, G. C. (1988). Inhibitors of collagenase IV and cell adhesion reduce the invasive activity of malignant tumour cells. *In* "Metastasis" (J. Whelan, ed.), pp. 193–210. Wiley, Chichester, U.K.

Reynolds, C. P., Tomayko, M. M., Donner, L., Helson, L., Seeger, R. C., Triche, T. J., and Brodeur, G. M. (1988). Biological classification of cell lines derived from human extra-cranial neural tumors. *In* "Advances in Neuroblastoma Research" (A. E. Evans, G. J. D'Angio, A. G. Knudson, and R. C. Seeger, eds.), Vol. 2, pp. 291–307. Alan R. Liss, New York.

Rich, A. M., Pearlstein, E., Weissmann, G., and Hoffstein, S. T. (1981). Cartilage proteoglycans inhibit fibronectin-mediated adhesion. *Nature (London)* **293**, 224–226.

Robertson, N. P., Starkey, J. R., Hamner, S., and Meadows, G. G. (1989). Tumor cell invasion of three-dimensional matrices of defined composition: Evidence for a specific role for heparan sulfate in rodent cell lines. *Cancer Res.* **49**, 1816–1823.

Rollins, B. J., Cathcart, M. K., and Culp, L. A. (1982). Fibronectin:proteoglycan binding as the molecular basis for adhesion of fibroblasts to extracellular matrices. *In* "The Glycoconjugates" (M. I. Horowitz, ed.), pp. 289–329. Academic Press, New York.

Roos, E., and Van de Pavet, I. V. (1987). Inhibition of lymphoma invasion and liver metastasis formation by pertussis toxin. *Cancer Res.* **47**, 5439–5444.

Rosen, J. J., and Culp, L. A. (1977). Morphology and cellular origins of substrate-attached material from mouse fibroblasts. *Exp. Cell Res.* **107**, 139–149.

Ruoslahti, E. (1988a). Fibronectin and its receptors. *Annu. Rev. Biochem.* **57**, 375–413.

Ruoslahti, E. (1988b). Structure and biology of proteoglycans. *Annu. Rev. Cell Biol.* **4**, 229–255.

Ryan, U. S. (1988). "Endothelial Cells," Vol. II. CRC Press, Boca Raton, Florida.

Saiki, I., Iia, J., Murata, J., Ogawa, R., Nishi, N., Sugimura, K., Tokura, S., and Azuma, I. (1989). Inhibition of the metastasis of murine malignant melanoma by synthetic polymeric peptides containing core sequences of cell-adhesive molecules. *Cancer Res.* **49**, 3815–3822.

Sanes, J. R., Rubenstein, J. L. R., and Nicolas, J.-F. (1986). Use of a recombinant retrovirus to study postimplantation cell lineage in mouse embryos. *EMBO J.* **5**, 3133–3142.

Sargent, N. S. E., Price, J. E., Darling, D. L., Flynn, M. P., and Tarin, D. (1987). Effects of altering surface glycoprotein composition on metastatic colonization potential of murine mammary tumour cells. *Br. J. Cancer* **55**, 21–28.

Saunders, S., and Bernfield, M. (1988). Cell-surface proteoglycan binds mouse mammary epithelial cells to fibronectin and behaves as a receptor for interstitial matrix. *J. Cell Biol.* **106**, 423–430.

Schlimok, G., Funke, I., Holzmann, B., Gottlinger, G., Schmidt, G., Hauser, H., Swierkot, S., Warnecke, H. H., Schneider, B., Koprowski, H., and Riethmuller, G. (1987). Micrometastatic cancer cells in bone marrow: *In vitro* detection with anticytokeratin and *in vivo* labeling with anti–17-1A monoclonal antibodies. *Proc. Natl. Acad. Sci. U.S.A.* **84**, 8672–8676.

Schmidt, G., Robenek, H., Harrach, B., Glossl, J., Nolte, V., Hormann, H., Richter, H., and Kresse, H. (1987). Interaction of small dermatan sulfate proteoglycan from fibroblasts with fibronectin. *J. Cell Biol.* **104**, 1683–1691.

Schultz, R. M., Silberman, S., Persky, B., Bajkowski, A. S., and Carmichael, D. F. (1988). Inhibition by human recombinant tissue inhibitor of metalloproteinases of human amnion invasion and lung colonization by murine B16-F10. *Cancer Res.* **48**, 5539–5545.

Schwab, M., Alitalo, K., Klempnauer, K.-H., Varmus, H. E., Bishop, J. M., Gilbert, F., Brodeur, G., Goldstein, M., and Trent, J. (1983). Amplified DNA with limited homology to *myc* cellular oncogene is shared by human neuroblastoma tumour. *Nature (London)* **305**, 245–247.

Schwarzbauer, J. E., Mulligan, R. C., and Hynes, R. O. (1987). Efficient and stable expression of recombinant fibronectin polypeptides. *Proc. Natl. Acad. Sci. U.S.A.* **84**, 754–758.

Sher, B. T., Bargatze, R., Holzmann, B., Gallatin, W. M., Matthews, D., Wu, N., Picker, L., Butcher, E. C., and Weissman, I. L. (1988). Homing receptors and metastasis. *Adv. Cancer Res.* **51**, 361–390.

Sheth, N. A., Doctor, V. M., Sampat, M. B., Grade, S. V., Arbatti, N. J., and Sheth, A. R. (1987). Inhibin-like material—an immunohistologic marker for prostatic origin of metastases. *Cancer Lett.* **36**, 93–98.

Skubitz, A. P. N., McCarthy, J. B., Charonis, A. S., and Furcht, L. T. (1988). Novel synthetic heparin-binding peptides of laminin and fibronectin which promote the adhesion of melanoma cells. *Invasion Metastasis* **9**, 89–101.

Springer, T. A., Thompson, W. S., Miller, L. J., Schmalsteig, F. C., and Anderson, D. C. (1984). Inherited deficiency of the Mac-1, LFA-1, p150,95 glycoprotein family and its molecular basis. *J. Exp. Med.* **160**, 1901–1918.

Staroselsky, A., Pathak, S., and Fidler, I. J. (1990). Changes in clonal composition during *in vivo* growth of mixed subpopulations derived from the murine k-1735 melanoma. *Anticancer Res.* **10**, 291–296.

Talmadge, C., Tanio, Y., Meeker, A., Talmadge, J., and Zbar, B. (1987). Tumor cells transfected with the neomycin resistance gene (neo) contain unique genetic markers useful for identification of tumor recurrence and metastasis. *Invasion Metastasis* **7**, 197–207.

Tarin, D., and Price, J. E. (1981). Influence of microenvironment and vascular anatomy on "metastatic" colonization potential of mammary tumors. *Cancer Res.* **41**, 3604–3609.

Tarin, D., Price, J. E., Kettlewell, M. G. W., Souter, R. G., Vass, A. C. R., and Crossley, B. (1984). Mechanisms of human tumor metastasis studied in patients with peritoneovenous shunts. *Cancer Res.* **44**, 3584–3592.

Tarone, G., Cirillo, D., Giancotti, F. G., Comoglio, P. M., and Marchisio, P. C. (1985). Rous sarcoma virus–transformed fibroblasts adhere primarily at discrete protrusions on the ventral membrane called podosomes. *Exp. Cell Res.* **159**, 141–157.

Terranova, V. P., Liotta, L. A., Russo, R. G., and Martin, G. R. (1982). Role of laminin in the attachment and metastasis of murine tumor cells. *Cancer Res.* **42**, 2265–2269.

Terranova, V. P., Williams, J. E., Liotta, L. A., and Martin, G. R. (1984). Modulation of the metastatic activity of melanoma cells by laminin and fibronectin. *Science* **226**, 982–984.

Thompson, L. K., Horowitz, P. M., Bentley, K. L., Thomas, D. D., Alderete, J. F., and Klebe, R. J. (1986). Localization of the ganglioside-binding site of fibronectin. *J. Biol. Chem.* **261**, 5209–5214.

Thorgeirsson, U. P., Turpeenniemi-Hujanen, T., Williams, J. E., Westin, E. H., Heilman, C. A., Talmadge, J. E., and Liotta, L. A. (1985). NIH/3T3 cells transfected with human tumor DNA containing activated *ras* oncogenes express the metastatic phenotype in nude mice. *Mol. Cell. Biol.* **5**, 259–262.

Tobey, S. L., McClelland, K. J., and Culp, L. A. (1985). Neurite extension by neuroblastoma cells on substratum-bound fibronectin's cell-binding fragment but not on the heparan sulfate–binding protein, platelet factor-4. *Exp. Cell Res.* **158**, 395–412.

Tomaselli, K. J., Damsky, C. H., and Reichardt, L. F. (1987). Interactions of a neuronal cell line (PC12) with laminin, collagen IV, and fibronectin: Identification of integrin-related glycoproteins involved in attachment and process outgrowth. *J. Cell Biol.* **105**, 2347–2358.

Tsokos, M., Ross, R. A., and Triche, T. J. (1985). Neuronal, Schwannian and melanocytic differentiation of human neuroblastoma cells *in vitro*. *In* "Advances in Neuroblastoma Research" (A. E. Evans, G. J. D'Angio, and R. C. Seeger, eds.), Vol. 1, pp. 55–68. Alan R. Liss, New York.

Turpeenniemi-Hujanen, T., Thorgeirsson, U. P., Rao, C. N., and Liotta, L. A. (1986). Laminin increases the release of type IV collagenase from malignant cells. *J. Biol. Chem.* **261**, 1883–1889.

Ugen, K. E., Mahalingam, M., Klein, P. A., and Kao, K.-J. (1988). Inhibition of tumor cell-induced platelet aggregation and experimental tumor metastasis by the synthetic Gly-Arg-Gly-Asp-Ser peptide. *J. Natl. Cancer Inst.* **80**, 1461–1466.

Vallen, E. A., Eldridge, K. A., and Culp, L. A. (1988). Heparan sulfate proteoglycans in the substratum adhesion sites of human neuroblastoma cells: Modulation of affinity binding to fibronectin. *J. Cell. Physiol.* **135**, 200–212.

Vogelstein, B., Fearon, E. R., Kern, S. E., Hamilton, S. R., Preisinger, A. C., Nakamura, Y., and White, R. (1989). Allelotype of colorectal carcinomas. *Science* **244**, 207–211.

Wagner, D. D., Ivatt, R., Destree, A. T., and Hynes, R. O. (1981). Similarities and differences between the fibronectins of normal and transformed hamster cells. *J. Biol. Chem.* **256**, 11708–11715.

Waite, K. A., Mugnai, G., and Culp, L. A. (1987). A second cell-binding domain on fibronectin (RGDS-independent) for neurite extension of human neuroblastoma cells. *Exp. Cell Res.* **169**, 311–327.

Wayner, E. A., Garcia-Pardo, A. Humphries, M. J., McDonald, J. A., and Carter, W. G. (1989). Identification and characterization of the T lymphocyte adhesion receptor for an alternative cell attachment domain (CS-1) in plasma fibronectin. *J. Cell Biol.* **109**, 1321–1330.

Weiss, L. (1990). Metastatic inefficiency. *Adv. Cancer Res.* **54**, 159–211.

Weiss, L., Orr, F. W., and Honn, K. V. (1989). Interactions between cancer cells and the microvasculature: A rate-regulator for metastasis. *Clin. Exp. Metastasis* **7**, 127–167.

Welch, D. R., Schissel, D. J., Howrey, R. P., and Aeed, P. A. (1989). Tumor-elicited polymorphonuclear cells, in contrast to "normal" circulating polymorphonuclear cells, stimulate invasive and metastatic potentials of rat mammary adenocarcinoma cells. *Proc. Natl. Acad. Sci. U.S.A.* **86**, 5859–5863.

Wells, R. S., Campbell, E. W., Swartzendruber, K. E., Holland, L. M., and Kraemer, P. M. (1982). Role of anchorage in the expression of tumorigenicity of untransformed mouse cell lines. *J. Natl. Cancer Inst.* **69**, 415–423.

Yamada, K. M., and Kennedy, D. W. (1984). Dualistic nature of adhesive protein function: Fibronectin and its biologically active peptide fragments can autoinhibit fibronectin function. *J. Cell Biol.* **99**, 29–36.

Yamada, K. M., Kennedy, G. R., Grotendorst, G. R., and Momoi, T. (1981). Glycolipids: Receptors for fibronectin? *J. Cell. Physiol.* **109**, 343–351.

Yamagata, M., Suzuki, S., Akiyama, S. K., Yamada, K. M., and Kimata, K. (1989). Regulation of cell-substrate adhesion by proteoglycans immobilized on extracellular substrates. *J. Biol. Chem.* **264**, 8012–8018.

Zardi, l., Carnemolla, B., Siri, A., Petersen, T. E., Paolella, G., Sebastio, G., and Baralle, F. E. (1987). Transformed human cells produce a new fibronectin isoform by preferential alternative splicing of a previously unobserved exon. *EMBO J.* **6**, 2337–2342.

Zeidman, I. (1957). Metastasis: A review of recent advances. *Cancer Res.* **17**, 157–162.

Chapter 5

Structural and Functional Characteristics of Human Melanoma

ULLRICH GRAEVEN,* DOROTHEA BECKER,[†,1] AND MEENHARD HERLYN*

*The Wistar Institute of Anatomy and Biology, Philadelphia, Pennsylvania, 19104 and
†Department of Tumor Biology, The University of Texas M. D. Anderson Cancer Center, Houston, Texas 77030*

I. Introduction

Proliferation and differentiation of normal cells is the result of a complex and as yet only partly understood, balance between stimulatory and inhibitory factors. Tumor cell proliferation may represent the escape of a single cell which, in a stepwise fashion, gains emancipation and independence from regulatory control(s) and thus interferes with the overall balance of the host organism. Foulds has defined this process, composed of several qualitatively different stages leading to a final phenotypic endpoint, as tumor progression (Foulds, 1954). Support for the theory of stepwise tumor progression comes from histologic, cytogenetic, and experimental *in vitro* studies showing that spontaneously occurring human cancer represents a multistep process based on the clonal evolution of cells with increasingly selective growth advantage (Nowell, 1976; Klein *et al.*, 1985).

[1]Present address: Department of Medicine, Division of Medical Oncology, University of Pittsburgh, Pittsburgh, Pennsylvania 15261

BIOCHEMICAL AND MOLECULAR ASPECTS
OF SELECTED CANCERS, VOL. 1

The human melanocytic system appears to be ideal for the study of tumor progression in a naturally occurring human malignancy. In contrast to other malignancies, cells from normal tissue, benign and/or precursor as well as malignant lesions, are easily obtained, and recent progress in tissue culture techniques allows cultivation of these cells under defined conditions. Consequently, human malignant melanoma represents one of the best clinically and experimentally studied human solid-tumor systems. Melanocytes from different stages of tumor progression have been extensively characterized with regard to their morphology, response to and production of growth factors, as well as their antigen expression. With increasing knowledge of the biochemical and molecular structures of many of these antigens, monoclonal antibodies (MAbs) against tumor-associated antigens have become important tools to delineate structural and/or functional changes during tumor progression.

Following a brief discussion of the similarities between clinical–pathological defined stages of melanoma progression and tumor progression of normal melanocytes and melanoma cells, as analyzed *in vitro,* we will focus on defined molecular and biochemical changes during melanoma progression and their possible functional implications.

II. Tumor Progression in the Human Melanocytic System

A. Tumor Progression *In Vivo*

Normal mature melanocytes are neuroectoderm-derived cells, which are interspersed between basal keratinocytes in the epidermis and are responsible for pigment (melanin) production. It has been proposed that melanocyte maturation and differentiation involves several stages, including melanoblasts and early and intermediate premelanocytes, with increasing competence for melanin synthesis. Mature melanocytes are the endpoint of differentiation (Bennett *et al.,* 1985; Valyi-Nagy *et al.,* 1990). Along this maturation pathway, each cell may transform to either nevus or melanoma cells.

Extensive histopathological and clinical studies of spontaneously occurring melanomas have allowed the delineation of five defined lesional stages of tumor progression in the melanocytic system (Clark *et al.,* 1984, 1986) (Table I). The earliest proliferative melanocytic lesion, the common acquired nevus, shows no architectural or cytological atypia and is composed of nests of otherwise mature melanocytes. Subsequent steps in tumor progression exhibit increasing levels of cytological and architectural atypias and gain the capacity to invade surrounding tissue. These steps include the dysplastic nevus showing aberrant differentiation, followed by the radial growth phase (RGP) primary melanoma, which has acquired growth autonomy but not metastatic potential, the vertical growth phase

TABLE I
TUMOR PROGRESSION IN THE HUMAN MELANOCYTIC SYSTEM

Step	Melanocytic lesions
1	Common acquired and congenital nevus
2	Dysplastic nevus
3	Radial growth phase (RGP) of primary melanoma
4	Vertical growth phase (VGP) of primary melanoma
5	Metastatic melanoma

(VGP) primary melanoma with competence for metastasis, and the final stage, metastatic melanoma.

B. *IN VITRO* TUMOR PROGRESSION IN HUMAN MELANOCYTES

The development of improved tissue-culture techniques for normal melanocytes and for cells derived from melanocytic lesions has allowed the cultivation and *in vitro* characterization of melanocytes from each step of the above outlined stages of tumor progression. These cells have become a most valuable tool in understanding mechanisms underlying the clinically and pathologically observed tumor progression.

1. *Normal Melanocytes*

Normal melanocytes in culture have a finite life span. For *in vitro* growth, melanocytes require a set of growth factors including insulin and basic fibroblast growth factor (bFGF); inducers of cyclic adenosine monophosphate (cAMP), such as α-melanocyte stimulating hormone (α-MSH); and protein kinase C activators, such as 12-0-tetradecanoylphorbol-13-acetate (TPA) (Eisinger and Marko, 1982; Gilchrest *et al.*, 1984; Halaban *et al.*, 1987; Herlyn *et al.*, 1987a, 1988) (Table II). Under these conditions, melanocytes are rich in melanosomes and have a high tyrosinase activity, both of which are essential for melanin production and serve as markers for melanocyte maturation (Mancianti and Herlyn, 1989). In contrast to melanocytes *in situ*, cultured melanocytes express several *melanoma-associated* antigens, most likely reflecting their proliferative state as opposed to their nonmitotic state *in situ*. Karyotypic analysis revealed no chromosomal abnormalities in melanocytes during *in vitro* culture (Balaban *et al.*, 1986). Melanocytes do not grow anchorage independently, as determined by colony formation in soft agar, and do not develop tumors in nude mice (Herlyn *et al.*, 1987a). Taken together, the growth characteristics of cultured normal

TABLE II
GROWTH REQUIREMENTS FOR MELANOCYTES *in vitro*

	Growth factor or mitogen			
Melanocyte	α-MSH	bFGF	IGF-I/ Insulin	TPA
Normal melanocytes	$+ + +$[a]	$+ + +$	$+ + +$	$+ + +$
Nevus cells	$+ + +$	$+ +$[b]	$+ + +$	$+ +$
Primary melanoma cells	O[c]	O	$+ +$	$\varnothing$[d]
Metastatic melanoma cells	O	O	O	$\varnothing$

[a] Essential.
[b] Mitogenic, but not required in all cultures.
[c] Not mitogenic.
[d] Inhibitory.

melanocytes are in good agreement with their normal and nontransformed phenotype *in situ*.

2. *Congenital and Common Acquired Nevus Cells*

Nevus cells, like normal melanocytes, show a finite life span *in vitro*, but are less dependent on growth promoters like TPA and bFGF (Table II). Although nevus cells have some capacity for anchorage-independent growth in soft agar, they are nontumorigenic in nude mice and demonstrate no sign of spontaneous malignant transformation during *in vitro* cultivation (Mancianti and Herlyn, 1989; Mancianti *et al.*, 1988, 1990). Common acquired and congenital nevi do not show chromosomal aberrations (Balaban *et al.*, 1984, 1986); however, the presence of abnormal clones in a small portion of examined compound nevi has been reported (Richmond *et al.*, 1986). These results indicate that nevus cells isolated from common acquired and congenital nevi, when grown *in vitro*, have characteristics of both normal and malignant cells.

3. *Dysplastic Nevus Cells*

Owing to difficulties in their isolation and the fact that dysplastic nevus cells often represent only a fraction of all the cells of a given nevus, little information is available on pure dysplastic nevus cell cultures. Therefore, dysplastic nevus cells studied to date resemble either common acquired nevus cells or early primary melanoma cells (Herlyn *et al.*, 1987a).

4. Radial Growth Phase Primary Melanoma Cells

Like dysplastic nevus cells, RGP primary melanoma cells are difficult to isolate and to maintain in culture. Most of the established RGP primary melanoma cell lines display a morphology similar to that of nevus cell lines, and share their prolonged but finite life span and inability to form tumors in nude mice (Herlyn et al., 1985a). Some cell lines, however, exhibit characteristics similar to VGP primary malignant melanoma. It has yet to be determined whether these cells represent unique RGP melanoma cells or a subpopulation within the tumor specimen that has already acquired true VGP characteristics and therefore has a growth advantage.

5. Vertical Growth Phase Primary Melanoma Cells

Cells from VGP primary melanomas have been successfully cultured as permanent cell lines in about 60% of the examined specimens (Kath et al., 1989). These cell lines have a remarkably reduced requirement for growth factors as compared to normal melanocytes, and in contrast to the latter, are inhibited by protein kinase C (PKC) activators (Herlyn et al., 1990). Although VGP cells are still responsive to the addition of growth factors to the medium, they are capable of growing under serum-free conditions (Rodeck et al., 1987b) (Table II). Along with their invasive and metastatic capacity in situ, cells from VGP primary melanoma grow in soft agar with relative high efficiency, and form tumors when injected into nude mice (Herlyn et al., 1987a, 1987b).

Karyotypic abnormalities found in these cell lines include hyperdiploidy and nonrandom numerical as well as structural clonal abnormalities predominantly involving chromosomes 1, 6, 7, 9, and 11 (Becher et al., 1983; Balaban et al., 1984; Parmiter et al., 1986). Chromosome analyses performed on freshly isolated cells and on cells cultivated for short and long periods revealed similar aberrations, thus indicating that these aberrations most likely represent genuine abnormalities and are not attributable to in vitro artifacts (Herlyn et al., 1985b).

6. Metastatic Melanoma Cells

Metastatic melanoma cells represent the final step in tumor progression; corresponding to their in situ characteristics, cells isolated from metastases exhibit under in vitro conditions the most advanced malignant phenotype, such as high efficiency of anchorage-independent growth in soft agar, rapid tumor formation in nude mice, growth at high cellular density without contact inhibition, and the capacity to proliferate in the absence of exogenously added growth factors (Herlyn et al., 1990) (Table II). Metastatic melanoma cell lines and metastatic melanoma specimens are characterized by the same chromosomal abnormalities

involving chromosomes 1, 6, 7, 9, and 11 as reported for VGP primary melanoma cells (Becher *et al.*, 1983, Parmiter *et al.*, 1986, Balaban *et al.*, 1984,
Trent *et al.*, 1990).

The *in vitro* reproducibility of the proposed clinical and histopathological
model of tumor progression within the melanocytic system is in support of its
biological significance, and the close resemblance between histopathologically
defined stages and their *in vitro* counterparts has proved valuable for the analysis
of mechanisms involved in tumor progression.

III. Changes in Growth Regulation during Tumor Progression

Many of the results we will discuss below were achieved by comparing the
growth requirements and characteristics of cultured normal melanocytes and melanocytes of different progression stages, particularly metastatic melanoma cells.
Additional important information was obtained from extensive studies utilizing
monoclonal antibodies (MAbs) against melanoma-associated antigens expressed
by melanoma cells, and by comparing their distribution among different stages
of tumor progression, and most recently, by analyzing the structure and function
of these antigens.

A. GROWTH FACTORS AND GROWTH FACTOR RECEPTORS

1. *Growth Factors*

Cell proliferation and differentiation rely on extensive communication between
cells. In addition, cells are subjected to external signals that have stimulatory or
inhibitory effects. Polypeptide growth factors that bind specifically to membrane
receptors exert an important role in this regulatory process. By producing a particular growth factor and its receptor, cells can gain the potential for autocrine
growth. It has been proposed that this type of autocrine growth stimulation may
be important for uncontrolled tumor cell growth (De Larco *et al.*, 1978).

Normal melanocytes grown *in vitro* display little or no detectable production
of growth factors (Rodeck *et al.*, submitted), and thus depend on exogenous
growth factors like bFGF and insulin for their proliferation. In contrast, malignant melanocytes obtained from advanced stages of tumor progression synthesize
a variety of growth factors and growth factor receptors. Among the growth factors produced by melanoma cells are transforming growth factor (TGF)-α (Marquard and Todaro, 1982), TGF-β (De Larco *et al.*, 1985), platelet-derived
growth factor (PDGF)-A and PDGF-B chains (Westermark *et al.*, 1986), interleukin (IL)-1 (Köck *et al.*, 1989; Bennicelli *et al.*, 1989), melanoma growth–

stimulatory activity (MGSA) (Richmond *et al.*, 1988), bFGF (Halaban *et al.*, 1988) and melanoma-derived melanocyte growth factor (Ogata *et al.*, 1987).

MGSA is identical to the protein encoded by the human gro gene (Anisowicz *et al.*, 1987) and belongs to the macrophage-inflammatory protein 2 family. MGSA was shown to promote growth of the producing melanoma cell line Hs0294, suggesting a role as an autocrine growth factor for melanoma cells (Lawson *et al.*, 1987). The exact biological function of MGSA/gro and the properties of its receptor are presently unknown.

In a recent study, constitutive bFGF production was detected in all melanoma cell lines tested, whereas the patterns of expression for other growth factors was highly variable (Rodeck *et al.*, submitted). Despite the fact that bFGF lacks a signal lead sequence (Abraham *et al.*, 1986), bFGF appears to be important for autocrine growth stimulation of melanoma cells. Studies utilizing antisense oligonucleotides and monoclonal antibodies to bFGF, upon addition to malignant melanoma cells, resulted in growth inhibition of melanoma cells (Becker *et al.*, 1989; Halaban *et al.*, 1988). Data obtained from transfection experiments of bFGF cDNA clones into normal murine melanocytes also suggest a crucial function for bFGF during tumor development, since the transformed melanocytes demonstrated growth autonomy, but no competence for tumor formation, upon injection into athymic mice (Dotto *et al.*, 1989). Further indication of the importance of bFGF as an autocrine growth factor lies in the fact that bFGF production can already be monitored at the stage of nevus cells (Mancianti and Herlyn, unpublished data).

For a number of growth factors, secreted by melanoma cells, that lack an unequivocal autostimulatory effect, a paracrine function has to be considered in addition to their sole autocrine effects. TGF-β, for example, is known to stimulate the production of extracellular matrix proteins in fibroblasts, and thereby can help to create a microenvironment suitable for melanocyte growth (Sporn *et al.*, 1987). The production of IL-1 may be relevant for the metastatic process, since coinjection of IL-1 with human melanoma cells enhanced the capacity of melanoma cells to form metastases in nude mice (Giavazzi *et al.*, 1990). In agreement with this notion, Lauri *et al.* (1990) and Rice *et al.* (1989) demonstrated that IL-1 increases tumor cell adhesion to endothelial cells, which is believed to be an important step during the metastatic cascade. Paracrine effects may also be hypothesized for PDGF, which is secreted by most melanoma cells as PDGF-A homodimer, and less frequently, if at all, as PDGF-B, which is homologous to the oncogene v-*sis* (Waterfield *et al.*, 1983). In contrast, expression of the PDGF receptor on melanoma cells represents a rare event (Rodeck *et al.*, submitted). Since PDGF can stimulate the proliferation of fibroblasts, PDGF may have important paracrine functions for the formation of the tumor stroma (Heldin and Westermark, 1990).

2. Growth Factor Receptors

Growth factor receptors expressed by melanocytes include the epidermal growth factor (EGF)/TGF-α receptor (Koprowski et al., 1985), nerve growth factor (NGF) receptor (Ross et al., 1985), FGF receptor (Becker and Herlyn, unpublished data), insulin-like growth factor (IGF)-I receptor (Rodeck et al., 1987a), PDGF-β receptor (Rodeck et al., submitted), and MSH receptor (Tatro et al., 1990) (Table III). The EGF receptor gene maps to human chromosome 7 (p12-p13), and the internal domain of the EGF receptor is homologous to the c-erbB protooncogene (Downward et al., 1984). Koprowski et al. (1985) presented evidence that in culture, only melanoma cells that have an extra copy of chromosome 7p express the EGF receptor. Structural rearrangements or additional copies of chromosome 7p are detected in metastatic melanoma, but not in nevi or RGP melanoma (Balaban et al., 1984). Thus, the EGF receptor/c-erbB gene might be of biological significance for advanced stages of melanocyte tumor progression. This is further supported by in situ studies showing EGF receptor expression most promi-

TABLE III
GROWTH FACTORS AND GROWTH FACTOR RECEPTORS
DETECTED ON HUMAN MELANOMA CELLS in vitro

Growth factor production[a]	Growth factor	Receptor expression[b]
+ + + +	bFGF	+
O	EGF	+
O	IGF-I/II	+
+	IL-1 α	+
+ +	IL-1 β	+
+	α-MSH	+
+ +	MGSA/gro	ND[c]
O	NGF	+ +
+ + +	PDGF-A	(+)[d]
+	PDGF-B	(+)[d]
+ + +	TGF-α	+
+ + +	TGF-β	+

[a]Relative quantities of growth factor production (O, +, + +, + + +, + + + +) confirmed by Northern blot hybridization using cDNA probes encoding the respective growth factors and/or by detection of proteins in cells and supernatants.

[b]Relative density of growth factor expression as determined by binding of radiolabeled ligand or monoclonal antibodies.

[c]Not determined.

[d]Few cell lines only.

nently on metastatic melanomas and VGP primary melanomas, but only weakly on dysplastic and RGP primary melanomas, and a lack of expression on mature nevi and normal melanocytes (Elder *et al.*, 1989). Additional evidence for the importance of the EGF receptor comes from studies on melanoma formation in the fish *Xiphophorus*, which have shown that the dominant tumor-inducing oncogene Tu encodes a receptor tyrosine kinase that displays significant similarities to the human EGF receptor (Wittbrodt *et al.*, 1989). However, the exact function of the EGF receptor remains to be determined, given the observation that metastatic melanoma cells adapted to growth *in vitro* respond poorly to the mitogenic activity of EGF (Rodeck *et al.*, 1987b), whereas freshly isolated metastatic melanoma cells are stimulated by EGF, even in the presence of serum (Singletary *et al.*, 1987).

The NGF receptor, encoded on chromosome 17 (Huebner *et al.*, 1986), is expressed on cultured cells from all stages of melanoma tumor progression and on normal melanocytes (Ross *et al.*, 1985). The only difference between normal and malignant cells lies in the number of receptor sites per cell, which ranges from 1×10^4 to 2×10^6 for melanoma cells, and 10 to 1×10^4 for normal melanocytes. These results correlate with *in situ* findings showing an increase in NGF-receptor expression with tumor progression (Elder *et al.*, 1989). Apart from these data, information concerning the biological function of the NGF receptor during melanoma progression is not yet available. NGF by itself has no growth-inducing function on melanocytes (Halaban, 1988).

Expression of the FGF receptor can be detected on melanoma cells (Becker and Herlyn, unpublished data). Since the exact mechanisms of bFGF release from melanoma cells are unknown, it remains to be elucidated whether cell-surface expression of the bFGF receptor is required for autocrine growth stimulation. In addition to bFGF, other members of the FGF family, such as the oncogene int-2, which is expressed in a small portion of melanomas (Theillet *et al.*, 1989; Adelaide *et al.*, 1988), may also act as ligands for the bFGF receptor.

Melanoma cells express IGF-I receptor, which reacts with insulin or IGF-I (Rodeck *et al.*, 1987a). Insulin and IGF-I exert a strong growth-stimulatory effect on melanocytes from all stages of tumor progression. Early primary melanomas require at least IGF-I or insulin for growth *in vitro*. Metastatic melanoma cells, although growth factor–independent, still respond to the addition of insulin or IGF-I (Rodeck *et al.*, 1987b). An autocrine role for IGF-I for melanoma growth is most unlikely, since none of the examined normal melanocytes and melanoma cells showed secretion of IGF-I or IGF-II, and no IGF-I transcripts were detected (Rodeck *et al.*, submitted).

Expression of the α-MSH receptors has been described for melanoma cells *in vitro* and *in situ* (Siegrist *et al.*, 1989; Tatro *et al.*, 1990). Normal human melanocytes and nevus cells are responsive to α-MSH and depend on exogenous α-MSH for *in vitro* growth in serum-free medium. Various effects of α-MSH on cultured human melanocytes have been reported, including changes in tyrosinase activity (Legros *et al.*, 1981), cytoplasmic granule accumulation (Packard, 1987) and the stimulation of cytoplasmic cAMP accumulation (Ranson *et al.*, 1988). However, the biological role of MSH and its receptor for melanoma tumor progression awaits further experimental analysis.

Expression of mRNA transcripts for the PDGF-β receptor, which binds PDGF-B homodimers and PDGF-AB heterodimers but no PDGF-A homodimers, was detected in 1 out of 4 melanoma cell lines tested (Rodeck *et al.*, submitted). Since melanoma cells predominantly secrete the PDGF-A homodimer, the level of PDGF-α receptor expression remains to be determined in order to elicit the function of PDGF for melanoma growth.

A protein detected by three different MAbs (ME491, LS62, and NKI/C-3) (Atkinson *et al.*, 1984; Sikora *et al.*, 1987; Mackie *et al.*, 1984), termed neuroglandular antigen (NGA), is expressed during early stages of melanoma tumor progression. Normal tissue melanocytes are negative, and dysplastic nevi and RGP primary melanomas are strongly positive, whereas further advanced stages of melanoma exhibit weaker or no expression of NGA (Atkinson *et al.*, 1984). NGA reveals a granular intracellular distribution and has been localized by electronmicroscopy to melanosomes, vacuoles, and the plasma membrane (Dixon *et al.*, 1990). The gene encoding NGA has been cloned, and the nucleotide sequence analysis has suggested that NGA is a membrane-bound protein with four transmembrane regions (Hotta *et al.*, 1988). The biological function of NGA remains undefined, yet supportive evidence suggests a role in growth regulation, probably as growth factor receptor for a yet undefined ligand (Hotta *et al.*, 1988; Rakowicz-Szulczynska *et al.*, 1989).

B. Signal Transduction

Regardless of the type of external regulatory factor, signals controlling DNA replication and selective gene expression have to be transmitted from the cell surface to the effector site, usually located inside the nucleus. Consequently, the mechanisms for signal transduction from the cell membrane via the cytoplasm to the nucleus are of great importance to cellular growth control. Thus, deregulation of this pathway may play a pivotal role in the development of neoplastic disorders (Macara, 1989). As with growth factors and receptors, several oncogenes have been found to encode proteins that resemble normal products of protooncogenes with key functions for signal transduction. Structural and functional alterations of three of the major proteins responsible for signal transduction have been reported for melanoma cells. In particular, these changes involve PKC, cAMP-dependent protein kinases (PKA), and guanine nucleotide-binding proteins (G proteins).

A recent study demonstrated that cultured normal human melanocytes fail to express PKC-α, PKC-β, or PKC-γ, in spite of the presence of TPA, an activator of PKC (Becker *et al.*, 1990). This result may be due to down-regulation of PKC after prolonged exposure of cells to TPA, or to expression of PKC-related genes other than PKC-α, PKC-β, or PKC-γ. In contrast, some primary and metastatic melanoma cells express PKC-α, but not PKC-β, or PKC-γ (Becker *et al.*, 1990). Phorbolester-induced activation of membrane-bound PKC in mouse B16 melanoma cells increases their capacity for hematogenous metastasis, whereas activation of cytosolic PKC without membrane association does not result in an increase in metastasis (Gopalakrishna and Barsky, 1988).

The investigation of PKA expression in cells from different stages of melanoma progression revealed expression of the PKA specific subunits C-α and RI-α in VGP primary and metastatic melanoma cells, but not in normal melanocytes (Becker *et al.*, 1990). In light of the recent observations that bFGF represents a substrate for phosphorylation by PKA (Feige and Baird, 1989), and given the fact that bFGF acts as an autocrine growth factor for melanoma cell proliferation, one may speculate that phosphorylation of bFGF by PKA may play an integral role in the progression of normal melanocytes to malignant melanomas.

C. ONCOGENES

Several studies have addressed the question of *ras* oncogene activation in human malignant melanomas. The oncogenes H-*ras*, K-*ras*, and N-*ras* encode similar proteins with molecular weights of 21,000 (p21). *Ras* oncogenes are closely related to the family of G proteins, membrane-bound guanine nucleotide-binding proteins, that are activated in response to extracellular signals and play an important role in the regulation of second messengers. Mutational analysis of *ras*-oncoproteins detected amino acid alterations at codons 12, 13, and 61, with the result that these mutant *ras*-encoded proteins are constitutively activated and thus give rise to uncontrolled second-messenger production (Bos, 1989; Hall, 1990). Expression of all three *ras* oncogenes has been detected in melanoma cells. Upon transfection of melanoma DNAs into NIH/3T3 cells, activated N-*ras* and H-*ras* genes were detected in 4 of 30 different melanomas tested (Albino *et al.*, 1984). Albino *et al.* (1989) found N-*ras* and H-*ras* displaying mutations at codon 61, but no K-*ras* expression, in about 24% of cultured melanoma cells. Metastatic melanoma cells in culture, expressing mutated N-*ras* and H-*ras*, had a very similar phenotype, characterized by high expression of EGF receptor and class II histocompatibility antigens, lack of pigmentation, and a epitheloid–spindle type morphology (Albino *et al.*, 1989). Noncultured melanomas had the mutated *ras* genes in 5 to 6% of the specimens. Interestingly, *ras* gene expression was not detected in specimens from normal and dysplastic nevi (Albino *et al.*, 1989). We have detected activated N-*ras* genes in 3 of 19 (16%) metastatic melanomas analyzed, but in none of 6 VGP primary melanomas tested (Becker, Parmiter, and Herlyn, unpublished). The results presented in Fig. 1 demonstrate the activation of N-*ras* genes, indicated by the presence of an 8.8 kb fragment, in secondary NIH/3T3 transformants derived from three independent metastases of the same patient. In a recent study, N-*ras* mutations were detected exclusively in tumor samples obtained from sun-exposed locations of

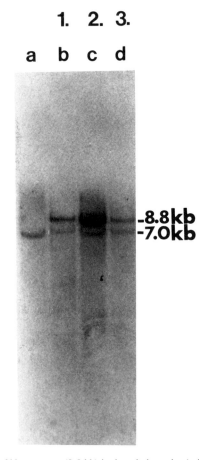

FIG. 1.   Detection of N-*ras* genes (8.8 kb) in three independently isolated metastases obtained from the same patient. Lanes a. NIH 3T3 DNA; b. secondary NIH WM 806 transformant; c. secondary NIH WM 852 transformant; d. secondary NIH WM 310 transformant. The endogenous mouse N-*ras* EcoR1 fragment is at 7.0 kb.

the body, suggesting a close correlation between UV irradiation and the type of *ras* mutation (Van't Veer *et al.*, 1989). In contrast to the former studies, Shukla *et al.* (1989) detected mutations of the K-*ras* gene at codon 12 in 20% of the examined genomic DNA samples from melanoma specimens. These mutations were also found in benign nevi and primary melanomas, suggesting the importance of *ras* activation during early events of melanoma development. However, these results are in contrast to those of Albino *et al.* (1989), which indicate that *ras* mutations are a late phenomenon. Although mutated *ras* oncogenes have reportedly clear effects on normal diploid melanocytes, including changes in their growth characteristics (Albino *et al.*, 1986), and *ras* oncogenes represent the family of oncogenes most constantly and frequently expressed in human malignant melanomas, their exact biological function remains to be determined.

A possible association between the c-*src* oncogene, a nonreceptor membrane-associated tyrosine kinase, and melanoma needs further confirmation, since elevated levels of pp60[c-src] kinase were detected in cell extracts of human melanomas (Barnekow *et al.*, 1987), but a comparison between normal melanocytes and melanoma cell lines did not reveal differences in the level or size of c-*src* transcripts (Albino, 1988).

Alterations of nuclear protooncogenes have so far been reported only for the *myb* oncogene. In 1 of 30 analyzed melanoma cell lines, Linnenbach *et al.* (1988) found rearrangements of c-*myb* in connection with a 6q22 chromosomal abnormality. Further analysis revealed that this rearrangement leads to a deletion in the 3'-end of the c-*myb* locus and concomitant translocation of a portion of chromosome 12 to chromosome 6 (Dasgupta *et al.*, 1989).

IV. Cell-Surface Structures on Melanoma Cells

Cell–cell and cell–substratum adhesive interactions have great importance for cell development and growth coordination within differentiated organs and tissues. Changes within the network of regulatory stimuli between adhesion receptors and their ligands can render cells irresponsive to these control mechanisms and thereby enable them to grow more independently or to survive in an otherwise hostile environment. About 60% of the antigenic determinants detected by MAbs against melanoma-associated cell-surface antigens are related to cell–cell or cell–substratum interactions.

A. Cell-to-Cell Interaction

Human lymphocyte antigens (HLA) class I and class II are important for the cellular immune response against tumors. Changes in the expression of both antigen groups have been detected during melanocytic tumor progression. Since

HLA class I are responsible for antigen presentation to cytotoxic T lymphocytes, changes in HLA class I expression may help tumor cells escape immune surveillance. In agreement with this notion is the finding that metastatic melanoma cells compared to primary melanoma cells have decreased HLA class I levels, and thereby may become less susceptible to destruction by cytotoxic T lymphocytes (Natali *et al.*, 1984; Holzmann *et al.*, 1987). On the other hand, natural killer cell–mediated nonspecific cytotoxicity can be stimulated by a decrease in HLA–class I expression, and therefore, melanoma cells with a reduced HLA–class I expression may become good targets for natural killer cells (Tanigushi *et al.*, 1985). Few data are available concerning the immunological relevance of differential expression of HLA class I. Studies on autologous cytotoxic T lymphocytes against melanoma cells indicate that HLA-A2 in particular is important for HLA-restricted antigen presentation to cytotoxic lymphocytes (Darrow *et al.*, 1989; Natali *et al.*, 1989). Furthermore, Versteeg *et al.* (1989) reported that expression of c-*myc* in melanoma cells selectively down-regulates the class I HLA-B locus expression, resulting in an increased susceptibility of c-*myc*–expressing melanoma cells to lysis by natural killer cells.

The expression of HLA class II exhibits a certain degree of correlation to the stage of melanoma progression, with highest levels detected in metastatic melanomas (Real *et al.*, 1985). Cytokines such as tumor necrosis factor and the interferons (IFN) α and γ can up-regulate HLA–class II expression in melanoma cells (Guerry *et al.*, 1987; Maio *et al.*, 1989). Up-regulation of HLA–class II expression has also been reported after transfection of melanocytes with the v-*ras* oncogene (Albino *et al.*, 1986). The significance of these antigenic changes remains obscure at present.

Another adhesion molecule responsible for tumor cell–lymphocyte interaction is the intercellular adhesion molecule-1 (Makgoba *et al.*, 1988), which binds to the lymphocyte function–related antigen-1. Intercellular adhesion molecule-1, shown to correlate with tumor progression and the risk of metastasis (Johnson *et al.*, 1989; Natali *et al.*, 1990), can be modulated by IL-1, IFN-γ, and tumor necrosis factor-α (Maio *et al.*, 1989; Yohn *et al.*, 1990). Johnson *et al.* (1989) propose that the expression of intercellular adhesion molecule-1, through attracting T lymphocytes, does not primarily induce immunological reactions, but enables single melanoma cells to dissociate from the primary tumor after binding to migrating leukocytes.

Muc 18, a melanoma-associated antigen that discriminates between normal and malignant melanocytes and also shows correlation with tumor progression (Lehmann *et al.*, 1987), is closely related to the neural-cell adhesion molecule (Lehmann *et al.*, 1989). Muc 18 belongs to the family of carcinoembryonic antigen–related proteins that share sequence homologies with the immunoglobulin gene superfamily (Oikawa *et al.*, 1987).

B. CELL SUBSTRATUM ADHESION

1. *Cellular Adhesion Proteins*

One feature of tumor progression is the ability to invade local tissue stroma and to metastasize to distant sites after migration. A prerequisite to this process is the ability of tumor cells to interact with different sets of extracellular matrix proteins. A group of cellular adhesion proteins that has particular importance for this interaction is the group of integrin molecules. Integrins are heterodimers composed of noncovalently bound α- and β-subunits and are subclassified according to the type of a common β-subunit associated with variable α-subunits (Albelda and Buck, 1990). In culture, normal melanocytes and melanoma cells express the vitronectin receptor (α_V/β_3) and all members of the β_1 family (α_1/β_1 to α_6/β_1) that bind to collagen, laminin, and fibronectin (Albelda *et al.*, 1990). No consistent difference between normal melanocytes and melanocytes from different stages of melanoma progression was detected. However, Albelda *et al.* (1990) have found a differential *in situ* expression of integrins on melanocytes representing different stages of tumor progression. Melanocytes from VGP primary melanoma and metastatic melanoma lesions had significantly higher expression levels of the α_4 subunit as compared to melanocytes from nevi and RGP primary melanomas, which primarily expressed the α_2 and α_3 subunits. Expression of the β_3 subunit was restricted exclusively to melanoma cells with metastatic potential. The functional importance of integrin-mediated tumor cell adhesion for metastasis is further supported by experiments that have shown that synthetic peptides containing the amino acid sequence Arg-Gly-Asp (RGD) (derived from one of the cell-binding domains of fibronectin) can inhibit the binding between integrins and extracellular matrix proteins containing the RGD-sequence (Ruoslahti and Pierschbacher, 1987). Using this approach, it was possible to inhibit the movement of human melanoma cells through an amniotic basement membrane in an experimental invasion model (Gehlsen *et al.*, 1988), and to reduce the number of metastatic nodules in the lungs of mice following injection of B16F10 melanoma cells together with RDG peptides (Humphries *et al.*, 1988).

Gangliosides may also play a critical role in cell attachment as GD2 and GD3 interact with cell-surface receptors for vitronectin and fibronectin. This is further supported by the fact that MAbs to GD2 and GD3 can block attachment of cells to substrate as well as inhibit invasion of cells through basement membranes (Cheresh *et al.*, 1986; Iliopulos *et al.*, 1989). Melanoma cells are rich in gangliosides GD2, GD3, acetylated GD3, GM2, and GM3. In cultured melanocytic cells, GD3 and acetylated GD3 seem to be up-regulated with tumor progression (Carubia *et al.*, 1984), and GD2 is expressed only on cells with metastatic potential (Thurin *et al.*, 1986). Transformation of normal melanocytes with v-*ras* leads to a marked increase of GD3 expression (Albino *et al.*, 1986).

Proteoglycans are proteins characterized by one or more glycosaminoglycan side chains. Several functions have been reported for this group of proteins, including mediation of cell binding to the extracellular matrix and capture of soluble factors such as growth factors. The functional characteristics of proteoglycans are determined by the type of glycosaminoglycan as well as the core protein. A large-molecular-weight complex, referred to as melanoma chondroitin sulfate proteoglycan (mCSP), composed of a 240 to 280-kDa core protein with chondroitin sulfate glycosaminoglycan side chains, can be detected on melanocytes and cells from nevi and melanoma in culture (Morgan *et al.*, 1981; Hellström *et al.*, 1983; Ross *et al.*, 1983). *In situ,* normal melanocytes show little expression of mCSP. Adhesion plaques deposited along the cell membrane of melanoma cells contain high amounts of mCSP. MAbs to mCSP inhibit colony formation of melanoma cells in soft agar, indicating an additional function of mCSP in cell–cell interactions (Harper and Reisfeld, 1983).

2. *Extracellular Matrix Proteins*

Melanoma cells secrete a variety of extracellular matrix (ECM) proteins, including collagen type IV, laminin (Natali *et al.*, 1985) and fibronectin (Herlyn *et al.*, 1987a), for which they also express the appropriate integrin receptor (Albelda *et al.*, 1990). The ability to produce particular ECM proteins may make melanocytes less dependent upon surrounding cells, i.e., fibroblasts, which are the main source of ECM proteins. Another ECM protein secreted by melanoma cells but not normal melanocytes is tenascin. This protein is expressed at restricted sites during embryogenesis and wound healing (Chiquet-Ehrismann, 1990). Experimental data indicate that tenascin is involved in cellular migration by locally reducing cellular binding to fibronectin (Lightner and Erickson, 1990). In agreement with this notion is the finding that normal melanocytes and melanoma cells do not bind to tenascin (Graeven and Herlyn, unpublished data). The secretion of tenascin by melanoma cells may therefore facilitate tumor cell migration.

C. TRANSPORT PROTEINS

Melanoma cells *in vitro* and *in situ* express several cation-binding and cation-transport proteins. The melanoma-associated antigen p97 reveals structural resemblance to transferrin and was thus named melanotransferrin (Rose *et al.*, 1986). P97 binds iron and shows internalization with subsequent reexpression after binding to anti-p97 MAbs (Richardson and Baker, 1990). Melanoma cells also express the transferrin receptor, and its expression appears to be correlated with tumor progression (van Muijen *et al.*, 1990).

The calcium-binding protein, S-100, has been identified on melanoma cells, and recent studies reported a growth-stimulatory effect of purified S-100 on human melanoma cell lines (van Eldik *et al.*, 1982; Klein *et al.*, 1989).

The common acute lymphoblastic leukemia antigen, expressed on hematopoietic cells, gliomas, and melanoma cells (Carrel *et al.*, 1983) represents a zinc-binding metallopeptidase identical to neutral endopeptidase (Jongeneel *et al.*, 1989). Neutral endopeptidase is present on the cell surface with its active site oriented toward the extracellular site. Neutral endopeptidase is capable of hydrolyzing and inactivating a wide range of proteins, including IL-1β (Pierat *et al.*, 1988). The expression of the common acute lymphoblastic leukemia antigen may render melanoma cells unresponsive to the influence of regulatory peptides released by surrounding normal cells, such as keratinocytes and fibroblasts. The biological relevance of such an interaction for melanoma progression remains to be determined.

V. Melanogenesis in Melanoma

Melanin production is the main function of normal melanocytes located in the epidermis. The number of melanosomes (the specific secretory granules of melanocytes) and the level of melanin production increase with melanocyte maturation. Melanocytes cultured in TPA-containing medium retain their mature phenotype. Melanoma cells present all grades of pigmentation from a seemingly normal pigment content to an amelanotic appearance. Consequently, much attention was focused on functional and structural changes of melanogenesis during melanocytic tumor progression.

One of the key enzymes for melanin synthesis is tyrosinase. Tyrosinase hydroxylates tyrosine and oxidizes dopa and 5, 6-dihydroxyindole. Using a MAb against human tyrosinase, McEwan *et al.* (1988) did not detect a significant correlation between tyrosinase levels and melanoma tumor progression; even amelanotic melanomas had detectable tyrosinase activity.

Malignant melanoma cells synthesize melanosomes that are disarranged in their melanosomal matrix protein composition (Jimbow *et al.*, 1984). Several MAbs have been generated against structural proteins of melanosomes in melanoma cells. Among these MAbs, HMSA 1, HMSA 2, HMSA 3, and HMSA 4 are reactive only with melanoma cells and not with normal melanocytes (Maeda *et al.*, 1987; Akutsu and Jimbow, 1986).

Another protein of importance for melanin production is GP 75. GP 75 demonstrates homology with the mouse b (BROWN) gene (Vijayasaradhi *et al.*, 1990) and has catalase activity (catalase B) (Halaban and Moellmann, 1990). Expression of this protein correlates with pigmentation of melanocytes and melanoma cells in culture (Thomson *et al.*, 1988).

VI. Summary

Human malignant melanoma provides an excellent model system for studying mechanisms of transformation and tumor progression. The fact that normal melanocytes and cells from different stages of melanoma progression can be cultured under defined conditions has facilitated the determination, and thus the correlation, of their biological characteristics to melanoma progression *in vivo*. Changes in growth-factor requirements have been defined, and the increasing growth-factor independence of melanocytes from advanced melanomas as compared to normal melanocytes has been studied in detail. Although melanoma cells produce a variety of growth factors and growth-factor receptors, only bFGF appears to have a clear autocrine role. Additional paracrine functions may be considered, especially for those growth factors that show no autocrine growth stimulation.

The ability to change the confirmation of cell–cell and cell–matrix interactions is another feature of melanoma cells. With increasing tumor progression, melanoma cells gain more competence for ECM protein production and adhesion-molecule expression, allowing interaction with a variety of different ECM compositions. Differential expression of cell-surface structures, like MHC molecules, may enable melanoma cells to circumvent the mechanisms of immune surveillance. The role of oncogenes and corresponding protooncogenes for melanoma development is still inconclusive and thus far, only activated *ras* genes have been identified with some consistency in up to 25% of advanced-stage melanomas.

Changes affecting intracellular signal transduction and gene regulation have only lately been addressed in the human melanocytic system. Further studies are required to understand the importance of signal transduction and the interaction of cytoplasmic and nuclear (proto-) oncogenes in the development of human melanoma.

Acknowledgments

These studies were supported, in part, by Grants CA-25874, CA-44877, CA-47159, and CA-10815 from the National Institutes of Health.

References

Abraham, J. M., Whang, J. L., Tumolo, A., Mergia, A., Friedmann, J., Gospodarowicz, D., and Fiddess, J. C. (1986). Human basic fibroblast growth factor: Nucleotide sequence and genome organization. *EMBO J.* **5,** 2523–2528.

Adelaide, J., Mattei, M.-G., Marcis, I., Raybaud, F., Planche, J., De Laperyiere, O., and Birnbaum, D. (1988). Chromosomal localization of the *hst* oncogene and its coamplification with the *int*-2 oncogene in a human melanoma. *Oncogene* **2,** 413–416.

Akutsu, Y., and Jimbow, K. (1986). Development and characterization of a mouse monoclonal antibody, MoAb HMSA-1, against a melanosomal fraction of human malignant melanoma. *Cancer Res.* **46,** 2904–2911.

Albelda, S. M., and Buck, C. A. (1990). Integrins and other cell adhesion molecules. *FASEB J.* **4,** 2868–2880.

Albelda, S. M., Mette, S. A., Elder, D. E., Stewart, R., Damjanovich, L., Herlyn, M., and Buck, C. A. (1990). Integrin distribution in malignant melanoma: Association of the beta 3 subunit with tumor progression. *Cancer Res.* **50,** 6757–6764.

Albino, A. P., Le Strange, R., Oliff, A. I., Furth, M. E., and Old, L. J. (1984). Transforming *ras* genes from human melanoma: A manifestation of tumour heterogeneity? *Nature (London)* **308,** 69–72.

Albino, A. P., Houghton, A. N., Eisinger, M., Lee, J. S., Kantor, R. R. S., Oliff, A. I., and Old, L. J. (1986). Class II histocompatibility antigen expression in human melanocytes transformed by Harvey sarcoma virus (Ha-MSV) and Kirsten MSV retroviruses. *J. Exp. Med.* **164,** 1710–1722.

Albino, A. P. (1988). The status of oncogenes in malignant melanoma. *In* "Advances in pigment cell research" (J. T. Bagnara, ed.), pp. 361–390. Alan R. Liss, New York.

Albino, A. P., Nanus, D. M., Mentle, I. R., Cordon-Cardo, C., McNutt, N. S., Bressler, J., and Andreeff, M. (1989). Analysis of *ras* oncogenes in malignant melanoma and precursor lesions: Correlation of point mutations with differentiation phenotype. *Oncogene* **4,** 1363–1374.

Anisowicz, A., Bardwell, L., and Sager, R. (1987). Constitutive overexpression of a growth-regulated gene in transformed Chinese hamster and human cells. *Proc. Natl. Acad. Sci. U.S.A.* **84,** 7188–7192.

Atkinson, B., Ernst, C. S., Ghrist, B. F. D., Herlyn, M., Blaszcyk, M., Ross, A. H., Herlyn, D., Maul, G., Steplewski, Z., and Koprowski, H. (1984). Identification of melanoma-associated antigens using fixed tissue screening of antibodies. *Cancer Res.* **44,** 2577–2581.

Balaban, G., Herlyn, M., Guerry, D., IV, Bartolo, R., Koprowski, H., Clark, W. H., Jr., and Nowell, P. C. (1984). Cytogenetics of human malignant melanoma and premalignant lesions. *Cancer Genet. Cytogenet.* **11,** 429–439.

Balaban, G. B., Herlyn, M., Clark, W. H., Jr., and Nowell, P. C. (1986). Karyotypic evolution in human malignant melanoma. *Cancer Genet. Cytogenet.* **19,** 113–122.

Barnekow, A., Paul, E., and Schartl, M. (1987). Expression of the c-*src* protooncogene in human skin tumors. *Cancer Res.* **47,** 235–240.

Becher, R., Gibas, Z., and Sandberg, A. A. (1983). Chromosome 6 in malignant melanoma. *Cancer Genet. Cytogenet.* **9,** 173–174.

Becker, D., Meier, C. B., and Herlyn, M. (1989). Proliferation of human malignant melanomas is inhibited by antisense oligodeoxynucleotides targeted against basic fibroblast growth factor. *EMBO J.* **8,** 3685–3691.

Becker, D., Beebe, S. J., and Herlyn, M. (1990). Differential expression of protein kinase C and cAMP-dependent protein kinase in normal human melanocytes and malignant melanomas. *Oncogene* **5,** 1133–1139.

Bennett, D. C., Bridges, K., and McKay, I. A. (1985). Clonal separation of mature melanocytes from premelanocytes in a diploid human cell strain: Spontaneous and induced pigmentation of premelanocytes. *J. Cell Sci.* **77,** 167–183.

Bennicelli, J. L., Elias, J., Kern, J., and Guerry, D. IV. (1989). Production of interleukin 1 activity by cultured human melanoma cells. *Cancer Res.* **49,** 930–935.

Bos, J. L. (1989). *Ras* oncogene in human cancer: A review. *Cancer Res.* **49,** 4682–4689.

Carrel, S., Schmidt-Kessen, A., Mach, J. P., Heumann, D., and Giradet, C. (1983). Expression of common acute lymphoblastic leukemia antigen (CALLA) on human malignant melanoma cells. *J. Immunol.* **130,** 2456–2460.

Carubia, J. M., Yu, R. K., Macala, L. J., Kirkwood, J. M., and Varga, J. M. (1984). Gangliosides of normal and neoplastic human melanocytes. *Biochem. Biophys. Res. Comm.* **120,** 500–504.

Cheresh, D. A., Pierschbacher, M. D., Herzig, M. A., and Mujoo, K. (1986). Disialoganglioside GD2 and GD3 are involved in the attachment of human melanoma and neuroblastoma cells to extracellular matrix proteins. *J. Cell Biol.* **102,** 688–696.

Chiquet-Ehrismann, R. (1990). What distinguishes tenascin from fibronectin? *FASEB J.* **4,** 2598–2604.

Clark, W. H., Jr., Elder, D. E., Guerry, D. IV, Epstein, M. N., Greene, M. H., and Van Horn, M. (1984). A study of tumor progression: The precursor lesions of superficial spreading and nodular melanoma. *Hum. Pathol.* **15,** 1147–1165.

Clark, W. H., Jr., Elder, D. E., and Van Horn, M. (1986). The biologic forms of malignant melanoma. *Hum. Pathol.* **17,** 443–450.

Darrow, T. L., Slingluff, C. L., and Seigler, H. F. (1989). The role of HLA Class I antigens in recognition of melanoma cells by tumor-specific cytotoxic T lymphocytes. *J. Immunol.* **142,** 3329–3335.

Dasgupta, P., Linnenbach, A. J., Giaccia, A. J., Stamato, T. D., and Reddy, E. P. (1989). Molecular cloning of the breakpoint region on chromosome 6 in cutaneous malignant melanoma: Evidence for deletion in the c-*myb* locus and translocation of a segment of chromosome 12. *Oncogene* **4,** 1201–1205.

De Larco, J. E., and Todaro, G. J. (1978). Growth factors from murine sarcoma virus–transformed cells. *Proc. Natl. Acad. Sci. U.S.A.* **75,** 4001–4005.

De Larco, J. E., Pigott, D. A., and Lazarus, J. A. (1985). Ectopic peptides released by a human melanoma cell line that modulate transformed phenotype. *Proc. Natl. Acad. Sci. U.S.A.* **82,** 5015–5019.

Dixon, W. T., Demetrick, D. J., Ohyama, K., Sikora, L. K. J., and Jerry, L. M. (1990). Biosynthesis, glycosylation, and intracellular processing of the neuroglandular antigen, a human melanoma–associated antigen. *Cancer Res.* **50,** 4557–4565.

Dotto, G. P., Moellmann, G., Ghosh, S., Edwards, M., and Halaban, R. (1989). Transformation of murine melanocytes by basic fibroblast growth factor cDNA and oncogenes and selective suppression of the transformed phenotype in a reconstituted cutaneous environment. *J. Cell Biol.* **109,** 3115–3128.

Downward, J., Yarden, Y., Mayes, E., Scarce, G., Totty, N., Stockwell, P., Ullrich, A., Schlessinger, J., and Waterfield, M. D. (1984). Close similarity of epidermal growth factor receptor and v-*erb*B oncogene protein sequences. *Nature (London)* **307,** 521–527.

Eisinger, M., and Marko, O. (1982). Selective proliferation of normal human melanocytes *in vitro* in the presence of phorbol ester and cholera toxin. *Proc. Natl. Acad. Sci. U.S.A.* **79,** 2018–2022.

Elder, D. E., Rodeck, U., Thurin, J., Cardillo, F., Clark, W. H., Stewart, R., and Herlyn, M. (1989). Antigenic profile of tumor progression in human melanocytic nevi and melanomas. *Cancer Res.* **49,** 5091–5096.

Feige, J. J., and Baird, A. (1989). Basic fibroblast growth factor is a substrate for protein phosphorylation and is phosphorylated by capillary endothelial cells in culture. *Proc. Natl. Acad. Sci. U.S.A.* **86,** 2683–2687.

Foulds, L. (1954). The experimental study of tumor progression: A review. *Cancer Res.* **14,** 327–339.

Gehlsen, K. R., Argraves, W. S., Pierschbacher, M. D., and Ruoslahti, E. (1988). Inhibition of *in vitro* tumor cell invasion by Arg-Gly-Asp-containing synthetic peptides. *J. Cell Biol.* **106,** 925–930.

Giavazzi, R., Garofalo, A., Bani, M. R., Abbate, M., Ghezzi, P., Boraschi, D., Mantovani, A., and Dejana, E. (1990). Interleukin 1–induced augmentation of experimental metastases from a human melanoma in nude mice. *Cancer Res.* **50,** 4771–4775.

Gilchrest, B. A., Vrabel, M. A., Flynn, E., and Szabo, G. (1984). Selective cultivation of human melanocytes from newborn and adult epidermis. *J. Invest. Dermatol.* **83,** 370–376.

Gopalakrishna, R., and Barsky, S. H. (1988). Tumor promoter–induced membrane-bound protein kinase C regulates hematogenous metastasis. *Proc. Natl. Acad. Sci. U.S.A.* **85,** 612–616.

Guerry, D., IV, Alexander, M. A., Elder, D. E., and Herlyn, M. (1987). Interferon-gamma regulates the T-cell response to precursor nevi and biologically early melanoma. *J. Immunol.* **139,** 305–312.

Halaban, R., Ghosh, S., and Baird, A. (1987). bFGF is the putative natural growth factor for human melanocytes. *In Vitro Cell Dev. Biol.* **23,** 47–52.

Halaban, R. (1988). Responses of cultured melanocytes to defined growth factors. *Pigment Cell Res.* [*Suppl.*] **1,** 18–26.

Halaban, R., Kwon, B. S., Ghosh, S., Delli-Bovi, P., and Baird, A. (1988). bFGF as an autocrine growth factor for human melanomas. *Oncogene Res.* **3,** 177–186.

Halaban, R., and Moellmann, G. (1990). Murine and human b-locus pigmentation genes encode a glycoprotein (gp75) with catalase activity. *Proc. Natl. Acad. Sci. U.S.A.* **87,** 4809–4813.

Hall, A. (1990). The cellular functions of small GTP-binding proteins. *Science* **249,** 635–640.

Harper, J. R., and Reisfeld, R. A. (1983). Inhibition of anchorage-independent growth of human melanoma cells by a monoclonal antibody to a chondroitin sulfate proteoglycan. *J. Natl. Cancer Inst.* **71,** 259–264.

Heldin, C.-H., and Westermark, B. (1990). Platelet-derived growth factor: Mechanism of action and possible *in vivo* function. *Cell Regulation* **1,** 555–566.

Hellström, I., Garrigues, H. J., Cabasco, L., Mosley, G. H., Brown, J. P., and Hellström, K. E. (1983). Studies of a high-molecular-weight, human melanoma–associated antigen. *J. Immunol.* **130,** 1467–1472.

Herlyn, M., Balaban, G., Bennicelli, J., Guerry, D., Halaban, R., Herlyn, D., Elder, D. E., Maul, G. G., Steplewski, Z., Nowell, P. C., Clark, W. H., and Koprowski, H. (1985a). Primary melanoma cells of the vertical growth phase: Similarities to metastatic cells. *J. Natl. Cancer Inst.* **74,** 283–289.

Herlyn, M., Thurin, J., Balaban, G., Bennicelli, J. L., Herlyn, D., Elder, D. E., Bondi, E., Guerry, D., Nowell, P., Clark, W. H., and Koprowski, H. (1985b). Characteristics of cultured human melanocytes isolated from different stages of tumor progression. *Cancer Res.* **45,** 5670–5676.

Herlyn, M., Clark, W. H., Rodeck, U., Mancianti, M. L., Jambrosic, J., and Koprowski, H. (1987a). Biology of disease. Biology of tumor progression in human melanocytes. *Lab. Invest.* **56,** 461–474.

Herlyn, M., Rodeck, U., Mancianti, M. L., Cardillo, F. M., Lang, A., Ross, A. H., Jambrosic, J., and Koprowski, H. (1987b). Expression of melanoma-associated antigens in rapidly dividing human melanocytes in culture. *Cancer Res.* **47,** 3057–3061.

Herlyn, M., Mancianti, M. L., Jambrosic, J., Bolen, J. B., and Koprowski, H. (1988). Regulatory factors that determine growth and phenotype of normal human melanocytes. *Exp. Cell Res.* **179,** 322–331.

Herlyn, M., Kath, R., Williams, N., Valyi-Nagy, I., and Rodeck, U. (1990). Growth regulatory factors for normal, premalignant, and malignant human cells. *Adv. Cancer Res.* **54,** 213–234.

Holzmann, B., Broecker, E. B., Lehman, J. M., Ruiter, D. J., Sorg, C., Riethmüller, G., and Johnson, J. P. (1987). Tumor progression in human malignant melanoma: Five stages defined by their antigeneic phenotypes. *Int. J. Cancer* **39,** 466–471.

Hotta, H., Ross, A. H., Huebner, K., Isobe, M., Wendeborn, S., Chao, M. V., Ricciardi, R. P., Tsujimoto, Y., Croce, C. M., and Koprowski, H. (1988). Molecular cloning and characterization of an antigen associated with early stages of melanoma tumor progression. *Cancer Res.* **48**, 2955–2962.

Huebner, K., Isobe, M., Chao, M., Bothwell, M., Ross, A. H., Finan, J., Hoxie, J. A., Sehgal, A., Buck, C. R., Lanahan, A., Nowell, P. C., Koprowski, H., and Croce, C. M. (1986). The nerve growth factor receptor gene is at human chromosome region 17q12–17q22, distal to the chromosome 17 breakpoint in acute leukemias. *Proc. Natl. Acad. Sci. U.S.A.* **83**, 1403–1407.

Humphries, M. J., Yamada, K. M., and Olden, K. (1988). Investigation of the biological effects of anti–cell adhesion synthetic peptides that inhibit experimental metastasis of B16-F10 murine melanoma cells. *J. Clin. Invest.* **81**, 782–790.

Iliopoulos, D., Ernst, C., Steplewski, Z., Jambrosic, J. A., Rodeck, U., Herlyn, M., Clark, W. H., Jr., Koprowski, H., and Herlyn, D. (1989). Inhibition of metastases of a human melanoma xenograft by monoclonal antibody to the GD2/GD3 gangliosides. *J. Natl. Cancer Inst.* **81**, 440–444.

Jimbow, K., Miyake, Y., Homma, K., Yasuda, K., Izumi, Y., Tsutsumi, A., and Ito, S. (1984). Characterization of melanogenesis and morphogenesis of melanosomes by physicochemical properties of melanin and melanosomes in malignant melanoma. *Cancer Res.* **44**, 1128–1134.

Johnson, J. P., Stade, B. G., Holzmann, B., Schwäble, W., and Riethmüller, G. (1989). *De novo* expression of intercellular-adhesion molecule 1 in melanoma correlates with increased risk of metastasis. *Proc. Natl. Acad. Sci. U.S.A.* **86**, 641–644.

Jongeneel, C. V., Quakenbush, E. J., Ronco, P., Verroust, P., Carrel, S., and Letarte, M. (1989). Common acute lymphoblastic leukemia antigen expressed on leukemia and melanoma cell lines has neutral endopeptidase activity. *J. Clin. Invest.* **83**, 713–717.

Kath, R., Rodeck, U., Menssen, H. D., Mancianti, M. L., Linnenbach, A. J., Elder, D. E., and Herlyn, M. (1989). Tumor progression in the human melanocytic system. *Anticancer Res.* **9**, 865–872.

Klein, G., and Klein, E. (1985). Evolution of tumors and the impact of molecular oncology. *Nature (London)* **315**, 190–195.

Klein, J. R., Hoon, D. S. B., Nangauyan, J., Okun, E., and Cochran, A. J. (1989). S-100 protein stimulates cellular proliferation. *Cancer Immunol. Immunother.* **29**, 133–138.

Koprowski, H., Herlyn, M., Balaban, G., Parmiter, A., Ross, A., and Nowell, P. C. (1985). Expression of the receptor for epidermal growth factor correlates with increased dosage of chromosome 7 in malignant melanoma. *Somat. Cell Mol. Genet.* **11**, 297–302.

Köck, A., Schwarz, T., Urbanski, A., Peng, Z., Vetterlein, M., Miksche, M., Ansel, J. C., Kung, H. F., and Luger, T. A. (1989). Expression and release of interleukin-1 by different human melanoma cell lines. *J. Natl. Cancer Inst.* **81**, 36–42.

Lauri, D., Bertomeu, M. C., Orr, F. W., Bastida, E., Sauder, D., and Buchanan, M. R. (1990). Interleukin-1 increases tumor cell adhesion to endothelial cells through an RGD-dependent mechanism: *In vitro* and *in vivo* studies. *Clin. Exp. Metastasis* **8**, 27–32.

Lawson, D. H., Thomas, H. G., Roy, R. G. B., Gordon, D. S., Chawla, R. K., Nixon, D. W., and Richmond, A. (1987). Preparation of a monoclonal antibody to a melanoma growth–stimulatory activity released into serum-free culture medium by Hs0294 malignant melanoma cells. *J. Cell. Biochem.* **34**, 169–185.

Legros, P. J., Coel, J., Doyen, A., Hanson, P., Van Tieghem, N., Vercammen-Grandjean, A., Fruhling, J., and Lejeune, F. J. (1981). Melanocyte–stimulating hormone binding and biologic activity in a melanoma cell line. *Cancer Res.* **41**, 1539–1544.

Lehmann, J. M., Holzmann, B., Breitbart, E. W., Schmiegelow, P., Riethmüller, G., and Johnson, J. P. (1987). Discrimination between benign and malignant cells of melanocytic lineage by two novel antigens, a glycoprotein with a molecular weight of 113,000 and a protein with a molecular weight of 76,000. *Cancer Res.* **47**, 841–845.

Lehmann, J. M., Riethmüller, G., and Johnson, J. P. (1989). MUC 18, a marker of tumor progression in human melanoma, shows sequence similarity to the neural cell adhesion molecules of the immunglobulin superfamily. *Proc. Natl. Acad. Sci. U.S.A.* **86,** 9891–9895.

Lightner, V. A., and Erickson, H. P. (1990). Binding of hexabrachion (tenascin) to the extracellular matrix and substratum and its effect on cell adhesion. *J. Cell Biol.* **95,** 263–277.

Linnenbach, A. J., Huebner, K., Reddy, E. P., Herlyn, M., Parmiter, A., Nowell, P. C., and Koprowski, H. (1988). Structural alteration in the MYB protooncogene and deletion within the gene encoding alpha-type protein kinase C in human melanoma cell lines. *Proc. Natl. Acad. Sci. U.S.A.* **85,** 74–78.

Macara, I. G. (1989). Oncogenes and cellular signal transduction. *Physiol. Rev.* **69,** 797–820.

Mackie, R. M., Cambell, I., and Turbitt, M. L. (1984). Use of NKI C3 monoclonal antibody in the assessment of benign and malignant melanocytic lesions. *J. Clin. Pathol.* **37,** 367–372.

Maeda, K., Yamada, K., and Jimbow, K. (1987). Development of MoAb HMSA-3 and HMSA-4 against human melanoma melanosomes and their reactivities on formalin-fixed melanoma tissue. *J. Invest. Dermatol.* **89,** 588–593.

Maio, M., Gulwani, B., Morgano, A., and Ferrone, S. (1989). Differential modulation by tumor necrosis factor and immune interferon of HLA class-II antigens expressed by melanoma cells. *Int. J. Cancer* **44,** 554–559.

Makgoba, M. W., Sanders, M. E., Luce, G. E. G., Dustin, M. L., Springer, T. A., Clark, E. A., Mannoni, P., and Shaw, S. (1988). ICAM-1, the ligand for LFA-1–dependent adhesion of B, T, and myeloid cells. *Nature (London)* **331,** 86–88.

Mancianti, M. L., and Herlyn, M. (1989). Tumor progression in melanoma: The biology of epidermal melanocytes *in vitro. In* "Skin Tumors: Experimental and Clinical Aspects" (C. J. Conti, T. J. Slaga, and A. J. P. Klein-Szanto, eds.), pp. 369–386. Raven Press, New York.

Mancianti, M. L., Clark, W. H., Jr., Hayes, F. A., and Herlyn, M. (1990). Malignant melanoma simultans arising in congenital melanocytic nevi do not show experimental evidence for a malignant phenotype. *Am. J. Pathol.* **136,** 817–829.

Mancianti, M. L., Herlyn, M., Weil, D., Jambrosic, J., Rodeck, U., Becker, D., Diamond, L., Clark, W. H., Jr., and Koprowski, H. (1988). Growth and phenotypic characteristics of human nevus cells in culture. *J. Invest. Dermatol.* **90,** 134–141.

Marquard, H., and Todaro, G. (1982). Human transforming growth factor production by a melanoma cell line; purification and initial characterization. *J. Biol. Chem.* **257,** 5220–5227.

McEwan, M., Parsons, P. G., and Moss, D. J. (1988). Monoclonal antibody against human tyrosinase and reactive with melanocytic and amelanotic melanoma cells. *J. Invest. Dermatol.* **90,** 515–519.

Morgan, A. C., Jr., Galloway, D. R., and Reisfeld, R. A. (1981). Production and characterization of monoclonal antibody to a melanoma-specific glycoprotein. *Hybridoma* **1,** 27–36.

Natali, P. G., Bigotti, A., Nicosta, M. R., Viora, M., and Ferrone, S. (1984). Phenotyping of lesions of melanocytic origin with monoclonal antibodies to melanoma-associated antigens and to the HLA-antigens. *J. Natl. Cancer Inst.* **73,** 13–24.

Natali, P. G., Nicotra, M. R., Bellocci, M., Cavaliere, R., and Bigotti, A. (1985). Distribution of laminin and collagen type IV in benign and malignant lesions of melanocytic origin. *Int. J. Cancer* **35,** 461–467.

Natali, P. G., Nicotra, M. R., Bigotti, A., Venturo, I., Marcenaro, L., Giacomini, P., and Russo, C. (1989). Selective changes in expression of HLA class I polymorphic determinants in human solid tumors. *Proc. Natl. Acad. Sci. U.S.A.* **86,** 6719–6723.

Natali, P., Nicotra, M. R., Cavaliere, R., Bigotti, A., Romano, G., Temponi, M., and Ferrone, S. (1990). Differential expression of intercellular adhesion molecule 1 in primary and metastatic melanoma lesions. *Cancer Res.* **50,** 1271–1278.

Nowell, P. C. (1976). The clonal evolution of tumor cell populations. *Science* **194,** 23–28.

Ogata, S., Furuhashi, Y., and Eisinger, M. (1987). Growth stimulation of human melanocytes:

Identification and characterization of melanoma-derived melanocyte growth factor (M-McGF). *Biochem. Biophys. Res. Commun.* **146**, 1204–1211.

Oikawa, S., Imajo, S., Noguchi, T., Kosaki, G., and Nakazato, H. (1987). The carcinoembryonic antigen (CEA) contains multiple immunglobulin-like domains. *Biochem. Biophys. Res. Commun.* **144**, 634–642.

Packard, B. S. (1987). Identification of a synthetic nonapeptide sequence that inhibits motility in culture of a melanoma subclone that possesses a high metastatic potential. *Proc. Natl. Acad. Sci. U.S.A.* **84**, 9015–9019.

Parmiter, A. H., Balaban, G., Herlyn, M., Clark, W. H., Jr., and Nowell, P. C. (1986). A t(1;19) chromosome translocation in three cases of human malignant melanoma. *Cancer Res.* **46**, 1526–1529.

Pierat, M. E., Najdovski, T., Appelboom, T. E., and Deschodt-Lanckman, M. M. (1988). Effect of human endopeptidase 24.11 ("enkephalinase") on IL-1-induced thymocyte proliferation assay. *J. Immunol.* **140**, 3808–3811.

Rakowicz-Szulczynska, E. M., and Koprowski, H. (1989). Nuclear uptake of monoclonal antibody to a surface glycoprotein and its effect on transcription. *Arch. Biochem. Biophys.* **268**, 366–379.

Ranson, M., Posen, S., and Mason, R. S. (1988). Human melanocytes as a target tissue for hormones: *In vitro* studies with 1-alpha-25, dihydroxyvitamin D_3, alpha-melanocyte stimulating hormone, and beta-estradiol. *J. Invest. Dermatol.* **91**, 593–598.

Real, F. X., Houghton, A. N., Albino, A. P., Cordon-Cardo, C., Melamed, M. R., Oettgen, H. F., and Old, L. J. (1985). Surface antigens of melanomas and melanocytes defined by mouse monoclonal antibodies: Specificity analysis and comparison of antigen expression in cultured cells and tissues. *Cancer Res.* **45**, 4401–4411.

Rice, G. E., and Bevilacqua, M. P. (1989). An inducible endothelial cell-surface glycoprotein mediates melanoma adhesion. *Science* **246**, 1303–1306.

Richardson, D. R., and Baker, E. (1990). The uptake of iron and transferrin by the human malignant melanoma cell. *Biochem. Biophys. Acta* **1053**, 1–12.

Richmond, A., Fine, R., Murray, D., Lawson, D. H., and Priest, J. H. (1986). Growth factor and cytogenetic abnormalities in cultured nevi and malignant melanomas. *J. Invest. Dermatol.* **86**, 295–302.

Richmond, A., Balentien, E., Thomas, H. G., Flaggs, G., Barton, D. E., Spiess, J., Bordoni, R., Francke, U., and Derynck, R. (1988). Molecular characterization and chromosomal mapping of melanoma growth stimulatory activity, a growth factor structurally related to beta-thromboglobulin. *EMBO J.* **7**, 2025–2033.

Rodeck, U., Herlyn, M., and Koprowski, H. (1987a). Interactions between growth factor receptors and corresponding monoclonal antibodies in human tumors. *J. Cell Biochem.* **35**, 315–320.

Rodeck, U., Herlyn, M., Menssen, H. D., Furlanetto, R. W., and Koprowski, H. (1987b). Metastatic but not primary melanoma cells grow *in vitro* independently of exogenous growth factors. *Int. J. Cancer* **40**, 687–690.

Rodeck, U., Melber, K., Kath, R., Menssen, H. D., Varello, M., Atkinson, B., and Herlyn, M. (1990). Heterogeneity of growth factor and cytokine production by melanoma cells. *Cancer Res.*, submitted.

Rose, T. M., Plowman, G. D., Teplow, D. B., Dreyer, W. J., Hellström, K. E., and Brown, J. P. (1986). Primary structure of the human melanoma–associated antigen p97 (melanotransferrin) deduced from the mRNA sequence. *Proc. Natl. Acad. Sci. U.S.A.* **83**, 1261–1265.

Ross, A. H., Cossu, G., Herlyn, M., Bell, J. R., Steplewski, Z., and Koprowski, H. (1983). Isolation and chemical characterization of a melanoma-associated proteoglycan antigen. *Arch. Biochem. Biophys.* **225**, 370–383.

Ross, A. H., Herlyn, M., Maul, G. G., Koprowski, H., Bothwell, M., Chao, M., Pleasure, D., and

Sonnenfield, K. H. (1985). The nerve growth–factor receptor in normal and transformed neural crest cells. *Ann. N.Y. Acad. Sci.* **486,** 115–123.

Ruoslahti, E., and Pierschbacher, M. D. (1987). New perspectives in cell adhesion: RDG and integrins. *Science* **238,** 491–497.

Shukla, V. K., Hughes, D. C., McCormick, F., and Padua, R. A. (1989). *Ras* mutations in human melanotic lesions: K-*ras* activation is a frequent and early event in melanoma development. *Oncogene Res.* **5,** 121–127.

Siegrist, W., Solca, F., Stutz, S., Giuffre, S., Carrel, J., Girard, J., and Eberle, A. N. (1989). Characterization of receptors for alpha-melanocyte-stimulating hormone on human melanoma cells. *Cancer Res.* **49,** 6352–6358.

Sikora, L. K. J., Pinto, A., Demetrick, D. J., Dixon, W. T., Urbanski, S. J., Temple, W., and Jerry, L. M. (1987). Characterization of a novel neuroglandular antigen (NGA) expressed on abnormal human melanocytes. *Int. J. Cancer* **39,** 138–145.

Singletary, S. E., Baker, F. L., Spitzer, G., Tucker, S. L., Tomasovic, B., Brock, W. A., Ajani, J. A., and Kelly, A. M. (1987). Biologic effect of epidermal growth factor on the *in vitro* growth of human tumors. *Cancer Res.* **47,** 403–406.

Sporn, M. B., Roberts, A. B., Wakefield, L. M., and de Crombrugghe, B. (1987). Some recent advances in the chemistry and biology of transforming growth factor-beta. *J. Cell Biol.* **105,** 1039–1045.

Tanigushi, K., Kärre, K., and Klein, G. (1985). Lung colonization and metastasis by disseminated B16 melanoma cells: H-2 associated control at the level of the host and the tumor cell. *Int. J. Cancer* **36,** 503–510.

Tatro, J. B., Atkins, M., Mier, J. W., Hardarson, S., Wolfe, H., Smith, T., Entwistle, M. L., and Reichlin, S. (1990). Melanotropin receptors demonstrated *in situ* in human melanoma. *J. Clin. Invest.* **85,** 1825–1832.

Theillet, C., Le Roy, X., De Lapeyriere, O., Grosgeorges, J., Adname, J., Raynaud, S. D., Simony-Lafontaine, J., Goldfarb, M., Escot, C., Birnbaum, D., and Gaudray, P. (1989). Amplification of FGF-related genes in human tumors: Possible involvement of HST in breast carcinomas. *Oncogene* **4,** 915–922.

Thomson, T. M., Real, F. X., Murakami, S., Cordon-Cardo, C., Old, L. J., and Houghton, A. N. (1988). Differentiation antigens of melanocytes and melanoma: Analysis of melanosome and cell-surface markers of human pigmented cells with monoclonal antibodies. *J. Invest. Dermatol.* **90,** 459–466.

Thurin, J., Thurin, M., Herlyn, M., Elder, D. E., Steplewski, Z., Clark, W. H., Jr., and Koprowski, H. (1986). GD2 ganglioside biosynthesis is a distinct biochemical event in human melanoma tumor progression. *FEBS Lett.* **208,** 17–22.

Trent, J. M., Meyskens, F. L., Salmon, S. E., Ryschon, K., Leong, S. P. L., Davis, J. R., and McGee, D. L. (1990). Relation of cytogenetic abnormalities and clinical outcome in metastatic melanoma. *N. Engl. J. Med.* **322,** 1508–1511.

Valyi-Nagy, I., and Herlyn, M. (1991). Regulation of growth and phenotype of normal human melanocytes in culture. *In* "Melanoma research: Genetics, growth factors, metastases, and antigens" (L. Nathanson, ed.), pp. 85–101. Kluwer Academic Publishers, Boston, MA.

van Eldik, L. J., Zendegin, J. G., Marshak, D. R., and Watterson, D. M. (1982). Calcium-binding proteins and molecular basis of calcium action. *Int. Rev. Cytol.* **77,** 1–61.

van Muijen, G. N. P., Ruiter, D. J., Hoefakker, S., and Johnson, J. P. (1990). Monoclonal antibody PAL-M1 recognizes the transferrin receptor and is a progression marker in melanocytic lesions. *J. Invest. Dermatol.* **95,** 65–69.

Van't Veer, L. J., Burgering, B. M. T., Versteeg, R., Boot, A. J. M., Ruiter, D. J., Osanto, S., Schrier, P. I., and Bos, J. L. (1989). N-*ras* mutations in human cutaneous melanoma from sun-exposed body sites. *Mol. Cell. Biol.* **9,** 3114–3116.

Versteeg, R., Pletenburg, L. T. C., Plomp, A. C., and Schrier, P. (1989). High expression of the c-*myc* oncogene renders melanoma cells prone to lysis by natural killer cells. *J. Immunol.* **143,** 4331–4337.

Vijayasaradhi, S., Bouchard, B., and Houghton, A. N. (1990). The melanoma antigen gp 75 is the human homologue of the mouse b (BROWN) locus gene product. *J. Exp. Med.* **171,** 1375–1380.

Waterfield, M. D., Scarce, G. T., Whittle, N., Stroobant, P., Johnsson, A., Wasteson, A., Westermark, B., Heldin, C.-H., Huang, J. S., and Deuel, T. F. (1983). Platelet-derived growth factor is structurally related to the putative transforming protein p²⁸ *sis* of simian sarcoma virus. *Nature* **304,** 35–39.

Westermark, B., Johnsson, A., Paulsson, Y., Betsholtz, C., Heldin, C.-H., Herlyn, M., Rodeck, U., and Koprowski, H. (1986). Human melanoma cell lines of primary and metastatic origin express the genes encoding the chains of platelet-derived growth factor (PDGF) and produce a PDGF-like growth factor. *Proc. Natl. Acad. Sci. U.S.A.* **83,** 7197–7200.

Wittbrodt, J., Adam, D., Malitschek, B., Mäueler, W., Raulf, F., Telling, A., Robertson, S. M., and Schartl, M. (1989). Novel putative receptor tyrosine kinase encoded by the melanoma-inducing Tu locus in *Xiphophorus*. *Nature (London)* **341,** 415–421.

Yohn, J. J., Critelli, M., Lyons, M. B., and Norris, D. A. (1990). Modulation of melanocyte intercellular adhesion molecule-1 by immune cytokines. *J. Invest. Dermatol.* **90,** 233–237.

Chapter 6

Glutathione Transferases in Normal, Preneoplastic, and Neoplastic Tissues: Forms and Functions

Kiyomi Sato and Shigeki Tsuchida

Second Department of Biochemistry, Hirosaki University School of Medicine, Hirosaki 036, Japan

I. Introduction

The glutathione transferases (glutathione *S*-transferases, GSTs; EC 2.5.1.18) are a family of multifunctional proteins, which act as enzymes and also as binding (carrier) proteins in various detoxication processes (see reviews by Jakoby, 1978; Chasseaud, 1979; Mannervik, 1985; Mannervik and Danielson, 1988; Coles and Ketterer, 1990), although recent studies have also shown that some glutathione and cysteine conjugates, mostly of halogenated hydrocarbons, can be of toxicological concern (Inskeep and Guengerich, 1984; Kim and Guengerich, 1990; see also reviews by Pickett and Lu, 1989; Coles and Ketterer, 1990). Glutathione transferases catalyze the nucleophilic attack of the sulfur atom of reduced glutathione by electrophilic groups in a second substrate; thus, they catalyze the first step in the mercapturic acid pathway, which is one of the most important detoxication processes in phase II drug metabolism.

Many molecular forms of glutathione transferase have been identified from various organs in a variety of species (see reviews by Mannervik, 1985; Mannervik and Danielson, 1988; Sato, 1989; Pickett and Lu, 1989; Coles and Ketterer, 1990). In particular, rat, human, and mouse glutathione transferases have been

BIOCHEMICAL AND MOLECULAR ASPECTS
OF SELECTED CANCERS, VOL. 1

TABLE I
MOLECULAR FORMS OF RAT GLUTATHIONE TRANSFERASE

Class[a]	Nomenclature		pI as dimer		Subunit M_r		Gene[b]		
	c	d	e	f	g	h	Exon	Intron	Size (kb)
Alpha	1-1	YaYa	10	(9.8)	25,000	25,434/25,474 (221)[i]	7	6	10
	1-2	YaYc	9.9	(9.7)					
	2-2	YcYc	9.8	(9.6)	28,000	25,209 (220)			
	8-8	YkYk	6.1	(5.8)	24,500				
	10-10[j]		9.6		25,500				
	?	YsYs[k]		(5.8)	26,000				
Mu	3-3	Yb_1Yb_1	8.9	(8.8)	26,500	25,806/25,802 (217)	8	7	5
	3-4	Yb_1Yb_2	8.0	(8.4)					
	4-4	Yb_2Yb_2	6.9	(8.2)	26,500	25,592 (217)	8	7	5
	6-6	$Yn_1Yn_1(Yb_3Yb_3)$		(6.2)	26,000	25,549 (217)			
	6-9	Yn_1Yn_2	5.8	(5.7)	26,000				
	3-6	Yb_1Yn_1	?	(8.3)					
	4-6	Yb_2Yn_1	?	(6.2)					
	9-9	Yn_2Yn_2	?	(5.4)	26,000				
	11-11[j]	YoYo	5.2		27,000				
Pi	7-7(P)[l]	YfYf,YpYp[l]	7.0	(8.3)	24,000	23,307 (209)	7	6	3
Theta	5-5		7.3		26,500				
	12-12[m]		?		26,000				
	?	YrsYrs[n]	7.9		26,000				
Microsomal[o]			10.1		14,000	17,430 (154)			

[a] Mannervik et al. (1985a).
[b] Pickett and Lu (1989).
[c] Jakoby et al. (1984).
[d] Mannervik (1985), and Hayes and Mantle (1986a).
[e] By isoelectric focusing.
[f] By chromatofocusing.
[g] Subunit molecular weight by SDS-gel electrophoresis (Mannervik, 1985; Sato, 1989).
[h] Subunit molecular weight deduced from cDNA (Mannervik and Danielson, 1988; Sato, 1989).
[i] In parenthesis, number of amino acid residues excluding NH₂-terminal methionine.
[j] Kispert et al. (1989).
[k] Tsuchida and Sato (1990).
[l] Sato et al. (1984a,b).
[m] Meyer et al. (1991).
[n] Hiratsuka et al. (1990).
[o] Morgenstern and DePierre (1983).

extensively investigated. Although particulate-bound glutathione transferases are known, most of the purified forms are localized in the cytosol as homodimeric or heterodimeric proteins, and they can be grouped in a species-independent classification (Mannervik *et al.*, 1985).

Glutathione transferases, including ligandin (a mixture of GSTs 1-1 and 1-2, shown in Table I), first identified as a binding protein for steroid hormones, bilirubin, and azodyes (Litwack *et al.*, 1971), have multipotential detoxifying functions. Many investigators of chemical carcinogenesis, therefore, have been stimulated to study changes in molecular forms and their roles in the metabolism of carcinogens (see reviews by Smith *et al.*, 1977; Jakoby, 1978; Chasseaud, 1979; Sato, 1989; Coles and Ketterer, 1990).

Recently, glutathione transferases have been investigated for elucidation of the mechanisms of chemoprevention of chemical carcinogenesis and (multi)-anticancer drug resistance (Hayes *et al.*, 1990a). Furthermore, some of the forms such as rat GST-P (7-7) and human GST-π have drawn attention as reliable preneoplastic or neoplastic marker enzymes, the existence of which facilitates analysis of carcinogenic processes and provides the basis for new methods of screening for carcinogens and carcinogenic modifiers. Their mechanisms of expression are current topics in relation to oncogene activation.

This chapter focuses on changes in molecular forms of glutathione transferase in preneoplastic and neoplastic tissues in the rat, mouse and man; their functions are also reviewed (see also the earlier review by Sato, 1989).

II. Molecular Forms of Glutathione Transferase and Their Expression and Functions in Normal Tissues

A. IDENTIFICATION AND CLASSIFICATION OF MOLECULAR FORMS

1. *Purification*

Most of the known cytosolic glutathione transferases can be highly purified by S-hexylglutathione–bound Sepharose affinity chromatography (Guthenberg and Mannervik, 1979) followed by isoelectric focusing (Hales *et al.*, 1978; Awasthi *et al.*, 1980) or chromatofocusing (Mannervik and Jensson, 1982), which allow separation of individual forms. A few forms, such as rat GST-E or (5-5) (Meyer *et al.*, 1984) and GST-YkYk (8-8) (Hayes, 1986; Jensson *et al.*, 1986) are not adsorbed on the above affinity column, but the latter is adsorbed on glutathione-bound Sepharose columns (Hayes, 1986). Some forms, such as rat GST-P (7-7), are not easily separable from other forms by isoelectric focusing or chromatofocusing, but have been purified in combination with ion-exchange chromatography (Satoh *et al.*, 1985b). Fast protein liquid chromatography is also useful for the separation of glutathione transferases (Alin *et al.*,

1985; Ketterer *et al.*, 1986; Tateoka *et al.*, 1987). A new rat form, GST-YrsYrs, described by Hiratsuka *et al.* (1990), was not at all adsorbed on an S-hexylglutathione-Sepharose column, but could be purified using a combination of several steps, including ion-exchange chromatography, chromatofocusing, blue Sepharose column chromatography, and gel filtration high-performance liquid chromatography. A mouse form ($Ya_1 Ya_1$, later corrected as $Ya_1 Ya_2$), which did not bind to either S-hexylglutathione– or glutathione–Sepharose columns, was purified using bromosulfophthalein-glutathione-Sepharose (McLellan and Hayes, 1989, 1990).

1-Chloro-2,4-dinitrobenzene (CDNB) has been used as a universal substrate for many glutathione transferase isoenzymes. However, rat GSTs 5-5/12-12 and GST-YrsYrs, all of which may belong to a new class, have exceptionally negligible activity toward CDNB, but have high activity toward certain alkyl epoxides [e.g., 1,2-epoxy-3-(p-nitrophenoxy)propane] and arylmethyl sulfates, respectively (Meyer *et al.*, 1991; Hiratsuka *et al.*, 1990).

2. Identification of Subunit Composition

The subunits of glutathione transferases have been separated into monomers under denaturing conditions by sodium dodecyl sulfate (SDS)–polyacrylamide gel electrophoresis (Bass *et al.*, 1977); these subunits were named Ya, Yb and Yc, in order of increasing apparent molecular weight. Subunits are also separable by isoelectric focusing in polyacrylamide gel or two-dimensional polyacrylamide gel electrophoresis (Kitahara *et al.*, 1983a, 1984; Satoh *et al.*, 1985a). Recently, reverse-phase, high-performance liquid chromatography has been used for isolation of subunits of this enzyme (Ostlund-Farrants *et al.*, 1987; see also a review by Coles and Ketterer, 1990). Following SDS-polyacrylamide electrophoresis or two-dimensional polyacrylamide electrophoresis, the immuno-(Western) blotting method is effective for identification of subunits and comparison of immunochemical properties between a new form and previously identified ones. Primary structures (whole amino acid sequences) of GST subunits obtained from base sequences of the cDNAs supply more precise information on homology or diversity among the subunits in the same and different species.

3. Species-Independent Classification

Mannervik *et al.* (1985) demonstrated that the major isoenzymes of cytosolic glutathione transferases from the rat, mouse, and man share structural catalytic properties, on the basis of which they proposed a species-independent classification. Isoenzymes from these species were grouped with respect to NH_2-terminal amino acid sequences, substrate specificities, sensitivities to inhibitors and immunological crossreactivities by immunodiffusion or immunoblotting into three Alpha, Mu and Pi classes. Each of the three mammalian animal species contains at least one isoenzyme of each class. The efficacy of this classification has been confirmed by other groups and is now being used for comparative identification and classification of new forms. A new class (family) Theta, which includes rat GST 5-5 and 12-12 (Meyer *et al.*, 1991) and also probably GST-YrsYrs (Hiratsuka *et al.*, 1990), has been proposed by Meyer *et al.* (1991) (see Table I).

B. RAT GLUTATHIONE TRANSFERASES

1. *Molecular Forms*

Rat glutathione transferases have been most extensively investigated. Most of the rat glutathione transferases are localized in the cytosol of various tissues, with the exception of one form purified from rat microsomal fractions (see the review by Morgenstern and DePierre, 1988). An as yet unidentified form, involved in the synthesis of leukotriene C_4, which catalyzes glutathione conjugation of leukotriene A_4, has also been reported to be present in membrane fractions of leukemia cells (Jakschik *et al.*, 1982; Bach *et al.*, 1984; Yoshimoto *et al.*, 1985). Prostaglandin-H D-isomerase (EC 5.3.99.2), with glutathione transferase activity toward CDNB, was purified from the cytosol fraction of rat spleen (Christ-Hazelhof and Nugteren, 1979; Urade *et al.*, 1987), and was found to differ immunologically from other known cytosolic glutathione transferases. Tsuchida *et al.* (1990) also identified a new form, YsYs in the Alpha class, from rat spleen. Hiratsuka *et al.* (1990) identified a unique form from rat cytosol, which is one of the three forms possessing only glutathione conjugation activity toward arylmethyl sulfates, reactive metabolites of carcinogenic arylmethanols. GST-E, which was named GST 5-5 in a new nomenclature (Jakoby *et al.*, 1984), but recently suggested to be not identical with 5-5 (Meyer *et al.*, 1991), GST 12-12, and probably also GST-YrsYrs, belong to a new class (Theta). GST 12-12 is different from GST-YrsYrs in the NH_2-terminal amino acid sequence; the thirteenth amino acid residue of subunit Yrs is serine, while that of subunit 12 is cysteine (Hiratsuka *et al.*, 1990; Meyer *et al.*, 1991). GST 11-11 is a labile form in the Mu class, which was purified from rat testis (Kispert *et al.*, 1989).

At least 19 molecular forms of cytosolic glutathione transferase and 14 different subunits have been identified from rat tissues (see Table I), and new forms continue to be reported.

Rat glutathione transferases have been given several different names (see review by Sato, 1989), but can be defined by their isoelectric points, subunit molecular weights on SDS–polyacrylamide gel electrophoresis and immunological properties using the immunoblot method (Hayes and Mantle, 1986a,b; Tsuchida *et al.*, 1987). The double immunodiffusion test, however, is still used for distinguishing between immuno-related forms (Tsuchida *et al.*, 1987). Hybridization between different subunits is also useful for detection of structural relationships between glutathione transferases (Kitahara and Sato, 1981; Ishikawa *et al.*, 1988).

Molecular weights of subunits were estimated by SDS–polyacrylamide gel electrophoresis according to the various marker proteins used (Sato, 1989). However, the value varies dependent on the acrylamide composition of the resolving gel (Hayes and Mantle, 1986b). Recently, NH_2-terminal amino acid sequencing was used for the identification of new forms, based on the suggestion of Mannervik *et al.* (1985).

In the nomenclature proposed by Jakoby *et al.* (1984), rat GST subunits have been assigned a number that refers to the order in which they were isolated and characterized (Table I). One form (GST 6-6), a major form in the rat testis, however, was corrected to GST 6-9, after the finding that it is in fact a heterodimer, $Yn_1 Yn_2$ (Tsuchida *et al.*, 1987; Ishikawa *et al.*, 1988). A homodimer GST-$Yn_1 Yn_1$ (6-6) with high leukotriene C_4 synthase activity was found in brain cytosol (Tsuchida *et al.*, 1987) and seems identical with $Yb_3 Yb_3$ deduced from cDNA (Abramovitz and Listowsky, 1987). Names such as Ya Ya (see Table I), which were first used by Bass *et al.* (1977) to indicate the subunit composition based on separation by SDS–polyacrylamide gel electrophoresis, are still used.

Subunits 1 and 8 have each been described to be separable into two distinct forms by high-performance liquid chromatography analysis (Coles and Ketterer, 1990; Hayes *et al.*, 1990b). Heterogeneity in subunit 1 has also been observed in cDNA clones (Pickett *et al.*, 1984a; Lai *et al.*, 1984).

2. Tissue Distribution

Tissue-specific expression of rat GST subunits has been described (Mannervik, 1985; Hayes and Mantle, 1986a; Tu and Qian, 1987; Pickett and Lu, 1989; Sato, 1989). Liver and kidney are the only tissues in which subunit 1 is abundantly expressed; it contributes to high glutathione transferase activity. In the kidney, the Alpha class (Subunits 1, 2, and 8) is abundantly expressed, while the Mu class (subunits 3 and 4) occurs at a low level. In the lung, subunits 2 and 8 (Alpha class) and 3 and 4 (Mu class) are expressed, but subunit 1 is undetectable. In some tissues one subunit predominates; e.g., subunit 7 in the small intestine, subunit 2 in the lactating mammary gland and the adrenal gland. Immunohistochemically, although subunits 1, 2, 3, and 4 are detectable in all hepatocytes in the normal liver, they are more abundant around the central vein than in the periportal region (Tatematsu *et al.*, 1985). Developmental changes in the isoenzyme composition in the liver are well known (McCusker *et al.*, 1989; Coles and Ketterer, 1990). In the late fetal liver, subunit 10 (YcYfetus) with subunit 2 is representative of the Alpha class, having high Se-independent glutathione peroxidase activity (Scott and Kirsch, 1987). Subunit Yk (8) is constantly expressed at relatively high levels during fetal and adult periods. Subunit Yf (7) is expressed only in the fetal liver (McCusker *et al.*, 1989).

Sex differences in the subunit composition in the liver have also been described (Igarashi et al., 1985, Igarashi and Satoh, 1989). In males, subunits 3 and 4 in the Mu class are the most abundant, followed by subunits 1 and 2 in the Alpha class, while subunits 3 and 4 are the lowest in females.

3. Induction by Drugs

Rat glutathione transferase subunits are preferentially induced by various drugs, including carcinogens and anticarcinogenic agents such as butylated hydroxyanisole (BHA), as summarized in Table II. Subunits 1 and 3 are inducible by almost all drugs examined. The glutathione transferase isoenzymes are known to be induced in a different manner by treatment with phenobarbital (PB) and 3-methylcholanthrene (3-MC), which are well-known enzyme inducers having different properties regarding induction of drug-metabolizing enzymes. The induction of subunit 3 (Yb_1) by 3-MC or β-naphthoflavone (β-NF) is not remark-

TABLE II
INDUCTION OF RAT HEPATIC GLUTATHIONE TRANSFERASES BY DRUGS

Inducer	Subunit				
	1	2	3	4	7
3'-Me-DAB[a,b]	↑	→	↑	→	→
AAF[a]	↑	→	↑	→	→
BHA[a,c,d]	↑	→	↑	→	↑[m]
Ethoxyquin[e,f]	↑	→	↑	→	↑[m]
Phenobarbital[b,g]	↑	→	↑	→	→
3-Methylcholanthrene[g]	↑	→	→	→	→
β-Naphthoflavone[h]	↑				
trans-Stilbene oxide[i]	↑	→	↑	→	↑
Oltipraz[j]	↑		↑		
Selenium deficiency[k]	↑	↑	→	→	
Lead nitrate[l]					↑ ↑

[a]Kitahara et al., 1984.
[b]Satoh et al., 1985b.
[c]Sato et al., 1984b.
[d]Tatematsu et al., 1985.
[e]Kensler et al., 1986.
[f]Thamavit et al., 1985.
[g]Igarashi et al., 1987.
[h]Pickett and Lu, 1989.
[i]Tahir et al., 1989.
[j]Davidson et al., 1990.
[k]Chang et al., 1990.
[l]Sato, 1988.
[m]Detected by immunohistochemistry.

able at the protein level, but is significant at the mRNA level (Pickett and Lu, 1989). Talalay *et al.* (1988) have suggested a common chemical signal (an electrophilic olefin or related electron-deficient center) regulating the induction of Phase II enzymes, including glutathione transferase, that protect against chemical carcinogenesis.

4. *Gene Structure and Regulation*

cDNAs of rat glutathione transferase subunits 1 (Ya) (Pickett *et al.*, 1984a; Lai *et al.*, 1984), 2 (Yc) (Telakowski-Hopkins *et al.*, 1985), 3 (Yb_1) (Ding *et al.*, 1985; Lai *et al.*, 1986), 4 (Yb_2) (Lai and Tu, 1986; Ding *et al.*, 1986), Yb_3 (Abramovitz and Listowsky, 1987), which may be identical with Yn_1 (subunit 6) (Ishikawa *et al.*, 1988), and 7 (Yp) (Suguoka *et al.*, 1985; Pemble *et al.*, 1986) and genomic DNAs of subunits 1 (Telakowski *et al.*, 1986), 3 (Morton *et al.*, 1990), 4 (Lai *et al.*, 1988) and 7 (Okuda *et al.*, 1987) have been cloned (Table I) (see also reviews by Mannervik and Danielson, 1988; Pickett and Lu, 1989; Sato, 1989). The cDNA of a rat microsomal glutathione transferase has also been cloned (DeJong *et al.*, 1988b). The primary structures of subunits can be deduced from respective cDNA base sequences. Molecular weights and numbers of amino acid residues, not including NH_2-terminal methionine, are shown in Table I. Within a class (family), even among different species, protein-coding regions are highly homologous (70–80%), while the 5' and 3' untranslated regions are very divergent. A small amino acid region (a 70–95 amino acid sequence from the NH_2-terminus) of the Ya subunit, which is encoded by exon 4 of the Ya structural gene, was found to be conserved between the Ya and Yc (Tu and Quian, 1986) and was suggested to be the glutathione-binding domain (Pickett and Lu, 1989).

Two Ya cDNA clones have been isolated: pGTB38 (Pickett *et al.*, 1984a) and pGTR261 (Lai *et al.*, 1984). Recently, Hayes *et al.* (1990b) isolated two Ya-type subunits, Ya_1 and Ya_2, and suggested that these subunits are encoded by pGTR261 and pGT38, respectively.

Pickett and his colleagues have investigated the mechanisms of regulation of glutathione transferases, especially of subunit 1 (Ya) (Telakowski-Hopkins *et al.*, 1988; see reviews by Pickett, 1987; Pickett and Lu, 1989). Rushmore *et al.* (1990) have identified three regulatory regions in the 5'-flanking sequence of the Ya subunit gene; the first region located from -867 to -857 contributing to the maximum basal level of the Ya gene, the second localized from -908 to -899 being the xenobiotic-response element (XRE), which is also found in 5' flanking region of cytochrome P-450IA1 gene, and the third localized -722 to -682 (β-naphthoflavone–responsive element) being important for β-naphthoflavone–inducible expression. The mechanisms of regulation of GST-P gene expression will be described later.

5. *Functions*

Functions of glutathione transferases as enzymes and binding (presumable carrier) proteins have been investigated mainly for rat forms. Glutathione transferases basically catalyze the glutathione conjugation reaction of electrophilic compounds, which are produced from many exogenous xenobiotics by biotransformation (Chasseaud, 1979; Coles and Ketterer, 1990), but also arise from endogenous substances (Mannervik, 1985; Igwe, 1986; Mannervik and Danielson, 1988). The glutathione conjugation reaction is the first step of the mercapturic acid pathway (Booth *et al.*, 1961; Boyland and Chasseaud, 1969; Chasseaud, 1979; Pickett and Lu, 1989), which is one of the most important detoxication processes. The second step of this pathway is catalyzed by γ-glutamyltransferase (EC 2.3.2.2), which has been used as one of the markers for putative preneoplastic hepatic foci in the rat (Sato, 1989). Ligandin (GST 1-1) has Δ^5-3-keto-steroid isomerase activity toward Δ^5-androstene-3,17-dione (Benson *et al.*, 1977). In addition, certain forms, such as rat GSTs 1-2, 2-2, 5-5, and 7-7, are known to possess selenium-independent glutathione peroxidase activity toward lipid peroxides (Kitahara *et al.*, 1983b; Meyer *et al.*, 1985; see reviews by Ketterer, 1986 and Ketterer *et al.*, 1987, 1989). GST 8-8 has high activity toward 4-hydroxynonenal, which is one of the most potent aldehyde products of lipid peroxidation (Jensson *et al.*, 1986; Danielson *et al.*, 1987). Some cytosolic glutathione transferases are also known to be involved in leukotriene (e.g., GST 6-6) and prostaglandin (GST 1-1) metabolism in the rat (Sato, 1989).

In addition, since ligandin was first identified as a basic form of glutathione transferase (Habig *et al.*, 1974), this and other forms have similarly been demonstrated to act as binding or carrier proteins for several dyes (bilirubin, bromosulfophthalein, and indocyanine green), cholic acid, steroid hormones, hematin (heme), and carcinogens (azodyes, 3-methylcholanthrene) (Smith *et al.*, 1977; Jakoby, 1978; Smith and Litwack, 1980; Maruyama and Listowsky, 1984; Senjo *et al.*, 1985; Homma *et al.*, 1986; Listowsky *et al.*, 1988), and for leukotriene C_4 (Sun *et al.*, 1986). Each GST subunit may perform particular functions as enzyme and/or binding protein independent of the other subunit composing the same molecular form (Sato, 1989). Specific activities and functions of respective forms toward activated carcinogen metabolites will be described below.

C. HUMAN GLUTATHIONE TRANSFERASES

1. *Molecular Forms*

Human glutathione transferases have been divided into basic, neutral, and acidic groups. However, the recent discovery of several new forms makes this classification inappropriate. So far at least 14 forms have been isolated from the cytosol and classified into the Alpha, Mu, and Pi classes (see Table III). In the

TABLE III

MOLECULAR FORMS OF HUMAN GLUTATHIONE TRANSFERASE

Class	Nomenclature			Subunit (M_r)	pI	Tissue distribution
Alpha	B_1B_1[a],	2-type 1[b]		26,000	9.1–8.9	Liver, kidney
	B_1B_2,	2-type 2-1		26,000	8.7	
	B_2B_2,	2-type 2		26,000	8.4	
	2-2[c]			28,500	9.9	Skin
	ω[d]			26,000	5.0	Liver
Mu	μ[e],	1-type 2	M_3M_3[f]	27,000	6.6	Liver
		1-type 2-1		27,000	?	
	ψ[g],	1-type 1		27,000	5.5	
		4[h,i]	N_2N_2	26,500	5.3	Muscle, heart
			M_3N_2	27,000, 26,500	5.6	Heart, brain
			M_1M_2	27,000, 27,000	8.3	Aorta
			M_2N_1	27,000, 26,500	6.6	Aorta
		5.2[j]		27,000	5.2	Testis
Pi	π[k],	3	ρ[l], λ[m]	24,500	4.8	Placenta, kidney, lung
Microsomal[n]				17,300	?	Liver

[a]Stockman et al., 1985.
[b]Board, 1981.
[c]del Boccio et al., 1987.
[d]Singhal et al., 1990.
[e]Warholm et al., 1981, 1983.
[f]Tsuchida et al., 1990.
[g]Singh et al., 1987b.
[h]Laisney et al., 1984.
[i]Board et al., 1988.
[j]Campbell et al., 1990.
[k]Guthenberg and Mannervik, 1981.
[l]Marcus et al., 1978.
[m]Hayes, 1986.
[n]McLellan et al., 1989.

Alpha class, five forms with pI values of 9.0 to 7.5 (α–ε) were resolved from human liver by Kamisaka et al. (1975), but the subunit structures were not clarified. Stockman et al. (1985) identified two basic homodimers and one heterodimer consisting of two subunits, B_1 and B_2, with the same molecular weights, but with different pIs and enzymatic properties. These two subunits were also reported by Soma et al. (1986). A basic form (pI 9.9) detected in the skin was homologous with rat GST 2-2 and grouped into this class (Del Boccio et al., 1987). Singhal et al. (1990) have reported that GST-ω, with a pI of 5.0, is a member of the Alpha class.

So far, eight molecular forms have been identified in the Mu class. GST-μ (pI 6.6), a homodimer with a subunit molecular weight of 27,000, has been reported as a neutral form (Warholm *et al.*, 1981), which is present in about 60% of adult human livers. GST-ψ, which is immunologically related to GST-μ but more acidic (pI 5.5), has also been reported (Awasthi *et al.*, 1980; Singh *et al.*, 1987b). On the other hand, Board (1981) separated three GST bands by starch gel electrophoresis: GST 1-type 2, 1-type 2-1, and 1-type 1, and thus demonstrated genetic polymorphism for GST-1. GST-μ and GST-ψ seem to correspond to GST 1-type 2 and 1-type 1, respectively, GST 1-type 2-1 being a heterodimer of GST-μ and GST-ψ. GST-4, noted in human muscle on starch gel electrophoresis (Laisney *et al.*, 1984), is a homodimer with a subunit molecular weight of 26,500, slightly smaller than that of GST-μ (Board *et al.*, 1988). The presence of a heterodimer consisting of GST-μ and GST-4 subunits, suggested by Laisney *et al.* (1984), has been demonstrated as GST-M_3N_2 by Tsuchida *et al.* (1990). This heterodimer may be identical with GST-5 since the two forms have very similar mobilities on electrophoresis (Laisney *et al.*, 1984). GST-M_1M_2 and GST-M_2N_1, with denitration activity toward nitroglycerin, have been isolated from the human aorta (Tsuchida *et al.*, 1990), suggesting that they are involved in vasodilation by this compound. Tsuchida *et al.* (1990) have identified five subunits: M_1, M_2, M_3, N_1, and N_2. M_1 to M_3 have the same molecular weight but different pIs; N_1 and N_2 also have different pIs. GST-5.2 has been isolated from the human testis and brain, the subunit molecular weight being slightly larger than that of GST-μ (Campbell *et al.*, 1990).

GST-π, found to be very similar to the acidic GST-ρ isolated from human erythrocytes (Marcus *et al.*, 1978), was purified from the placenta (Guthenberg and Mannervik, 1981), this being the only form of the Pi class demonstrated so far. However, the presence of multiple forms has been suggested (Singh *et al.*, 1988; Ahmad *et al.*, 1990).

Among these multiple forms, cDNAs encoding five GST subunits have been cloned, and their primary structures have been deduced; two subunits of GST-α (Tu and Qian, 1986; Rhoads *et al.*, 1987; Board and Webb, 1987), GST-μ (DeJong *et al.*, 1988a; Seidegard *et al.*, 1988), the testis GST-5.2 (Campbell *et al.*, 1990) and GST-π (Kano *et al.*, 1987). Two GST forms, expressed in *Escherichia coli* from two cDNA clones, λGTH1 and λGTH2, encoding GST-α subunits, showed different specific activities toward cumene hydroperoxide (Chow *et al.*, 1988) and different specificities in the conversion of prostaglandin H_2 to $F_{2\alpha}$ or D_2 (Burgess *et al.*, 1989). The form from λGTH2, possessing high activity toward cumene hydroperoxide, is similar to GST-B_2B_2 (Stockman *et al.*, 1987), suggesting that λGTH2 may encode the B_2 subunit. The deduced amino acid sequence from λGTH1 is identical to that from the pGST2-3 (Board and Webb, 1987), which encodes the B_1 subunit (Lewis *et al.*, 1988a).

Chromosome mapping revealed the GST-α gene to be located at 6p12 (Board and Webb, 1987), GST-μ at 1p31 (DeJong *et al.*, 1988a), and GST-π at 11q13 (Moscow *et al.*, 1988).

2. *Tissue Distribution*

As described above, several forms of glutathione transferase in the liver have been reported by many investigators, although their results have, in some cases, differed considerably from one another regarding expression of the various iso-enzymes. These discrepancies are partly due to interindividual differences in expression of GST-μ (Warholm *et al.*, 1981; Hussey *et al.*, 1986) or GST-α (Board, 1981; Strange *et al.*, 1984). Affinity ligands used for purification may also be involved in the generation of different glutathione transferase profiles in the liver. Some investigators (Stockman *et al.*, 1985; Soma *et al.*, 1986) utilized *S*-hexylglutathione-Sepharose (Guthenberg and Mannervik, 1979), while others (Singh *et al.*, 1985; Vander Jagt *et al.*, 1985) applied glutathione-Sepharose (Simons and Vander Jagt, 1977). This may be of importance since the presence of human glutathione transferase forms exhibiting preferential affinity for gluta-thione-Sepharose, such as the rat GST 8-8, have been described (Tsuchida *et al.*, 1990).

The distribution of glutathione transferases has been also studied in extra-hepatic organs including the kidney (Tateoka *et al.*, 1987; Singh *et al.*, 1987c), lung (Koskelo *et al.*, 1981), brain (Theodore *et al.*, 1985), intestine (Peters *et al.*, 1989), adrenal (Sherman *et al.*, 1983), testis (Aceto *et al.*, 1989), prostate (Tew *et al.*, 1987), and uterus (Di Ilio *et al.*, 1988a). These studies revealed expression to be tissue-specific (Laisney *et al.*, 1984). Forms in the Alpha class are expressed in the liver, kidney, and intestine, while GST-π is expressed as a major form in many organs other than the adult liver. GST-π is also expressed in fetal liver (Guthenberg *et al.*, 1986; Hiley *et al.*, 1988). Developmental change in expression of other forms has also been noted in several tissues (Faulder *et al.*, 1987).

3. *Functions*

The functions of the various human glutathione transferases have not been so clearly defined as those of rat GST forms (see reviews by Mannervik and Dan-ielson, 1988; Sato, 1989). However, human forms are presumed to have activi-ties similar to the equivalent rat forms. GST-α-ε possesses binding activity to bilirubin (Kamisaka *et al.*, 1975; Vander Jagt *et al.*, 1985), and GST-ε (B_1B_1) possesses Δ^5-androstene-3, 17-dione isomerase (Benson *et al.*, 1977) and pros-taglandin $F_{2\alpha}$ reductase activities (Burgess *et al.*, 1989). As described above, GST-B_2B_2 shows high peroxidase activity toward cumene hydroperoxide (Stock-man *et al.*, 1987), and also prostaglandin D_2-isomerase activity (Burgess *et al.*,

1989). Glutathione conjugation of benzo[a]pyrene derivatives is catalyzed by GST-μ (Warholm *et al.*, 1981) and GST-π (Robertson *et al.*, 1986b).

D. GLUTATHIONE TRANSFERASES IN THE MOUSE AND OTHER SPECIES

1. *Mouse Glutathione Transferases*

So far at least three, one, and two forms of mouse cytosolic glutathione transferase have been identified in the Alpha, Pi, and Mu classes, respectively, as summarized in Table IV. Gupta *et al.* (1990) described three forms with different pIs in the Mu class, but subunit structures have not yet been clarified. The major forms in the liver, GSTs M I, M II and M III, are all homodimers with different molecular weights. Mouse GST M II in the Pi class is related to rat GST 7-7 (GST-P) and human GST-π, but GST M II is basic, and rat GST 7-7 is neutral and human GST-π is acidic. The amino acid sequence of GST M II deduced from the base sequence of cDNA was found to share 92% and 85% identity with GST-P and GST-π, respectively, (Hatayama *et al.*, 1990). The amounts of these forms in liver, however, considerably differ among the three species. In particular, GST M II is a major form in adult male mouse liver (Hatayama *et al.*, 1986; McLellan and Hayes, 1987), and, though present in significant levels as a minor form in adult female liver, was found to be further inducible by injection of testosterone to females (Hatayama *et al.*, 1986) or by administration of various drugs, including BHA. On the other hand, following castration of male mice, the levels were reduced to the lower levels of female mice (Hatayama *et al.*, 1986). The levels of GSTs M I and M III were hardly affected by castration or

TABLE IV
MOLECULAR FORMS OF MOUSE GLUTATHIONE TRANSFERASE

Class	Nomenclature					
	a	pI	Subunit M_r	pI[b]	c	Subunit M_r
Alpha (3 forms)	M I	9.7	25,500	10.6 10.3	Ya$_3$Ya$_3$	25,800
					Ya$_1$Ya$_2$	25,600
Mu (2 forms)	M III	8.5	27,000	8.8 9.3	YbYb	26,400
Pi (1 form)	M II	8.7	24,000	9.0	YfYf	24,800

[a] Warholm *et al.*, 1986; Hatayama *et al.*, 1986.
[b] Benson *et al.*, 1989. Molecular form named by its pI.
[c] McLellan and Hayes, 1990.

TABLE V
INDUCTION OF MOUSE GLUTATHIONE TRANSFERASES BY DRUGS[a]

| | | Molecular forms | | | | | |
| | | Alpha | | | Pi | Mu | |
Inducer[b] sex		10.6 (MI)	10.3	Ya₁Ya₂	9.0 (M II)	8.7 (M III)	9.3
BHA[c,d]	F	→	↑ ↑	↑ ↑ ↑	↑	↑ ↑	↑ ↑ ↑
	M	→	↑ ↑	↑ ↑ ↑	→	↑ ↑	↑ ↑
BEX[c]	F	→	↑ ↑		↑	↑	↑ ↑ ↑
	M	↑	↑ ↑		→	↑	↑ ↑ ↑
BNF[d,e]	F	→		↑	↑	↑	↑
	M	→		↑	→	↑	
PB[e,f]	F		↑			↑	↑
	M	→			→	↑	

[a] Single, double and triple upward arrows indicate slight (within 5-fold), moderate (5-fold to 10-fold) and strong (above 10-fold) induction, respectively. A horizontal arrow indicates no change.
[b] BHA, tert-butylhydroxyanisole; BEX, bisethylxanthogen; BNF, β-naphthoflavone; PB, phenobarbital.
[c] Benson et al., 1989.
[d] McLellan and Hayes, 1990.
[e] Sisk and Pearson, 1990.
[f] Di Simplicio et al., 1989.

by administration of testosterone, but GST M III was influenced by administration of various drugs (Table V).

Mouse liver glutathione transferases have attracted attention with regard to the antioxidant-associated chemoprevention of carcinogenesis in the liver and other organs (Wattenberg, 1972; Benson et al., 1978, 1979, 1984; Pearson et al., 1983; Dock et al., 1984; see reviews by Wattenberg, 1985; Wattenberg et al., 1986). The major forms induced by BHA have been identified as GST-9.3 in the Mu class and Ya₁Ya₂ in the Alpha class, the latter being undetectable in normal liver (McLellan and Hayes, 1988) (Table V). GST Ya₃Ya₃ (probably MI), which is constitutively expressed in normal liver, was not significantly induced (McLellan and Hayes, 1989). 3-Methylcholanthrene did not induce any mouse hepatic forms (Di Simplicio et al., 1989), and β-naphthoflavone, which is suggested to act through the Ah receptor, and phenobarbital are not strong inducers for any forms of mouse glutathione transferases. In mouse lung, six isoenzymes have been isolated, and GSTs with pI 8.7 and pI 7.9, respectively, in the Mu class were preferentially induced by BHA and bound with benzo[a]pyrene

(B[a]P) metabolites, indicating antineoplastic activity of BHA against B[a]P-induced neoplasia in mouse lung (Singh *et al.*, 1987a).

Mouse GST cDNAs have been cloned: M I (Ya) (Daniel *et al.*, 1987; Pearson *et al.*, 1988), M II (Hatayama *et al.*, 1990), M III (8.7) (Pearson *et al.*, 1988) and M III (9.3) (Pearson *et al.*, 1988). A genomic DNA of M I was also cloned (Daniel *et al.*, 1987).

2. *Molecular Forms in Other Species*

Multimolecular forms have also been identified in other species: five forms in rhesus monkey (Asaoka *et al.*, 1977), three (Smith *et al.*, 1980), six (Jensen and Mackay, 1990) or seven forms (Inaba, 1987) in hamster liver, four forms in guinea pig liver (Oshino *et al.*, 1990; Kamei *et al.*, 1990) and five (Wiener, 1986) or four (Igarashi *et al.*, 1988) forms in dog liver. Dog liver has three major forms, all of which are immunologically related to rat GST-P (7-7) (Igarashi *et al.*, 1988).

III. Glutathione Transferases Increased in (Pre)neoplastic Tissues

A. RAT GLUTATHIONE TRANSFERASES INCREASED IN CHEMICAL HEPATOCARCINOGENESIS

Several groups have investigated changes in glutathione transferase isoenzymes during rat chemical hepatocarcinogenesis. First, rat basic forms in class Alpha such as GSTs 1-1 (YaYa) and 1-2 (YaYc) known as ligandin and in the Mu class such as GSTs 3-3 (Yb$_1$Yb$_1$) and 3-4 (Yb$_1$Yb$_2$), earlier, respectively named GSTs A and C (Kitahara *et al.*, 1983a), were noticed to be increased (see reviews by Pickett, 1987; Coles and Ketterer, 1990). From 1983 to 1985, attention was concentrated on GST-P or GST 7-7, identified as a good marker for rat hepatic preneoplastic and neoplastic lesions by our and other laboratories (see review by Sato, 1989).

1. *Rat GST-P (7-7) as a Preneoplastic Marker*

A new neutral form (pI 6.7 or 6.8), almost the only form in the rat placenta, was purified and named the placental form (GST-P) (Sato *et al.*, 1984a,b). Although GST-P was undetectable in normal rat liver, it was found to be markedly increased in hyperplastic nodule-bearing livers (Kitahara *et al.*, 1984), allowing its purification and preparation of polyclonal antibody in rabbits (Satoh *et al.*, 1985b). Ketterer and his colleagues similarly noted an unidentified form in primary hepatoma induced by N,N'-dimethyl-4-aminoazobenzene (Ketterer *et al.*,

1983) and later determined this to be GST 7-7 (Meyer *et al.*, 1985). Guthenberg *et al.* (1986) and Robertson *et al.* (1986a), using GST-P antibody, demonstrated that their new form (GST 7-7), purified from rat kidney and lung, is immunologically identical to GST-P. GST-YfYf, purified from the kidney by Hayes (1988), is identical with GST 7-7.

GST-P (7-7) characteristically has the smallest molecular weight and a neutral *pI* (see Table I), and while it is not immunologically crossreactive with any other forms, there is considerable crossreactivity among species, including rat, mouse, hamster, dog, horse, and man (Satoh *et al.*, 1985b; see reviews by Sato, 1988, 1989).

GST-P levels in normal rat tissues, including placenta, fetal, and adult livers, are generally very low (Satoh *et al.*, 1985b). The kidney (proximal and distal tubules), lung (bronchiolar epithelial cells), pancreas (ductular cells), small intestine (columnar epithelial cells), skin (epithelial cells), and brain (astroglia cells) contain significant amounts (see review by Sato, 1989). GST-P is ubiquitous but is often found only in small amounts. It is especially very low in adult rat livers, but significant in fetal liver (McCusker *et al.*, 1989), though first described to be negligible by several groups (see review by Sato, 1989).

a. Expression during Chemical Hepatocarcinogenesis.   It was first found by double immunodiffusion studies that GST-P is markedly increased in rat liver bearing hyperplastic nodules induced by the Solt and Farber model (Solt and Farber, 1976). This was confirmed using two-dimensional electrophoresis followed by immunoblotting (Sato *et al.*, 1984a, Kitahara *et al.*, 1984; Satoh *et al.*, 1985b; Sato, 1988). Sugioka *et al.* (1985) also noted similar polypeptides expressed in rat hyperplastic nodules and primary and transplantable hepatocarcinomas and confirmed to be GST-P. Eriksson *et al.* (1983) further reported the appearance of a polypeptide (M_r 21,000, so named p21) detectable by SDS-polyacrylamide slab gel electrophoresis in isolated hyperplastic nodules induced by six different models, including the Solt and Farber model. This polypeptide (later renamed p26) was also immunologically identified to be the GST-P subunit (Roomi *et al.*, 1985b; Rushmore *et al.*, 1987, 1988). A glutathione transferase form named GST 7-7 was also reported to be increased in hyperplastic nodules (Jensson *et al.*, 1985).

The amount of GST-P protein increases 30-fold or more during the early stage of hepatocarcinogenesis induced by the Solt and Farber model. The levels of GST-P in hyperplastic nodule-bearing livers and in primary and transplantable (Morris 5123D) hepatomas induced by different carcinogens are 10-fold higher than in normal liver but negligible in transplantable Yoshida ascites hepatoma AH 130 (Satoh *et al.*, 1985b), indicating that GST-P tends to decrease with dedifferentiation in hepatomas, as is the case for many drug-metabolizing enzymes. However, rat Zajdela ascites hepatoma cells have been reported to have a significant amount of only the GST 7-7 form, inducible up to twofold by i.p. injection of *trans*-stilbene oxide (Tahir *et al.*, 1989).

Immunohistochemically GST-P was demonstrated to be localized in enzyme-altered foci that are also detectable by γ-glutamyltransferase (GGT) activity (Sato *et al.*, 1984a). However, a proportion of GST-P–positive foci are not positive for GGT staining (Tatematsu *et al.*, 1985, 1987). The foci are inducible with a large number of different protocols using a variety of carcinogens [diethylnitrosamine (DEN), dimethylnitrosamine (DMN), 2-acetylaminofluorene (AAF), aflatoxin B_1 (AfB_1), heterocyclic amines, etc.] (see review by Sato, 1989). Hepatomas induced by DEN, AAF, AfB_1, 3'-methyl-4-dimethylamino-azobenzene (3'-Me-DAB), and other genotoxic carcinogens also usually strongly express GST-P. Sex differences are observed in the development of GST-P–positive foci induced by some carcinogens; for example, the areas of GST-P–positive lesions induced in the Solt and Farber model are far larger in male rats than in females (Sato, 1989), and strain differences are also observed (Asamoto *et al.*, 1989). GST-P is expressed not only in putative preneoplastic hepatic foci induced by chemicals, but also in spontaneous lesions. Examples include spontaneous *altered cell foci* in the livers of aged Fisher 344 rats (Mitaka and Tsukada, 1987) or in the livers of LEC rats without administration of any exogenous carcinogens (Oyamada *et al.*, 1988; Masuda *et al.*, 1989), in both cases particularly in males.

Immunohistochemical staining further revealed that very small GST-P–positive foci or even single cells, appearing 1 or 2 weeks after a single administration of initiator (Moore *et al.*, 1986, 1987a; Sato, 1988) or in one model even within 48 hr of single doses of DEN, DMN, or AfB_1 (Moore *et al.*, 1987a), are detectable before an increase in GST-P content is biochemically apparent (Sato, 1988). The numbers of these cells increase with increasing doses of initiator (e.g., DEN) and are not induced by promoters of liver carcinogenesis such as phenobarbital, 3-methylcholanthrene, polychlorinated biphenyls and isosafrole (Moore *et al.*, 1987a). Therefore, GST-P is considered to be an accurate marker for very early *initiated cells,* indicating a clonal origin of GST-P–positive foci and hepatomas. GST-P–positive small foci (minifoci) persist for a long time (at least 6 mo) after a single injection of DEN, 200mg/kg (Satoh *et al.*, 1989) or even 10mg/kg (Takahashi *et al.*, 1987), showing that these lesions are to a great extent irreversible and develop into large foci after feeding AAF for 2 or 3 weeks accompanied by partial hepatectomy (selection pressure) (Satoh *et al.*, 1989).

b. Inducibility by Drugs.   Unlike the majority of drug-metabolizing enzymes, GST-P is not inducible by administration of a large variety of hepatocarcinogenic promoters or modulators (3-methylcholanthrene, α-hexachlorocyclohexane, carbon tetrachloride, cyproterone acetate, phenobarbital, polychlorinated biphenyls) or even by hepatocarcinogens (DEN, AAF, 3'-Me-DAB, AfB_1, choline- and methionine-deficient diet, ethionine, clofibrate) without the appearance of pre-neoplastic foci and hyperplastic nodules (Roomi et al., 1985b; Satoh et al., 1985b), or additional drugs (Ito et al., 1988). GST-P did prove slightly inducible with antioxidants, BHA and butylated hydroxytoluene (BHT) (Tatematsu et al., 1985, 1987, 1988b) and by ethoxyquin (Thamavit et al., 1985; Manson et al., 1987) in periportal areas. The expression of GST-P after administration of these drugs, however, does not interfere with the detection of GST-P–positive foci, whereas γ-glutamyltransferase is so strongly induced by these drugs that en-zyme-altered foci are no longer recognizable (Tatematsu et al., 1985).

Among the other drugs examined, lead nitrate proved exceptional in inducing significant levels of GST-P throughout the whole rat liver with no zonal prefer-ence (Roomi et al., 1986, 1987; Columbano et al., 1990). In this case, expres-sion of GST-P, which is transient and reversible within 2 weeks (Sato, 1988), appears to be part of a general biochemical pattern involving drug-metabolizing enzymes very similar to those exhibited by hepatic nodules (Roomi et al., 1986). Although lead nitrate is a hepatic mitogen, lead nitrate–associated hyperplasia cannot replace compensatory cell proliferation after hepatectomy or carbon tetra-chloride poisoning in the development of GST-P–positive foci (Columbano et al., 1987a,b, 1990).

In contrast to some other known rat hepatic preneoplastic markers, such as glucose-6-phosphatase, adenosine triphosphatase, γ-glutamyltransferase and glucose-6-phosphate dehydrogenase, GST-P appears to be more stable after withdrawal of carcinogens from the diet (Tatematsu et al., 1988a), although its expression is slowly reversible. Ease of visualization and this advantage have established GST-P as one of the best markers for detection of early liver lesions, now widely used for analysis of hepatocarcinogenesis (Xu et al., 1990a,b; Hase-gawa et al., 1989; Imaida et al., 1989; Yokota et al., 1990) and in rapid bioassay methods for carcinogens and modifiers of hepatocarcinogenesis (see review by Ito et al., 1989).

GST-P is also elevated in acinar cell lesions of rat pancreas induced by hy-droxyaminoquinoline 1-oxide (Moore et al., 1987b) and in squamous metapla-sias and squamous cell carcinomas in rat lung induced by N-nitrosobis(2-hy-droxypropyl)amine (Yamamoto et al., 1988).

c. Hepatic Preneoplasia Not Expressing GST-P.   It has been reported by Reddy and colleagues (see reviews by Reddy and Rao, 1986, and Rao and Reddy, 1987) and other groups (Numoto et al., 1984; Glauert et al., 1986; Greaves et al., 1986; Hendrich et al., 1987; Wirth et al., 1987) that a new class of carcinogens (nongenotoxic), including the peroxisome-proliferating hypolipidemic agents such as clofibrate, nafenopin, ciprofibrate, Wy-14643, tibric acid and di-(2-ethylhexyl)phthalate, can induce GST-P–negative and/or GGT-negative foci and hepatomas. Glutathione transferase activity is known to be inhibited by clofibrate

(Foliot *et al.*, 1986), but this cannot account for the preceding observations, because the mRNAs of GST-P, γ-glutamyltransferase, and α-fetoprotein are not expressed in foci and hepatomas induced by peroxisome-proliferating agents (Rao *et al.*, 1988). However, ethionine, which is another proposed nongenotoxic agent, does induce GST-P–positive foci and hepatomas (Ogiso *et al.*, 1985).

Peroxisome proliferators have been considered to be nongenotoxic, because these agents are negative for the Ames test, but recent studies by Nishimura and his colleagues have shown that the adduct 8-hydroxyguanosine is elevated in the DNA of the liver and kidney of rats given di-(2-ethylhexyl)phthalate and di-(2-ethylhexyl)adipate. This suggests the involvement of oxidative DNA damage in hepatocarcinogenesis by peroxisome proliferators (Takagi *et al.*, 1990).

d. GST-P Gene Expression and Relation to Oncogene Activation.   The structure of GST-P and the mechanisms underlying regulation of its expression during chemical hepatocarcinogenesis have been investigated by Muramatsu and his colleagues (1987). They cloned a rat GST-P cDNA (pGP5) from a cDNA library prepared from poly(A)$^+$ RNA of 2-acetylaminofluorene–induced rat hepatocellular carcinoma (hepatoma) by screening with synthetic DNA probes deduced from a partial amino acid sequence of GST-P subunit and determined the complete amino acid sequence (Suguoka *et al.*, 1985). The molecular weight of the rat GST-P subunit was calculated to be 23,307, not including the methionine at the NH$_2$-terminus. They also showed by Northern blot and dot-blot analysis, using their cDNA probe (pGP5), that GST-P mRNA (about 750 nucleotides) is abundant in hyperplastic nodules, in Morris 5123D, 7316A, and 7794A, and in chemically induced hepatomas, but is barely detectable in normal liver, in fetal liver, and in an undifferentiated hepatoma, AH 130. Lower levels of mRNA were detected in lung, testis, kidney, spleen, and placenta, approximately in this order (Muramatsu *et al.*, 1987). Thus, they suggested that the amount of GST-P in a tissue is for the most part, if not totally, regulated at the transcription level. Pemble *et al.* (1986, 1987) and Taylor *et al.* (1987) also cloned a cDNA (pGSTr7) of GST 7-7 by using poly(A)$^+$ RNA isolated from *N,N'*-dimethyl-4-aminoazobenzene–induced rat hepatoma. The amino acid sequence of the GST 7-7 was also identical with that reported by Suguoka *et al.* (1985). Okuda *et al.* (1987) have isolated the GST-P gene from a phage library using their GST-P cDNA clone (pGP5). They demonstrated that it is about 3000 bp long and consists of seven exons and six introns, with the initiator codon being split between the first and second exons. The cap site was mapped 70 nucleotides upstream from the translation initiation site and the promoter "TATA" box was found 27 bp upstream from this putative cap site. Sequences 200 bp upstream from the cap site were rich in G + C residues (61%). They also analyzed the cis-acting regulatory DNA elements of the rat GST-P gene using the chloramphenicol acetyltransferase (CAT) activity assay method (Muramatsu *et al.*, 1987; Sakai *et al.*, 1988).

Various regions of the 5'-flanking sequence were fused with a bacterial CAT gene, and the transcriptional activity of each construct was determined by transient expression assay after introduction into a hepatoma cell line (dRLh84). Two enhancing elements (GPEI and GPEII) were located 2500 and 2200 bp upstream from the transcription initiation site (Sakai et al., 1988). GPEII contained two simian virus 40 and one polyoma enhancer core-like sequences. A silencing element was found 400 bp upstream from the cap site. 12-0-Tetradecanoylphorbol-13-acetate (TPA) response element (TRE)-like sequences (TGATTCAG) were present in the GPEI and in position -16 (Sakai et al., 1988; Okuda et al., 1989). Furthermore, they found GPEI to be an imperfect palindrome composed of two TRE-like sequences (*GTCAGTCA* CTA*TGATTCAG*), each having no activity by itself but rather acting synergistically to form a strong enhancer, which is active even at the low level of AP-1 (an oncogene c-*jun* product) activity in F9 embryonic stem cells. They also isolated a rat c-*jun* clone (Sakai et al., 1989) and demonstrated that the product (AP-1) and a related protein (c-*fos* product) are trans-acting on the enhancing elements (Sakai et al., 1988; Okuda et al., 1989, 1990). It is currently thought that nuclear oncogene c-*jun* and c-*fos* products form a heterodimer and trans-act to amplify TRE-containing genes (Rausher et al., 1988). Indeed, c-*jun* and c-*fos* are expressed in livers bearing GST-P–positive foci induced by the Solt-Farber model (Sato et al., 1990), and sex differences are observed in the expression of c-*fos* and c-*myc* (Porsch-Hallstrom et al., 1989). GST-P was also demonstrated to be highly expressed with malignant transformation *in vitro* of primary hepatocytes either by transfection with *ras* oncogenes or by treatment with activated aflatoxin B_1 (Power et al., 1987). Transformation of rat liver epithelial cells with v-H-*ras* or v-*raf* also caused expression of GST-P and MDR-1, independent of chemical exposure, resulting in multidrug resistance (Burt et al., 1988). Li et al. (1988) demonstrated that the expression of a metallothionein-*ras* fusion gene (MTrasT24) specifically increases mRNA levels of γ-glutamyltransferase and GST-P in cultured rat liver epithelial cells, in which these genes have been shown to be expressed together. However, recent studies have suggested that GST-P and γ-glutamyltransferase are regulated differently (Pitot et al., 1989; Winokur and Lieberman, 1990).

The GST-P gene is located on rat chromosome 1 at band q43 (Masuda et al., 1986).

e. Functions.   The actual role(s) and function(s) of GST-P in preneoplastic cells also await clarification. There is no evidence that carcinogens inducing GST-P–positive foci are detoxified via glutathione conjugation by GST-P, and although AAF and 3'-Me-DAB are known to be conjugated with glutathione, the process is nonenzymatic (Ketterer et al., 1983, 1986). As mentioned above, it is known that putative preneoplastic foci are resistant to cytotoxic agents, including hepatocarcinogens. Among the basic forms, GSTs 1-1, 1-2, and 2-2 have large capacities to bind bilirubin, heme, and cholic acids, but they markedly lose glutathione transferase activities through binding to these compounds; the activities of GSTs 3-3, 3-4, and 4-4 are less affected (Fukai *et al.,* 1989). GST-P activity, in contrast, is almost unaffected by binding to such endogenous compounds (Sato, 1988), suggesting that the increased levels of GST-P in foci might allow replacement of basic forms with regard to glutathione transferase activity. Among the substrates examined so far, it was pointed out by Mannervik *et al.* (1985) that GST 7-7 and other class Pi forms in common are unique in possessing a high activity toward ethacrynic acid, but other particular substrate specificities have not yet been noted. Recently, Gopalan *et al.* (1990) described GST 7-7 with significant activity toward aflatoxin B_1-8,9-oxide. GST 7-7 purified from rat lung stereoselectively exerts the highest activity toward the carcinogenic (+)-7β,8α-dihydroxy-9α,10α-oxy-7,8,9,10-tetrahydrobenzo[a]pyrene (Robertson *et al.,* 1986a), suggesting that the various glutathione transferases may have different stereoselectivities toward the same substances and that GST-P may have unique properties. Furthermore, GST 7-7 purified from hepatomas possessed selenium-independent glutathione peroxidase activity toward lipid hydroperoxides, especially toward arachidonate and linoleate hydroperoxides (Meyer *et al.,* 1985), and also toward thymine hydroperoxide (Tan *et al.,* 1986). Thus, GST-P (7-7) expression may be related to the prevention of lipid peroxidation, the latter process being considered to play an important role(s) during tumor promotion. GST 7-7 may also be concerned with drug-resistant mechanisms of preneoplastic foci (Ketterer, 1986; Ketterer *et al.,* 1986). Lipid hydroperoxides produced by some promotion regimens can be removed by a series of coupled reactions: glutathione peroxidase activity (selenium-independent) of GST 7-7 and other forms, followed by reduction of oxidized glutathione by glutathione reductase [NAD(P)H] with NADPH supplied from the pentose phosphate pathway (Sato, 1989). The fact that glutathione reductase, NADPH-generating glucose-6-phosphate dehydrogenase and the total and reduced glutathione levels are all increased in enzyme-altered foci and hyperplastic nodules supports the possibility that the above-described reactions might be operating (Sato, 1989).

On the other hand, it has recently been noted that some forms of glutathione transferase, especially in the Pi class, are irreversibly inactivated with sulfhydryl(SH)-blocking reagents such as N-ethylmaleimide (NEM) and iodoacetamide; e.g., the human erythrocyte form (Hirrell *et al.,* 1987), the bovine placental Pi form (Schaffer *et al.,* 1988) and the horse erythrocyte Pi form (Ricci *et al.,* 1989). Rat GST-P (7-7), human GST-π and mouse GST M II, all in class Pi, are irreversibly inactivated by NEM (Sato *et al.,* 1989, 1990), and only one cysteine residue, the 47th, in the NH$_2$-terminal, which is common to all three, is involved in this inactivation (Tamai *et al.,* 1990). The Pi class forms are also reversibly inactivated with hydrogen peroxide (H_2O_2) or oxidized glutathione (GSSG) (Schaffer *et al.,* 1988; Sato *et al.,* 1989), while other forms in the other

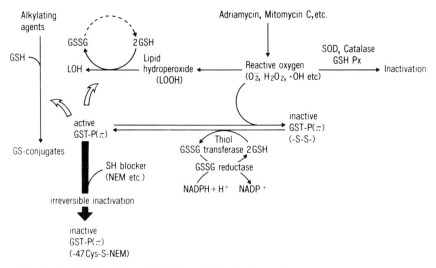

FIG. 1.   Possible functions of GST-P or GST-π in drug resistance. NEM, N-ethylmaleimide; SOD, superoxide dismutase; GSH Px, glutathione peroxidase.

classes are hardly affected; the microsomal form and Mu class forms are known to be activated by active oxygen species (Aniya and Anders, 1989; Murata *et al.*, 1990). In this inactivation, intra- or intersubunit disulfide bonds between the 47th cysteine residue and other cysteine residue(s) are involved (H. Shen, K. Tamai, K. Satoh, I. Hatayama, S. Tsuchida, and K. Sato, unpublished results). Thus, the thiol redox state, which is influenced by active oxygen metabolites, might regulate the Pi class forms, as shown in Fig. 1, and also, as pointed out, certain key enzymes of other metabolic pathways (see review by Ziegler, 1985).

2. *Other Forms and Their Functions*

Among the major forms of glutathione transferase in rat liver, those containing subunits 1 (Ya) and 3 (Yb$_1$), in particular, are inducible by several drugs (Table II), and their elevated activities may prevent or modify chemical carcinogenesis in the liver and other organs. In the Alpha class, subunit 1 (Ya) is known to have glutathione conjugation activity toward benzo[*a*]pyrene-7,8-diol-9,10-oxide (Jernstrom *et al.*, 1985) and aflatoxin B$_1$-8,9-oxide (Coles *et al.*, 1985), while subunit 8 (Yk) acts on 4-hydroxynonenal (Jensson *et al.*, 1986). In the Mu class, subunit 3 (Yb$_1$) has activity toward aflatoxin B$_1$-8,9-epoxide (Gopalan *et al.*, 1990) and subunit 4 (Yb$_2$) toward benzo[*a*]pyrene-7,8-diol-9,10-oxide (Robertson and Jernstrom, 1986) and *trans*-stilbene oxide (Seidegard *et al.*, 1988), and denitrosation activity toward 1,3-bis(2-chloroethyl)-1-nitrosourea (BCNU) (Smith *et al.*, 1989) and 1-methyl-2-nitro-1-nitrosoguanidine (MNNG) (Jensen *et al.*, 1990). Subunits 5 and 12 have specific high activity toward particular epoxides (Meyer *et al.*, 1991), and Yrs toward arylmethyl sulfate (Hiratsuka *et al.*, 1990), as described above.

Microsome-mediated aflatoxin B_1 binding to DNA is well known to be modulated by cytosolic glutathione transferase in rat livers and to be reduced when glutathione transferases (mainly GSTs 1-1 and 3-3) are induced by BHA or PB (Lotlikar *et al.*, 1984, 1989; Jhee *et al.*, 1989). Coles *et al.* (1985) reported that GSTs in the Alpha class have most activity against aflatoxin B_1-8,9-epoxide, while recently Gopalan *et al.* (1990) described GST 3-3 in the Mu class to be most active toward this metabolite.

In chemical hepatocarcinogenesis, the basic subunits 1/2 (Ya/Yc) and 3/4 (Yb_1/Yb_2), in addition to GST-P (7-7), are increased in foci and nodules as well as in surrounding hepatocytes and may perform multiple detoxication functions as enzymes and binding proteins in the resistance of these lesions to cytotoxic agents (Pickett *et al.*, 1984b; see reviews by Pickett and Lu, 1989; Coles and Ketterer, 1990). In these foci and nodules, a large range of enzymes are changed, some finding application as marker enzymes for these lesions (see a review by Sato, 1989). Among the drug-metabolizing enzymes, phase I species are reduced while phase II forms including glutathione transferases are increased, such a deviation pattern of drug-metabolizing enzymes being considered to be responsible for the resistance of these lesions to cytotoxic agents. Since Farber and his co-workers (Farber, 1982, 1984; Farber and Cameron, 1980) pointed out that enzyme-altered foci and hyperplastic nodules induced by different carcinogens in rat liver have pleiotropic resistance to structurally unrelated agents, they were termed *resistant foci and nodules*. In aflatoxin B_1–induced hyperplastic nodules, the Ya_2 subunit in the Alpha class was found to be increased, and was suspected to endow resistance of these cells to this carcinogen (Hayes *et al.*, 1990b; Harrison *et al.*, 1990b). It was also noted that subunit Yk (8) with a high activity toward 4-hydroxynonenal, a lipid peroxide metabolite, was also increased in hyperplastic nodules (Harrison *et al.*, 1990b).

B. HUMAN GLUTATHIONE TRANSFERASES AND FUNCTIONS

Since the identification of GST-P as a good marker for rat hepatocarcinogenesis (Sato *et al.*, 1984a,b; Satoh *et al.*, 1985b), the expression of the human equivalent form, GST-π, has been examined in many cancer tissues. For example, Soma *et al.* (1986) reported a significant increase of GST-π levels in metastatic liver tumors originating from the gallbladder, stomach, and colon. Immunohistochemical studies revealed that both colon carcinomas and squamous cell carcinomas of the uterine cervix express GST-π (Kodate *et al.*, 1986; Shiratori *et al.*, 1987). Other investigators have further reported increased levels

TABLE VI
Expression of Glutathione Transferase Forms in Human Cancer Tissues

Cancer	Activity[a] (nmol/min/ mg protein)	Form	Reference
Colon	130 ± 30	GST-π	Kodate et al., 1986; Tsuchida et al., 1989.
Breast	70 ± 50	GST-π (GST-α)[b]	Moscow et al., 1988, 1989a; Lewis et al., 1989; Howie et al., 1989
Stomach		GST-π	Tsutsumi et al., 1987.
Ovary		GST-π	Moscow et al., 1989a.
Kidney	327 ± 130	GST-π	Di Ilio et al., 1987; Harrison et al., 1990a.
Bladder	200 ± 50	GST-π	Lewis et al., 1989; Lafuente et al., 1990.
Lung	205 ± 131	GST-π	Di Ilio et al., 1988b; Eimoto et al., 1988.
Uterine cervix	260 ± 190	GST-π	Shiratori et al., 1987.
Esophagus	230 ± 160	GST-π	Tsuchida et al., 1989.
Head and Neck		GST-π	Moscow et al., 1989a.
Malignant melanoma	400	GST-π	Mannervik et al., 1987.
Leukemia		GST-π	McQuaid et al., 1989.

[a] GST activity toward 1-chloro-2,4-dinitrobenzene.
[b] In some breast cancer, GST-α is expressed as a minor form.

of GST-π in several tumors by immunohistochemical or Northern blotting methods. Table VI summarizes the types of human primary cancers expressing GST-π. GST activity toward 1-chloro-2,4-dinitrobenzene is increased 2-fold to 10-fold in cancer tissues as compared to the respective control tissue values (Shiratori et al., 1987; Di Ilio et al., 1987; Tsuchida et al., 1989). More than 70–90% of the GST activity in cancer tissues is due to GST-π. However, cancers originating from the liver or kidney, both of which are organs normally possessing high GST activity, show less activity than the respective control tissues (Mouelhi et al., 1987; Di Ilio et al., 1987).

GST-π is expressed as the major form in many cell lines established from colon (CX-1, HT29), breast (MX-1), ovary (PE04), bladder (HT1376, EJ, SCaBER), lung (NCI H358, PC13), uterine cervix (CaSki), and head and neck cancers (SCC-25). However, a few cell lines from breast (MCF-7, ZR 75-1) and lung cancers (SW2-105, NCI H69) do not express GST-π in significant amounts (Batist et al., 1986; Shea et al., 1988; Awasthi et al., 1988; Nakagawa et al., 1988; Tsuchida et al., 1989; Lewis et al., 1989; Singh et al., 1990). A pronounced increase of GST-π expression in MCF-7 cells resistant to doxorubicin will be described below in Section III,C.

The expression in various tumor tissues (Table VI) and in cell lines indicates that GST-π may be a useful marker for a wide range of cancers. Many lesions expressing GST-π have been histologically classified as adenocarcinomas or squamous cell carcinomas. In lung tumors, GST-π is expressed in both adeno-carcinomas and squamous cell carcinomas, but not in small cell lung cancers (Di Ilio *et al.*, 1988b; Eimoto *et al.*, 1988; Awasthi *et al.*, 1988; Nakagawa *et al.*, 1988). In spite of the striking expression of GST-P in rat hepatocarcinogenesis, GST-π is hardly expressed in human primary hepatocellular carcinomas. Ket-terer and his colleagues reported that GST-P and GST-π genes share a TPA-responsive element as a promoter, but the expression of the two genes may be regulated by different mechanisms (Cowell *et al.*, 1988; Dixon *et al.*, 1989).

GST-π is expressed not only in cancers, but also in preneoplastic tissues such as colon adenomas (Kodate *et al.*, 1986), dysplasia of the uterine cervix and esophagus (Shiratori *et al.*, 1987), and the cirrhotic liver (Sato *et al.*, 1987; Hayes *et al.*, 1987). GST-π expression has been noted in cervical dysplasia accompanying koilocytosis, which suggests infection by human papilloma virus (Shiratori *et al.*, 1987). Chan *et al.* (1990) have reported a strong correlation between infection with cancer-associated human papilloma virus (types 16/18 and 31/33/35) and GST-π expression. Thus, GST-π may be a useful marker not only for various cancers but also for high-risk precancerous lesions. Colorectal tumorigenesis has been considered to proceed through a series of genetic alter-ations, including *ras* gene activation and loss of putative tumor-suppressor genes (see the review by Fearon and Vogelstein, 1990). Human colon adenomas will provide a good model for studying the relationship between GST-π expression and *ras* gene activation or other genetic alterations.

Investigation of the levels of GST-π in sera of patients with tumors such as stomach and esophagus cancers has revealed significant elevation (Tsuchida *et al.*, 1989; Niitsu *et al.*, 1989). In addition, these high serum values decreased to the normal range after surgical removal of tumors, suggesting that follow-up of serum GST-π levels may be useful for monitoring such patients during the course of treatment.

Alterations of other glutathione transferase forms in cancers remain to be clari-fied. Glutathione transferases in the Alpha class are down-regulated in renal car-cinomas (Di Ilio *et al.*, 1987).

GST-μ has high conjugating activity toward *trans*-stilbene oxide, and its ex-pression is less frequent in patients with lung cancer than in normal controls, suggesting that loss of GST-μ is a possible marker for development of lung cancer (Seidegard *et al.*, 1985, 1986, 1987). Hereditary differences in the ex-pression of this form are attributable to deletion of the gene (Seidegard *et al.*, 1988). While a correlation between GST-μ deficiency and sister chromatid ex-change induction by *trans*-stilbene oxide has been demonstrated (Weincke *et al.*,

1990), the frequencies of GST-μ expression in patients with breast or colon cancers are not significantly different from those in normal controls (Peters *et al.*, 1990).

An enzyme involved in the formation of fatty acid ethyl esters in extrahepatic organs, previously identified as cytotoxic metabolites from alcohol, has been shown to be a form of glutathione transferase similar to GST-π in isoelectric point and NH$_2$-terminal amino acid sequence (Bora *et al.*, 1989), indicating that both alcohol and xenobiotic metabolism is catalyzed by this form. This result suggests that carcinogen metabolism may be influenced by alcohol, providing experimental support for high incidences of some cancers in patients with alcohol abuse (Bora *et al.*, 1989).

C. ROLES OF GLUTATHIONE TRANSFERASES AND GLUTATHIONE IN DRUG RESISTANCE

1. *Glutathione Transferases*

Many anticancer agents as well as carcinogens have been considered to be detoxified by conjugation with glutathione (reviews by Arrick and Nathan, 1984; Tew and Clapper, 1987; Hayes and Wolf, 1988; Moscow and Cowan, 1988; Tew, 1989). Melphalan has been shown to be conjugated with glutathione by GST (Dulik *et al.*, 1986), and GST-π was found to increase after acquisition of doxorubicin resistance by a human breast cancer cell line, MCF-7 (Batist *et al.*, 1986). Since then, the relationship between drug resistance and the expression of glutathione transferase forms has been extensively studied in many cancer cell lines (Table VII), indicating a two- to fivefold increase of activity due mainly to the Pi class in cell lines resistant to alkylating agents, doxorubicin, or cisplatin. In the cell line, PE04, crossresistant to cisplatin, chlorambucil, and 5-fluorouracil, GST-π expression is enhanced (Lewis *et al.*, 1988b). Furthermore, the direct involvement of glutathione transferase in drug resistance has been demonstrated by the increased resistance to several drugs in cell lines transfected with cDNAs encoding GST forms (Manoharan *et al.*, 1987; Nakagawa *et al.*, 1990; Miyazaki *et al.*, 1990; Puchalski and Fahl, 1990; Black *et al.*, 1990), and also by the reduced resistance of cell lines treated with inhibitors of GST forms (Tew *et al.*, 1988; Hall *et al.*, 1989). However, transfection of MCF-7 cells with GST-π cDNA did not result in resistance to doxorubicin (Moscow *et al.*, 1989b), indicating that GST-π may not be involved in the resistance, but rather that P-glycoprotein is responsible in this case (Fairchild *et al.*, 1990). In general, glutathione transferase activity is not increased in cell lines exhibiting the phenotypes of typical multidrug resistance, which include resistance to *Vinca* alkaloids (Yusa *et al.*, 1988; Kramer *et al.*, 1988; Medh *et al.*, 1990).

In drug-resistant cell lines, particular glutathione transferase forms are in

TABLE VII

Activities and Molecular Forms of Glutathione Transferase in Cancer Cell Lines Resistant to Anticancer Drug

Cell line (origin)	Resistant drug	Activity[a]	Form	Reference
MCF-7 (human breast cancer)	Doxorubicin	161 (4)[b]	GST-π	Batist et al., 1986.
16C (mouse mammary carcinoma)	Doxorubicin	48 (10)		Lee et al., 1989.
Walker 256 (rat mammary carcinoma)	Chlorambucil	53 (17)	GST 2-2	Buller et al., 1987.
CHO (Chinese hamster ovary cell)	Chlorambucil	650 (240)	Alpha (Ya,Yc)	Lewis et al., 1988a; Robson et al., 1987.
CHO	Cisplatin		Pi	Saburi et al., 1989.
PE04 (human ovarian carcinoma)	Cisplatin Chlorambucil 5-Fluorouracil	215 (74)	GST-π	Lewis et al., 1988b.
SCC-25 (human squamous cell carcinoma)	Cisplatin	447 (231)	GST-π	Teicher et al., 1987.
P-388 (mouse leukemia)	Doxorubicin	14 (9)	Pi	Deffie et al., 1988.
P-388	Doxorubicin	97 (54)	Pi	Singh et al., 1989.
8226 (human myeloma)	Doxorubicin	1 (1)	no	Bellamy et al., 1989.
HS-Sultan (human myeloma)	Melphalan	118 (77)	GST-π	Gupta et al., 1989.
9L (rat gliosarcoma)	Nitrogen mustard	75 (30)	GST-P	Evans et al., 1987.
9L-2 (rat gliosarcoma)	BCNU	30 (30)	GST 4-4	Smith et al., 1989.
G3361 (human malignant melanoma)	Cisplatin	283 (52)	GST-π	Wang et al., 1989.
G3361	Melphalan	257	GST-π	
G3361	BCNU	178	GST-π	
G3361	4-hydroperoxycyclophosphamide	163	GST-π	

[a]GST activity toward 1-chloro-2, 4-dinitrobenzene.

[b]GST activity in sensitive cell lines in parentheses.

duced that are suitable for detoxification of respective anticancer agents. For example, rat GST 4-4, expressed in a 1,3-bis(2-chloroethyl)-1-nitrosourea-resistant cell line, has been shown to detoxify the drug by a denitrosation reaction (Smith *et al.*, 1989), and rat GST 2-2 as well as 1-1, expressed in chlorambucil-resistant cell lines, is also considered to detoxify the drug by glutathione conjugation from its structural similarity to melphalan (Buller *et al.*, 1987; Robson *et al.*, 1987). The finding that the Pi class forms are expressed in many cell lines resistant to structurally unrelated agents is analogous to the expression of rat GST-P in hepatocarcinogenesis induced by many genotoxic carcinogens (Sato, 1988, 1989). The actual role of the Pi class forms in drug-resistant cell lines, however, remains to be clarified. The fact of reversible inactivation by active oxygen species including hydrogen peroxide and superoxide anion (Tamai *et al.*, 1990; Murata *et al.*, 1990) suggests that the Pi class forms may function like scavengers to remove active oxygen metabolites escaping from metabolism by the superoxide dismutase, catalase, or selenium(Se)-dependent glutathione peroxidase, which are usually depressed in cancer tissues (Fig. 1). Since cytotoxicity of doxorubicin has been suggested to be dependent on the formation of free radicals (Mimnaugh *et al.*, 1989), this possible scavenger function as well as the glutathione peroxidase activity of Pi class forms toward lipid hydroperoxides (Meyer *et al.*, 1985) may be important as mechanisms of doxorubicin-resistance (Fig. 1). There is no evidence yet that specific anticancer agents inducing expression of the Pi class forms are detoxified via glutathione conjugation by these forms, although GST-π has been shown to be involved in demethylation of methyl parathion (Radulovic *et al.*, 1986). While doxorubicin also possesses a similar methyl ester in its structure, the question of whether GST-π is involved in demethylation of doxorubicin remains to be clarified.

As mentioned above, glutathione transferase activities are not increased or detectable in some resistant cell lines. In such cell lines, other mechanisms may be involved in acquisition of multidrug resistance. These include increased drug output (efflux) due to changes in transport mechanisms (in which the P-glycoprotein of 170 kDa and the *mdr* genes are active) (see Chapter 11, this volume); decreased activation of prodrugs (in phase I); alteration in drug target enzymes; and alterations in cellular metabolism and repair mechanisms such as topoisomerases and increased inactivating enzymes in phase II (see reviews by Moscow and Cowan, 1988; Hayes *et al.*, 1990a). However, the finding of high amounts of GST-π in most human colon and other cancers before treatment (Table IV) suggests that glutathione transferases may play important roles, not only in acquired resistance, but also in natural resistance. Since the modulation of glutathione transferase forms with inhibitors has been shown to be promising for overcoming this resistance in experimental models, the effectiveness of similar approaches should be evaluated in clinical fields.

2. *Glutathione and Glutathione-related Enzymes*

The relationship between intracellular glutathione levels and drug or radiation resistance of cancer cells has been studied extensively (reviews by Ozols *et al.*, 1988; Mitchell *et al.*, 1989), glutathione metabolism being revealed as one of the major determinants of therapeutic efficacy. Figure 2 illustrates the pathways involved in glutathione conjugation of drugs and in the glutathione peroxidase reaction. Glutathione synthesis is regulated by γ-glutamylcysteine synthetase, an inhibitor of which, buthionine sulfoximine, has been widely used to examine the effect of glutathione depletion on drug resistance (Griffith, 1989). Lipid hydroperoxides, produced via active oxygen metabolites from some anticancer drugs, are reduced by glutathione peroxidase and also by some forms of glutathione transferase. Glutathione conjugates of drug (GS-X) and oxidized glutathione (GSSG) are pumped out by a particular ATPase species, whose activity is dependent on GS-X or GSSG and Mg^{2+}. The presence of this ATPase has been demonstrated in human red blood cells (Kondo *et al.*, 1987), rat liver (Inoue *et al.*, 1984), and heart (Ishikawa, 1989).

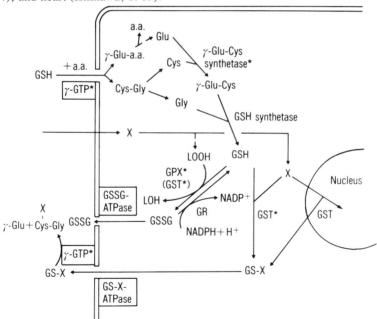

FIG. 2.   Metabolic pathways involved in glutathione conjugation of drugs and in the glutathione peroxidase reaction. Asterisks indicate the enzymes that are increased in drug-resistant cancer cell lines. GSH, reduced glutathione; GSSG, oxidized glutathione; X, drug; GPX, Se-dependent glutathione peroxidase; GR, glutathione reductase; γ-GTP, γ-glutamyltranspeptidase; γ-Glu-Cys synthetase, γ-glutamylcysteine synthetase; LOOH, lipid hydroperoxide; a. a., amino acid.

Among the glutathione-related enzymes, γ-glutamyltranspeptidase, γ-glutamylcysteine synthetase, and glutathione peroxidase have also been reported to be increased in some resistant cell lines (Ahmad *et al.*, 1987; Evans *et al.*, 1987; Lewis *et al.*, 1988a; Carmichael *et al.*, 1988; Lee *et al.*, 1989; Howie *et al.*, 1990). Whether the increase of GS-X–dependent ATPase occurs in drug resistance remains to be clarified. This enzyme is similar to P-glycoprotein, a product of the *mdr* 1 gene, regarding the property of ATP-dependent pumping of drugs. Although glutathione conjugation is not required for P-glycoprotein action and its subunit molecular weight (about 170,000) is different from that of GSSG-dependent ATPase from red blood cells (85,000 and 65,000, Kondo *et al.*, 1987), the exact relationship between GS-X–dependent ATPase and P-glycoprotein awaits further study (West, 1990). In this connection, the finding that reduction of intracellular glutathione levels results in increased retention of daunorubicin (Lutzky *et al.*, 1989) is interesting.

IV. Concluding Remarks

Although some glutathione conjugates are known to be cytotoxic, mutagenic, and even carcinogenic (Pickett and Lu, 1989), glutathione transferases have attracted a great deal of attention as important detoxicating enzymes during chemical carcinogenesis. Multimolecular forms are known, as with other drug-metabolizing enzymes (e.g., cytochrome P-450, UDP-glucuronosyl transferases, sulfotransferases), this multiplicity extending between tissues, sexes, and species, and in inducibility by drugs as described in this chapter. Thus, the variety of forms that exist in normal tissues is not always sufficient to detoxify all the electrophiles from a xenobiotic, protection by constitutive glutathione transferases is imperfect, and cytotoxic or genotoxic damage occurs in such tissues. Glutathione transferases, which are known to act toward electrophiles derived from known carcinogens, are limited to several forms, such as those composing subunits 1, 3, 5, and 7 in the rat. As polyaromatic hydrocarbon epoxides (those from benzo[*a*]pyrene and 3-methylcholanthrene) are good substrates for these forms, abundant in rat liver, these carcinogens are generally not hepatocarcinogenic. Similarly, the newly described GST-YrsYrs group is unique in possessing activity only toward arylmethyl sulfates, which are known to be carcinogenic in rat skin but not in the liver, where these isoenzymes are abundant. So far, no glutathione transferase forms have been identified that act on aromatic amines such as *N*-acetylaminofluorene and 3′-methyl-4-dimethylaminoazobenzene, these compounds being typical hepatocarcinogens, although they are conjugated with glutathione by nonenzymatic reactions. For some carcinogens such as aflatoxin B_1, the amounts of the specific glutathione transferase forms (rat GSTs 1-1 or 3-3) present in normal liver are not sufficient to detoxify the electrophiles derived from these compounds; thus these are highly hepatocarcinogenic. However, when sufficient isoenzymes are induced by drugs such as antioxidants, detoxification is enhanced, and thus inducers may act to prevent or modify hepatocarcinogenesis. On the other hand, some forms observed to be increased within hepatic preneoplastic lesions have been suggested to participate in the acquired resistance mechanisms of these cells to cytotoxic agents by detoxifying or inactivating these agents, thus helping *promotion* of these cells. Forms that exist in normal hepatocytes and are further inducible by drugs can participate in the above mechanisms, but newly expressed forms in the foci, such as GST-P (7-7), may also be involved. GST-P (7-7) has also become established as one of the best positive markers for early detection of putative preneoplastic cells during chemically induced hepatocarcinogenesis. Although it is not expressed in lesions induced by some nonmutagenic hepatocarcinogens, the fact that this isoenzyme is not induced by many drugs, in contrast to other drug-metabolizing enzyme species, has particular advantage for its use in screening carcinogens and modifiers of carcinogenesis (promoters and inhibitors). Interest has focused on the regulation of GST-P gene expression associated with activation of oncogenes, such as c-*jun* and c-*fos,* or a connection with protein kinase C through TPA stimulation. Other glutathione transferases in the Pi class, such as human GST-π, have also been found in increased levels in preneoplastic and neoplastic lesions in a wide variety of organs in man and in other species. They have been investigated to clarify their participation in the mechanism underlying (multi)drug resistance in experimental and human tumors, but much remains to be clarified. So far, the functions of glutathione transferases have been studied mainly in relation to the metabolism of xenobiotics, including carcinogens. More recently this has been extended to include the metabolism of endogenous substances such as lipid and nucleotide peroxides and active oxygen species. Further investigation of this enzyme family is clearly warranted in the interests of better cancer prevention and therapy.

References

Abramovitz, M., and Listowsky, I. (1987). Selective expression of a unique glutathione *S*-transferase Yb₃ gene in rat brain. *J. Biol. Chem.* **262**, 7770–7773.

Aceto, A., Di Ilio, C., Angelucci, S., Felaco, M., and Federici, G. (1989). Glutathione transferase isoenzymes from human testis. *Biochem. Pharmacol.* **38**, 3653–3660.

Ahmad, S., Okine, L., Le, B., Najarian, P., and Vistica, D. T. (1987). Elevation of glutathione in phenylalanine mustard-resistant murine L1210 leukemia cells. *J. Biol. Chem.* **262**, 15048–15053.

Ahmad, H., Wilson, D. E., Fritz, R. R., Singh, S. V., Medh, R. D., Nagle, G. T., Awasthi, Y. C., and Kurosky, A. (1990). Primary and secondary structural analyses of glutathione *S*-transferase π from human placenta. *Arch. Biochem. Biophys.* **278**, 398–408.

Alin, P., Jensson, H., Guthenberg, C., Danielson, U. H., Tahir, M. K., and Mannervik, B. (1985).

Purification of major basic glutathione transferase isoenzymes from rat liver by use of affinity chromatography and fast protein liquid chromatofocusing. *Anal. Biochem.* **146**, 313–320.

Aniya, Y., and Anders, M. W. (1989). Activation of rat liver microsomal glutathione S-transferase by reduced oxygen species. *J. Biol. Chem.* **264**, 1998–2002.

Arrick, B. A., and Nathan, C. F. (1984). Glutathione metabolism as a determinant of therapeutic efficacy: A review. *Cancer Res.* **44**, 4224–4232.

Asamoto, M., Tsuda, H., Kagawa, M., Camargo, J. L. V., Ito, N., and Nagase, S. (1989). Strain differences in susceptibility to 2-acetylaminofluorene and phenobarbital promotion of rat hepatocarcinogenesis in a medium-term assay system: Quantitation of glutathione S-transferase P-positive foci development. *Jpn. J. Cancer Res.* **80**, 939–944.

Asaoka, K., Ito, H., and Takahashi, K. (1977). Monkey glutathione S-aryltransferases. I. Tissue distribution and purification from the liver. *J. Biochem.* **82**, 973–981.

Awasthi, Y. C., Dao, D. D., and Saneto, R. P. (1980). Interrelationship between anionic and cationic forms of glutathione S-transferases of human liver. *Biochem. J.* **191**, 1–10.

Awasthi, Y. C., Singh, S. V., Ahmad, H., Moller, P. C., and Gupta, V. (1988). Expression of glutathione S-transferase isoenzymes in human small-cell lung cancer cell lines. *Carcinogenesis (London)* **9**, 89–93.

Bach, M. K., Brashler, J. R., and Morton, D. R., Jr. (1984). Solubilization and characterization of the leukotriene C_4 synthetase of rat basophil leukemia cells: A novel, particulate glutathione S-transferase. *Arch. Biochem. Biophys.* **230**, 455–465.

Bass, N. M., Kirsch, R. E., Tuff, S. A., Marks, I., and Saunders, S. J. (1977). Ligandin heterogeneity: Evidence that the two nonidentical subunits are the monomers of two distinct proteins. *Biochim. Biophys. Acta* **492**, 163–175.

Batist, G., Tulpule, A., Sinha, B. K., Katki, A. G., Meyers, C. E., and Cowan, K. H. (1986). Overexpression of a novel anionic glutathione transferase in multidrug-resistant human breast cancer cells. *J. Biol. Chem.* **261**, 15544–15549.

Bellamy, W. T., Dalton, W. S., Meltzer, P., and Dorr, R. T. (1989). Role of glutathione and its associated enzymes in multidrug-resistant human myeloma cells. *Biochem. Pharmacol.* **38**, 787–793.

Benson, A. M., Talalay, P., Keen, J. H., and Jakoby, W. B. (1977). Relationship between the soluble glutathione-dependent Δ^5-3-ketosteroid isomerase and the glutathione S-transferases of the liver. *Proc. Natl. Acad. Sci. U.S.A.* **74**, 158–162.

Benson, A. M., Batzinger, R. P., Ou, S.-Y. L., Bueding, E., Cha, Y. N., and Talalay, P. (1978). Elevation of hepatic glutathione S-transferase activities and protection against mutagenic metabolites of benzo(a)pyrene by dietary antioxidants. *Cancer Res.* **38**, 4486–4495.

Benson, A. M., Cha, Y.-N., Bueding, E., Heine, H. S., and Talalay, P. (1979). Elevation of extrahepatic glutathione S-transferase and epoxide hydratase activities by 2(3)-*tert*-butyl-4-hydroxyanisole. *Cancer Res.* **39**, 2971–2977.

Benson, A. M., Hunkeler, M. J., and Morrow, J. F. (1984). Kinetics of glutathione transferase, glutathione transferase messenger RNA, and reduced nicotinamide adenine dinucleotide (phosphate): Quinone reductase induction by 2(3)-*tert*-butyl-4-hydroxyanisole in mice. *Cancer Res.* **44**, 5256–5261.

Benson, A. M., Hunkeler, M. J., and York, J. L. (1989). Mouse hepatic glutathione transferase isoenzymes and their differential induction by anticarcinogens. *Biochem. J.* **261**, 1023–1029.

Black, S. M., Beggs, J. D., Hayes, J. D., Bartoszek, A., Muramatsu, M., Sakai, M., and Wolf, C. R. (1990). Expression of human glutathione S-transferases in *Saccharomyces cerevisiae* confers resistance to the anticancer drugs adriamycin and chlorambucil. *Biochem. J.* **268**, 309–315.

Board, P. G. (1981). Biochemical genetics of glutathione-S-transferase in man. *Am. J. Hum. Genet.* **33**, 36–43.

Board, P. G., and Webb, G. C. (1987). Isolation of a cDNA clone and localization of human glutathione S-transferase 2 genes to chromosome band 6p12. *Proc. Natl. Acad. Sci. U.S.A.* **84,** 2377–2381.

Board, P. G., Suzuki, T., and Shaw, D. C. (1988). Human muscle glutathione S-transferase (GST-4) shows close homology to human liver GST-1. *Biochim. Biophys. Acta.* **953,** 214–217.

Booth, J., Boyland, E., and Sims, P. (1961). An enzyme from rat liver catalysing conjugation with glutathione. *Biochem. J.* **79,** 516–524.

Bora, P. S., Spilburg, C. A., and Lange, L. G. (1989). Metabolism of ethanol and carcinogens by glutathione transferases. *Proc. Natl. Acad. Sci. U.S.A.* **86,** 4470–4473.

Boyland, E., and Chasseaud, L. F. (1969). The role of glutathione and glutathione S-transferases in mercapturic acid biosynthesis. *Adv. Enzymol.* **32,** 173–219.

Buller, A. L., Clapper, M. L., and Tew, K. D. (1987). Glutathione S-transferases in nitrogen mustard–resistant and –sensitive cell lines. *Mol. Pharmacol.* **31,** 575–578.

Burgess, J. R., Chow, N-W. I., Reddy, C. C., and Tu, C-P. D. (1989). Amino acid substitutions in the human glutathione S-transferases confer different specificities in the prostaglandin endoperoxide conversion pathway. *Biochem. Biophys. Res. Commun.* **158,** 497–502.

Burt, R. K., Garfield, S., Johnson, K., and Thorgeirsson, S. S. (1988). Transformation of rat liver epithelial cells with v-H-*ras* or v-*raf* causes expression of MDR-1, glutathione-S-transferase-P and increased resistance to cytotoxic chemicals. *Carcinogenesis (London)* **9,** 2329–2332.

Campbell, E., Takahashi, Y., Abramovitz, M., Peretz, M., and Listowsky, I. (1990). A distinct human testis and brain μ-class glutathione S-transferase. *J. Biol. Chem.* **265,** 9188–9193.

Carmichael, J., Forrester, L. M., Lewis, A. D., Hayes, J. D., Hayes, P. C., and Wolf, C. R. (1988). Glutathione S-transferase isoenzymes and glutathione peroxidase activity in normal and tumour samples from human lung. *Carcinogenesis (London)* **9,** 1617–1621.

Chan, S. Y., Shih, P., Davis, J. M., Longo, D., and Kantor, R. R. S. (1990). Glutathione S-transferase-Pi (GST-Pi), an early marker for human papillomavirus (HPV)-induced cervical neoplasm. *Proc. Am. Assoc. Cancer Res.* **31,** 166.

Chang, M., Burgess, J. R., Scholz, R. W., and Reddy, C. C. (1990). The induction of specific rat liver glutathione S-transferase subunits under inadequate selenium nutrition causes an increase in prostaglandin $F_{2\alpha}$ formation. *J. Biol. Chem.* **265,** 5418–5423.

Chasseaud, L. F. (1979). The role of glutathione and glutathione S-transferases in the metabolism of chemical carcinogens and other electrophilic agents. *Adv. Cancer Res.* **29,** 175–274.

Chow, N-W. I., Whang-Peng, J., Kao-Shan, C-S., Tam, M. F., Lai, H-C. J., and Tu, C-P. D. (1988). Human glutathione S-transferases. *J. Biol. Chem.* **263,** 12797–12800.

Christ-Hazelhof, E., and Nugteren, D. H. (1979). Purification and characterisation of prostaglandin endoperoxide D-isomerase, a cytoplasmic, glutathione-requiring enzyme. *Biochim. Biophys. Acta* **572,** 43–51.

Coles, B., and Ketterer, B. (1990). The role of glutathione and glutathione transferases in chemical carcinogenesis. *CRC Crit. Rev. Biochem. Mol. Biol.* **25,** 47–70.

Coles, B., Meyer, D. J., Ketterer, B., Stanton, C. A., and Garner, R. C. (1985). Studies on the detoxication of microsomally activated aflatoxin B_1 by glutathione and glutathione transferases *in vitro. Carcinogenesis (London)* **6,** 693–697.

Columbano, A., Ledda-Columbano, G. M., Coni, P., and Pani, P. (1987a). Failure of mitogen-induced cell proliferation to achieve initiation of rat liver carcinogenesis. *Carcinogenesis (London)* **8,** 345–347.

Columbano, A., Ledda-Columbano, G. M., Lee, G., Rajalakshmi, S., and Sarma, D. S. R. (1987b). Inability of mitogen-induced liver hyperplasia to support the induction of enzyme-altered islands induced by liver carcinogens. *Cancer Res.* **47,** 5557–5559.

Columbano, A. Ledda-Columbano, G. M., Ennas, M. G., Curto, M., Chelo, A., and Pani, P. (1990). Cell proliferation and promotion of rat liver carcinogenesis: Different effect of hepatic regeneration and mitogen-induced hyperplasia on the development of enzyme-altered foci. *Carcinogenesis (London)* **11**, 771–776.

Cowell, I. G., Dixon, K. H., Pemble, S. E., Ketterer, B., and Taylor, J. B. (1988). The structure of the human glutathione S-transferase π gene. *Biochem. J.* **255**, 79–83.

Daniel, V., Sharon, R., Tichauer, Y., and Sarid, S. (1987). Mouse glutathione S-transferase Ya subunit: Gene structure and sequence. *DNA* **6**, 317–324.

Danielson, U. H., Esterbauer, H., and Mannervik, B. (1987). Structure-activity relationships of 4-hydroxyalkenals in the conjugation catalysed by mammalian glutathione transferases. *Biochem. J.* **247**, 707–713.

Davidson, N. E., Egner, P. A., and Kensler, T. W. (1990). Transcriptional control of glutathione S-transferase gene expression by the chemoprotective agent 5-(2-pyrazinyl)-4-methyl-1,2-dithiole-3-thione (oltipraz) in rat liver. *Cancer Res.* **50**, 2251–2255.

Deffie, A. M., Alam, T., Seneviratne, C., Beenken, S. W., Batra, J. K., Shea, T. C., Henner, W. D., and Goldenberg, G. J. (1988). Multifactorial resistance to adriamycin: Relationship of DNA repair, glutathione transferase activity, drug efflux, and P-glycoprotein in cloned cell lines of adriamycin-sensitive and -resistant P388 leukemia. *Cancer Res.* **48**, 3595–3602.

DeJong, J. L., Chang, C-M., Whang-Peng, J., Knutsen, T., and Tu, C-P. D. (1988a). The human liver glutathione S-transferase gene superfamily: Expression and chromosome mapping of an Hb subunit cDNA. *Nucleic Acids Res.* **16**, 8541–8554.

DeJong, J. L., Morgenstern, R., Jornvall, H., DePierre, J. W., and Tu, C-P. D. (1988b). Gene expression of rat and human microsomal glutathione S-transferases. *J. Biol. Chem.* **263**, 8430–8436.

Del Boccio, G., Di Ilio, C., Alin, P., Jornvall, H., and Mannervik, B. (1987). Identification of a novel glutathione transferase in human skin homologous with class alpha glutathione transferase 2-2 in the rat. *Biochem. J.* **244**, 21–25.

Di Ilio, C., Del Boccio, G., Aceto, A., and Federici, G. (1987). Alteration of glutathione transferase isoenzyme concentrations in human renal carcinoma. *Carcinogenesis (London)* **8**, 861–864.

Di Ilio, C., Aceto, A., Del Boccio, G., Casalone, E., Pennelli, A., and Federici, G. (1988a). Purification and characterization of five forms of glutathione transferase from human uterus. *Eur. J. Biochem.* **171**, 491–496.

Di Ilio, C., Del Boccio, G., Aceto, A., Casaccia, R., Mucilli, F., and Federici, G. (1988b). Elevation of glutathione transferase activity in human lung tumor. *Carcinogenesis (London)* **9**, 335–340.

Di Simplicio, P., Jensson, H., and Mannervik, B. (1989). Effects of inducers of drug metabolism on basic hepatic forms of mouse glutathione transferase. *Biochem. J.* **263**, 679–685.

Ding, G. J.-F., Lu, A. Y. H., and Pickett, C. B. (1985). Rat liver glutathione S-transferases. Nucleotide sequence analyses of a Yb₁ cDNA clone and prediction of the complete amino acid sequence of the Yb₁ subunit. *J. Biol. Chem.* **260**, 13268–13271.

Ding, G. J.-F., Ding, V. D.-H., Rodkey, J. A., Bennett, C. D., Lu, A. Y. H., and Pickett, C. B. (1986). DNA sequence analysis of a Yb₂ cDNA clone and regulation of the Yb₁ and Yb₂ mRNAs by phenobarbital. *J. Biol. Chem.* **261**, 7952–7957.

Dixon, K. H., Cowell, I. G., Xia, C. L., Pemble, S. E., Ketterer, B., and Taylor, J. B. (1989). Control of expression of the human glutathione S-transferase π gene differs from its rat orthologue. *Biochem. Biophys. Res. Commun.* **163**, 815–822.

Dock, L., Martinez, M., and Jernstrom, B. (1984). Induction of hepatic glutathione S-transferase activity by butylated hydroxyanisole and conjugation of benzo[a]pyrene diolepoxide. *Carcinogenesis (London)* **5**, 841–844.

Dulik, D. M., Fenselau, C., and Hilton, J. (1986). Characterization of melphalan-glutathione adducts whose formation is catalyzed by glutathione transferases. *Biochem. Pharmacol.* **35**, 3405–3409.

Eimoto, H., Tsutsumi, M., Nakajima, A., Yamamoto, K., Takashima, Y., Maruyama, H., and

Konishi, Y. (1988). Expression of the glutathione S-transferase placental form in human lung carcinomas. *Carcinogenesis (London)* **9,** 2325–2327.

Eriksson, L. C., Sharma, R. N., Roomi, M. W., Ho, R. K., Farber, E., and Murray, R. K. (1983). A characteristic electrophoretic pattern of cytosolic polypeptides from hepatocyte nodules generated during liver carcinogenesis in several models. *Biochem. Biophys. Res. Commun.* **117,** 740–745.

Evans, C. G., Bodell, W. J., Tokuda, K., Doane-Setzer, P., and Smith, M. T. (1987). Glutathione and related enzymes in rat brain tumor cells resistance to 1,3-bis(2-chloroethyl)-1-nitrosourea and nitrogen mustard. *Cancer Res.* **47,** 2525–2530.

Fairchild, C. R., Moscow, J. A., O'Brien, E. E., and Cowan, K. H. (1990). Multidrug resistance in cells transfected with human genes encoding a variant P-glycoprotein and glutathione S-transferase-π. *Mol. Pharmacol.* **37,** 801–809.

Farber, E. (1982). Chemicals, evolution, and cancer development. *Am. J. Pathol.* **108,** 270–275.

Farber, E. (1984). Cellular biochemistry of the stepwise development of cancer with chemicals. *Cancer Res.* **44,** 5463–5474.

Farber, E., and Cameron, R. (1980). The sequential analysis of cancer development. *Adv. Cancer Res.* **31,** 125–226.

Faulder, C. G., Hirrell, P. A., Hume, R., and Strange, R. C. (1987). Studies of the development of basic, neutral, and acidic isoenzymes of glutathione S-transferase in human liver, adrenal, kidney, and spleen. *Biochem. J.* **241,** 221–228.

Fearon, E. R., and Vogelstein, B. (1990). A genetic model for colorectal tumorigenesis. *Cell* **61,** 759–767.

Foliot, A., Touchard, D., and Mallet, L. (1986). Inhibition of liver glutathione S-transferase activity in rats by hypolipidemic drugs related or unrelated to clofibrate. *Biochem. Pharmacol.* **35,** 1685–1690.

Fukai, F., Yatomi, S., Morita, T., Nishizawa, S., Nagai, T., and Katayama, T. (1989). Protection of glutathione S-transferase from bilirubin inhibition. *J. Biochem.* **105,** 968–973.

Glauert, H. P., Beer, D., Rao, M. S., Schwarz, M., Xu, Y.-D., Goldsworthy, T. L., Coloma, J., and Pitot, H. C. (1986). Induction of altered hepatic foci in rats by the administration of hypolipidemic peroxisome proliferators alone or following a single dose of diethylnitrosamine. *Cancer Res.* **46,** 4601–4606.

Gopalan, P., Jensen, D. E., and Lotlikar, P. D. (1990). Glutathione conjugation of synthetic and microsome-mediated aflatoxin B_1-8,9-epoxide by purified glutathione S-transferase from rats. *Proc. Am. Assoc. Cancer Res.* **31,** 111.

Greaves, P., Irisarri, E., and Monro, A. M. (1986). Hepatic foci of cellular and enzymatic alteration and nodules in rats treated with clofibrate or diethylnitrosamine followed by phenobarbital: Their rate of onset and their reversibility. *J. Natl. Cancer Inst.* **76,** 475–484.

Griffith, O. W. (1989). L-Buthionine-S, R-sulfoximine: Mechanism of action, resolution of diastereomers, and use as a chemotherapeutic agent. *In* "Glutathione Centennial" (N. Taniguchi, T. Higashi, Y. Sakamoto, and A. Meister, eds.), pp. 285–299. Academic Press, New York.

Gupta, V., Singh, S. V., Ahmad, H., Medh, R. D., and Awasthi, Y. C. (1989). Glutathione and glutathione S-transferases in a human plasma cell line resistant to melphalan. *Biochem. Pharmacol.* **38,** 1993–2000.

Gupta, S., Medh, R. D., Leal, T., and Awasthi, Y. C. (1990). Selective expression of the three classes of glutathione S-transferase isoenzymes in mouse tissues. *Toxicol. Appl. Pharmacol.* **104,** 533–542.

Guthenberg, C., and Mannervik, B. (1979). Purification of glutathione S-transferases from rat lung by affinity chromatography. *Biochem. Biophys. Res. Commun.* **86,** 1304–1310.

Guthenberg, C., and Mannervik, B. (1981). Glutathione S-transferase (Transferase π) from human placenta is identical or closely related to glutathione S-transferase (Transferase ρ) from erythrocytes. *Biochim. Biophys. Acta* **661**, 255–260.

Guthenberg, C., Warholm, M., Rane, A., and Mannervik, B. (1986). Two distinct forms of glutathione transferase from human foetal liver. *Biochem. J.* **235**, 741–745.

Habig, W. H., Pabst, M. J., Fleischner, G., Gatmaitan, Z., Arias, I. M., and Jakoby, W. B. (1974). The identity of glutathione S-transferase B with ligandin, a major binding protein of liver. *Proc. Natl. Acad. Sci. U.S.A.* **71**, 3879–3882.

Hales, B. F., Jaeger, V., and Neims, A. H. (1978). Isoelectric focusing of glutathione S-transferases from rat liver and kidney. *Biochem. J.* **175**, 937–943.

Hall, A., Robson, C. N., Hickson, I. D., Harris, A. L., Proctor, S. J., and Cattan, A. R. (1989). Possible role of inhibition of glutathione S-transferase in the partial reversal of chlorambucil resistance by indomethacin in a Chinese hamster ovary cell line. *Cancer Res.* **49**, 6265–6268.

Harrison, D. J., Hallam, L., and Lauder, J. (1990a). Glutathione S-transferase expression in fetal kidney and Wilms' tumour. *Br. J. Cancer.* **61**, 836–840.

Harrison, D. J., May, L., Hayes, J. D., and Neal, G. E. (1990b). Glutathione S-transferase localization in aflatoxin B_1-treated rat. *Carcinogenesis (London)* **11**, 927–931.

Hasegawa, R., Mutai, M., Imaida, K., Tsuda, H., Yamaguchi, S., and Ito, N. (1989). Synergistic effects of low-dose hepatocarcinogens in induction of glutathione S-transferase P-positive foci in the rat liver. *Jpn. J. Cancer Res.* **80**, 945–951.

Hatayama, I., Satoh, K., and Sato, K. (1986). Developmental and hormonal regulation of the major form of hepatic glutathione S-transferase in male mice. *Biochem. Biophys. Res. Commun.* **140**, 581–588.

Hatayama, I., Satoh, K., and Sato, K. (1990). A cDNA sequence coding a class Pi glutathione S-transferase of mouse. *Nucleic Acids Res.* **18**, 4606.

Hayes, J. D. (1986). Purification and physical characterization of glutathione S-transferase K. *Biochem. J.* **233**, 789–798.

Hayes, J. D. (1988). Selective elution of rodent glutathione S-transferases and glyoxalase I from the S-hexylglutathione-Sepharose affinity matrix. *Biochem. J.* **255**, 913–922.

Hayes, J. D., and Mantle, T. J. (1986a). Use of immunoblot techniques to discriminate between the glutathione S-transferase Yf, Yk, Ya, Yn/Yb, and Yc subunits and to study their distribution in extrahepatic tissues. *Biochem. J.* **233**, 779–788.

Hayes, J. D., and Mantle, T. J. (1986b). Anomalous electrophoretic behaviour of the glutathione S-transferase Ya and Yk subunits isolated from man and rodents. *Biochem. J.* **237**, 731–740.

Hayes, J. D., and Wolf, C. R. (1988). Role of glutathione transferase in drug resistance. *In* "Glutathione Conjugation" (B. Ketterer and H. Sies, eds.), pp 316–356. Academic Press, London.

Hayes, P. C., Portmann, B., Aldis, P. M., Williams, R., and Hayes, J. D. (1987). Glutathione S-transferases and human pathology. *In* "Glutathione S-transferases and Carcinogenesis" (T. J. Mantle, C. B. Pickett, and J. D. Hayes, eds.), pp. 175–187. Taylor & Francis, London.

Hayes, J. D., Pickett, C. B., and Mantle, T. J. (1990a). "Glutathione S-transferases and Drug Resistance," pp. 1–459. Taylor & Francis, London.

Hayes, J. D., Kerr, L. A., Harrison, D. J., Cronshaw, A. D., Ross, A. G., and Neals, G. E. (1990b). Preferential overexpression of the class alpha rat Ya_2 glutathione S-transferase subunit in livers bearing aflatoxin-induced preneoplastic nodules. *Biochem. J.* **268**, 295–302.

Hendrich, S., Campbell, H. A., and Pitot, H. C. (1987). Quantitative stereological evaluation of four histochemical markers of altered foci in multistage hepatocarcinogenesis in the rat. *Carcinogenesis (London)* **8**, 1245–1250.

Hiley, C., Fryer, A., Bell, J., Hume, R., and Strange, R. C. (1988). The human glutathione S-transferases. *Biochem. J.* **254**, 255–259.

Hiratsuka, A., Sebata, N., Kawashima, K., Okuda, H., Ogura, K., Watabe, T., Satoh, K., Hatayama, I., Tsuchida, S., Ishikawa, T., and Sato, K. (1990). A new class of rat glutathione S-transferase Yrs-Yrs inactivating reactive sulfate esters as metabolites of carcinogenic arylmethanols. *J. Biol. Chem.* **265**, 11973–11981.

Hirrell, P. A., Collins, M. F., Nimmo, I. A., and Strange, R. C. (1987). The human glutathione *S*-transferases. Studies on the kinetic stability, and inhibition characteristics of the erythrocyte enzyme. *Biochim. Biophys. Acta* **913**, 92–96.

Homma, H., Maruyama, H., Niitsu, Y., and Listowsky, I. (1986). A subclass of glutathione *S*-transferases as intracellular high-capacity and high-affinity steroid-binding proteins. *Biochem. J.* **235**, 763–768.

Howie, A. F., Miller, W. R., Hawkins, R. A., Hutchinson, A. R., and Beckett, G. J. (1989). Expression of glutathione *S*-transferase B1, B2, Mu, and Pi in breast cancers and their relationship to oestrogen-receptor status. *Brit. J. Cancer.* **60**, 834–837.

Howie, A. F., Forrester, L. M., Glancey, M. J., Schlager, J. J., Powis, G., Beckett, G. J., Hayes, J. D., and Wolf, C. R. (1990). Glutathione *S*-transferase and glutathione peroxidase expression in normal and tumour human tissues. *Carcinogenesis (London)* **11**, 451–458.

Hussey, A. J., Stockman, P. K., Beckett, G. J., and Hayes, J. D. (1986). Variations in the glutathione *S*-transferase subunits expressed in human livers. *Biochim. Biophys. Acta* **874**, 1–12.

Igarashi, T., Satoh, T., Iwashita, K., Ono, S., Ueno, K., and Kitagawa, H. (1985). Sex difference in subunit composition of hepatic glutathione *S*-transferase in rats. *J. Biochem (Tokyo)* **98**, 117–123.

Igarashi, T., Irokawa, N., and Ono, S. (1987). Difference in the effects of phenobarbital and 3-methylcholanthrene treatment on subunit composition of hepatic glutathione *S*-transferase in male and female rats. *Xenobiotica* **17**, 127–137.

Igarashi, T., Namba, E., Sagami, F., Tsukidate, K., Fukuda, T., Horie, T., Satoh, T., and Kitagawa, H. (1988). Dog liver glutathione *S*-transferase and its strong immunoreactivity with rat transferase P(7-7). *Biochem. Pharmacol.* **37**, 4713–4718.

Igarashi, T., and Satoh, T. (1989). Sex and species differences in glutathione *S*-transferase activities. *Drug Metab. Drug Interact.* **7**, 191–212.

Igwe, O. J. (1986). Biologically active intermediates generated by the reduced glutathione conjugation pathway. *Biochem. Pharmcol.* **35**, 2987–2994.

Imaida, K., Tatematsu, M., Kato, T., Tsuda, H., and Ito, N. (1989). Advantages and limitations of stereological estimation of placental glutathione *S*-transferase–positive rat liver cell foci by computerized three-dimensional reconstruction. *Jpn. J. Cancer Res.* **80**, 326–330.

Inaba, Y. (1987). Subunit-structural and immunological characterization of glutathione *S*-transferase molecular forms in hamster liver: Comparison with rat forms. *Hirosaki Med. J.* **39**, 58–69.

Inoue, M., Akerboom, T. P. M., Sies, H., Kinne, R., Thao, T., and Arias, I. M. (1984). Biliary transport of glutathione *S*-conjugate by rat liver canalicular membrane vesicles. *J. Biol. Chem.* **259**, 4998–5002.

Inskeep, P. B., and Guengerich, F. P. (1984). Glutathione-mediated binding of dibromoalkanes to DNA: Specificity of rat glutathione-*S*-transferases and dibromoalkane structure. *Carcinogenesis (London)* **5**, 805–808.

Ishikawa, T. (1989). ATP/Mg^{2+}-dependent cardiac transport system for glutathione *S*-conjugates. *J. Biol. Chem.* **264**, 17343–17348.

Ishikawa, T., Tsuchida, S., Satoh, K., and Sato, K. (1988). The subunit structure of a major glutathione *S*-transferase form (M_T) in rat testis: Evidence for a heterodimer consisting of subunits with different isoelectric points. *Eur. J. Biochem.* **176**, 551–557.

Ito, N., Tsuda, H., Tatematsu, M., Inoue, T., Tagawa, Y., Aoki, T., Uwagawa, S., Kagawa, M., Ogiso, T., Masui, T., Imaida, K., Fukushima, S., and Asamoto, M. (1988). Enhancing effect of various hepatocarcinogens on induction of preneoplastic glutathione *S*-transferase placental form positive foci in rats—an approach for a new medium-term bioassay system. *Carcinogenesis (London)* **9**, 387–394.

Ito, N., Imaida, K., Hasegawa, R., and Tsuda, H. (1989). Rapid bioassay methods for carcinogens and modifiers of hepatocarcinogenesis. *CRC Crit. Rev. Toxicol.* **19**, 385–415.

Jakoby, W. B. (1978). The glutathione *S*-transferases: A group of multifunctional detoxification proteins. *Adv. Enzymol.* **46**, 383–414.

Jakoby, W. B., Ketterer, B., and Mannervik, B. (1984). Glutathione transferases: Nomenclature. *Biochem. Pharmacol.* **33**, 2539–2540.

Jakschik, B. A., Harper, T., and Murphy, R. C. (1982). Leukotriene C_4 and D_4 formation by particulate enzymes. *J. Biol. Chem.* **257**, 5346–5349.

Jensen, D. E., and Mackay, R. L. (1990). Rat, mouse, and hamster isozyme specificity in the glutathione transferase–mediated denitrosation of nitrosoguanidinium compounds. *Cancer Res.* **50**, 1440–1448.

Jensson, H., Eriksson, L. C., and Mannervik, B. (1985). Selective expression of glutathione transferase isoenzymes in chemically induced preneoplastic rat hepatocyte nodules. *FEBS Lett.* **187**, 115–120.

Jensson, H., Guthenberg, C., Alin, P., and Mannervik, B. (1986). Rat glutathione transferase 8-8, an enzyme efficiently detoxifying 4-hydroxyalk-2-enals. *FEBS Lett.* **203**, 207–209.

Jernstrom, B., Martinez, M., Meyer, D. J., and Ketterer, B. (1985). Glutathione conjugation of the carcinogenic and mutagenic electrophile ($\pm$)-7β,8α-dihydroxy-9α,10α-oxy-7,8,9,10-tetrahydro-benzo(a)pyrene catalyzed by purified rat liver glutathione transferases. *Carcinogenesis (London)* **6**, 85–89.

Jhee, E.-C., Ho, L. L., Tsuji, K., Gopalan, P., and Lotlikar, P. D. (1989). Effect of butylated hydroxyanisole pretreatment of aflatoxin B_1-DNA binding and aflatoxin B_1-glutathione conjugation in isolated hepatocytes from rats. *Cancer Res.* **49**, 1357–1360.

Kamei, K., Oshino, R., and Hara, S. (1990). Amino acid sequence of glutathione *S*-transferase b from guinea pig liver. *J. Biochem.* **107**, 111–117.

Kamisaka, K., Habig, W. H., Ketley, J. N., Arias, I. M., and Jakoby, W. B. (1975). Multiple forms of human glutathione *S*-transferase and their affinity for bilirubin. *Eur. J. Biochem.* **60**, 153–161.

Kano, T., Sakai, M., and Muramatsu, M. (1987). Structure and expression of a human class π glutathione *S*-transferase messenger RNA. *Cancer Res.* **47**, 5626–5630.

Kensler, T. W., Egner, P. A., Davidson, N. E., Roebuck, B. D., Pikul, A., and Groopman, J. D. (1986). Modulation of aflatoxin metabolism, aflatoxin-N[7]-guanine formation, and hepatic tumorigenesis in rats fed ethoxyquin: Role of induction of glutathione *S*-transferases. *Cancer Res.* **46**, 3924–3931.

Ketterer, B. (1986). Detoxication reactions of glutathione and glutathione transferases. *Xenobiotica* **16**, 957–973.

Ketterer, B., Coles, B., and Meyer, D. J. (1983). The role of glutathione in detoxication. *Environ. Health Perspect.* **49**, 59–69.

Ketterer, B., Meyer, D. J., Coles, B., Taylor, J. B., and Pemble, S. (1986). Glutathione transferases and carcinogenesis. *In* "Antimutagenesis and Anticarcinogenesis Mechanisms" (D. M. Shankel, P. E. Hartman, T. Kada, and A. Hollaender, eds.), pp. 103–126. Plenum, New York.

Ketterer, B., Tan, K. H., Meyer, D. J., and Coles, B. (1987). Glutathione transferases: A possible role in the detoxication of DNA and lipid hydroperoxides. *In* "Glutathione *S*-transferases and Carcinogenesis" (T. J. Mantle, C. B. Pickett, and J. D. Hayes, eds.), pp. 149–163. Taylor & Francis, London.

Ketterer, B., Taylor, J. B., Meyer, D. J., Coles, B., Pemble, S., Cowell, I. G., and Dixon, K. (1989). Glutathione *S*-transferases: Structure and function. *In* "Glutathione Centennial. Molecular Perspectives and Clinical Implications" (N. Taniguchi, T. Higashi, Y. Sakamoto, and A. Meister, eds.), pp. 241–257. Academic Press, London.

Kim, D-H., and Guengerich, F. P. (1990). Formation of the DNA adduct S-[2-(N[7]-guanyl)ethyl]glutathione from ethylene dibromide: Effects of modulation of glutathione and glutathione S-transferase levels and lack of a role for sulfation. *Carcinogenesis (London)* **11**, 419–424.

Kispert, A., Meyer, D. J., Lalor, E., Coles, B., and Ketterer, B. (1989). Purification and characterization of a labile rat glutathione transferase of the Mu class. *Biochem. J.* **260**, 789–793.

Kitahara, A., and Sato, K. (1981). Immunological relationships among subunits of glutathione S-transferases A, AA, B and ligandin and hybrid formation between AA and ligandin by guanidine hydrochloride. *Biochem. Biophys. Res. Commun.* **103**, 943–950.

Kitahara, A., Satoh, K., and Sato, K. (1983a). Properties of the increased glutathione S-transferase A form in rat preneoplastic hepatic lesions induced by chemical carcinogenesis. *Biochem. Biophys. Res. Commun.* **112**, 20–28.

Kitahara, A., Yamazaki, T., Ishikawa, T., Camba, E. A., and Sato, K. (1983b). Changes in activities of glutathione peroxidase and glutathione reductase during chemical hepatocarcinogenesis. *Jpn. J. Cancer Res. (Gann)* **74**, 649–655.

Kitahara, A., Satoh, K., Nishimura, K., Ishikawa, T., Ruike, K., Sato, K., Tsuda, H., and Ito, N. (1984). Changes in molecular forms of rat hepatic glutathione S-transferase during chemical hepatocarcinogenesis. *Cancer Res.* **44**, 2698–2703.

Kodate, C., Fukushi, A., Narita, T., Kudo, H., Soma, Y., and Sato, K. (1986). Human placental form of glutathione S-transferase (GST-π) as a new immunohistochemical marker for human colonic carcinoma. *Jpn. J. Cancer Res. (Gann)* **77**, 226–229.

Kondo, T., Kawakami, Y., Taniguchi, N., and Beutler, E. (1987). Glutathione disulfide–stimulated Mg^{2+}-ATPase of human erythrocyte membranes. *Proc. Natl. Acad. Sci. U.S.A.* **84**, 7373–7377.

Koskelo, K., Valmet, E., and Tenhunen, R. (1981). Purification and characterization of an acid glutathione S-transferase from human lung. *Scand. J. Clin. Lab. Invest.* **41**, 683–689.

Kramer, R. A., Zakher, J., and Kim, G. (1988). Role of the glutathione redox cycle in acquired and *de novo* multidrug resistance. *Science* **241**, 694–697.

Lafuente, A., Giralt, M., Cervello, I., Pujol, F., and Mallol, J. (1990). Glutathione-S-transferase activity in human superficial transitional cell carcinoma of the bladder. *Cancer* **65**, 2064–2068.

Lai, H.-C. J., and Tu, C.-P. D. (1986). Rat glutathione S-transferases supergene family: Characterization of an anionic Yb subunit cDNA clone. *J. Biol. Chem.* **261**, 13793–13799.

Lai, H.-C. J., Li, N.-Q., Weiss, M. J., Reddy, C. C., and Tu, C.-P. D. (1984). The nucleotide sequence of a rat liver glutathione S-transferase subunit cDNA clone. *J. Biol. Chem.* **259**, 5536–5542.

Lai, H.-C. J., Grove, G., and Tu, C.-P. D. (1986). Cloning and sequence analysis of a cDNA for a rat liver glutathione S-transferase Yb subunit. *Nucleic Acids Res.* **14**, 6101–6114.

Lai, H.-C. J., Qian, B., Grove, G., and Tu, C.-P. D. (1988). Gene expression of rat glutathione S-transferases. Evidence for gene conversion in the evolution of the Yb multigene family. *J. Biol. Chem.* **263**, 11389–11395.

Laisney, V., Cong, N. V., Gross, M. S., and Frezal, J. (1984). Human genes for glutathione S-transferases. *Hum. Genet.* **68**, 221–227.

Lee, F. Y. F., Sciandra, J., and Siemann, D. W. (1989). A study of the mechanism of resistance to adriamycin *in vivo*. *Biochem. Pharmacol.* **38**, 3697–3705.

Lewis, A. D., Hickson, I. D., Robson, C. N., Harris, A. L., Hayes, J. D., Griffiths, S. A., Manson, M. M., Hall, A. E., Moss, J. E., and Wolf, C. R. (1988a). Amplification and increased expression of alpha class glutathione S-transferase–encoding genes associated with resistance to nitrogen mustards. *Proc. Natl. Acad. Sci. U.S.A.* **85**, 8511–8515.

Lewis, A. D., Hayes, J. D., and Wolf, C. R. (1988b). Glutathione and glutathione-dependent enzymes in ovarian adenocarcinoma cell lines derived from a patient before and after the onset of drug resistance: Intrinsic differences and cell cycle effects. *Carcinogenesis (London)* **9**, 1283–1287.

Lewis, A. D., Forrester, L. M., Hayes, J. D., Wareing, C. J., Carmichael, J., Harris, A. L.,

Mooghen, M., and Wolf, C. R. (1989). Glutathione S-transferase isoenzymes in human tumours and tumour-derived cell lines. *Br. J. Cancer* **60**, 327–331.

Li, Y., Seyama, T., Godwin, A. K., Winokur, T. S., Lebovitz, R. M., and Lieberman, M. W. (1988). MTrasT24, a metallothionein-ras fusion gene, modulates expression in cultured rat liver cells of two genes associated with *in vivo* liver cancer. *Proc. Natl. Acad. Sci. U.S.A.* **85**, 344–348.

Listowsky, I., Abramovitz, M., Homma, H., and Niitsu, Y. (1988). Intracellular binding and transport of hormones and xenobiotics by glutathione-S-transferases. *Drug Metab. Rev.* **19**, 305–318.

Litwack, G., Ketterer, B., and Arias, I. M. (1971). Ligandin: A hepatic protein which binds steroids, bilirubin, carcinogens, and a number of exogenous organic anions. *Nature (London)* **234**, 466–467.

Lotlikar, P. D., Jhee, E. C., Insetta, S. M., and Clearfield, M. S. (1984). Modulation of microsome-mediated aflatoxin B_1 binding to exogenous and endogenous DNA by cytosolic glutathione S-transferases in rat and hamster livers. *Carcinogenesis (London)* **5**, 269–276.

Lotlikar, P. D., Raj, H. G., Bohm, L. S., Ho, L. L., Jhee, E-C., Tsuji, K., and Gopalan, P. (1989). A mechanism of inhibition of aflatoxin B_1-DNA binding in the liver by phenobarbital pretreatment of rats. *Cancer Res.* **49**, 951–957.

Lutzky, J., Astor, M. B., Taub, R. N., Baker, M. A., Bhalla, K., Gervasoni, J. E. Jr., Rosado, M., Stewart, V., Krishna, S., and Hindenburg, A. A. (1989). Role of glutathione and dependent enzymes in anthracycline-resistant HL60/AR cells. *Cancer Res.* **49**, 4120–4125.

Mannervik, B. (1985). The isoenzymes of glutathione transferase. *Adv. Enzymol.* **57**, 357–417.

Mannervik, B., and Jensson, H. (1982). Binary combinations of four protein subunits with different catalytic specificities explain the relationship between six basic glutathione S-transferases in rat liver cytosol. *J. Biol. Chem.* **257**, 9909–9912.

Mannervik, B., and Danielson, U. H. (1988). Glutathione transferases—structure and catalytic activity. *CRC Crit. Rev. Biochem. Mol. Biol.* **23**, 283–337.

Mannervik, B., Alin, P., Guthenberg, C., Jensson, H., Tahir, M. K., Warholm, M., and Jornvall, H. (1985). Identification of three classes of cytosolic glutathione transferase common to several mammalian species: Correlation between structural data and enzymatic properties. *Proc. Natl. Acad. Sci. U.S.A.* **82**, 7202–7206.

Mannervik, B., Castro, V. M., Danielson, U. H., Tahir, M. K., Hansson, J., and Ringborg, U. (1987). Expression of class pi glutathione transferase in human malignant melanoma cells. *Carcinogenesis (London)* **8**, 1929–1932.

Manoharan, T. H., Puchalski, R. B., Burgess, J. A., Pickett, C. B., and Fahl, W. E. (1987). Promoter-glutathione S-transferase Ya cDNA hybrid genes. *J. Biol. Chem.* **262**, 3739–3745.

Manson, M. M., Green, J. A., and Driver, H. E. (1987). Ethoxyquin alone induces preneoplastic changes in rat kidney whilst preventing induction of such lesions in liver by aflatoxin B_1. *Carcinogenesis (London)* **8**, 723–728.

Marcus, C. J., Habig, W. H., and Jakoby, W. B. (1978). Glutathione transferase from human erythrocytes: Nonidentity with the enzymes from liver. *Arch. Biochem. Biophys.* **188**, 287–293.

Maruyama, H., and Listowsky, I. (1984). Preferential binding of steroids by anionic forms of rat glutathione S-transferase. *J. Biol. Chem.* **259**, 12449–12455.

Masuda, R., Yoshida, M. C., Sasaki, M., Okuda, A., Sakai, M., and Muramatsu, M. (1986). Localization of the gene for glutathione S-transferase P on rat chromosome 1 at band q43. *Jpn. J. Cancer Res.(Gann)* **77**, 1055–1058.

Masuda, R., Yoshida, M. C., and Sasaki, M. (1989). Gene expression of placental glutathione S-transferase in hereditary hepatitis and spontaneous hepatocarcinogenesis of LEC strain rats. *Jpn. J. Cancer Res.* **80**, 1024–1027.

McCusker, F. M. G., Boyce, S. J., and Mantle, T. J. (1989). The development of glutathione S-transferase subunits in rat liver. Sensitive detection of the major subunit forms of rat glutathione S-transferase by using an ELISA method. *Biochem. J.* **262**, 463–467.

McLellan, L. I., and Hayes, J. D. (1987). Sex-specific constitutive expression of the preneoplastic marker glutathione S-transferase, YfYf, in mouse liver. *Biochem. J.* **245,** 399–406.

McLellan, L. I., and Hayes, J. D. (1989). Differential induction of class alpha glutathione S-transferases in mouse liver by the anticarcinogenic antioxidant butylated hydroxyanisole. *Biochem. J.* **263,** 393–402.

McLellan, L. I., and Hayes, J. D. (1990). Differential regulation of murine glutathione S-transferases by xenobiotics. *In* "Glutathione S-transferases and Drug Resistance" (J. D. Hayes, C. B. Pickett, and T. J. Mantle, eds)., pp. 196–211. Taylor & Francis, London.

McLellan, L. I., Wolf, C. R., and Hayes, J. D. (1989). Human microsomal glutathione S-transferase. Its involvement in the conjugation of hexachlorobuta-1,3-diene with glutathione. *Biochem J.* **258,** 87–93.

McQuaid, S., McCann, S., Daly, P., Lawlor, E., and Humphries, P. (1989). Observations on the transcriptional activity of the glutathione S-transferase π gene in human haematological malignancies and in the peripheral leucocytes of cancer patients under chemotherapy. *Br. J. Cancer.* **59,** 540–543.

Medh, R. D., Gupta, V., Zhang, Y., Awasthi, Y. C., and Belli, J. A. (1990). Glutathione S-transferase and P-glycoprotein in multidrug-resistant Chinese hamster cells. *Biochem. Pharmacol.* **39,** 1641–1645.

Meyer, D. J., Christodoulides, L. G., Tan, K. H., and Ketterer, B. (1984). Isolation, properties, and tissue distribution of rat glutathione transferase E. *FEBS Lett.* **173,** 327–330.

Meyer, D. J., Beale, D., Tan, K. H., Coles, B., and Ketterer, B. (1985). Glutathione transferase in primary rat hepatomas: The isolation of a form with GSH peroxidase activity. *FEBS Lett.* **184,** 139–143.

Meyer, D. J., Coles, B., Gilmore, K. S., and Ketterer, B. (1991). Theta, a new class of glutathione transferases purified from rat and man. *Biochem. J.* **274,** 409–414.

Mimnaugh, E. G., Dusre, L., Atwell, J., and Myers, C. E. (1989). Differential oxygen radical susceptibility of adriamycin-sensitive and -resistant MCF-7 human breast tumor cells. *Cancer Res* **49,** 8–15.

Mitaka, T., and Tsukada, H. (1987). Sexual difference in histochemical characteristics of "altered cell foci" in the liver of aged Fisher 344 rats. *Jpn. J. Cancer Res. (Gann)* **78,** 785–790.

Mitchell, J. B., Cook, J. A., DeGraff, W., Glatstein, E., and Russo, A. (1989). Glutathione modulation in cancer treatment: Will it work? *Int. J. Radiat. Oncol. Biol. Phys.* **16,** 1289–1295.

Miyazaki, M., Kohno, K., Saburi, Y., Matsuo, K., Ono, M., Kuwano, M., Tsuchida, S., Sato, K., Sakai, M., and Muramatsu, M. (1990). Drug resistance to *cis*-diamminedichloroplatinum (II) in Chinese hamster ovary cell lines transfected with glutathione S-transferase pi gene. *Biochem. Biophys. Res. Commun.* **166,** 1358–1364.

Moore, M. A., Nakamura, T., and Ito, N. (1986). Immunohistochemically demonstrated glucose-6-phosphate dehydrogenase, γ-glutamyl transpeptidase, ornithine decarboxylase and glutathione S-transferase enzymes: Absence of direct correlation with cell proliferation in rat liver putative preneoplastic lesions. *Carcinogenesis (London)* **7,** 1419–1424.

Moore, M. A., Nakagawa, K., Satoh, K., Ishikawa, T., and Sato, K. (1987a). Single GST-P positive liver cells—putative initiated hepatocytes. *Carcinogenesis (London)* **8,** 483–486.

Moore, M. A., Makino, T., Tsuchida, S., Sato, K., Ichihara, A., Amelizad, Z., Oesch, F., and Konishi, Y. (1987b). Altered drug-metabolizing potential of acinar cell lesions induced in rat pancreas by hydroxyaminoquinoline 1-oxide. *Carcinogenesis (London)* **8,** 1089–1094.

Morgenstern, R., and DePierre, J. W. (1983). Microsomal glutathione transferase. Purification in unactivated form and further characterization of the activation process, substrate specificity, and amino acid composition. *Eur. J. Biochem.* **134,** 591–597.

Morgenstern, R., and DePierre, J. W. (1988). Membrane-bound glutathione transferases. *In* "Glutathione Conjugation" (H. Sies, and B. Ketterer, eds.), pp. 157–174. Academic Press, London.

Morton, M. R., Bayney, R. M., and Pickett, C. B. (1990). Isolation and characterization of the rat glutathione S-transferase Yb₁ subunit gene. *Arch. Biochem. Biophys.* **277**, 56–60.

Moscow, J. A., and Cowan, K. H. (1988). Multidrug resistance. *J. Natl. Cancer Inst.* **80**, 14–20.

Moscow, J. A., Townsend, A. J., Goldsmith, M. E., Whang-Peng, J., Vickers, P. J., Poisson, R., Legault-Poisson, S., Myers, C. E., and Cowan, K. H. (1988). Isolation of the human anionic glutathione S-transferase cDNA and the relation of its gene expression to estrogen-receptor content in primary breast cancer. *Proc. Natl. Acad. Sci. U.S.A.* **85**, 6518–6522.

Moscow, J. A., Fairchild, C. R., Madden, M. J., Ransom, D. T., Wieand, H. S., O'Brien, E. E., Poplack, D. G., Cossman, J., Myers, C. E., and Cowan, K. H. (1989a). Expression of anionic glutathione-S-transferase and P-glycoprotein genes in human tissues and tumors. *Cancer Res.* **49**, 1422–1428.

Moscow, J. A., Townsend, A. J., and Cowan, K. H. (1989b). Elevation of π class glutathione S-transferase activity in human breast cancer cells by transfection of the GST-π gene and its effect on sensitivity to toxins. *Mol. Pharmacol.* **36**, 22–28.

Mouelhi, M. E., Didolkar, M. S., Elias, E. G., Guengerich, F. P., and Kauffman, F. C. (1987). Hepatic drug-metabolizing enzymes in primary and secondary tumors of human liver. *Cancer Res.* **47**, 460–466.

Muramatsu, M., Okuda, A., Kano, T., and Sakai, M. (1987). Structure and regulation of rat glutathione S-transferase P (GST-P) gene. *In* "Glutathione S-transferases and Carcinogenesis" (T. J. Mantle, C. B. Pickett, and J. D. Hayes, eds.), pp. 111–119. Taylor & Francis, London.

Murata, T., Hatayama, I., Satoh, K., Tsuchida, S., and Sato, K. (1990). Activation of rat glutathione transferase in class mu by active oxygen species. *Biochem. Biophys. Res. Commun.* **171**, 845–851.

Nakagawa, K., Yokota, J., Wada, M., Sasaki, Y., Fujiwara, Y., Sakai, M., Muramatsu, M., Terasaki, T., Tsunokawa, Y., Terada, M., and Saijo, N. (1988). Levels of glutathione S-transferase π mRNA in human lung cancer cell lines correlate with the resistance to cisplatin and carboplatin. *Jpn. J. Cancer Res. (Gann)* **79**, 301–304.

Nakagawa, K., Saijo, N., Tsuchida, S., Sakai, M., Tsunokawa, Y., Yokota, J., Muramatsu, M., Sato, K., Terada, M., and Tew, K. D. (1990). Glutathione-S-transferase π as a determinant of drug resistance in transfectant cell lines. *J. Biol. Chem.* **265**, 4296–4301.

Niitsu, Y., Takahashi, Y., Saito, T., Hirata, Y., Arisato, N., Maruyama, H., Kohgo, Y., and Listowsky, I. (1989). Serum glutathione-S-transferase-π as a tumor marker for gastrointestinal malignancies. *Cancer* **63**, 317–323.

Numoto, S., Furukawa, K., Furuya, K., and Williams, G. M. (1984). Effects of the hepatocarcinogenic peroxisome-proliferating hypolipidemic agents clofibrate and nafenopin on the rat liver cell membrane enzymes γ-glutamyltranspeptidase and alkaline phosphatase and on the early stages of liver carcinogenesis. *Carcinogenesis (London)* **5**, 1603–1611.

Ogiso, T., Tatematsu, M., Tamano, S., Tsuda, H., and Ito, N. (1985). Comparative effects of carcinogens on the induction of placental glutathione S-transferase–positive liver nodules in a short-term assay and of hepatocellular carcinomas in a long-term assay. *Toxicol. Pathol.* **13**, 257–273.

Okuda, A., Sakai, M., and Muramatsu, M. (1987). The structure of the rat glutathione S-transferase-P gene and related pseudogenes. *J. Biol. Chem.* **262**, 3858–3863.

Okuda, A., Imagawa, M., Maeda, Y., Sakai, M., and Muramatsu, M. (1989). Structural and functional analysis of an enhancer GPEI having a phorbol 12-0-tetradecanoate 13-acetate responsive element-like sequence found in the rat glutathione transferase P gene. *J. Biol. Chem.* **264**, 16919–16926.

Okuda, A., Imagawa, M., Sakai, M., and Muramatsu, M. (1990). Functional cooperativity between two TPA-responsive elements in undifferentiated F9 embryonic stem cells. *EMBO J.* **9**, 1131–1135.

Oshino, R., Kamei, K., Nishioka, M., and Shin, M. (1990). Purification and characterization of glutathione S-transferases from guinea pig liver. *J. Biochem.* **107,** 105–110.

Ostlund-Farrants, A-K., Meyer, D. J., Coles, B., Southan, C., Aitken, A., Johnson, P. J., and Ketterer, B. (1987). The separation of glutathione transferase subunits by using reverse-phase high-pressure liquid chromatography. *Biochem. J.* **245,** 423–428.

Oyamada, M., Dempo, K., Fujimoto, Y., Takahashi, H., Satoh, M. I., Mori, M., Masuda, R., Yoshida, M. C., Satoh, K., and Sato, K. (1988). Spontaneous occurrence of placental glutathione S-transferase-positive foci in the livers of LEC rats. *Jpn. J. Cancer Res. (Gann)* **79,** 5–8.

Ozols, R. F., Masuda, H., and Hamilton, T. C. (1988). Mechanisms of cross-resistance between radiation and antineoplastic drugs. *Natl. Cancer Inst. Monogr.* **6,** 159–165.

Pearson, W. R., Windle, J. J., Morrow, J. F., Benson, A. M., and Talalay, P. (1983). Increased synthesis of glutathione S-transferases in response to anticarcinogenic antioxidant. Cloning and measurement of mRNA. *J. Biol. Chem.* **258,** 2052–2062.

Pearson, W. R., Reinhart, J., Sisk, S. C., Anderson, K. S., and Adler, P. N. (1988). Tissue-specific induction of murine glutathione transferase mRNAs by butylated hydroxyanisole. *J. Biol. Chem.* **263,** 13324–13332.

Pemble, S. E., Taylor, J. B., and Ketterer, B. (1986). Tissue distribution of rat glutathione transferase subunit 7, a hepatoma marker. *Biochem. J.* **240,** 885–889.

Pemble, S. E., Taylor, J. B., Dixon, K. H., Cowell, I. G., and Ketterer, B. (1987). Tissue expression of glutathione transferase subunit 7: A possible multigene family. *In* "Glutathione S-transferases and Carcinogenesis" (T. J. Mantle, C. B. Pickett, and J. D. Hayes, eds.), pp. 121–123. Taylor & Francis, London.

Peters, W. H. M., Roelofs, H. M. J., Nagengast, F. M., and Van Tongeren, J. H. M. (1989). Human intestinal glutathione S-transferases. *Biochem. J.* **257,** 471–476.

Peters, W. H. M., Kock, L., Nagengast, F. M., and Roelofs, H. M. J. (1990). Immunodetection with a monoclonal antibody of glutathione S-transferase mu in patients with and without carcinomas. *Biochem. Pharmacol.* **39,** 591–597.

Pickett, C. B. (1987). Structure and regulation of glutathione S-transferase genes. *Essays Biochem.* **23,** 116–143.

Pickett, C. B., and Lu, A. Y. H. (1989). Glutathione S-transferases: Gene structure, regulation, and biological function. *Annu. Rev. Biochem.* **58,** 743–764.

Pickett, C. B., Telakowski-Hopkins, C. A., Ding, G. J.-F., Algenbright, L., and Lu, A. Y. H. (1984a). Rat liver glutathione S-transferases. Complete nucleotide sequence of a glutathione S-transferase mRNA and the regulation of the Ya, Yb, and Yc mRNAs by 3-methylcholanthrene and phenobarbital. *J. Biol. Chem.* **259,** 5182–5188.

Pickett, C. B., Williams, J. B., Lu, A. Y. H., and Cameron, R. G. (1984b). Regulation of glutathione transferase and DT-diaphorase mRNAs in persistent hepatocyte nodules during chemical hepatocarcinogenesis. *Proc. Natl. Acad. Sci. U.S.A.* **81,** 5091–5095.

Pitot, H. C., Goodspeed, D., Dunn, T., Hendrich, S., Maronpot, R. R., and Moran, S. (1989). Regulation of the expression of some genes for enzymes of glutathione metabolism in hepatotoxicity and hepatocarcinogenesis. *Toxicol. Appl. Pharmacol.* **97,** 23–34.

Porsch-Hallstrom, L., Blanck, A., Eriksson, L. C., and Gustafsson, J-A. (1989). Expression of the c-*myc*, c-*fos* and c-*ras*[Ha] protooncogenes during sex-differentiated rat liver carcinogenesis in the resistant hepatocyte model. *Carcinogenesis (London)* **10,** 1793–1800.

Power, C., Sinha, S., Webber, C., Manson, M. M., and Neal, G. E. (1987). Transformation related expression of glutathione-S-transferase P in rat liver cells. *Carcinogenesis (London)* **8,** 797–801.

Puchalski, R. B., and Fahl, W. E. (1990). Expression of recombinant glutathione S-transferase π, Ya, or Yb₁ confers resistance to alkylating agents. *Proc. Natl. Acad. Sci. U.S.A.* **87,** 2443–2447.

Radulovic, L. L., Laferla, J. J., and Kulkarni, A. P. (1986). Human placental glutathione S-transferase–mediated metabolism of methylparathion. *Biochem. Pharmacol.* **35,** 3473–3480.

Rao, M. S., and Reddy, J. J. (1987). Peroxisome proliferation and hepatocarcinogenesis. *Carcinogenesis (London)* **8,** 631–636.

Rao, M. S., Nemali, M. R., Usuda, N., Scarpelli, D. G., Makino, T., Pitot, H. C., and Reddy, J. K. (1988). Lack of expression of glutathione-*S*-transferase P, γ-glutamyl transpeptidase, and α-fetoprotein mRNAs in liver tumors induced by peroxisome proliferators. *Cancer Res.* **48,** 4919–4925.

Rauscher, F. J., III, Sambucetti, L. C., Curran, T., Distel, R. J., and Spiegelman, B. M. (1988). A common DNA binding site for *fos* protein complexes and transcription factor AP-1. *Cell* **52,** 471–480.

Reddy, J. K., and Rao, S. (1986). Peroxisome proliferators and cancer: Mechanisms and implications. *Trends Pharmacol. Sci.* **7,** 438–443.

Rhoads, D. M., Zarlengo, R. P., and Tu, C-P, D. (1987). The basic glutathione *S*-transferases from human livers are products of separate genes. *Biochem. Biophys. Res. Commun.* **145,** 474–481.

Ricci, G., Del Boccio, G., Pennelli, A., Aceto, A., Whitehead, E. P., and Federici, G. (1989). Nonequivalence of the two subunits of horse erythrocyte glutathione transferase in their reaction with sulfhydryl reagents. *J. Biol. Chem.* **264,** 5462–5467.

Robertson, I. G. C., and Jernstrom, B. (1986). The enzymatic conjugation of glutathione with bay-region diol-epoxides of benzo(a)pyrene, benz(a)anthracene and chrysene. *Carcinogenesis (London)* **7,** 1633–1636.

Robertson, I. G. C., Jensson, H., Mannervik, B., and Jernstrom, B. (1986a). Glutathione transferases in rat lung: The presence of transferase 7-7, highly efficient in the conjugation of glutathione with the carcinogenic (+)-7β,8α-dihydroxy-9α,10α-oxy-7,8,9,10-tetrahydrobenzo[a]pyrene. *Carcinogenesis (London)* **7,** 295–299.

Robertson, I. G. C., Guthenberg, C., Mannervik, B., and Jernstrom, B. (1986b). Differences in stereoselectivity and catalytic efficiency of three human glutathione transferases in the conjugation of glutathione with 7β, 8α-dihydroxy-9α, 10α-oxy-7,8,9,10-tetrahydrobenzo(a)pyrene. *Cancer Res.* **46,** 2220–2224.

Robson, C. N., Lewis, A. D., Wolf, C. R., Hayes, J. D., Hall, A., Proctor, S. J., Harris, A. L., and Hickson, I. D. (1987). Reduced levels of drug-induced DNA cross-linking in nitrogen mustard-resistant Chinese hamster ovary cells expressing elevated glutathione *S*-transferase activity. *Cancer Res.* **47,** 6022–6027.

Roomi, M. W., Satoh, K., Sato, K., and Farber, E. (1985a). Natural distribution of placental glutathione S-transferase and its modulation by chemicals. *Fed. Proc.* **44,** 521.

Roomi, M. W., Satoh, K., Sato, K., and Farber, E. (1985b). Identification of P-21 polypeptide from rat hepatocyte nodule as placental glutathione *S*-transferase. *Proc. Am. Assoc. Cancer Res.* **26,** 77.

Roomi, M. W., Columbano, A., Ledda-Columbano, G. M., and Sarma, D. S. R. (1986). Lead nitrate induces certain biochemical properties characteristic of hepatocyte nodules. *Carcinogenesis (London)* **7,** 1643–1646.

Roomi, M. W., Columbano, A., Ledda-Columbano, G. M., and Sarma, D. S. R. (1987). Induction of the placental form of glutathione *S*-transferase by lead nitrate administration in rat liver. *Toxicol. Pathol.* **15,** 202–205.

Rushmore, T. H., Sharma, R. N. S., Roomi, M. W., Harris, L., Satoh, K., Sato, K., Murray, R. K., and Farber, E. (1987). Identification of a characteristic cytosolic polypeptide of rat preneoplastic hepatocyte nodules as placental glutathione *S*-transferase. *Biochem. Biophys. Res. Commun.* **143,** 98–103.

Rushmore, T. H., Harris, L., Nagai, M., Sharma, R. N., Hayes, M. A., Cameron, R. G., Murray, R. K., and Farber, E. (1988). Purification and characterization of P-52 (glutathione *S*-transferase-P or 7-7) from normal liver and putative preneoplastic liver nodules. *Cancer Res.* **48,** 2805–2812.

Rushmore, T. H., King, R. G., Paulson, K. E., and Pickett, C. B. (1990). Regulation of glutathione

S-transferase Ya subunit gene expression: Identification of a unique xenobiotic-responsive element controlling inducible expression by planar aromatic compounds. *Proc. Natl. Acad. Sci. U.S.A.* **87**, 3826–3830.

Saburi, Y., Nakagawa, M., Ono, M., Sakai, M., Muramatsu, M., Kohno, K., and Kuwano, M. (1989). Increased expression of glutathione S-transferase gene in *cis*-diamminedichloroplatinum(II)-resistant variants of a Chinese hamster ovary cell line. *Cancer Res.* **49**, 7020–7025.

Sakai, M., Okuda, A., and Muramatsu, M. (1988). Multiple regulatory elements and phorbol 12-O-tetradecanoate 13-acetate responsiveness of the rat placental glutathione transferase gene. *Proc. Natl. Acad. Sci. U.S.A.* **85**, 9456–9460.

Sakai, M., Okuda, A., Hatayama, I., Sato, K., Nishi, S., and Muramatsu, M. (1989). Structure and expression of the rat c-*jun* messenger RNA: Tissue distribution and increase during chemical hepatocarcinogenesis. *Cancer Res.* **49**, 5633–5637.

Sato, K. (1988). Glutathione S-transferases and hepatocarcinogenesis. *Jpn. J. Cancer Res. (Gann)* **79**, 556–572.

Sato, K. (1989). Glutathione transferases as markers of preneoplasia and neoplasia. *Adv. Cancer Res.* **52**, 205–255.

Sato, K., Kitahara, A., Satoh, K., Ishikawa, T., Tatematsu, M., and Ito, N. (1984a). The placental form of glutathione S-transferase as a new marker protein for preneoplasia in rat chemical hepatocarcinogenesis. *Jpn. J. Cancer Res. (Gann)* **75**, 199–202.

Sato, K., Kitahara, A., Yin, Z., Waragai, F., Nishimura, K., Hatayama, I., Ebina, T., Yamazaki, T., Tsuda, H., and Ito, N. (1984b). Induction by butylated hydroxyanisole of specific molecular forms of glutathione S-transferase and UDP-glucuronyltransferase and inhibition of development of γ-glutamyl transpeptidase-positive foci in rat liver. *Carcinogenesis* (London) **5**, 473–477.

Sato, K., Satoh, K., Hatayama, I., Tsuchida, S., Soma, Y., Shiratori, Y., Tateoka, N., Inaba, Y., and Kitahara, A. (1987). Placental glutathione S-transferase as a marker for (pre)neoplastic tissues. *In* "Glutathione S-transferases and Carcinogenesis" (T. J. Mantle, C. B. Pickett, and J. D. Hayes, eds.), pp. 127–137. Taylor & Francis, London.

Sato, K., Tsuchida, S., Satoh, K., Hatayama, I., Ishikawa, T., and Tamai, K. (1989). Properties and functions of neutral and acidic glutathione S-transferases. *In* "Glutathione Centennial. Molecular Perspectives and Clinical Implications" (N. Taniguchi, T. Higashi, Y. Sakamoto, and A. Meister, eds.), pp. 259–270. Academic Press, San Diego.

Sato, K., Satoh, K., Tsuchida, S., Hatayama, I., Tamai, K., and Shen, H. (1990). Glutathione S-transferases and (pre)neoplasia. *In* "Glutathione S-transferases and Drug Resistance" (J. D. Hayes, C. B. Pickett, and T. J. Mantle, eds.), pp. 389–398. Taylor & Francis, London.

Satoh, K., Kitahara, A., and Sato, K. (1985a). Identification of heterogeneous and microheterogeneous subunits of glutathione S-transferase in rat liver cytosol. *Arch. Biochem. Biophys.* **242**, 104–111.

Satoh, K., Kitahara, A., Soma, Y., Inaba, Y., Hatayama, I., and Sato, K. (1985b). Purification, induction, and distribution of placental glutathione transferase: A new marker enzyme for preneoplastic cells in the rat chemical hepatocarcinogenesis. *Proc. Natl. Acad. Sci. U.S.A.* **82**, 3964–3968.

Satoh, K., Hatayama, I., Tateoka, N., Tamai, K., Shimizu, T., Tatematsu, M., Ito, N., and Sato, K. (1989). Transient induction of single GST-P–positive hepatocytes by DEN. *Carcinogenesis* (London) **10**, 2107–2111.

Schaffer, J., Gallay, O., and Ladenstein, R. (1988). Glutathione transferase from bovine placenta. Preparation, biochemical characterization, crystallization, and preliminary crystallographic analysis of a neutral class pi enzyme. *J. Biol. Chem.* **263**, 17405–17411.

Scott, T. R., and Kirsch, R. E. (1987). The isolation of a fetal rat liver glutathione S-transferase isoenzyme with high glutathione peroxidase activity. *Biochim. Biophys. Acta* **926**, 264–269.

Seidegard, J., DePierre, J. W., and Pero, R. W. (1985). Hereditary interindividual differences in the glutathione transferase activity towards *trans*-stilbene oxide in resting human mononuclear leukocytes are due to a particular isoenzyme(s). *Carcinogenesis (London)* **6**, 1211–1216.

Seidegard, J., Pero, R. W., Miller, D. G., and Beattie, E. J. (1986). A glutathione transferase in human leukocytes as a marker for the susceptibility to lung cancer. *Carcinogenesis* (London) **7**, 751–753.

Seidegard, J., Guthenberg, C., Pero, R. W., and Mannervik, B. (1987). The *trans*-stilbene oxide-active glutathione transferase in human mononuclear leukocytes is identical with the hepatic glutathione transferase μ. *Biochem. J.* **246**, 783–785.

Seidegard, J., Vorachek, W. R., Pero, R. W., and Pearson, W. R. (1988). Hereditary differences in the expression of the human glutathione transferase active on *trans*-stilbene oxide are due to a gene deletion. *Proc. Natl. Acad. Sci. U.S.A.* **85**, 7293–7297.

Senjo, M., Ishibashi, T., and Imai, Y. (1985). Purification and characterization of cytosolic liver protein facilitating heme transport into apocytochrome b_5 from mitochondria. Evidence for identifying the heme transfer protein as belonging to a group of glutathione *S*-transferases. *J. Biol. Chem.* **260**, 9191–9196.

Shea, T. C., Kelley, S. L., and Henner, W. D. (1988). Identification of an anionic form of glutathione transferase present in many human tumors and human tumor cell lines. *Cancer Res.* **48**, 527–533.

Sherman, M., Titmuss, S., and Kirsch, R. E. (1983). Glutathione *S*-transferase in human organs. *Biochem. Int.* **6**, 109–118.

Shiratori, Y., Soma, Y., Maruyama, H., Sato, S., Takano, A., and Sato, K. (1987). Immunohistochemical detection of the placental form of glutathione *S*-transferase in dysplastic and neoplastic human uterine cervix lesions. *Cancer Res.* **47**, 6806–6809.

Simons, P. C., and Vander Jagt, D. L. (1977). Purification of glutathione *S*-transferases from human liver by glutathione-affinity chromatography. *Anal. Biochem.* **82**, 334–341.

Singh, S. V., Dao, D. D., Partridge, C. A., Theodore, C., Srivastava, S. K., and Awasthi, Y. C. (1985). Different forms of human liver glutathione *S*-transferases arise from dimeric combinations of at least four immunologically and functionally distinct subunits. *Biochem. J.* **232**, 781–790.

Singh, S. V., Creadon, G., Das, M., Mukhtar, H., and Awasthi, Y. C. (1987a). Glutathione *S*-transferases of mouse lung. Selective binding of benzo[a]pyrene metabolites by the subunits which are preferentially induced by t-butylated hydroxyanisole. *Biochem. J.* **243**, 351–358.

Singh, S. V., Kurosky, A., Awasthi, Y. C. (1987b). Human liver glutathione *S*-transferase ψ. Chemical characterization and secondary-structure comparison with other mammalian glutathione S-transferases. *Biochem. J.* **243**, 61–67.

Singh, S. V., Leal, T., Ansari, G. A. S., and Awasthi, Y. C. (1987c). Purification and characterization of glutathione *S*-transferases of human kidney. *Biochem. J.* **246**, 179–186.

Singh, S. V., Ahmad, H., Kurosky, A., and Awasthi, Y. C. (1988). Purification and characterization of unique glutathione *S*-transferases from human muscle. *Arch. Biochem. Biophys.* **264**, 13–22.

Singh, S. V., Nair, S., Ahmad, H., Awasthi, Y. C., and Krishan, A. (1989). Glutathione *S*-transferases and glutathione peroxidases in doxorubicin-resistant murine leukemic P 388 cells. *Biochem. Pharmacol.* **38**, 3505–3510.

Singh, S. V., Ahmad, H., and Krishan, A. (1990). Expression of glutathione-related enzymes in human bladder cancer cell lines. *Biochem. Pharmacol.* **39**, 1817–1820.

Singhal, S. S., Gupta, S., Ahmad, H., Sharma, R., and Awasthi, Y. C. (1990). Characterization of a novel α-class anionic glutathione *S*-transferase isozyme from human liver. *Arch. Biochem. Biophys.* **279**, 45–53.

Sisk, S. C., and Pearson, W. R. (1990). Induction of murine glutathione transferases by BHA and other xenobiotics. *In* "Glutathione *S*-transferases and Drug Resistance" (J. D. Hayes, C. B. Pickett, and T. J. Mantle, eds.), pp. 222–231. Taylor & Francis, London.

Smith, G. J., and Litwack, G. (1980). Roles of ligandin and the glutathione S-transferases in binding steroid metabolites, carcinogens, and other compounds. *Rev. Biochem. Toxicol.* **2**, 1–47.

Smith, G. J., Ohl, V. S., and Litwack, G. (1977). Ligandin, the glutathione S-transferases, and chemically induced hepatocarcinogenesis: A review. *Cancer Res.* **37**, 8–14.

Smith, G. J., Ohl, V. S., and Litwack, G. (1980). Purification and properties of hamster liver ligandins, glutathione S-transferases. *Cancer Res.* **40**, 1787–1790.

Smith, M. T., Evans, C. G., Doane-Setzer, P., Castro, V. M., Tahir, M. K., and Mannervik, B. (1989). Denitrosation of 1,3-bis(2-chloroethyl)-1-nitrosourea by class mu glutathione transferases and its role in cellular resistance in rat brain tumor cells. *Cancer Res.* **49**, 2621–2625.

Solt, D., and Farber, E. (1976). New principle for the analysis of chemical carcinogenesis. *Nature (London)* **263**, 701–703.

Soma, Y., Satoh, K., and Sato, K. (1986). Purification and subunit-structural and immunological characterization of five glutathione S-transferases in human liver, and the acidic form as a hepatic tumor marker. *Biochim. Biophys. Acta* **869**, 247–258.

Strange, R. C., Faulder, C. G., Davis, B. A., Hume, R., Brown, J. A. H., Cotton, W., and Hopkinson, D. A. (1984). The human glutathione S-transferases: Studies on the tissue distribution and genetic variation of the GST1, GST2, and GST3 isozymes. *Ann. Hum. Genet.* **48**, 11–20.

Stockman, P. K., Beckett, G. J., and Hayes, J. D. (1985). Identification of a basic hybrid glutathione S-transferase from human liver. Glutathione S-transferase δ is composed of two distinct subunits (B1 and B2). *Biochem. J.* **227**, 457–465.

Stockman, P. K., McLellan, L. I., and Hayes, J. D. (1987). Characterization of the basic glutathione S-transferase B1 and B2 subunits from human liver. *Biochem. J.* **244**, 55–61.

Sugioka, Y., Fujii-Kuriyama, Y., Kitagawa, T., and Muramatsu, M. (1985). Changes in polypeptides pattern of rat liver cells during chemical hepatocarcinogenesis. *Cancer Res.* **45**, 365–378.

Suguoka, Y., Kano, T., Okuda, A., Sakai, M., Kitagawa, T., and Muramatsu, M. (1985). Cloning and the nucleotide sequence of rat glutathione S-transferase-P cDNA. *Nucleic Acid Res.* **13**, 6049–6057.

Sun, F. F., Chau, L-Y., Spur, B., Corey, E. J., Lewis, R. A., and Austen, K. F. (1986). Identification of a high-affinity leukotriene C_4-binding protein in rat liver cytosol as glutathione S-transferase. *J. Biol. Chem.* **261**, 8540–8546.

Tahir, M. K., Guthenberg, C., and Mannervik, B. (1989). Glutathione transferases in rat hepatoma cells. Effects of ascites cells on the isoenzyme pattern in liver and induction of glutathione transferases in the tumour cells. *Biochem. J.* **257**, 215–220.

Takagi, A., Sai, K., Umemura, T., Hasegawa, R., and Kurokawa, Y. (1990). Significant increase of 8-hydroxydeoxyguanosine in liver DNA of rats following short-term exposure to the peroxisome proliferators di(2-ethylhexyl)phthalate and di(2-ethylhexyl)adipate. *Jpn. J. Cancer Res.* **81**, 213–215.

Takahashi, S., Tsutsumi, M., Nakae, D., Denda, A., Kinugasa, T., and Konishi, Y. (1987). Persistent effect of a low dose of preadministered diethylnitrosamine on the induction of enzyme-altered foci in rat liver. *Carcinogenesis (London)* **8**, 509–513.

Talalay, P., De Long, M., and Prochaska, H. J. (1988). Identification of a common chemical signal regulating the induction of enzymes that protect against chemical carcinogenesis. *Proc. Natl. Acad. Sci. U.S.A.* **85**, 8261–8265.

Tamai, K., Satoh, K., Tsuchida, S., Hatayama, I., Maki, T., and Sato, K. (1990). Specific inactivation of glutathione S-transferases in class pi by SH-modifiers. *Biochem. Biophys. Res. Commun.* **167**, 331–338.

Tan, K. H., Meyer, D. J., Coles, B., and Ketterer, B. (1986). Thymine hydroperoxide, a substrate for rat Se-dependent glutathione peroxidase and glutathione transferase isoenzymes. *FEBS Lett.* **207**, 231–233.

Tatematsu, M., Mera, Y., Ito, N., Satoh, K., and Sato, K. (1985). Relative merits of immunohistochemical demonstrations of placental, A, B, and C forms of glutathione S-transferase and histochemical demonstration of γ-glutamyl transferase as markers of altered foci during liver carcinogenesis in rats. *Carcinogenesis (London)* **6**, 1621–1626.

Tatematsu, M., Tsuda, H., Shirai, T., Masui, T., and Ito, N. (1987). Placental glutathione S-transferase (GST-P) as a new marker for hepatocarcinogenesis: *In-vivo* short-term screening for hepatocarcinogens. *Toxicol. Pathol.* **15**, 60–68.

Tatematsu, M., Mera, Y., Inoue, T., Satoh, K., Sato, K., and Ito, N. (1988a). Stable phenotypic expression of glutathione S-transferase placental type and unstable phenotypic expression of γ-glutamyltransferase in rat liver preneoplastic and neoplastic lesions. *Carcinogenesis (London)* **9**, 215–220.

Tatematsu, M., Aoki, T., Kagawa, M., Mera, Y., and Ito, N. (1988b). Reciprocal relationship between development of glutathione S-transferase positive liver foci and proliferation of surrounding hepatocytes in rats. *Carcinogenesis (London)* **9**, 221–225.

Tateoka, N., Tsuchida, S., Soma, Y., and Sato, K. (1987). Purification and characterization of glutathione S-transferases in human kidney. *Clin. Chim. Acta* **166**, 207–218.

Taylor, J. B., Pemble, S. E., Cowell, I. G., Dixon, K. H., and Ketterer, B. (1987). Molecular biology of glutathione transferases. *Biochem. Soc. Trans.* **15**, 578–581.

Teicher, B. A., Holden, S. A., Kelley, M. J., Shea, T. C., Cucchi, C. A., Rosowsky, A., Henner, W. D., and Frei, E. III. (1987). Characterization of a human squamous carcinoma cell line resistant to *cis*-diamminedichloroplatinum (II). *Cancer Res.* **47**, 388–393.

Telakowski-Hopkins, C. A., Rodkey, J. A., Bennett, C. D., Lu, A. Y. H., and Pickett, C. B. (1985). Rat liver glutathione S-transferases. Construction of a cDNA clone complementary to a Yc mRNA and prediction of the complete amino acid sequence of a Yc subunit. *J. Biol. Chem.* **260**, 5820–5825.

Telakowski-Hopkins, C. A., Rothkopf, G. S., and Pickett, C. B. (1986). Structural analysis of a rat liver glutathione S-transferase Ya gene. *Proc. Natl. Acad. Sci. U.S.A.* **83**, 9393–9397.

Telakowski-Hopkins, C. A., King, R. G., and Pickett, C. B. (1988). Glutathione S-transferase Ya subunit gene: Identification of regulatory elements required for basal level and inducible expression. *Proc. Natl. Acad. Sci. U.S.A.* **85**, 1000–1004.

Tew, K. D. (1989). The involvement of glutathione S-transferases in drug resistance. *Anticancer Drugs* **191**, 103–112.

Tew, K. D., and Clapper, M. L. (1987). Glutathione S-transferases and anticancer drug resistance. *In* "Mechanisms of Drug Resistance in Neoplastic Cells" (P. V. Woolley and K. D. Tew, eds.), pp. 141–159. Academic Press, New York.

Tew, K. D., Clapper, M. L., Greenberg, R. E., Weese, J. L., Hoffman, S. J., and Smith, T. M. (1987). Glutathione S-transferases in human prostate. *Biochim. Biophys. Acta* **926**, 8–15.

Tew, K. D., Bomber, A. M., and Hoffman, S. J. (1988). Ethacrynic acid and piriprost as enhancers of cytotoxicity in drug-resistant and -sensitive cell lines. *Cancer Res.* **48**, 3622–3625.

Thamavit, W., Tatematsu, M., Ogiso, T., Mera, Y., Tsuda, H., and Ito, N. (1985). Dose-dependent effects of butylated hydroxyanisole, butylated hydroxytoluene, and ethoxyquin in induction of foci of rat liver cells containing the placental form of glutathione S-transferase. *Cancer Lett.* **27**, 295–303.

Theodore, C., Singh, S. V., Hong, T. D., and Awasthi, Y. C. (1985). Glutathione S-transferases of human brain. *Biochem. J.* **225**, 375–382.

Tsuchida, S., and Sato, K. (1990). Rat spleen glutathione transferases. A new acidic form belonging to the alpha class. *Biochem. J.* **266**, 461–465.

Tsuchida, S., Izumi, T., Shimizu, T., Ishikawa, T., Hatayama, I., Satoh, K., and Sato, K. (1987). Purification of a new acidic glutathione S-transferase, GST-Yn_1Yn_1, with a high leukotriene-C_4 synthase activity from rat brain. *Eur. J. Biochem.* **170**, 159–164.

Tsuchida, S., Sekine, Y., Shineha, R., Nishihira, T., and Sato, K. (1989). Elevation of the placental glutathione S-transferase form (GST-π) in tumor tissues and the levels in sera of patients with cancer. *Cancer Res.* **49**, 5225–5229.

Tsuchida, S., Maki, T., and Sato, K. (1990). Purification and characterization of glutathione transferases with an activity toward nitroglycerin from human aorta and heart. *J. Biol. Chem.* **265**, 7150–7157.

Tsutsumi, M., Sugisaki, T., Makino, T., Miyagi, N., Nakatani, K., Shiratori, T., Takahashi, S., and Konishi, Y. (1987). Oncofetal expression of glutathione S-transferase placental form in human stomach carcinomas. *Jpn. J. Cancer Res. (Gann)* **78**, 631–633.

Tu, C.-P. D., and Qian, B. (1986). Human liver glutathione S-transferases: Complete primary sequence of an Ha subunit cDNA. *Biochem. Biophys. Res. Commun.* **141**, 229–237.

Tu, C.-P. D., and Qian, B. (1987). Nucleotide sequence of the human liver glutathione S-transferase subunit 1 cDNA. *Biochem. Soc. Trans.* **15**, 734–736.

Urade, Y., Fujimoto, N., Ujihara, M., and Hayaishi, O. (1987). Biochemical and immunological characterization of rat spleen prostaglandin D synthetase. *J. Biol. Chem.* **262**, 3820–3825.

Vander Jagt, D. L., Hunsaker, L. A., Garcia, K. B., and Royer, R. E. (1985). Isolation and characterization of the multiple glutathione S-transferases from human liver. Evidence for unique heme-binding sites. *J. Biol. Chem.* **260**, 11603–11610.

Wang, Y., Teicher, B. A., Shea, T. C., Holden, S. A., Rosbe, K. W., Al-Achi, A., and Henner, W. D. (1989). Crossresistance and glutathione-S-transferase π levels among four human melanoma cell lines selected for alkylating agent resistance. *Cancer Res.* **49**, 6185–6192.

Warholm, M., Guthenberg, C., Mannervik, B., and von Bahr, C. (1981). Purification of a new glutathione S-transferase (transferase μ) from human liver having high activity with benzo(α)pyrene-4,5-oxide. *Biochem. Biophys. Res. Commun.* **98**, 512–519.

Warholm, M., Guthenberg, C., and Mannervik, B. (1983). Molecular and catalytic properties of glutathione transferase μ from human liver: An enzyme efficiently conjugating epoxides. *Biochemistry* **22**, 3610–3617.

Warholm, M., Jensson, H., Tahir, M. K., and Mannervik, B. (1986). Purification and characterization of three distinct glutathione transferases from mouse liver. *Biochemistry* **25**, 4119–4125.

Wattenberg. L. W. (1972). Inhibition of carcinogenic and toxic effects of polycyclic hydrocarbons by phenolic antioxidants and ethoxyquin. *J. Natl. Cancer Inst.* **48**, 1425–1430.

Wattenberg, L. W. (1985). Chemoprevention of cancer. *Cancer Res.* **45**, 1–8.

Wattenberg, L. W., Hanley, A. B., Barany, G., Sparnins, V. L., Lam, L. K. T., and Fenwick, G. R. (1986). Inhibition of carcinogenesis by some minor dietary constituents. *In* "Diet, Nutrition and Cancer" (Y. Hayashi, M. Nagao, T. Sugimura, S. Takayama, L. Tomatis, L. W. Wattenberg, and G. N. Wogan, eds.), pp. 193–203. Japan Sci. Soc. Press, Tokyo/VNU Sci. Press, Utrecht.

West, I. C. (1990). What determines the substrate specificity of the multidrug-resistance pump? *T.I.B.S.* **15**, 42–46.

Wiencke, J. K., Kelsey, K. T., Lamela, R. A., and Toscano, W. A., Jr. (1990). Human glutathione S-transferase deficiency as a marker of susceptibility to epoxide-induced cytogenetic damage. *Cancer Res.* **50**, 1585–1590.

Wiener, H. (1986). Heterogeneity of dog-liver glutathione S-transferases. Evidence for a unique temperature dependence of catalytic process. *Eur. J. Biochem.* **157**, 351–363.

Winokur, T. S., and Lieberman, M. W. (1990). Immunofluorescent analysis of γ-glutamyl transpeptidase and glutathione-S-transferarase-P during the initial phase of experimental hepatocarcinogenesis. *Carcinogenesis (London)* **11**, 365–369.

Wirth, P. J., Rao, M. S., and Evarts, R. P. (1987). Coordinate polypeptide expression during hepatocarcinogenesis in male F-344 rats: Comparison of the Solt-Farber and Reddy models. *Cancer Res.* **47**, 2839–2851.

Xu, Y-H., Maronpot, R., and Pitot, H. C. (1990a). Quantitative stereologic study of the effects of varying the time between initiation and promotion on four histochemical markers in rat liver during hepatocarcinogenesis. *Carcinogenesis (London)* **11**, 267–272.

Xu, Y-H., Campbell, H. A., Sattler, G. L., Hendrich, S., Maronpot, R., Sato, K., and Pitot, H. C. (1990b). Quantitative stereological analysis of the effects of age and sex on multistage hepatocarcinogenesis in the rat by use of four cytochemical markers. *Cancer Res.* **50**, 472–479.

Yamamoto, K., Yokose, Y., Nakajima, A., Eimoto, H., Shiraiwa, K., Tamura, K., Tsutsumi, M., and Konishi, Y. (1988). Comparative histochemical investigation of the glutathione *S*-transferase placental form and γ-glutamyltranspeptidase during N-nitrosobis(2-hydroxypropyl)amine–induced lung carcinogenesis in rats. *Carcinogenesis (London)* **9**, 399–404.

Yokota, K., Singh, U., and Shinozuka, H. (1990). Effects of a choline-deficient diet and a hypolipidemic agent on single glutathione *S*-transferase placental form-positive hepatocytes in rat liver. *Jpn. J. Cancer Res.* **81**, 129–134.

Yoshimoto, T., Soberman, R. J., Lewis, R. A., and Austen, K. F. (1985). Isolation and characterization of leukotriene C₄ synthetase of rat basophilic leukemia cells. *Proc. Natl. Acad. Sci. U.S.A.* **82**, 8399–8403.

Yusa, K., Hamada, H., and Tsuruo, T. (1988). Comparison of glutathione S-transferase activity between drug-resistant and -sensitive human tumor cells: Is glutathione transferase associated with multidrug resistance? *Cancer Chemother. Pharmacol.* **22**, 17–20.

Ziegler, D. M. (1985). Role of reversible oxidation-reduction of enzyme thiols-disulfides in metabolic regulation. *Annu. Rev. Biochem.* **54**, 305–329.

Chapter 7

Steroid Hormones and Hormone Receptors in Neoplastic Diseases

Clark W. Distelhorst

Department of Medicine, Case Western Reserve University, and Ireland Cancer Center, University Hospitals of Cleveland, Cleveland, Ohio 44106

I. Introduction

The role of steroid hormones in promoting the growth of certain malignancies, most notably prostate carcinoma and breast carcinoma, has been recognized for many years (Beatson, 1896; Huggins and Clark, 1940; Huggins and Hodges, 1941). Likewise, endocrine manipulations such as orchiectomy for prostate cancer and ovariectomy or hypophysectomy for breast cancer were among the earliest successful approaches to treating cancer. Similarly, recognition that glucocorticosteroid hormones induce atrophy of normal lymphoid tissues led to the first successful use of these hormones in the treatment of malignant lymphomas over 40 years ago (Pearson *et al.*, 1949). These remarkable advances in clinical medicine occurred even though the molecular events involved in regulation of tumor cell growth by steroid hormones were not understood. The first description of the estradiol receptor by Jensen and colleagues in 1960 opened the door for increased understanding of the fundamental mechanisms by which steroid hormones interact with cells (Jensen, *et al.*, 1982). Recently, cloning of the genes for various steroid hormone receptors revealed that steroid hormone receptors are members of a large superfamily of ligand-regulated transcriptional regulatory

227

molecules and produced new insight into the potential oncogenic role of steroid hormones and their receptors.

This chapter focuses on steroid hormones and steroid hormone receptors in neoplastic disease.

II. Molecular Mechanisms of Steroid Hormone Action

According to current dogma, all effects of steroid hormones on cells are mediated through specific proteins, referred to as receptors, which interact with DNA and regulate gene transcription. The structural and functional properties of steroid hormone receptors and the mechanisms through which they regulate gene transcription have been reviewed recently (Beato, 1989; Yamamoto, 1985; O'Malley et al., 1986; Gustaffsson et al., 1987; Evans, 1988; Litwack, 1988; Burnstein and Cidlowski, 1989; Distelhorst, 1989; Evans, 1989; Munck et al., 1990). Steroid hormone receptors are ligand-regulated transcriptional regulatory molecules that either induce or repress the transcription of target genes. In the absence of hormone, the receptor molecules are inactive; upon binding their hormonal ligand, the receptors are converted to an active form that interacts with specific enhancer sequences on DNA. Through interaction with these sequences, receptor molecules regulate the rate of transcription initiation from nearby promoters, causing an increase in the transcription of specific genes (Yamamoto, 1985). Glucocorticoid receptors can also cause decreased transcription of specific genes, although the mechanism of these negative effects has not yet been fully elucidated.

The genes for the steroid and thyroid hormone receptors are part of a large superfamily of genes that encode ligand-responsive transcription factors (Evans, 1988). Each of the members of this family share a high degree of homology (ranging from 42 to 94%) in a central-core sequence that is rich in cysteine, lysine, and arginine residues. This region, which constitutes the DNA-binding domain, appears to form a *zinc-finger* structural motif in which multiple cysteine- and histidine-rich repeating units fold into a fingered structure coordinated by a zinc ion. This finger of amino acids is proposed to interact with a half turn of DNA (Evans, 1988). The presence of a highly conserved sequence element corresponding to the DNA-binding domain initiated searches for cryptic receptor genes by low-stringency hybridization; through this technique, a number of new ligand-dependent transcription factors have been identified, including the gene that encodes the retinoic acid receptor and a gene that encodes a receptor closely related to the retinoic acid receptor that has been implicated in the etiology of hepatocellular carcinoma and therefore named HAP (see below) (Evans, 1988).

The mechanism through which the appropriate hormonal ligand converts the receptor from an inactive form to a form that is active in transcriptional regulation remains to be fully elucidated. Current evidence suggests that the unliganded hormone-binding region of steroid hormone receptors represses receptor activity; by binding to the receptor, hormonal ligand relieves this repressive activity, and the hormonal signal is transduced through the interaction of the receptor with DNA and the regulation of gene transcription (Yamamoto *et al.*, 1988), (Eilers *et al.*, 1989). Recent developments suggest that the repressor function of the hormone-binding domain may be mediated through interaction with the 90-kDa heat-shock protein, HSP90 (Yamamato *et al.*, 1988; Howard *et al.*, 1990).

As stated earlier, current dogma holds that all effects of steroid hormones on cells are mediated by receptors that interact with DNA and regulate gene transcription. This dogma may not hold true for long, as there is presently emerging evidence that steroid hormones may also bind to cell membrane receptors and exert effects on cells independent of regulation of gene transcription (Touchette, 1990).

III. Regulation of Steroid Hormone Receptor Levels in Cells

In general, the magnitude of a cell's response to a particular steroid hormone is determined by the intracellular concentration of the appropriate steroid hormone receptor. Perhaps the most convincing experimental evidence that this is the case was provided by the work of Vanderbilt and colleagues (Vanderbilt *et al.*, 1987), who constructed cell lines expressing different levels of glucocorticoid receptor and demonstrated that the extent of a structural alteration in the chromatin at a characterized glucocorticoid response element, as well as the magnitude of several transcriptional responses elicited by the receptor, was roughly proportional to the number of receptor molecules per cell. Thus, factors that may regulate the intracellular level of steroid hormone receptors in tumor cells may be important determinants of hormonal responsiveness *in vivo*.

There is considerable evidence that different classes of steroid hormone receptors in tumor cells are under autoregulatory control; thus, the dominant factor regulating steroid hormone receptor levels in tumor cells appears to be the cognate hormonal ligand itself. The effects of autoregulatory control on the intracellular content of different classes of steroid hormone receptors in tumor cells and the mechanisms of autoregulatory control are summarized here.

A. Estrogen and Progesterone Receptors

The autoregulatory control of estrogen and progesterone receptors has been extensively investigated. Whereas various growth factors were found to have very little effect on estrogen-receptor levels in breast cancer cell lines, the dominant factor regulating estrogen-receptor levels was found to be the steroid hormonal ligand itself (Read *et al.*, 1989). Whether estrogens up-regulate or down-regulate their own receptor is, however, dependent on the individual cell line. Thus, in one particular cell line, the T47D breast cancer line, estradiol induces a significant increase in the level of estrogen receptors; but in another cell line, the MCF-7 breast cancer line, estradiol induces a decrease in the level of estrogen receptors (Read *et al.*, 1989). In addition, estrogen receptors are regulated differently by different hormonal ligands. For example, in the T47D breast cancer cell line, estradiol induces a 2.5-fold increase in estrogen-receptor mRNA levels; in contrast, the progestin R5020 induces a marked decrease in estrogen-receptor mRNA levels (Read *et al.*, 1989). The mechanisms of differential autoregulatory control in different cell lines and by different ligands are not understood at present. In the MCF-7 cell line, the mechanism of estrogen-receptor down-regulation by estradiol is complex, and appears to involve inhibition of estrogen-receptor gene transcription at early times and a posttranslational effect on receptor mRNA at later times (Saceda *et al.*, 1988).

Progesterone receptors, like estrogen receptors, are also under autoregulatory control. In breast cancer cell lines, progesterone receptors are down-regulated by progestins (Read *et al.*, 1988) and up-regulated by estrogens (Nardulli *et al.*, 1988; Wei *et al.*, 1988). Receptor autoregulation is not unique to breast cancer cell lines, as progesterone has been found to down-regulate its own receptor in rat prostate carcinoma cells as well (Mobbs *et al.*, 1987). The mechanism of down-regulation by progestins involves both a decrease in the rate of receptor synthesis and a decrease in receptor half-life (Nardulli and Katzenellenbogen, 1988). The mechanism of up-regulation by estrogens involves an increase in the rate of receptor synthesis, rather than modulation of the rate of receptor degradation (Nardulli *et al.*, 1988).

B. GLUCOCORTICOID RECEPTORS

There is considerable evidence that glucocorticoid hormones down-regulate the level of their own receptor in cells (McIntyre and Samuels, 1985; Rosewicz *et al.*, 1988; Vedeckis *et al.*, 1989). A variety of mechanisms appear to be involved in glucocorticoid receptor autoregulation, including decreased rate of receptor gene transcription (Rosewicz *et al.*, 1988) and decreased receptor mRNA half-life (Vedeckis *et al.*, 1989). Intriguingly, the glucocorticoid receptor gene appears to contain several internal glucocorticoid receptor-binding regions that may be responsible for autoregulation of receptor transcription (Vedeckis *et al.*, 1989). In addition, in certain cell lines (McIntyre and Samuels, 1985), but not others (Distelhorst and Howard, 1989), glucocorticoids appear to induce a reduction in receptor half-life. Finally, it should be noted that regulation of the glucocorticoid receptor by its cognate ligand may be tissue specific; in certain cell lines, glucocorticoids up-regulate rather than down-regulate the level of their own receptor (Eisen *et al.*, 1988).

IV. Estrogens and Regulation of Tumor Cell Growth

The possibility that certain steroid hormones, mainly estrogens, play a role in both carcinogenesis and tumor progression has intrigued investigators for many years. Based upon both epidemiological and experimental studies, the length of estrogenic exposure of the mammary glands appears to be proportional to breast cancer risk (Henderson *et al.*, 1988). Thus, an increased incidence of breast cancer has been linked to diethylsilbestrol exposure during pregnancy (Greenberg *et al.*, 1984) and estrogen treatment for postmenopausal symptoms (Barrett-Connor, 1989), (Bergkvist *et al.*, 1989). Also, the risk of both localized and widespread endometrial cancer has been linked to long-term use of conjugated estrogens (Shapiro *et al.*, 1985). *In vitro*, estradiol stimulates the proliferation and invasiveness of the MCF-7 human breast cancer cell line (Thompson *et al.*, 1988; Thompson *et al.*, 1989). Endometrial cells also respond to estrogens with increased proliferation (Pavlik and Katzenellenbogen, 1978).

The mechanisms responsible for promotion of tumor cell growth and invasion by estrogens appear to be complex. Estrogens have a direct mitogenic effect on breast cancer cells and shorten the duration of their cell cycle (Kendra and Katzenellenbogen, 1987). Also, estrogens induce a large number of enzymes and other proteins involved in nucleic acid synthesis in isolated breast cancer cell lines including DNA polymerase, the c-*myc* protooncogene, thymidine and uridine kinases, thymidylate synthetase, carbamyl-phosphate synthetase, aspartate transcarbamylase, dihydroorotase, glucose-6-phosphate dehydrogenase, and dihydrofolate reductase (Lippman and Dickson, 1989). Also, a role for polyamines in estrogen-regulated breast cancer cell growth has been suggested by the observation that inhibition of polyamine synthesis in the MCF-7 breast cancer cell line inhibits estradiol-induced cell proliferation (Kendra and Katzenellenbogen, 1987). Each of these estrogenic effects could potentially contribute to direct stimulation of tumor cell growth by estrogens. More indirect effects related to the expression of various growth factors, and non–growth factor peptides appear to be involved in the promotion of breast cancer growth as well.

A. REGULATION OF GROWTH FACTORS BY ESTROGENS

Estrogenic stimulation plays a critical role in the differentiation and proliferation of normal mammary epithelium; thus, it is not surprising that neoplastic mammary epithelium should also respond to estrogenic stimulation, possibly through many of the same mechanisms. One way that estrogens control breast tumor growth is by inducing pituitary synthesis and secretion of prolactin or by allowing breast cancer cells to overcome growth-inhibiting agents in their environment (Lippman and Dickson, 1989). Another way that estrogens can control breast tumor growth is by inducing the synthesis and release from breast cancer cells of polypeptide growth factors that mediate growth of breast cancer cells in either an autocrine or paracrine fashion (Lippman and Dickson, 1989).

Among the growth factors implicated in regulating breast cancer growth in response to estrogens are transforming growth factor alpha (TGF-α), epidermal growth factor (EGF), insulin-like growth factors (IGF-I and IGF-II), transforming growth factor beta (TGF-β) and platelet-derived growth factor (PDGF). Both TGF-α and EGF act via the EGF receptor, a ligand-inducible tyrosine kinase; the EGF receptor is present on both normal and cancerous cell lines (Lippman and Dickson, 1989), and in certain cells, its transcription is increased by estradiol (Mukku and Stancel, 1985). Thus, estradiol may increase the responsiveness of tumor cells to TGF-α and EGF by inducing an increase in the expression of the EGF receptor. Estrogens may also promote proliferation of tumor cells by inducing the synthesis of TGF-α and EGF. For example, estradiol induces TGF-α and its mRNA in MCF-7 breast cancer cells, implicating TGF-α as an autocrine growth factor in breast cancer (Bates *et al.*, 1988). Also, EGF overexpression has been closely associated with poor prognosis in clinical breast cancer and with rapid tumor growth rate in experimental systems (Lippman and Dickson, 1989).

Another group of growth factors, the insulin-like growth factors, have also been implicated in hormonal stimulation of tumor cell growth. Virtually all breast cancer cell lines express mRNA for insulin receptors, IGF-I receptors, and IGF-II receptors (Cullen *et al.*, 1990). In MCF-7 breast cancer cells, antibody to the IGF-I receptor blocks the mitogenic effect of both IGF-I and IGF-II (Cullen *et al.*, 1990). Also, estrogen stimulates a threefold to sixfold induction of IGF-I–like growth factor in breast cancer cell lines, and secretion of IGF-1–related factors is inhibited by antiestrogens (Huff *et al.*, 1988). Thus, IGF-1–related factors appear to be autocrine growth factors for breast cancer cells.

Certain other growth factors, such as TGF-β, that normally inhibit rather than promote tumor cell growth, may be blocked by estrogens. For example, TGF-β secretion is inhibited by treatment of MCF-7 breast cancer cells with estrogen, whereas antiestrogens strongly stimulate its secretion (Lippman and Dickson, 1989). These observations suggest that one way in which estrogens promote breast cancer cell growth is through inhibition of TGF-β secretion. The effects of estrogen on TGF-β are dependent on individual cell type; thus in osteoblast-like osteosarcoma cells, estradiol induces rather than represses production of TGF-β (Komm *et al.*, 1988).

Another way in which growth factors may promote tumor progression in response to hormonal stimulation is by acting in a paracrine fashion on other cellular elements. For example, in breast cancer, estrogen-induced PDGF may act in a paracrine manner on fibroblasts and possibly other surrounding tissues; this could result in the production by fibroblasts of mediators such as IGF-I that might further enhance tumor growth (Lippman and Dickson, 1989). *In vivo,* growth factors and estrogen probably act in concert with other systemic mitogens (e.g., IGF-II), to promote tumor growth (Lippman and Dickson, 1989).

B. REGULATION OF NONGROWTH FACTOR PROTEINS BY ESTROGENS

Two-dimensional gel analysis of polypeptide patterns of MCF-7 breast cancer cells support the view that a few specific polypeptides are regulated by diverse tumorigenic stimuli in MCF-7 cells (Worland *et al.,* 1989). Both estrogens and antiestrogens alter the synthesis and/or secretion of several proteins by breast cancer cells; the role these proteins play in promoting breast cancer cell growth is not entirely clear. These proteins include various plasminogen activators and collagenolytic enzymes, as well as less well identified proteins of 24 kDa, 52 kDa, 160 kDa, 37–39 kDa, 32 kDa, and 7 kDa (Westley *et al.,* 1984; Lippman and Dickson, 1989). Two of these proteins, the 52-kDa protein, which has cathepsin D activity, and the 7-kDa protein, which has been identified as the product of the pS2 gene, are of particular interest and will be discussed in greater detail below. A 24-kDa protein is regulated by estrogen in human breast cancer cell lines and in human tumor biopsies; this protein has striking homology to low-molecular-weight heat-shock proteins of *Drosophila* and to mammalian alpha-crystallins (Fuqua *et al.,* 1989). A particularly intriguing observation is that estrogen induces the cell-surface receptor for laminin in MCF-7 breast cancer cells; since the laminin receptor mediates attachment of cells to basement membranes, the induction of this protein in breast cancer cells may contribute to tumor invasiveness (Lippman and Dickson, 1989). Interestingly, estrogens and antiestrogens have differential effects on protein expression in breast cancer cells. For example, the antiestrogen tamoxifen stimulates MCF-7 cells to produce a 37-kDa glycoprotein and secrete it into the culture medium, whereas estradiol stimulates increased synthesis of a 32-kDa secreted glycoprotein (Sheen and Katzenellenbogen, 1987). Thus, detailed characterization of peptides that are stimulated or repressed in response to estrogens and antiestrogens may provide significant clues as to the mechanisms of action of these important hormones in regulating tumor cell growth.

Of particular current interest is the observation that estrogens stimulate human breast cancer cells to synthesize and secrete pro-cathepsin D, the precursor of cathepsin D, a lysosomal acidic protease (Touitou *et al.,* 1989). Pro-cathepsin D is secreted more abundantly by cancer cells than by normal cells (Capony *et al.,* 1989); also, estradiol does not alter the level of cathepsin D in an endometrial cancer cell line (Touitou *et al.*, 1989). Thus, the estrogenic stimulation of cathepsin D appears to be relatively specific for breast cancer cells. In MCF-7 breast cancer cells, cathepsin D is induced by EGF and several other growth factors; the induction by growth factors is indirect, but the induction by estrogens is direct and at the transcriptional level (Cavailles *et al.*, 1989). Cathepsin D may play an important role in the pathogenesis of breast cancer both by promoting tumor invasiveness and by functioning as an autocrine growth stimulator. Cathepsin D can degrade extracellular matrices and proteoglycans (Thorpe *et al.*, 1989; Briozzo *et al.*, 1988). Thus, cathepsin D from breast cancer cells may degrade basement membranes and consequently facilitate tumor invasion when released into an acidic microenvironment. *In vitro* studies have demonstrated that the secreted pro-cathepsin D interacts with the mannose 6-phosphate/IGF II receptor on breast cancer cells via mannose 6-phosphate signals and displays an autocrine mitogenic activity for breast cancer cells (Capony *et al.*, 1989). That cathepsin D may play a role in the pathogenesis of breast cancer is supported by clinical studies in which high levels of cathepsin D in breast cancer cells have been found to be an important predictor of earlier relapse (Thorpe *et al.*, 1989).

Another estrogen-induced factor of considerable interest in breast cancer is pS2. pS2 mRNA encodes a small 84-amino acid, cysteine-rich secretory protein that is regulated at the transcriptional level by estrogens (Tomasetto *et al.*, 1990). pS2 is secreted into the medium of MCF-7 breast cancer cells, and its synthesis is induced by estradiol, but not by the antiestrogen, tamoxifen (Nunez *et al.*, 1987). Regulation of pS2 synthesis appears to occur at the transcriptional level (Cavailles *et al.*, 1989). pS2 is not expressed in normal breast tissue and is thought to be an autocrine or paracrine stimulator of breast tumor cell proliferation, as it is also induced by the tumor promotor TPA, by EGF, and by oncogenes *jun* or *ras* (Cavailles *et al.*, 1989; Tomasetto *et al.*, 1990). pS2 gene expression is an estrogen-dependent biochemical and immunocytochemical marker in breast cancer (Rio *et al.*, 1987); pS2 is expressed in 50% of primary human breast tumors, and its expression correlates with hormone-dependent status (Nunez *et al.*, 1989; Tomasetto *et al.*, 1990).

V. Oncogenic Potential of Steroid Hormones and Steroid Hormone Receptors

There is currently considerable speculation about the potential oncogenic role of steroid hormone receptors (Green and Chambon, 1986; Sluyser, 1990). This is based largely on recognition that steroid hormone receptors have structural homology with the avian erythroblastosis virus oncogene v-*erb*A, which has been shown to transform avian erythrocyte cells. The human c-*erb*A gene, the cellular counterpart of the viral oncogene v-*erb*A, represents the thyroid hormone receptor. The *erb*A genes encode a cysteine-rich domain that shows high homology with the DNA-binding domain of steroid hormone receptors. It has been proposed that loss of hormonal dependency of certain tumors might be attributed to the appearance of mutated or truncated steroid receptor–like proteins that act constitutively in the regulation of gene transcription (Green and Chambon, 1986; Sluyser, 1990). Interest in the potential oncogenic role of steroid hormone receptors has also been stimulated by the possible linkage between the progesterone receptor gene and the gene coding for the human homolog of the mouse mammary tumor virus integration site, int-2, which surrounds a proto-oncogene thought to be involved in the development of murine mammary cancers (Law *et al.*, 1987). Both genes map to human chromosome band 11q13; that these two genes share the same chromosomal location raises important questions about their possible linkage and about the relationship between the mammary-specific oncogene and the steroid hormone in development, growth, and hormone dependence of human cancers (Law *et al.*, 1987).

The oncogenic potential of the retinoic acid receptor, a member of the steroid hormone receptor superfamily, has been recently recognized. The retinoic acid receptor gene is normally silent in liver cells; but when hepatitis B virus integrates next to liver cell sequences encoding the retinoic acid receptor, the receptor becomes expressed (Dejean *et al.*, 1986; de-The *et al.*, 1987; Benbrook *et al.*, 1988). The discovery of the retinoic acid receptor gene apparently contributing to tumor development is surprising, inasmuch as vitamin A and other retinoids are generally considered to have antitumor activity; the gene, however, might contribute to tumor development when expressed erroneously in liver tissue, where it is normally silent (Sluyser, 1990).

In addition to intrinsic oncogenic potential, steroid hormone receptors may be involved in the pathogenesis of cancer through their interaction with environmental toxins. A prime example is the aryl hydrocarbon hydroxylase receptor, or Ah receptor. The Ah receptor is a member of the steroid hormone receptor superfamily of transcriptional regulatory proteins (Cuthill *et al.*, 1987; Gustafsson *et al.*, 1987; Perdew and Poland, 1988). Although its natural or physiologic ligand is currently unknown, the Ah receptor preferentially binds compounds known to induce microsomal aryl hydrocarbon hydroxylase (Gustafsson *et al.*, 1987). These compounds are polycyclic aromatic hydrocarbons (e.g. β-naphthoflavone, 3-methylcholanthrene, benzopyrene, and chlorinated hydrocarbons (e.g. 2,3,7,8-tetrachlorodibenzo-*p*-dioxin, or TCDD). In response to these ligands, the Ah receptor regulates the expression of a number of genes coding for enzymes involved in the metabolism of foreign compounds (cytochrome P450s, glutathione *S*-transferases, quinone reductases, etc.). The Ah receptor mediates tumor promotion, in addition to a variety of toxic responses, including epithelial hyperplasia and metaplasia, lymphoid involution, and teratogenesis, which are characteristic of TCDD exposure (Cuthill *et al.*, 1987; Gustafsson *et al.*, 1987;

Perdew and Poland, 1988). The TCDD-induced thymic hypoplasia in many respects appears to be similar to glucocorticoid-induced atrophy of the thymus (Gustafsson *et al.*, 1987). The Ah receptor is present in almost every tissue examined (Gustafsson *et al.*, 1987); thus, aberrant expression of the Ah receptor could potentially induce neoplasia in a variety of tissues, although the precise role of the Ah receptor in specific tumors remains to be explored.

VI. Mechanisms of Steroid Hormone-Induced Tumor Regression

It is remarkable that steroid hormones are implicated not only in promoting tumor cell growth but also in inducing tumor regression. This property is responsible for the widespread successful use of steroid hormones in the treatment of malignancy. The mechanisms involved in steroid hormone–induced regression are emphasized here.

While estradiol stimulates the proliferation of breast cancer cells through its interaction with the estrogen receptor, antiestrogens such as the triphenylethylene tamoxifen inhibit breast cancer cell growth (Miller and Katzenellenbogen, 1983; Katzenellenbogen *et al.*, 1987). Antiestrogen binding sites distinct from the estrogen receptor have been identified in breast cancer cell lines; although these sites selectively bind antiestrogens, they do not appear to function directly to mediate the growth-modulatory effects of antiestrogens on breast cancer cells (Sheen *et al.*, 1985). Rather, it appears that antiestrogen effects on breast cancer cells are mediated through interaction of antiestrogens with the estrogen receptor (Miller *et al.*, 1985). Thus, it has been demonstrated that antiestrogens bind to the estrogen receptor and antagonize the binding of estradiol, although equilibrium-binding analysis reveals that the antiestrogen tamoxifen interacts differently with the estrogen receptor than estradiol (Sasson and Notides, 1988). The precise mechanism through which antiestrogens inhibit tumor cell growth has not been defined; antiestrogens appear to act beyond the level of the tumor stem cell and thereby decrease the clonal growth of MCF-7 cells in soft agar colony assay, consistent with the view that antiestrogens are cytostatic rather than cytotoxic for breast cancer cells (Kodama *et al.*, 1985; Lippman and Dickson, 1989). The cytostatic effect of tamoxifen is, at least in part, due to inhibition of growth factor release from tumor cells (Bardon *et al.*, 1987).

The proliferation of breast cancer cells is inhibited by retinoic acid, as well as androgens and progestins (Lacroix and Lippman, 1980; Chambon *et al.*, 1989). Progestins and androgens induce triglyceride accumulation in T47D breast cancer cells; this suggests that progestins may induce commitment of cancer cells to a terminal differentiation program, explaining progestin action in treating progesterone receptor–positive breast cancer (Chambon *et al.*, 1989).

Another class of steroid hormones, the glucocorticosteroids, have an entirely different effect on tumor cells. Glucocorticosteroids inhibit the proliferation of lymphoid tumor cells and are actually cytotoxic to lymphoid tumor cells. This lympholytic property of glucocorticoids is largely responsible for the efficacy of glucocorticoids as therapeutic agents for lymphoid malignancies including non-Hodgkin's lymphomas and acute lymphoblastic leukemia. The mechanism of glucocorticoid action in lymphoid malignancies has been the subject of intense investigation but remains incompletely understood. Much has been learned about the cytostatic effect of glucocorticoids from studies of cell lines, such as the P1798 murine lymphoma cell line, which are not lysed by glucocorticoids but whose growth is suppressed by glucocorticoids (Thompson *et al.*, 1989). In these cells, glucocorticoids inhibit transcription of the gene encoding ribosomal RNA, through inhibition of an RNA polymerase I transcription initiation factor (Thompson *et al.*, 1989). The gene encoding thymidine kinase is regulated in a similiar manner. Thus, glucocorticoids appear to have the general property of regulating the synthesis of certain transcription factors. Glucocorticoids also regulate the translation of a certain class of mRNAs, including those that encode ribosomal proteins (Thompson *et al.*, 1989). The possibility that glucocorticoids may regulate lymphoid cell growth through effects on oncogene expression has also been investigated. Steady-state mRNA levels of c-*myc*, c-*myb*, and c-ki-*ras* are dramatically and rapidly decreased after glucocorticoid treatment of S49 mouse lymphoma cells; this may be the mechanism by which glucocorticoids inhibit cell-cycle progression of S49 cells (Eastman and Vedeckis, 1986). In another study, a variety of growth factors and oncogenes were investigated in a human lymphoid leukemia cell line and only c-*Myc* was found to be regulated by dexamethasone (Yuh and Thompson, 1989).

In regard to the mechanism of glucocorticoid-induced lymphocytolysis, it appears that lymphoid cells at immature stages of differentiation are programed to undergo an endogenous suicide process following exposure to pharmacologic concentrations of glucocorticoids. A variety of metabolic effects accompany glucocorticoid-induced lymphocytolysis, including inhibition of amino acid incorporation into protein due to a decreased rate of protein synthesis, coupled with increased free amino acid pools that result, at least in part, from an accelerated rate of intracellular protein degradation (MacDonald and Cidlowski, 1982). One of the earliest and most striking events in glucocorticoid-induced lymphocytolysis is nuclear pyknosis, which at the molecular level is characterized by internucleosomal DNA fragmentation, and which appears to precede overt cell death (Compton and Cidlowski, 1986). Glucocorticoid hormones induce the same pattern of DNA fragmentation in human acute lymphoblastic leukemia cells as previously described in mouse lymphoma cell lines and in normal rat thymocytes, suggesting a common mechanism of glucocorticoid-induced lymphocytolysis in different species (Distelhorst, 1988). Glucocorticoid-induced DNA damage in susceptible lymphoid cells is accompanied by decreases in cellular content of NAD and ATP secondary to activation of poly(ADP-ribose) polymerase; it has been proposed that the consequent depletion of NAD and ATP may essentially produce a state of metabolic depletion that leads to cell death (Berger et al., 1987).

The mechanism through which glucocorticoids induce DNA damage remains to be defined. In rat thymocytes, glucocorticoid-induced DNA damage is blocked by inhibitors of RNA and protein synthesis, suggesting that glucocorticoid regulation of a lysis gene(s) may be the initiating event in glucocorticoid-induced lymphocytolysis (Compton et al, 1988). The presence of a genetic locus that encodes a lysis function in lymphoid cells is also supported by cell fusion and complementation studies using different classes of steroid-resistant mouse lymphoma cells (Gasson and Bourgeois, 1983). There has been speculation that the lysis gene product might be an endonuclease that is responsible for DNA fragmentation observed after glucocorticoid treatment of lymphoid cells. This postulate appeared to be supported by recent evidence that glucocorticoids induce two major protein families in rat thymocytes that appear to have endonuclease activity (Compton and Cidlowski, 1987); however, more recent studies have cast doubt on these findings, and it is thus not yet firmly established that glucocorticoids actually induce endonuclease activities in lymphoid cells (Al-nemri and Litwack, 1989).

Although androgens promote the growth of prostate carcinoma cells, little is known about their mechanism of action, other than it is mediated through the androgen receptor. Recent studies are beginning to elucidate events that accompany prostatic atrophy that occurs upon androgen withdrawal. In studies of prostate gland atrophy following withdrawal of hormonal stimulation, novel RNAs and proteins are expressed in tissues during the period preceding cell death (Buttyan et al., 1989). The expression of one gene in particular, the TRPM-2 gene (testosterone-repressed prostate message-2 gene) is associated with the onset of cellular atrophy and death in many rodent tissues (e.g., in prostatic regression) (Buttyan et al., 1989). Further characterization of this gene and its product will likely lead to a much better understanding of the events that occur during programed cell death.

VII. Mechanisms of Steroid Hormone Unresponsiveness in Tumor Cells

During the natural course of human malignancy, many tumors that are initially responsive to steroid hormones become steroid hormone–resistant. For example, breast tumors frequently display estrogen-independent growth, and lymphoid malignancies frequently become resistant to the lympholytic effects of glucocorticoids. The mechanisms of hormonal unresponsiveness have been the subject of intense investigation and will be summarized here.

In breast cancer, the principal limitation to the utility of antiestrogens is the resistance that develops in tumors treated with these agents (Lippman and Dickson, 1989). Forty percent of patients with estrogen receptor–positive tumors fail to respond to antiestrogens; thus, the presence of estrogen receptors does not necessarily confer estrogen responsiveness (Miller et al., 1984). However, tamoxifen resistance may also be the result of estrogen receptor defects, as described in a tamoxifen-resistant variant of the MCF-7 breast cancer cell line (Nawata et al., 1981b). The functional properties of estrogen receptors from tamoxifen-resistant cells are often not different from those of estrogen receptors from wild-type, sensitive cells; thus, unresponsiveness to antiestrogens frequently may take place at steps beyond the initial interaction of ligand with intracellular receptor (Nawata et al., 1981a; Miller et al., 1984; Bronzert et al., 1985; Lippman and Dickson, 1989; Mullick and Chambon, 1990).

Hormonal unresponsiveness can result from a low-level or absent estrogen receptor expression in breast cancer cells. Recent studies have begun to shed light on genetic defects responsible for decreased estrogen-receptor expression in breast cancer cells. A restriction fragment–length polymorphism has been identified in the human estrogen-receptor gene using Pvu II; there appears to be an association between one particular allele and the failure of breast cancer cells to express estrogen receptors (Hill et al. 1989). Garcia et al. (1980) have reported a frequently occurring estrogen-receptor variant that carries two point mutations in the region of the gene encoding the amino-terminal domain of the protein. Analysis of human estrogen receptor mRNA performed on 71 human breast tumors using an RNase protection assay has revealed a detectable mismatch in the RNA coding for the amino-terminal domain of the estrogen receptor (Garcia et al., 1988). This mutation is associated with low levels of estrogen receptor and thus may have an indirect effect on the success of hormonal therapy (Garcia et al., 1988).

Glucocorticoid resistance occurs commonly in lymphoid malignancies and frequently limits the success of therapy. The effectiveness of glucocorticoid-mediated lymphocytolysis is contingent upon a variety of factors, including the cellular level of glucocorticoid receptors (Gruol et al., 1986; Gruol et al., 1989). Loss of cAMP-dependent protein kinase activity causes a measurable decrease of steroid sensitivity in murine T-lymphoma cells (Gruol et al., 1986; Gruol et al., 1989). Thus, cAMP-dependent protein kinase activity has the potential to modulate the steroid sensitivity of lymphoma cells by affecting the level of glucocorticoid receptors as well as the receptor's efficiency in producing a cytolytic response. Membrane permeability to steroid hormones may also be a determinant of dexamethasone resistance in murine thymoma cells (Johnson et al., 1984). A variety of defects in the glucocorticoid receptor have been shown to produce glucocorticoid resistance in mouse lymphoma cell lines (Yamamoto et al., 1976). Most frequently, glucocorticoid resistance is explained by a deficiency of glucocorticoid receptors; in some resistant clones, however, glucocorticoid resistance is due to mutations in the receptor coding sequence that give rise to receptors that function abnormally (Miesfeld *et al.*, 1984). Receptor defects have also been identified as causes of glucocorticoid resistance in human lymphoid leukemia cells (Harmon and Thompson, 1981; Harmon *et al.*, 1985; Thompson *et al.*, 1988; Harmon *et al.*, 1989). In certain mouse and human lymphoid cells, glucocorticoid resistance occurs in the presence of a normal complement of functional glucocorticoid receptors; cell fusion experiments suggest that glucocorticoid resistance in these cells is due to a defect(s) at another locus than the receptor (Gasson and Bourgeois, 1983; Zawydiwski *et al.*, 1983; Harmon *et al.*, 1985; Yuh and Thompson, 1987). These resistant mutants may have a mutation in the lysis gene (see above) or, alternatively, the lysis gene may be inactivated during differentiation, possibly through methylation of DNA (Gasson *et al.*, 1983).

An interesting and important observation is that glucocorticoid resistance may arise *in vivo* by different mechanisms than *in vitro*. This conclusion stems from the work of Thompson and colleagues (Lucas *et al.*, 1988; Wood and Thompson, 1984) who investigated the mechanism of glucocorticoid resistance in the P1798 murine lymphoma cell line. P1798 mouse lymphoma cells are functionally haploid; variants selected for dexamethasone resistance in culture have lost receptor, whereas selection for resistance to cytolysis *in vivo* is not associated with receptor mutations (Lucas *et al.*, 1988). Also, cells that are resistant to the cytolytic effects of glucocorticoids *in vivo* are sensitive to antiproliferative effects of glucocorticoids in culture; cells that are resistant to dexamethasone in culture undergo cytolysis when treated with dexamethasone *in vivo* (Wood and Thompson, 1984). Thus, different mechanisms may be involved in loss of glucocorticoid responsiveness *in vivo* and *in vitro*. These findings are particularly provacative as we attempt to understand the mechanism of glucocorticoid resistance in acute lymphoblastic leukemia and lymphoma in humans. Thus, *in vitro* assays for glucocorticoid resistance and mechanisms of glucocorticoid resistance *in vitro* may not pertain to the situation *in vivo*.

VIII. Steroid Hormone Receptors as Prognostic Markers

Because hormonal regulation of tumor cell growth is mediated through hormonal receptors, assays for steroid hormone receptors have proven to be useful prognostic markers and predictors of therapeutic responses to hormonal therapy. For example, estrogen and progesterone receptors have been investigated extensively as prognostic markers in breast cancer. Both biochemical assays and sensitive immunocytochemical assays have been employed and appear to give comparable results (King *et al.*, 1985; Berger *et al.*, 1989; Graham *et al.*, 1989b;

Kinsel *et al.*, 1989). In a series of primary breast cancers, 55% were positive for both progesterone and estrogen receptors, 26% were negative for both, 18% were positive for estrogen receptors but negative for progesterone receptors, and 2% were positive for progesterone receptors but negative for estrogen receptors (Berger *et al.*, 1989). Similar results have been obtained in other large series of patients (Allegra *et al.*, 1979). The presence of estrogen receptors in breast tumors is of significant prognostic importance; patients with estrogen receptor–positive tumors have a significantly better prognosis than patients with receptor-negative tumors (Kinsel *et al.*, 1989). Also, the presence of estrogen and progesterone receptors in breast tumors is an important predictor of hormonal responsiveness; thus, patients with advanced breast cancer in whom estrogen-receptor status is negative by immunocytochemical assay generally fail to respond to estrogen therapy (McClelland *et al.*, 1986; Benner *et al.*, 1988). Progesterone receptors are also a strong predictor of response to hormonal therapy in metastatic breast cancer (Graham *et al.*, 1989a).

Both estrogen and progesterone receptors are detectable in endometrial adenocarcinoma cells, where the level of these receptors correlates with the degree of cellular differentiation (Creasman *et al.*, 1985; Segreti *et al.*, 1989). Immunocytochemical assays of fresh frozen sections of endometrial carcinoma tissue demonstrate considerable heterogeneity in terms of the cellular distribution of estrogen and progesterone receptors (Bergeron *et al.*, 1988a; Bergeron *et al.*, 1988b). In general, estrogen-receptor content is low in tumor tissue compared to normal proliferative or hyperplastic endometrium (Bergeron *et al.*, 1988a). Estrogen and progesterone receptors are important prognostic markers in endometrial cancer. There is an inverse correlation between surgical stage and estrogen-receptor content of primary tumor specimens (Mutch *et al.*, 1987). In stages I and II endometrial cancer, estrogen and progesterone receptor status were found to be significant prognostic factors; prognosis was better for patients with tumors positive for estrogen and progesterone receptors than for patients with receptor-negative tumors (Creasman *et al.*, 1985). The presence of progesterone receptors in biopsy specimens, however, does not necessarily predict a therapeutic response to progesterone therapy; only 60% of cases positive for progesterone receptors respond to progesterone treatment (Bergeron *et al.*, 1988b).

The level of glucocorticoid receptors in human acute lymphoblastic leukemia cells varies according to the subtype of leukemia. T-cell acute lymphoblastic leukemia cells have, on the average, fewer glucocorticoid receptors than non-T, non-B cell acute lymphoblastic leukemia cells (Yarbro *et al.*, 1977). Although there is a correlation between presence of glucocorticoid receptors in human leukemia and lymphoma cells and both *in vitro* and *in vivo* response to treatment with glucocorticoids (Lippman *et al.*, 1978; Bloomfield *et al.*, 1980); the range of glucocorticoid receptors is sufficiently broad, and the overlap of receptor levels from responders and nonresponders is so great that measurement of glucocorticoid receptors in acute lymphoblastic leukemia or lymphoma samples has not become a reliable prognostic indicator. Although one mechanism of glucocorticoid resistance in human acute lymphoblastic leukemia is a deficiency of glucocorticoid receptors, this is a relatively uncommon mechanism; most glucocorticoid-resistant leukemia cells appear to have adequate levels of functional glucocorticoid receptors (Lippman *et al.*, 1973; Lippman *et al.*, 1974). Therefore, the presence of glucocorticoid receptors in a sample of leukemia cells does not guarantee glucocorticoid responsiveness (Lippman *et al.*, 1974).

IX. Summary and Conclusions

As is frequently the case, clinical observations and applications often precede basic understanding. Thus, clinical investigators have known for many decades that steroid hormones regulate tumor cell growth, are potentially oncogenic, and are useful in the treatment of certain malignancies; only recently has an understanding of the molecular mechanisms underlying these observations begun to emerge. It is highly likely that this understanding will in turn lead to new, innovative approaches to the diagnosis and treatment of cancer.

References

Allegra, J. C., Lippman, M. E., Thompson, E. B., Simon, R., Barlock, A., Green, L., Huff, K. K., Do, H. M., and Aitken, S. C. (1979). Distribution, frequency, and quantitative analysis of estrogen, progesterone, androgen, and glucocorticoid receptors in human breast cancer. *Cancer Res* **39**, 1447–1454.

Alnemri, E. S., and Litwack, G. (1989). Glucocorticoid-induced lymphocytolysis is not mediated by an induced endonuclease. *J. Biol. Chem.* **264**, 2636–2640.

Bardon, S., Vignon, F., Montcourrier, P., and Rochefort, H. (1987). Steroid receptor–mediated cytotoxicity of an antiestrogen and an antiprogestin in breast cancer cells. *Cancer Res.* **47**, 1441–1448.

Barrett-Conner, E. (1989). Postmenopausal estrogen replacement and breast cancer risk. *N. Engl. J. Med.* **321**, 319–320.

Bates, S. E., Davidson, N. E., Valverius, E. M., Freter, C. E., Dickson, R. B., Tam, J. P., Kudlow, J. E., Lippman, M. E., and Salomon, D. S. (1988). Expression of transforming growth factor alpha and its messenger ribonucleic acid in human breast cancer: Its regulation by estrogen and its possible functional significance. *Mol. Endocrinol.* **2**, 543–555.

Beato, M. (1989). Gene regulation by steroid hormones. *Cell* **56**, 335–344.

Beatson, G. T. (1896). On the treatment of inoperable cases of carcinoma of the mamma: Suggestions for a new method of treatment, with illustrative cases. *Lancet* **2**, 104–107.

Benbrook, D., Lemhardt, E., and Piahl, M. (1988). A new retinoic acid receptor identified from a hepatocellular carcinoma. *Nature* **333**, 669–672.

Benner, S. E., Clark, G. M., and McGuire, W. L. (1988). Steroid receptors, cellular kinetics, and lymph node status as prognostic factors in breast cancer. *Am. J. Med. Sci.* **296**, 59–66.

Berger, N. A., Berger, S. J., Sudar, D. C., and Distelhorst, C. W. (1987). Role of nicotinamide adenine dinucleotide and adenosine triphosphate in glucocorticoid-induced cytotoxicity in susceptible lymphoid cells. *J. Clin. Invest.* **79,** 1558–1563.

Berger, U., Wilson, P., Thethi, S., McClelland, R. A., Greene, G. L., and Coombes, R. C. (1989). Comparison of an immunocytochemical assay for progesterone receptor with a biochemical method of measurement and immunocytochemical examination of the relationship between progesterone and estrogen receptors. *Cancer Res.* **49,** 5176–5179.

Bergeron, C., Ferenczy, A., and Shyamala, G. (1988a). Distribution of estrogen receptors in various cell types of normal, hyperplastic and neoplastic human endometrial tissues. *Lab Invest.* **58,** 338–345.

Bergeron, C., Ferenczy, A., Toft, D. O., and Shyamala, G. (1988b). Immunocytochemical study of progesterone receptors in hyperplastic and neoplastic endometrial tissues. *Cancer Res.* **48,** 6132–6136.

Bergkvist, L., Adami, H. O., Persson, I., Hoover, R., and Schairer, C. (1989). The risk of breast cancer after estrogen and estrogen-progestin replacement. *N. Engl. J. Med.* **321,** 293–297.

Bloomfield, C. D., Peterson, B. A., Zaleskas, J., Frizzera, G., Smith, K.A., Hildebrandt, L., Gail-Peczalska, K. J., and Munck, A. (1980). *In-vitro* glucocorticoid studies for predicting response to glucocorticoid therapy in adults with malignant lymphoma. *Lancet* **1,** 1952–1956.

Briozzo, P., Morisset, M., Capony, F., Rougeot, C., and Rochefort, H. (1988). *In vitro* degradation of extracellular matrix with M_r 52,000 cathepsin D secreted by breast cancer cells. *Cancer Res.* **48,** 3688–3692.

Bronzert, D. A., Greene, G. L., and Lippman, M. E. (1985). Selection and characterization of a breast cancer cell line resistant to the antiestrogen LY 117018. *Endocrinology* **117,** 1409–1417.
    Burnstein, K.L., and Cidlowski, J. A. (1989). Regulation of gene expression by glucocorticoids. *Annu. Rev. Physiol.* **51,** 683–699.

Buttyan, R., Olsson, C. A., Pintar, J., Chang, C., Bandyk, M., Ng, P. Y., and Sawczuk, I. S. (1989). Induction of the TRPM-2 gene in cells undergoing programed death. *Mol. Cell. Biol.* **9,** 3473–3481.

Capony, F., Rougeot, C., Montcourrier, P., Cavailles, V., Salazar, G., and Rochefort, H. (1989). Increased secretion, altered processing, and glycosylation of pro-cathepsin D in human mammary cancer cells. *Cancer Res.* **49,** 3904–3909.

Cavailles, V., Garcia, M., and Rochefort, H. (1989) Regulation of cathepsin#-D and pS2 gene expression by growth factors in MCF7 human breast cancer cells. *Mol. Endocrinol.* **3,** 552–558.

Chambon, M., Rocheford, H., Vial, H. J., and Chalbos, D. (1989). Progestins and androgens stimulate lipid accumulation in T47D breast cancer cells via their own receptors. *J. Steroid Biochem.* **33,** 915–922.

Compton, M. M., and Cidlowski, J. A. (1986). Rapid *in vivo* effects of glucocorticoids on the integrity of rat lymphocyte genomic deoxyribonucleic acid. *Endocrinology* **118,** 38–45.

Compton, M. M., and Cidlowski, J. A. (1987). Identification of a glucocorticoid-induced nuclease in thymocytes. A potential "lysis gene" product. *J. Biol. Chem.* **262,** 8288–8292.

Compton, M. M., Haskill, J. S., and Cidlowski, J. A. (1988). Analysis of glucocorticoid actions on rat thymocyte deoxyribonucleic acid by fluorescence-activated flow cytometry. *Endocrinology* **122,** 2158–2164.

Creasman, W. T., Soper, J. T., McCarty, K. S. J., McCarty, K. S. S., Hinshaw, W., and Clarke, P. D. L. (1985). Influence of cytoplasmic steroid receptor content on prognosis of early stage endometrial carcinoma. *Am. J. Obstet. Gynecol.* **151,** 922–932.

Cullen, K. J., Yee, D., Sly, W. S., Perdue, J., Hampton, B., Lippman, M. E., and Rosen, N. (1990). Insulin-like growth factor receptor expression and function in human breast cancer. *Cancer Res.* **50,** 48–53.

Cuthill, S., Poellinger, L., and Gustafsson, J. A. (1987). The receptor for 2,3,7,8-tetrachlorodibenzo-*p*-dioxin in the mouse hepatoma cell line Hepa 1c1c7. A comparison with the glucocorticoid receptor and the mouse and rat hepatic dioxin receptors. *J. Biol. Chem.* **262**, 3477–3481.

de-The, H., Marchio, A., Tiollais, P., and Dejean, A. (1987). A novel steroid thyroid receptor gene inappropriately expressed in human hepatocellular carcinomas. *Nature* **330**, 667–670.

Dejean, A., Boulgueleret, L., Grzeschik, K. H., and Tiollais, P. (1986). Hepatitis B virus DNA integration in a sequence homologous to v-*erb*A and steroid receptor genes in a hepatocellular carcinoma. *Nature* **322**, 70–72.

Distelhorst, C. W. (1988). Glucocorticosteroids induce DNA fragmentation in human lymphoid leukemia cells. *Blood* **72**, 1305–1309.

Distelhorst, C. W. (1989). Recent insight into the structure and function of the glucocorticoid receptor. *J. Lab. Clin. Med.* **113**, 404–412.

Distelhorst, C. W., and Howard, K. J. (1989). Kinetic pulse-chase labeling study of the glucocorticoid receptor in mouse lymphoma cells. Effect of glucocorticoid and antiglucocorticoid hormones on intracellular receptor half-life. *J. Biol. Chem.* **264**, 13080–13085.

Eastman, R. S. B., and Vedeckis, W. V. (1986). Glucocorticoid inhibition of c-*myc*, c-*myb*, and c-Ki-*ras* expression in a mouse lymphoma cell line. *Cancer Res.* **46**, 2457–2462.

Eilers, M., Picard, D., Yamamoto, K. R., and Bishop, J. M. (1989). Chimaeras of *myc* oncoprotein and steroid receptors cause hormone-dependent transformation of cells. *Nature* **340**, 66–68.

Eisen, L. P., Elsasser, M. S., and Harmon, J. M. (1988). Positive regulation of the glucocorticoid receptor in human T cells sensitive to the cytolytic effects of glucocorticoids. *J. Biol. Chem.* **263**, 12044–12048.

Evans, R. M. (1988). The steroid and thyroid hormone receptor superfamily. *Science* **240**, 889–895.

Evans, R. M. (1989). Molecular characterization of the glucocorticoid receptor. *Recent Prog. Horm. Res.* **45**, 1–22.

Fuqua, S. A., Blum, S. M., and McGuire W. L. (1989). Induction of the estrogen-regulated "24K" protein by heat shock. *Cancer Res.* **49**, 4126–4129.

Garcia, T., Lehrer, S., Bloomer, W. D., and Schachter, B. (1988). A variant estrogen receptor messenger ribonucleic acid is associated with reduced levels of estrogen binding in human mammary tumors. *Mol. Endocrinol.* **2**, 785–791.

Garcia, T., Sanchez, M., Cox, J. L., Shaw, P. A., Ross, J. B., Lehrer, S., and Schachter, B. (1989). Identification of a variant form of the human estrogen receptor with an amino acid replacement. *Nucleic Acids Res.* **17**, 8364.

Gasson, J. C., and Bourgeois, S. (1983). A new determinant of glucocorticoid sensitivity in lymphoid cell lines. *J. Cell Biol.* **96**, 409–415.

Gasson, J. C., Ryden, T., and Bourgeois, S. (1983). Role of *de novo* DNA methylation in the glucocorticoid resistance of a T-lymphoid cell line. *Nature* **302**, 621–623.

Graham, M.L., II, Bunn, P. A. J., Jewett, P. B., Gonzalez, A. C., and Horwitz, K. B. (1989a). Simultaneous measurement of progesterone receptors and DNA indices by flow cytometry: Characterization of an assay in breast cancer cell lines. *Cancer Res.* **49**, 3934–3942.

Graham, M. L., II, Dalquist, K. E., and Horwitz, K. B. (1989b). Simultaneous measurement of progesterone receptors and DNA indices by flow cytometry: Analysis of breast cancer cell mixtures and genetic instability of the T47D line. *Cancer Res.* **49**, 3943–3949.

Green, S., and Chambon, P. (1986). A superfamily of potentially oncogenic hormone receptors [news]. *Nature* **324**, 615–617.

Greenberg, E. R., Barnes, A. B., Resseguie, L., Barrett, J. A., Burnside, S., Lanza, L. L., Neff, R. K., Stevens, M., Young, R. H., and Colton, T. (1984). Breast cancer in mothers given diethylstilbestrol in pregnancy. *N. Engl. J. Med.* **311**, 1394–1398.

Gruol, D. J., Ashby, M. N., Campbell, N. F., and Bourgeois, S. (1986). Isolation of new types of dexamethasone-resistant variants from a cAMP-resistant lymphoma. *J. Steroid Biochem.* **24**, 255–258.

Gruol, D. J., Rajah, F. M., and Bourgeois, S. (1989). Cyclic AMP–dependent protein kinase modulation of the glucocorticoid-induced cytolytic response in murine T-lymphoma cells *Mol. Endocrinol.* **3,** 2119–2127.

Gustafsson, J. A., Carlstedt, D. J., Poellinger, L., Okret, S., Wikstrom, A. C., Bronnegard, M., Gillner, M., Dong, Y., Fuxe, K., and Cintra, A. (1987). Biochemistry, molecular biology, and physiology of the glucocorticoid receptor. *Endocr. Rev.* **8,** 185–234.

Harmon, J. M., and Thompson, E. B. (1981). Isolation and characterization of dexamethasone-resistant mutants from human lymphoid cell line CEM-C7. *Mol. Cell. Biol.* **1,** 512–521.

Harmon, J. M., Thompson, E. B., and Baione, K. A. (1985). Analysis of glucocorticoid-resistant human leukemic cells by somatic cell hybridization. *Cancer Res.* **45,** 1587–1593.

Harmon, J. M., Elsasser, M. S., Eisen, L. P., Urda, L. A., Ashraf, J., and Thompson, E. B. (1989). Glucocorticoid receptor expression in receptorless mutants isolated from the human leukemic cell line CEM-C7. *Mol. Endocrinol.* **3,** 734–743.

Henderson, B. E., Ross, R., and Bernstein, L. (1988). Estrogen as a cause of human cancer-colon. The Richard and Hinda Rosenthal Foundation Award Lecture. *Cancer Res.* **48,** 246–253.

Hill, S. M., Fuqua, S. A., Chamness, G. C., Greene, G. L., and McGuire, W. L. (1989). Estrogen-receptor expression in human breast cancer assoicated with an estrogen-receptor gene restriction fragment–length polymorphism. *Cancer Res.* **49,** 145–148.

Howard, K. J., Holley, S. J., Yamamoto, K. R., and Distelhorst, C. W. (1990). Mapping the HSP90 binding region on the glucocorticoid receptor. *J. Biol. Chem.,* in press.

Huff, K. K., Knabbe, C., Lindsey, R., Kaufman, D., Bronzert, D., Lippman, M. E., and Dickson, R. B. (1988). Multihormonal regulation of insulin-like growth factor-I-related protein in MCF-7 human breast cancer cells. *Mol. Endocrinol.* **2,** 200–208.

Huggins, C. and Clark, P. J. (1940). Quantitative studies of prostatic secretion. II. The effect of castration and of estrogen injection on the normal and on the hyperplastic prostate glands of dogs. *J. Exp. Med.* **72,** 747–762.

Huggins, C., and Hodges, C. V. (1941). Studies on prostatic cancer. I. The effect of castration, of estrogen and of androgen injection on serum phosphatases in metastatic carcinoma of the prostate. *Cancer Res.* **1,** 293–297.

Jensen, E. V., Greene, G. L., Closs, L. E., DeSombre, E. R., and Nadji, M. (1982). Receptors reconsidered: A 20-year perspective. *Recent Prog. Horm. Res.* **38,** 1–40.

Johnson, D. M., Newby, R. F., and Bourgeois, S. (1984). Membrane permeability as a determinant of dexamethasone resistance in murine thymoma cells. *Cancer Res.* **44,** 2435–2440.

Katzenellenbogen, B. S., Kendra, K. L., Norman, M. J., and Berthois, Y. (1987). Proliferation, hormonal responsiveness, and estrogen-receptor content of MCF-7 human breast cancer cells grown in the short-term and long-term absence of estrogens. *Cancer Res.* **47,** 4355–4360.

Kendra, K. L., and Katzenellenbogen, B. S. (1987). An evaluation of the involvement of polyamines in modulating MCF-7 human breast cancer cell proliferation and progesterone-receptor levels by estrogen and antiestrogen. *J. Steroid Biochem.* **28,** 123–128.

King, W. J., DeSombre, E. R., Jensen, E. V., and Greene, G. L. (1985). Comparison of immuno-cytochemical and steroid-binding assays for estrogen receptor in human breast tumors. *Cancer Res.* **45,** 293–304.

Kinsel, L. B., Szabo, E., Greene, G. L., Konrath, J., Leight, G. S., and McCarty, K. S. J. (1989). Immunocytochemical analysis of estrogen receptors as a predictor of prognosis in breast cancer patients: Comparison with quantitative biochemical methods. *Cancer Res.* **49,** 1052–1056.

Kodama, F., Greene, G. L., and Salmon, S. E. (1985). Relation of estrogen-receptor expression to clonal growth and antiestrogen effects on human breast cancer cells. *Cancer Res.* **45,** 2720–2724.

Komm, B. S., Terpening, C. M., Benz, D. J., Graeme, K. A., Gallegos, A., Korc, M., Greene, G. L., OMalley, B. W., and Haussler, M. R. (1988). Estrogen binding receptor mRNA, and biologic response in osteoblast-like osteosarcoma cells. *Science* **241,** 81–84.

Lacroix, A., and Lippman, M. E. (1980). Biniding of retinoids to human breast cancer cell lines and their effects on cell growth. *J. Clin. Invest.* **65**, 586–591.

Law, M. L., Kao, F. T., Wei, Q., Hartz, J. A., Greene, G. L., Zarucki, S. T., Conneely, O. M., Jones, C., Puck, T. T., OMalley, B. W., *et al.* (1987). The progesterone receptor gene maps to human chromosome band 11q13, the site of the mammary oncogene int-2 [published erratum appears in *Proc. Natl. Acad. Sci. U. S. A.* (1988) **85** (24), 9688]. *Proc. Natl. Acad. Sci. U. S. A.* **84**, 2877–2881.

Lippman, M. E., Halterman, R. H., Leventhal, B. G., Perry, S., and Thompson, E. B. (1973). Glucocorticoid-binding proteins in human acute lymphoblastic leukemic blast cells. *J. Clin. Invest.* **52**, 1715–1725.

Lippman, M. E., Perry, S., and Thompson, E. B. (1974). Cytoplasmic glucocorticoid-binding proteins in glucocorticoid-unresponsive human and mouse leukemic cell lines. *Cancer Res.* **34**, 1572–1576.

Lippman, M. E., Yarbro, G. K., and Leventhal, B. G. (1978). Clinical implications of glucocorticoid receptors in human leukemia. *Cancer Res.* **38**, 4251–4256.

Litwack, G. (1988). The glucocorticoid receptor at the protein level. *Cancer Res.* **48**, 2636–2640.
Lippman, M. E. and Dickson, R. B. (1989). Mechanisms of growth control in normal and malignant breast epithelium. *Recent Prog. Horm. Res.* **45**, 383–435.

Lucas, K. L., Barbour, K. W., Housley, P. R., and Thompson, E. A. J. (1988). Biochemical and molecular characterization of the glucocorticoid receptor of lymphosarcoma P1798 variants. *Mol. Endocrinol.* **2**, 291–299.

MacDonald, R. G. and Cidlowski, J. A. (1982). Glucocorticoids inhibit precursor incorporation into protein in splenic lymphocytes by stimulating protein degradation and expanding intracellular amino acid pools. *Biochim. Biophys. Acta* **717**, 236–247.

McClelland, R. A., Berger, U., Miller, L. S., Powles, T. J., Jensen, E. V., and Coombes, R. C. (1986). Immunocytochemical assay for estrogen receptor: Relationship to outcome of therapy in patients with advanced breast cancer. *Cancer Res.* **46**, 4241s-4243s.

McIntyre, W. R., and Samuels, H. H. (1985). Triamcinolone acetonide regulates glucocorticoid-receptor levels by decreasing the half-life of the activated nuclear-receptor form. *J. Biol. Chem.* **260**, 418–427.

Miesfeld, R., Okret, S., Wikstrom, A. C., Wrange, O., Gustafsson, J. A., and Yamamoto, K. R. (1984). Characterization of a steroid hormone–receptor gene and mRNA in wild-type and mutant cells. *Nature* **312**, 779–781.

Miller, M. A., and Katzenellenbogen, B. S. (1983). Characterization and quantitation of antiestrogen binding sites in estrogen receptor–positive and –negative human breast cancer cell lines. *Cancer Res.* **43**, 3094–3100.

Miller, M. A., Lippman, M. E., and Katzenellenbogen, B. S. (1984). Antiestrogen binding in antiestrogen growth-resistant estrogen-responsive clonal variants of MCF-7 human breast cancer cells. *Cancer Res.* **44**, 5038–5045.

Miller, M. A., Mullick, A., Greene, G. L. and Katzenellenbogen, B. S. (1985). Characterization of the subunit nature of nuclear estrogen receptors by chemical cross-linking and dense amino acid labeling. *Endocrinology* **117**, 515–522.

Mobbs, B. G., Johnson, I. E., DeSombre, E. R., Toth, J. and Hughes, A. (1987). Regulation of estrogen and progestin receptor concentrations in an experimental rat prostatic carcinoma by estrogen, antiestrogen, and progesterone. *Cancer Res.* **47**, 2645–2651.

Mukku, V. R., and Stance, G. M. (1985). Regulation of epidermal growth factor receptor by estrogen. *J. Biol. Chem.* **260**, 9820–9824.

Mullick, A., and Chambon, P. (1990). Characterization of the estrogen receptor in two antiestrogen-resistant cell lines, LY2 and T47D. *Cancer Res.* **50**, 333–338.

Munck, A., Mendel, D. B., Smith, L. I., and Orti, E. (1990). Glucocorticoid receptors and actions. *Am. Rev. Respir. Dis.* **141**, PS2–10.

Mutch, D. G., Soper, J. T., Budwit, N. D. A., Cox, E. B., Creasman, W. T., McCarty, K. S. S., and McCarty, K. S. J. (1987). Endometrial adenocarcinoma estrogen-receptor content: Association of clinicopathologic features with immunohistochemical analysis compared with standard biochemical methods. *Am. J. Obstet. Gynecol.* **157,** 924–931.

Nardulli, A.M., Greene, G. L., OMalley, B. W., and Katzenellenbogen, B. S. (1988). Regulation of progesterone-receptor messenger ribonucleic acid and protein levels in MCF-7 cells by estradiol: Analysis of estrogen's effect on progesterone-receptor synthesis and degradation. *Endocrinology* **122,** 934–944.

Nardulli, A. M., and Katzenellenbogen, B. S. (1988). Progesterone-receptor regulation in T47D human breast cancer cells: Analysis by density labeling of progesterone-receptor synthesis and degradation and their modulation by progestin. *Endocrinology* **122,** 1532–1540.

Nawata, H., Bronzert, D., and Lippman, M. D. (1981a). Isolation and characterization of a tamoxifen-resistant cell line derived from MCF-7 breast cancer cells. *J. Biol. Chem* **256,** 5016–5021.

Nawata, H., Chong, M. T., Bronzert, D., and Lippman, M. E. (1981b). Estradiol-independent growth of a subline of MCF-7 human breast cancer cells in culture. *J. Biol. Chem.* **256,** 6859–6902.

Nunez, A. M., Berry, M., Imler, J. L., and Chambon, P. (1989). The 5′ flanking region of the pS2 gene contains a complex enhancer region responsive to oestrogens, epidermal growth factor, a tumour promoter (TPA), the c-Ha-*ras* oncoprotein and the c-*jun* protein. *EMBO J.* **8,** 823–829.

Nunez, A. M., Jakowlev, S., Briand, J. P., Gaire, M., Krust, A., Rio, M. C., and Chambon, P. (1987). Characterization of the estrogen-induced pS2 protein secreted by the human breast cancer cell line MCF-7. *Endocrinology* **121,** 1759–1765.

O'Malley, B. W., Schrader, W. T., and Tsai, M. J. (1986). Molecular actions of steroid hormones. *Adv. Exp. Med. Biol.* **196,** 1–10.

Pavlik, E. J, and Katzenellenbogen, B. S. (1978). Human endometrial cells in primary tissue culture: Estrogen interactions and modulation of cell proliferation. *J. Clin. Endocrinol. Metab.* **47,** 333–344.

Pearson, O. H., Eliel, L. P., Rawson, R. W., Dobriner, K., and Rhoades, C. P. (1949). ACTH and cortison-induced regression of lymphoid tumors in man: A preliminary report. *Cancer* **2,** 934–945.

Perdew, G. H., and Poland, A. (1988). Purification of the Ah receptor from C57BL/6J mouse liver. *J. Biol. Chem.* **263,** 9848–9852.

Read, L. D., Snider, C. E., Miller, J. S., Greene, G. L., and Katzenellenbogen, B. S. (1988). Ligand-modulated regulation of progesterone receptor messenger ribonucleic acid and protein in human breast cancer cell lines. *Mol. Endocrinol.* **2,** 263–271.

Read, L. D., Greene, G.L., and Katzenellenbogen, B. S. (1989). Regulation of estrogen receptor messenger ribonucleic acid and protein levels in human breast cancer cell lines by sex steroid hormones, their antagonists, and growth factors. *Mol. Endocrinol.* **3,** 295–304.

Rio, M. C., Bellocq, J. P., Gairard, B., Rasmussen, U. B., Krust, A., Koehl, C., Calderoli, H., Schiff, V., Renaud, R., and Chambon, P. (1987). Specific expression of the pS2 gene in subclasses of breast cancers in comparison with expression of the estrogen and progesterone receptors and the oncogene ERBB2. *Proc. Natl. Acad. Sci. U.S.A.* **84,** 9243–9247.

Rosewicz, S., McDonald, A. R., Maddux, B. A., Goldfine, I. D., and Miesfeld, R. L. (1988). Mechanism of glucocorticoid receptor down-regulation by glucocorticoids. *J. Biol. Chem.* **263,** 2581–2584.

Saceda, M., Lippman, M. E., Chambon, P., Lindsey, R. L., Ponglikitmongkol, M., Puente, M., and Martin, M. B. (1988). Regulation of the estrogen receptor in MCF-7 cells by estradiol. *Mol. Endocrinol.* **2,** 1157–1162.

Sasson, S., and Notides, A. C. (1988). Mechanism of the estrogen-receptor interaction with 4-hydroxytamoxifen. *Mol. Endocrinol.* **2,** 307–312.

Segreti, E. M., Novotny, D. B., Soper, J. T., Mutch, D. G., Creasman, W. T., and McCarty, K. S. (1989). Endometrial cancer: Histologic correlates of immunohistochemical localization of progesterone receptor and estrogen receptor. *Obstet Gynecol.*

Shapiro, S., Kelley, J. P., Rosenberg, L., Kaufman, D. W., Helmrich, S. P., Rosenshein, N. B., Lewis, J. L., Knapp, R. C., Stolley, P. D., and Schottenfeld, D. (1985). Risk of localized and widespread endometrial cancer in relation to recent and discontinued use of conjugated estrogens. *N. Engl. J. Med.* **313,** 969–972.

Sheen, Y. Y., Simpson, D. M., and Katzenellenbogen, B. S. (1985). An evaluation of the role of antiestrogen-binding sites in mediating the growth-modulatory effects of antiestrogens: Studies using t-butylphenoxyethyl diethylamine, a compound lacking affinity for the estrogen receptor. *Endocrinology* **117,** 561–564.

Sheen, Y. Y., and Katzenellenbogen, B. S. (1987). Antiestrogen stimulation of the production of a 37,000 molecular weight secreted protein and estrogen stimulation of the production of a 32,000 molecular weight secreted protein in MCF-7 human breast cancer cells. *Endocrinology* **120,** 1140–1151.

Sluyser, M. (1990). Steroid/thyroid receptor-like proteins with oncogenic potential: A review. *Cancer Res.* **50,** 451–458.

Thompson, E. A., Jr. (1989). Glucocorticoid inhibition of gene expression and proliferation of murine lymphoid cells *in vitro*. *Cancer Res.*

Thompson, E. B., Yuh, Y. S., Ashraf, J., Gametchu, B., Johnson, B., and Harmon, J. M. (1988a). Mechanisms of glucocorticoid function in human leukemic cells: Analysis of receptor gene mutants of the activation-labile type using the covalent affinity ligand dexamethasone mesylate. *J. Steroid Biochem.* **30,** 63–70.

Thompson, E. W., Reich, R., Shima, T. B., Albini, A., Graf, J., Martin, G. R., Dickson, R. B., and Lippman, M. E. (1988b). Differential regulation of growth and invasiveness of MCF-7 breast cancer cells by antiestrogens. *Cancer Res.* **48,** 6764–6768.

Thompson, E. W., Katz, D., Shima, T. B., Wakeling, A. E., Lippman, M. E., and Dickson, R. B. (1989). ICI 164,384, a pure antagonist of estrogen-stimulated MCF-7 cell proliferation and invasiveness. *Cancer Res.* **49,** 6929–6934.

Thorpe, S. M., Rochefort, H., Garcia, M., Freiss, G., Christensen, I. J., Khalaf, S., Paolucci, F., Pau, B., Rasmussen, B. B., and Rose, C. (1989). Association between high concentrations of 52,000 cathepsin D and poor prognosis in primary human breast cancer. *Cancer Res.* **49,** 6008–6014.

Tomasetto, C., Rio, M. C., Gautier, C., Wolf, C., Hareuverni, M., Chambon, P., and Lathe, R. (1990). hSP, the domain-duplicated homolog of pS2 protein, is coexpressed with pS2 in stomach but not in breast carcinoma. *EMBO J.* **9,** 407–414.

Touchette, N. (1990). Man bites dogma: A new role for steroid hormones. *J. N.I.H. Res.* **2,** 71–74.

Touitou, I., Cavailles, V., Garcia, M., Defrenne, A., and Rochefort, H. (1989). Differential regulation of cathepsin D by sex steroids in mammary cancer and uterine cells. *Mol. Cell. Endocrinol.* **66,** 231–238

Vanderbilt, J. N., Miesfeld, R., Maler, B. A., and Yamamoto, K. R. (1989). Intracellular receptor concentration limits glucocorticoid-dependent enhancer activity. *Mol. Endocrinol.* **1,** 68–74.

Vedeckis, W. V., Ali, M., and Allen, H. R. (1989). Regulation of glucocorticoid receptor protein and mRNA levels. *Cancer Res.* **49**(Suppl), 2295s-2302s.

Wei, L. L., Krett, N. L., Francis, M. D., Gordon, D. F., Wood, W. M., OMalley, B. W. and Horwitz, K. B. (1988). Multiple human progesterone receptor messenger ribonucleic acids and their autoregulation by progestin agonists and antagonists in breast cancer cells. *Mol. Endocrinol.* **2,** 62–72.

Westley, B., May, F. E., Brown, A. M., Krust, A., Chambon, P., Lippman, M. E., and Rochefort, H. (1984). Effects of antiestrogens on the estrogen-regulated pS2 RNA and the 52- and 160-

kilodalton proteins in MCF7 cells and two tamoxifen-resistant sublines. *J. Biol. Chem.* **259**, 10030–10035.

Wood, K. M., and Thompson, E. A. J. (1984). Isolation and characterization of lymphosarcoma P1798 variants selected for resistance to the cytolytic effects of glucocorticoids *in vivo* and in culture. *Mol. Cell. Endocrinol.* **37**, 169–180.

Worland, P. J., Bronzert, D., Dickson, R. B., Lippman, M. E., Hampton, L., Thorgeirsson, S. S., and Wirth, P. J. (1989). Secreted and cellular polypeptide patterns of MCF-7 human breast cancer cells following either estrogen stimulation or v-H-*ras* transfection. *Cancer Res.* **49**, 51–57.

Yamamoto, K. R., Gehring, U., Stampfer, M. R., and Sibley, C. H. (1976). Genetic approaches to steroid hormone action. *Recent Prog. Horm. Res.* **32**, 3–32.

Yamamoto, K. R. (1985). Steroid receptor–regulated transcription of specific genes and gene networks. *Annu. Rev. Genet.* **19**, 209–252.

Yamamoto, K. R, Godowski, P.J., and Picard, D. (1988). Ligand-regulated nonspecific inactivation of receptor function: A versatile mechanism for signal transduction. *Cold Spring Harb. Symp. Quant. Biol.* **2**, 803–811.

Yarbro, G. S., Lippman, M. E., Johnson, G. E., and Leventhal, B. G. (1977). Glucocorticoid receptors in subpopulations of childhood acute lymphocytic leukemia. *Cancer Res.* **37**, 2688–2695.

Yuh, Y. S., and Thompson, E. B. (1987). Complementation between glucocorticoid receptor and lymphocytolysis in somatic cell hybrids of two glucocorticoid-resistant human leukemic clonal cell lines. *Somat. Cell. Mol. Genet.* **13**, 33–45.

Yuh, Y. S., and Thompson, E. B. (1989). Glucocorticoid effect on oncogene/growth gene expression in human T-lymphoblastic leukemic cell line CCRF-CEM. Specific c-*myc* mRNA suppression by dexamethasone. *J. Biol. Chem.* **264**, 10904–10910.

Zawydiwski, R., Harmon, J. M., and Thompson, E. B. (1983). Glucocorticoid-resistant human acute lymphoblastic leukemia cell line with functional receptor. *Cancer Res.* **43**, 3865–3873.

Chapter 8

Patterns and Significance of Genetic Changes in Neuroblastomas

GARRETT M. BRODEUR

Department of Pediatrics, Washington University School of Medicine,
St. Louis, Missouri 63110

I. Introduction

Neuroblastoma, a tumor of postganglionic sympathetic neurons, is perhaps the most fascinating and enigmatic of childhood neoplasms from both clinical and biological viewpoints. Over 500 new cases are diagnosed in the United States each year, making this tumor the most common solid tumor in children (Young *et al.*, 1986). However, improvements in cancer treatment over the past 25 years have had relatively little impact on the long-term survival of children with neuroblastoma. Despite its resistance to conventional modalities of therapy, there are clues that neuroblastoma might be particularly susceptible to innovative approaches to treatment. These clues include the good prognosis for infants, even with disseminated disease, the propensity of the tumor to occasionally undergo

251

spontaneous regression in patients, and the ability to undergo spontaneous or induced differentiation to a benign ganglioneuroma. Thus, a better understanding of this disease at the biological level may suggest new and potentially more effective approaches to treatment.

A great deal of progress has been made in the past few years in advancing our knowledge of human neuroblastoma at the cellular and molecular level (Brodeur and Fong, 1989; Brodeur, 1990a; Brodeur, 1990b; Evans *et al.*, 1985; Evans *et al.*, 1988; Evans *et al.*, 1991). The genetic predisposition to this disease is becoming clarified; a specific oncogene amplified in neuroblastoma cells has prognostic significance; and the deletion of the short arm of chromosome 1 has been more precisely defined. These and other recent genetic observations have contributed to our understanding of tumor predisposition, tumorigenesis, genetic heterogeneity, tumor progression, and prognosis. This chapter will review the clinical and biological significance of these genetic changes.

II. Genetics of Human Neuroblastoma

A. HEREDITARY PREDISPOSITION TO NEUROBLASTOMA

A subset of patients exhibit a predisposition to develop neuroblastoma, and this predisposition follows an autosomal dominant pattern of inheritance. Indeed, Knudson and Strong (1972) have estimated that as many as 22% of all neuroblastomas could be the result of germinal mutation. Regression analysis of their data indicated that neuroblastoma fits the two-mutation hypothesis proposed by Knudson for the origin of childhood cancer (Knudson, 1971). According to this hypothesis, the nonhereditary form of neuroblastoma would result from two postzygotic (somatic) mutations in a single cell, causing malignant transformation of the cell, which then develops into a single tumor. Hereditary tumors would arise in individuals in whom the first mutation is acquired as a prezygotic (germinal) event, so it is present in all cells. Only one additional mutation in any cell of the target tissue would be needed to induce malignant transformation, so these individuals have a higher incidence of neuroblastoma with a peak incidence at an earlier age. In addition, they may develop tumors at multiple primary sites, either simultaneously or sequentially. If such persons survive, one half of their offspring should be carriers of the germinal mutation, with an estimated 63% chance of developing a neuroblastoma (Knudson and Strong, 1972).

The nature of the two mutations was not specified by Knudson, but Comings (1973) suggested that these mutations inactivated two alleles of a specific gene on homologous chromosomes. If the two-mutation hypothesis is correct for neuroblastoma, it has several important implications. First, the baseline incidence of this tumor may remain fairly stable, reflecting a constant rate of spontaneous mutation. However, an increase in exposure to environmental mutagens would cause an increase in both hereditary and nonhereditary forms. Second, all patients with a family history of neuroblastoma, those with multifocal primary tumors, and a subset of the remaining patients would be carriers of a germinal mutation. Obligate and suspected carriers could be screened regularly during early childhood when the risk of neuroblastoma is highest. The task of identifying predisposed individuals would be greatly simplified if the chromosomal location of the predisposition locus or loci were identified, and if informative probes were available for genetic counseling.

There have been a number of reports of familial neuroblastoma, as well as bilateral or multifocal disease. These are consistent with the existence of hereditary predisposition to neuroblastoma in some patients (Chatten and Voorhess, 1967; Wong *et al.*, 1971; Hardy and Nesbit, 1972; Arenson *et al.*, 1976; Wagget *et al.*, 1973). The topic of familial neuroblastoma was reviewed recently by Kushner and co-workers (Kushner *et al.*, 1986). The median age at diagnosis of unselected patients with neuroblastoma is 30 months, with about 25% of cases diagnosed within the first year of life. In contrast, the median age of patients with familial neuroblastoma is 9 months, and 60% are diagnosed by 1 year of age. At least 20% of patients with familial neuroblastoma have bilateral adrenal tumors or multifocal primary tumors. The concordance or discordance for neuroblastoma in monozygotic siblings was reviewed (Kushner and Helson, 1985). This study suggests that hereditary factors may be predominant in neuroblastoma diagnosed in infants, whereas random environmental mutations may be more important in older children. There have been a few reports of neuroblastoma associated with the fetal hydantoin and fetal alcohol syndromes (Seeler *et al.*, 1979; Allen *et al.*, 1980, Kinney *et al.*, 1980). While these reports suggest that prenatal exposure to hydantoins or ethanol may increase the risk of neuroblastoma, these associations have not been confirmed with certainty.

B. Constitutional Cytogenetic Abnormalities in Patients with Neuroblastoma

Retinoblastoma and Wilms' tumor are two common childhood neoplasms that fit the two-mutation model for hereditary neoplasms. Each is associated with characteristic congenital anomalies and specific constitutional chromosome abnormalities (Vogel, 1979; Matsunaga, 1981). The latter may represent an exaggerated form of the germinal mutation required for oncogenesis in hereditary cases. However, no one has identified as yet a constitutional cytogenetic predisposition syndrome or associated congenital anomaly with predisposition to the development of neuroblastoma (Brodeur, 1990b).

Neuroblastomas were reported in three patients with trisomy D (or trisomy 13) before banding analysis became routine (Feingold *et al.*, 1971; Nevin *et al.*,

1972), but this finding has not been reported since. Indeed, these cases were newborns who died in the first week of life, and two were found to have only microscopic (*in situ?*) neuroblastoma at autopsy. The association of trisomy 13 and neuroblastoma should be interpreted with caution, since microscopic foci of adrenal neuroblasts in a newborn might represent residual elements of normal development of the fetal adrenal medulla (Turkel and Itabashi, 1975; Ikeda *et al.*, 1981), rather than *in situ* neuroblastoma (Beckwith and Perrin, 1963).

Table I summarizes the cases of constitutional chromosome abnormalities, detected by banding, that have been reported in individuals with neuroblastoma, but no consistent pattern is evident (Pegelow *et al.*, 1975; Hecht and Kaiser-McCaw, 1981; Hecht *et al.*, 1982; Moorhead and Evans, 1980; Nagano *et al.*, 1980; Robinson and McCorquodale, 1981; Sanger *et al.*, 1984; Rudolph *et al.*, 1988). In one study by Moorhead and Evans (Moorhead and Evans, 1980), two of 37 patients with neuroblastoma, whose constitutional karyotypes were analyzed by banding, had balanced translocations. The other reports were of individual cases with constitutional chromosome abnormalities. The case originally reported by Pegelow and associates (Pegelow *et al.*, 1975) is particularly interesting. This child had two constitutional cytogenetic abnormalities, which were subsequently determined to be inv(11)(q21q23) and del(21)(p11)—one inherited from each parent (Hecht and Kaiser-McCaw, 1981). Both parents apparently had had children with neuroblastoma by other partners. Nevertheless, the child with both constitutional cytogenetic abnormalities was phenotypically normal and did not have obvious multifocal disease. Indeed, Hecht and co-workers (1982) have subsequently reported that neuroblastoma predisposition was not linked to either

TABLE I
CONSTITUTIONAL CHROMOSOME ABNORMALITIES IN PATIENTS WITH NEUROBLASTOMA[c]

Chromosome abnormality	Comments	References
Del(21)(p11); inv(11)(q21q23)	One from each parent	(Pegelow *et al.*, 1975)
		(Hecht and Kaiser-McCaw, 1981)
		(Hecht *et al.*, 1982)
t(4p;7p) balanced	Normal phenotype	(Moorhead and Evans, 1980)
t(11q;16q) balanced	Normal phenotype	(Moorhead and Evans, 1980)
Partial tri(2p) and mono(16p)	Congenital anomalies	(Nagano *et al.*, 1980)
Partial tri(3q) and mono(8p)	Congenital anomalies	(Nagano *et al.*, 1980)
Trisomy 18	Congenital anomalies	(Robinson and McCorquodale, 1981)
Partial tri(15q) and mono(13q)	Congenital anomalies	(Sanger *et al.*, 1984)
Fra(1)(p13.1)	Hereditary fragile site	(Rudolph *et al.*, 1988)

[a]Modified from Brodeur and Fong (1989).

the abnormal chromosome 11 or 21 in this family. Finally, Rudolph *et al.*, (1988) reported the occurrence of a fragile site on chromosome 1 (1p13.1) in lymphocytes from 9 of 20 patients with neuroblastoma. While this report is interesting with regard to the association of abnormalities of chromosome 1p in neuroblastoma cells, the region involved in these patients is quite proximal to the site usually deleted in the tumor cells (see below) and unlikely to be related.

Neuroblastoma has also been associated with neurofibromatosis and aganglionosis of the colon, suggesting that it might be an expression of neurocristopathy (Knudson and Strong, 1972; Knudson and Amromin, 1966; Knudson and Meadows, 1976; Witzleben and Landy, 1974; Kushner *et al.*, 1985). However, a recent analysis of the simultaneous occurrence of neuroblastoma and neurofibromatosis in the same patient suggests that the coincidence can be accounted for by chance alone (Kushner *et al.*, 1985). A variety of other congenital anomalies and genetic syndromes have been reported in association with neuroblastoma. These include tuberous sclerosis, Beckwith-Wiedemann syndrome, congenital heart disease, Friedreich ataxia, dermatomyositis, nesidioblastosis, cystic fibrosis, and asymmetric crying facies (Emery *et al.*, 1983; de la Monte *et al.*, 1985; Miller *et al.*, 1983; Kalmanti and Athanasiou, 1985; Barr *et al.*, 1986; Moss *et al.*, 1985; Grotting *et al.*, 1979; Lenarsky *et al.*, 1985). However, only one or a few patients with each association have been reported. Several studies have shown a general increase in the incidence of congenital anomalies in patients with neuroblastoma, but no specific congenital abnormality occurred with increased frequency (Miller and Fraumeni, 1968; Sy and Edmondson, 1968; Nakissa *et al.*, 1985).

Other malignant diseases have been observed in individuals with neuroblastoma following treatment, such as pheochromocytoma, renal cell carcinoma, astrocytoma, and acute leukemia (Fairchild *et al.*, 1979; Shah *et al.*, 1983; Secker-Walker *et al.*, 1985; Weh *et al.*, 1986; Meadows *et al.*, 1985). Interestingly, in a case of acute lymphoblastic leukemia, the malignant karyotype had a t(4;11)(q21;q23) translocation (Secker-Walker *et al.*, 1985), and another case with acute monoblastic leukemia had a t(9;11)(p21;q23) translocation (Weh *et al.*, 1986). The karyotypes seen in leukemias that occur as second malignant diseases in patients with neuroblastoma are identical to those seen in *de novo* leukemias. However, second cancers are not frequent in patients with neuroblastoma, and no particular second cancer has occurred with sufficient frequency to indicate a specific relationship with neuroblastoma (Meadows *et al.*, 1985).

III. Cytogenetic Abnormalities and Tumor Cell Ploidy in Neuroblastomas

A. DELETIONS AND PARTIAL MONOSOMY FOR CHROMOSOME 1_p

Deletion of the short arm of chromosome 1 (Fig. 1A) has emerged as the most characteristic cytogenetic abnormality in primary human neuroblastomas and

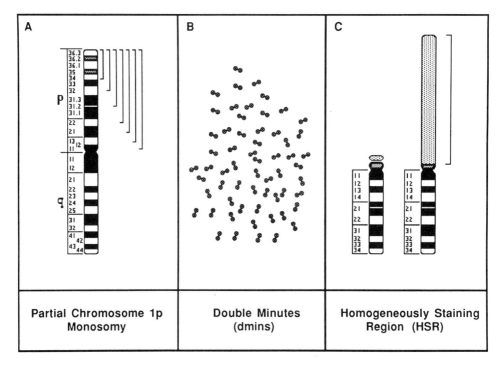

FIG. 1.   Common cytogenetic abnormalities in human neuroblastomas. Shown are diagrammatic representations of the three most common cytogenetic abnormalities seen in human neuroblastomas. (A) Deletions of the short arm of chromosome 1. The brackets indicate that the region deleted in different tumors is variable in terms of its proximal breakpoint, but the distal short arm appears to be deleted in all cases, resulting in partial 1p monosomy. (B) Extrachromosomal double-minute chromatin bodies (dmins). Dmins are seen in about 30% of primary neuroblastomas and a larger number of neuroblastoma cell lines. These are a cytogenetic manifestation of gene amplification, and in all cases analyzed so far, the amplification unit included the *MYCN* oncogene. (C) Homogeneously staining region (HSR). A representative HSR on the short arm of chromosome 13 is shown in this example, but HSRs in neuroblastomas have been identified on at least 18 of the 24 different human chromosomes (Brodeur and Seeger, 1986). HSRs are a cytogenetic manifestation of gene amplification in which the amplified sequences are chromosomally integrated. All neuroblastomas with HSRs studied to date have had *MYCN* amplification. (Reprinted from Brodeur 1990a with permission.)

tumor-derived cell lines (Brodeur and Fong, 1989; Brodeur *et al.*, 1977; Biedler *et al.*, 1980; Brodeur *et al.*, 1981; Gilbert *et al.*, 1984; Brodeur *et al.*, 1988). We reviewed the karyotypes of 60 near-diploid neuroblastomas and cell lines, with modal chromosome numbers between 44 and 53 (Brodeur and Fong, 1989). In this analysis, 50 of 60 (83%) had a deletion or rearrangement of the short arm of chromosome 1 (Table II). This was the only numerical or structural cytogenetic abnormality that occurred with statistically increased frequency ($p < 0.001$).

TABLE II
SELECTED CHROMOSOME ABNORMALITIES IN
NEAR-DIPLOID NEUROBLASTOMAS[a]

Tissue source	Del lp	Dmins	HSRs
Primary tumors	23/33 (70%)	15/33 (45%)	1/33 (3%)
Cell lines	23/27 (85%)	15/27 (56%)	14/27 (52%)
Total	46/60 (77%)	30/60 (50%)	15/60 (25%)

[a]Modified from Brodeur and Fong (1989).

However, it is notable that a substantial number of tumors karyotyped recently had modal chromosome numbers in the triploid range (Franke *et al.*, 1986; Hayashi *et al.*, 1986; Kaneko *et al.*, 1987; Christiansen and Lampert, 1988; Hayashi *et al.*, 1988). In contrast to the near-diploid tumors, the near-triploid tumors rarely if ever had deletion or rearrangements of the short arm of chromosome 1, or cytogenetic manifestations of gene amplification.

B. DMINS, HSRs, AND GENE AMPLIFICATION

A substantial number of neuroblastomas have either extrachromosomal double-minute chromatin bodies (dmins), chromosomally integrated homogeneously staining regions (HSRs), or both in subpopulations of cells (Fig. 1B,C). These two abnormalities are cytogenetic manifestations of gene amplification. Dmins in neuroblastomas were first described in neuroblastomas before chromosome banding was developed (Cox *et al.*, 1965). Subsequently, HSRs were identified in neuroblastoma cell lines (Biedler and Spengler, 1976a; Biedler and Spengler, 1976b), and it was suggested that these abnormalities might be cytogenetic manifestations of gene amplification. Dmins are the predominant form of amplified DNA in primary tumors, but dmins and HSRs are found with about equal frequency in neuroblastoma cell lines (Brodeur and Fong, 1989; Brodeur *et al.*, 1981; Gilbert *et al.*, 1984; Balaban-Malenbaum and Gilbert, 1980) (Table II). Indeed, either dmins or HSRs (or both in subsets of cells) occur in about 90% of neuroblastoma cell lines. Evidence suggests that there is selection *in vitro* for cell lines derived from tumors that have pre-existing dmins or HSRs, and there is no evidence to date that these abnormalities develop with time in culture, at least in neuroblastomas. It is unclear why HSRs are a more common form of amplified DNA in established cell lines than they are in primary tumors.

C. TUMOR CELL PLOIDY

Flow-cytometric analysis of the DNA content of human neuroblastoma cells was first reported in a series of 35 infants (Look *et al.*, 1984). In this analysis, abnormally high DNA content was associated with lower stages of tumor and a response to initial chemotherapy, whereas those with a "normal" DNA content were likely to have advanced stages of tumor (especially stage 4) and a poor response to chemotherapy. This latter group of tumors likely had subtle genetic abnormalities that were not detectable by flow cytometry, such as dmins or chromosome 1 deletions. Nevertheless, subsequent studies have confirmed the prognostic importance of flow cytometric measurement of DNA content (Gansler *et al.*, 1986; Taylor *et al.*, 1988; Oppedal *et al.*, 1988). This modality provides a complementary approach to the genetic analysis of human neuroblastomas, and it appears to provide important information in predicting response to therapy and outcome, at least in subsets of patients (Look *et al.*, 1990).

IV. Deletions, Loss of Heterozygosity (LOH), and Suppressor Genes

Two important classes of genes have been identified that appear to play an important role in malignant transformation (Brodeur, 1987). Oncogenes were the first class of cancer-related genes to be discovered. They compose a heterogeneous group and are activated usually by amplification, unregulated expression, or mutation. The second class is generally referred to as suppressor genes, and deletion or inactivation is associated with cancer predisposition or tumor development. Inactivation of both copies of the relevant suppressor gene may be required for malignant transformation. At least one oncogene has been identified that is characteristically activated, usually by gene amplification, in a subset of neuroblastomas. In addition, the location of one and possibly two suppressor genes has been found.

A. DELETION OR LOH OF CHROMOSOME 1p

Partial 1p monosomy is the most characteristic cytogenetic abnormality found in neuroblastomas (Brodeur and Fong, 1989; Brodeur *et al.*, 1977; Biedler *et al.*, 1980; Brodeur *et al.*, 1981; Gilbert *et al.*, 1984; Brodeur *et al.*, 1988), and the region most commonly deleted is between 1p32 and 1pter (Fig. 1A). This deletion is thought to represent the loss of a putative neuroblastoma suppressor gene (Brodeur and Fong, 1989; Brodeur *et al.*, 1981). Loss or inactivation of one or both copies of this gene may be an important step in the development of neuroblastoma. Although abnormalities of chromosome 1 have been reported in a variety of other malignant diseases (Douglass *et al.*, 1985; Atkin, 1986), most other cases have trisomy for the long arm of chromosome 1, not monosomy for the short arm. No chromosome-deletion syndrome has been identified as yet that predisposes to the development of neuroblastoma (Brodeur and Fong, 1989). The absence of any chromosome 1p deletion syndromes suggests that deletions large enough to be visible cytogenetically are incompatible with life, owing to the expression of embryonic lethal mutations. Nevertheless, there are reports of familial neuroblastoma inherited in an autosomal dominant manner, suggesting that there is a gene that confers predisposition to the development of this tumor in a subset of patients (Brodeur and Fong, 1989, Kushner *et al.*, 1986).

Partial monosomy of chromosome 1p is the most consistent cytogenetic abnormality found in human neuroblastomas, but its overall frequency cannot be determined from cytogenetic studies alone, because most studies reported to date have come from patients with advanced stages of disease or from established neuroblastoma cell lines. In addition, cytogenetic analysis of primary tumor tissue is not always successful, so there may be preferential reporting of tumors with near-diploid karyotypes. Therefore, we used a panel of chromosome 1–specific DNA probes that identify restriction fragment–length polymorphisms (RFLPs) along the short and long arms of chromosome 1 to assess chromosome deletion or somatic LOH (Brodeur *et al.*, 1988; Fong *et al.*, 1989). By comparing the pattern seen in normal DNA of heterozygous patients with that obtained in tumor DNA from the same patient, we could assess LOH, which is the molecular equivalent of a deletion (See Fig. 2 for example).

We studied pairs of human neuroblastoma DNA and constitutional DNA from 45 primary neuroblastomas and 2 tumor-derived cell lines (Fong *et al.*, 1989). Thirteen of the 47 cases (28%) showed LOH at two or more loci. Twelve of the 13 tumors revealed a pattern of LOH consistent with terminal deletions of chromosome 1p, whereas the remaining tumor apparently had an interstitial deletion. The common region of LOH in these 13 cases lies at the distal end of the short

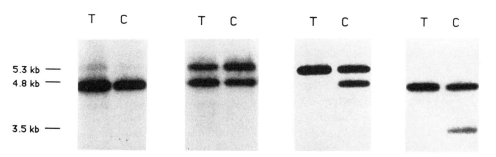

FIG. 2. Restriction fragment–length polymorphism (RFLP) and loss of heterozygosity (LOH). Southern hybridization with a hypervariable probe (pYNZ2 or D1S57) to normal and tumor DNA after digestion with the restriction enzyme *Taq*I. The first panel in the figure shows a case in which polymorphism was not seen in the constitutional DNA (C), so the case is uninformative with respect to allelic loss or LOH in the tumor DNA (T). The second panel shows a case in which polymorphism was seen in the constitutional DNA, so it was informative, and no LOH was seen in the tumor. On the other hand, the last two panels show cases in which the constitutional DNA was informative, and LOH was detected in the tumor, as demonstrated by the absence of the lower band in both cases. (Reprinted from Brodeur and Fong 1989 with permission.)

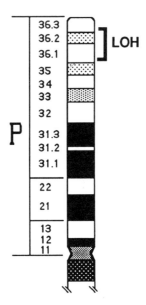

FIG. 3.   Consistent region of LOH on chromosome 1p in neuroblastomas. Shown is a diagram of
the short arm of chromosome 1, with the bands and subbands indicated on the left. Also shown is a
bracket indicating the region that is consistently deleted in human neuroblastomas, based on molecular analysis with polymorphic probes (Fong *et al.*, 1989; Weith *et al.*, 1989). At least one neuro-
blastoma-suppressor gene probably is encoded in this region.

arm of chromosome 1 from 1p36.1 to 1p36.3 (Fig. 3). Weith and co-workers
(1989) have studied 9 tumors from patients with advanced stages of disease and
identified a similar region that is consistently deleted. We postulate that loss or
inactivation of a gene (or genes) at this site is critical for the development or
progression of neuroblastoma, and so a putative neuroblastoma gene most likely
is located within this chromosomal region.

    Mutation in the critical 1p36 locus on one chromosome, followed by deletion
of the same region on the homologous chromosome (as manifested by LOH),
may be an important mechanism in the malignant transformation or progression
of some or all human neuroblastomas. In addition, deletion or somatic LOH in
the tumor tissue has been demonstrated at loci on distal chromosome 1p in some
melanomas, medullary thyroid carcinomas, and pheochromocytomas (Mathew
et al., 1987; Dracopoli *et al.*, 1989; Tsutsumi *et al.*, 1989). Since all four neoplasms are embryologically derived from neural crest cells, this suggests that
there may be a common mechanism underlying the formation or progression of
these embryologically related tumors.

B. LOH of Other Chromosomes

There is recent evidence that LOH for the long arm of chromosome 14 also occurs with increased frequency in neuroblastomas (Suzuki *et al.*, 1989). In this report, LOH for chromosome 14 was found in 6 of 12 informative cases, whereas LOH for chromosome 1p was found in 2 of 9 cases, and one case had LOH for both regions. In addition, they found LOH for chromosome 13q in 2 of 11 cases. While the exact frequency of these abnormalities and their association with other clinical and biological variables is not yet clear, the finding of LOH on other chromosomes besides 1p provides further evidence for genetic heterogeneity in this tumor.

V. Oncogene Amplification and Expression in Neuroblastomas

A. Identification of *MYCN* Amplification

Although cytogenetic analysis of human neuroblastomas frequently has revealed dmins or HSRs in primary tumors and cell lines (Brodeur and Fong, 1989; Brodeur *et al.*, 1981), the nature of the amplified sequences was not known until recently. Initially, evidence for amplification of genes associated with drug resistance was sought, but none was found. However, a study was undertaken to determine whether a protooncogene was amplified in a panel of neuroblastoma cell lines. An oncogene related to the viral oncogene v-*myc*, but distinct from *MYC* was amplified in 8 of the 9 neuroblastoma cell lines tested (Schwab *et al.*, 1983), and this finding has been confirmed independently in other laboratores (Kohl *et al.*, 1983; Montgomery *et al.*, 1983).

The amplified *MYCN* sequence was mapped to the HSRs on different chromosomes in neuroblastoma cell lines, and the normal single-copy locus was mapped to the distal short arm of chromosome 2 (Kohl *et al.*, 1983; Schwab *et al.*, 1984). This most likely indicates that a large region from this chromosome, which includes the *MYCN* locus, becomes amplified initially as extrachromosomal dmins (Brodeur and Seeger, 1986). In a small percentage of primary tumors and about half of established neuroblastoma cell lines, the amplified DNA occurs as an HSR that is linearly integrated into a chromosome. The size, structure, and organization of the amplified sequences is a subject of considerable interest and investigation (Kinzler *et al.*, 1986; Zehnbauer *et al.*, 1988; Shiloh *et al.*, 1985; Shiloh *et al.*, 1986; Amler and Schwab, 1989), which may shed light on the mechanisms involved in the amplification process.

B. Clinical Significance of *MYCN* Amplification

In collaboration with others, we began a study of primary tumors from untreated patients to determine whether *MYCN* amplification occurred. In our initial analysis of 63 primary tumors, amplification ranging from 3-fold to 300-fold per haploid genome was found in 24 tumors (38%) (Brodeur *et al.*, 1984). All cases with *MYCN* amplification in this initial study came from patients with advanced stages of disease (stages III and IV by the Evans staging system). Next, the progression-free survival of 89 patients was analyzed according to the stage of disease and *MYCN* copy number (Seeger *et al.*, 1985; Brodeur *et al.*, 1986). *MYCN* amplification clearly was associated with rapid tumor progression and a poor outcome, independent of the stage of the tumor. Two of 16 patients with less advanced disease (stage II) had amplification. Although in general, patients with stage II have a good prognosis, both patients with *MYCN* amplification had rapid tumor progression, compared to only one of the remaining 14 patients.

These studies were extended to over 800 patients with neuroblastoma enrolled in protocols of the Children's Cancer Study Group (CCSG) and the Pediatric Oncology Group (POG) (Brodeur and Fong, 1989; Brodeur *et al.*, 1988). Examples of *MYCN* amplification seen in some of the primary tumors are shown in Fig. 4. In general, the same pattern seen in our earlier studies has been borne out by the larger study (Table III). It is now clear that, among patients with less advanced stages of disease traditionally associated with a good prognosis, a minority (5–10%) have tumors with *MYCN* amplification (Brodeur and Fong, 1989; Brodeur *et al.*, 1988). Our data indicate that these patients are destined to have rapid tumor progression and a poor outcome, similar to their counterparts with advanced stages of disease. Over 30% of patients with more advanced tumor stages had *MYCN* amplification, and they also had an expectedly poor outcome. Our findings that *MYCN* amplification is associated with a poor outcome regardless of the clinical stage of tumor is supported by preliminary studies from Japan and Europe (Tsuda *et al.*, 1987; Nakagawara *et al.*, 1987; Bartram and Berthold, 1987).

We analyzed the *MYCN* copy number in multiple simultaneous or consecutive samples of neuroblastoma tissue from 60 patients (Brodeur *et al.*, 1987) to determine whether or not the presence or absence of *MYCN* was consistent in different tumor samples from a given patient, or if single-copy tumors ever developed amplification at the time of recurrence. Indeed, we found a consistent pattern of *MYCN* copy number (either amplified or unamplified) in different tumor samples taken from an individual patient, either simultaneously or consecutively (Brodeur *et al.*, 1987). These results suggest that *MYCN* amplification is an intrinsic biological property of a subset of neuroblastomas. Tumors that develop *MYCN* amplification generally do so by the time of diagnosis, and so far no case of neuroblastoma with a single copy (per haploid genome) of *MYCN* at the time of diagnosis have developed amplification subsequently.

C. *MYCN* EXPRESSION

About 25–30% of the children with neuroblastoma have *MYCN* amplification in their tumors, and virtually all of these children have rapidly progressive and

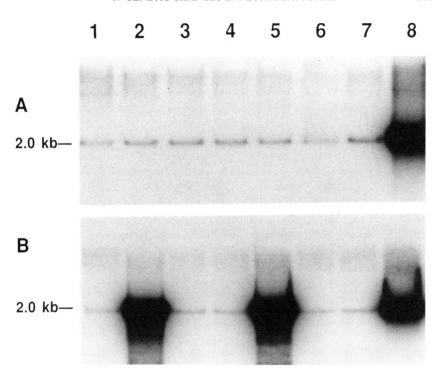

FIG. 4.   Southern blots showing MYCN amplification. Equal amounts of DNA were digested to completion with the restriction enzyme *Eco*RI, electrophoresed, blotted, and hybridized to a radioactive probe for the *MYCN* oncogene. In both rows, lane 1 represents DNA from a normal lymphoblastoid cell line as a single-copy control, and lane 8 represents DNA from the NGP cell line, with 150 copies of *MYCN* per haploid genome, as determined by serial dilution and laser densitometry. (A) Lanes 2–7 represent 6 neuroblastomas with a single copy of *MYCN* per haploid genome. (B) Lanes 2 and 5 show examples of tumors with *MYCN* amplification, whereas the other tumors have the normal single-copy signal. (Reprinted from Brodeur 1990a with permission.

TABLE III

CORRELATION OF *MYCN* COPY NUMBER AND STAGE
IN 817 PATIENTS WITH NEUROBLASTOMA [a]

Stage at diagnosis	Frequency of *MYCN* amplification
Benign ganglioneuromas	0/18 (0%)
Low stages (A, B; I, II)	9/213 (4%)
Stage D-S or IV-S	4/58 (7%)
Advanced stages (C,D: III, IV)	165/528 (32%)

[a]Modified from Brodeur and Fong (1989).

fatal disease. However, in patients with single-copy tumors, there is not yet a biological marker for or explanation why half of the remaining do not survive. A general correlation has been demonstrated between *MYCN* copy number and expression (Bartram and Berthold, 1987; Grady-Leopardi *et al.*, 1986; Seeger *et al.*, 1988; Nisen *et al.*, 1988; Slavc *et al.*, 1990), and the level of expression per gene may be activated relative to *MYCN* expression in nonneural tumors and tissues (Kohl *et al.*, 1984; Thiele *et al.*, 1987). It has been shown that a substantial number of tumors without *MYCN* amplification overexpress this gene, but a high level of *MYCN* expression in single-copy tumors does not appear to identify a subset with a particularly poor outcome (Bartram and Berthold, 1987; Grady-Leopardi *et al.*, 1986; Seeger *et al.*, 1988; Nisen *et al.*, 1988; Slavc *et al.*, 1990). It is still possible that activation of *MYCN* by mechanisms other than amplification or overexpression may play an important role. In addition, it is likely that either activation of other oncogenes, deletion of chromosome 1p, or other genetic lesions may contribute to the poor clinical outcome in these patients.

Since *MYCN* overexpression per se in single-copy tumors does not appear to be associated with a poor prognosis, some have raised questions as to whether or not *MYCN* is the critical gene expressed from the amplified domain in tumors with *MYCN* amplification. Indeed, it is a formal possibility that *MYCN* is just a fortuitous marker that allowed identification of the amplified domain, and it is linked to a nearby gene that ultimately confers a poor outcome. However, there is compelling evidence that *MYCN* is a potent transforming gene (Schwab *et al.*, 1985; Yancopoulos *et al.*, 1985; Small *et al.*, 1987), and to date no other gene has been identified that is consistently amplified and expressed in tumors with *MYCN* amplification. Another explanation for the apparent discrepancy between the prognosis of *MYCN* amplified tumors and single-copy expressing tumors is that there is a threshold of expression above which a poor outcome results, and this threshold is rarely if ever exceeded by single-copy tumors. The effect of the very high levels of expression in tumors with *MYCN* amplification could result from a saturation of all normal sites on DNA or proteins, or it could result in the interaction of *MYCN* with another substrate, which would not occur at usual levels of expression.

D. THE ASSOCIATION BETWEEN CHROMOSOME 1p LOH AND *MYCN* AMPLIFICATION

The presence of *MYCN* amplification in human neuroblastomas has been shown to correlate strongly with advanced clinical stage and poor prognosis (Brodeur and Fong, 1989; Brodeur *et al.*, 1988; Brodeur *et al.*, 1984; Seeger *et al.*, 1985; Brodeur *et al.*, 1986; Nakagawara *et al.*, 1987; Bartram and Berthold, 1987; Grady-Leopardi *et al.*, 1986; Seeger *et al.*, 1988; Nisen *et al.*, 1988; Slavc *et al.*, 1990). Our recent studies (Fong *et al.*, 1989) showed a very strong correlation between *MYCN* amplification and chromosome 1p LOH ($p < 0.001$), indicating that LOH was common in patients with amplification (8 of 9 patients, or 89%). Indeed, the correlation between these two abnormalities in neuroblastoma cell lines is almost 100% (Brodeur and Fong, 1989; Brodeur *et al.*, 1981). Both *MYCN* amplification and deletion of chromosome 1p (as detected by cytogenetic analysis) (Hayashi *et al.*, 1986; Kaneko *et al.*, 1987; Christiansen and Lampert, 1988; Hayashi *et al.*, 1988, Hayashi *et al.*, 1989) appear strongly correlated with a poor clinical outcome and with each other, but it is not yet clear whether they are independent prognostic variables. Nevertheless, they appear to characterize a genetically distinct subset of very aggressive neuroblastomas.

Cytogenetic evidence would suggest that deletion of chromosome 1p occurs in 70 to 80% of primary neuroblastomas, whereas our molecular studies demonstrated LOH for distal chromosome 1p in only 30 to 40%. There are several possible explanations why LOH was not seen in a higher proportion of tumors. First, many cytogenetic analyses have focused on near-diploid tumors with relatively few rearrangements, and these are usually from patients with advanced stages of disease. When all karyotypes are taken into consideration, the percentage of tumors with chromosome 1p abnormalities is closer to 40%. Also, it is possible that mutational events at the critical region on chromosome 1p in other neuroblastomas may be too small to be detectable with current techniques. Finally, it is possible that deletion of a gene or genes from chromosome 1p is restricted to a subset of patients, or alternatively it may be a secondary event associated with disease progression in a subset. Our data showing the consistency of *MYCN* copy number over time (Brodeur *et al.*, 1987) would suggest that *MYCN* amplification is an intrinsic biologic property of a subset of tumors, so it must occur relatively early in these cases. Since cases with *MYCN* amplification represent a subset of patients with chromosome 1p deletion, we suspect that the 1p deletion may precede the development of amplification.

E. STUDIES OF OTHER ONCOGENES IN NEUROBLASTOMAS

We have sought evidence for amplification of other oncogenes, including *MYC, MYCL, NRAS, HRAS, KRAS, EGR1, NGL, SIS, SRC, MYB, FOS*, and *ETS* in over 100 neuroblastomas, but none was found (Brodeur and Fong, 1989). Similarly, we investigated expression at the RNA level of the above oncogenes in 10 neuroblastoma cell lines and a subset of primary tumors, but marked overexpression was found only for *MYCN* in the cell lines and tumors with amplification of this gene (Brodeur and Fong, 1989). Although *NRAS* was first identified as the transforming gene of a human neuroblastoma cell line (Shimizu *et al.*, 1983; Taparowsky *et al.*, 1983), subsequent studies of primary neuroblastomas by us and others (Ballas *et al.*, 1988; Ireland, 1989; Moley *et al.*, 1991) indicate that *ras* activation by mutation of codons 12, 13, 59, or 61 is rare. Finally, there is a study of *HRAS* expression in neuroblastomas in which tumors with higher levels of expression had a better outcome (Tanaka *et al.*, 1988). Thus, in the subset of the patients lacking *MYCN* amplification, there is no consistent evidence to date correlating activation of an oncogene other than *MYCN* with poor outcome.

VI. Structural Analysis of the *MYCN*-Amplified Domain in Neuroblastomas

Estimates of the size of the amplified domain around the *MYCN* protooncogene in neuroblastomas have ranged from 300 kb to 3000 kb, based on physical, chemical, and electrophoretic measurements of the amplified DNA (Brodeur and Seeger, 1986). However, all these approaches to map the size of the amplified domain have been indirect. An attempt has been made to clone and map the amplified domain around *MYCN* in a representative neuroblastoma cell line (Kinzler *et al.*, 1986; Zehnbauer *et al.*, 1988). A region spanning 140 kb around the *MYCN* locus was mapped with cosmid and lambda clones, and additional amplified clones were identified that were not contained in the 140-kb contiguous region. The entire 140-kb contiguous locus was amplified in a panel of 12 primary neuroblastomas with *MYCN* amplification, whereas the non-contiguous fragments were amplified in subsets of them (Zehnbauer *et al.*, 1988). These data indicate that, although each tumor had a relatively unique pattern of amplified DNA fragments, there was considerable similarity among the amplification units of different tumors.

Amler and Schwab (1989) have analyzed the amplified domain of a series of neuroblastoma cell lines with *MYCN* amplification, most in the form of chromosomally integrated HSRs. They analyzed the amplified domain by pulsed-field gel electrophoresis and hybridization with DNA probes that represent the 5' and 3' ends of the *MYCN* gene. They confirmed the heterogeneity of size of the amplified domain seen in different neuroblastomas demonstrated by earlier studies (Kinzler *et al.*, 1986; Zehnbauer *et al.*, 1988; Shiloh *et al.*, 1985; Shiloh *et al.*, 1986). They also concluded that most amplified regions of DNA consisted of multiple tandem arrays of DNA segments ranging in size from 100 to 700 kb, and that *MYCN* was at or near the center of the amplified units. Nonetheless, their data were most consistent with both tandem and inverted repeats, and rearrangements were more commonly found in the cell lines with higher *MYCN* copy number (greater than 50–100 copies per haploid genome).

We have begun a structural analysis of the amplified domain in human neuroblastomas in order to determine the size and heterogeneity of this region in different tumors and cell lines, as well as its clinical implications. Because of the large size of the domain, we have used the yeast artificial chromosome (YAC) cloning vector system (Schneider *et al.*, 1991). To date, 16 YACs have been identified that contain segments of the amplified domain from a representative neuroblastoma cell line, and the YACs can be arranged in a contiguous linear map of ≥1 megabase (Schneider *et al.*, 1991). All the YAC clones are consistent with a single, linear map of the region, with few if any rearrangements identified thus far. Our data also indicate that the core of the domain amplified in different tumors is at least 500 kb. The very large size suggests that there may be other genes near *MYCN* whose expression is important in mediating the aggressive phenotype associated with *MYCN* amplification. Alternatively, the nearest origin(s) of replication may be a considerable distance from *MYCN*, requiring a large domain to be stably replicated as an extrachromosomal element.

Our data show greater uniformity of the amplified domain within a given tumor and are more consistent with the deletion model for the initial event in the development of gene amplification, as suggested by Wahl and others (Carroll *et al.*, 1988; Stark *et al.*, 1989; Wahl, 1989). This is also supported by recent data documenting excision of *MYCN* from one of the two chromosome 2 homologs (Hunt *et al.*, 1990). The deletion model suggests that a large region containing the selectable marker and an origin of replication is deleted and circularizes, forming an extrachromosomal episome (Fig. 5). This episome segregates randomly during cell division, but cells with more copies of the marker gene have a selective advantage and accumulate to a certain stable average number. Although there would inevitably be heterogeneity in the number of episomes per cell, the average number in a population should be relatively stable. Larger episomes or episome multimers would be visible with the light microscope, and called dmins. As a rare event, the episomes would integrate into a chromosome at an apparently random site, forming an HSR (Fig. 5). Due to the secondary recombinational events, the structure of the amplified domains from HSRs would likely be more rearranged and heterogeneous. This might explain the apparent discrepancies in results of amplified domain analysis seen between various laboratories.

VII. Genetics of Neuroblastomas Identified by Screening

Recent studies of the cytogenetic features of tumors identified as a result of mass screening of infants for neuroblastomas in Japan (Hayashi *et al.*, 1986; Hayashi *et al.*, 1988) suggest that the majority of patients identified have lower stages of disease, and virtually all of the tumors are in the hyperdiploid or triploid range. Flow-cytometric analyses of the DNA content of neuroblastomas,

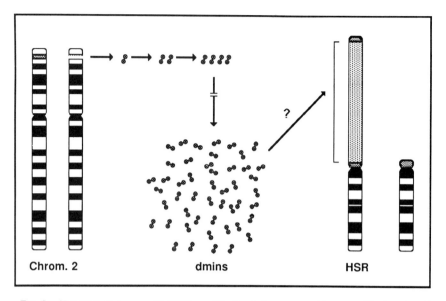

Fig. 5. Hypothetical process of MYCN amplification in human neuroblastomas. The location of
the normal *MYCN* gene is shown by the shaded band, chromosome 2p24 on the left. The current
data suggest that a large region of DNA containing the *MYCN* gene is deleted from one homolog of
chromosome 2 and forms an extrachromosomal element or episome, which is probably circular. It
must contain an origin of replication but lacks a centromere of kinetocore, so it does not segregate
evenly between daughter cells during mitosis. However, since it seems to provide a growth advantage
in vivo and *in vitro*, the episomes accumulate in a subset of cells but remain unstable and therefore
heterogeneously distributed among the cells in the population. If these episomes are large enough to
be seen in the light microscope, they are called dmins. As a rare event, particularly in cells *in vitro*
with pre-existing *MYCN* amplification, the dmins linearly integrate into a chromosome at a seemingly
random site.

as well as cytogenetic studies of modal chromosome number, have associated
hyperdiploid and triploid karyotypes with lower stages of disease and favorable
outcomes (Franke *et al.*, Hayashi *et al.*, 1986; Kaneko *et al.*, 1987; Christiansen
and Lampert, 1988; Hayashi *et al.*, 1988; Look *et al*, 1984; Gansler *et al.*, 1986;
Taylor *et al.*, 1988; Oppedal *et al.*, 1988). Therefore, the results of the screening
study have suggested at least two possibilities: either (1) all neuroblastomas begin
as tumors with a more favorable genotype and phenotype, and some evolve into
more aggressive tumors with adverse genetic features; or (2) there are at least
two different subsets of neuroblastoma, and the more favorable group presents
earlier and therefore is the predominant group detected by screening. Our data,
combined with those discussed above, are more consistent with the latter explanation (Brodeur and Fong, 1989; Fong *et al.*, 1989; Hayashi *et al.*, 1989).

VIII. Summary and Conclusions

Patterns are emerging, based on cytogenetic, molecular, and flow-cytometric analysis that suggest that neuroblastomas may be assigned to three genetically distinct groups (Table IV). The first comprises those with hyperdiploid or triploid modal karyotypes (or compatible DNA content by flow cytometry). Deletion of chromosome 1p, dmins, HSRs, or molecular evidence of *MYCN* amplification are rarely seen. These patients are more likely to be infants with low stages of disease (stages 1, 2, or 4S by the International Neuroblastoma Staging System) (Brodeur *et al.*, 1988), and they generally have a very favorable prognosis. Most of the infants detected by the neuroblastoma screening studies described above appear to fall into this category. The second group consists of tumors that are generally near-diploid or tetraploid modal chromosome number or DNA content. These tumors lack chromosome 1p deletion, dmins, HSRs, or *MYCN* amplification, and the patients are more likely to be over 1 year of age and have advanced stages of disease (stages 3 or 4). While their overall outcome is generally poor, their tumors respond at least initially to treatment, and they may survive for several years before they succumb ultimately to their disease. The third group consists of tumors that are also generally near-diploid or tetraploid, with chromosome 1p deletion (LOH), with or without dmins or HSRs (i.e., *MYCN* amplification). The patients also are more likely to be over 1 year of age and have advanced stages of disease (stages 3 or 4). In contrast to the second group, they generally respond to treatment only transiently, if at all, and they have rapid progression and die within months to a year or so. It remains to be determined whether tumors in one group ever evolve or "progress" into a less-unfavorable group, but current evidence would suggest that they are genetically distinct.

TABLE IV
CLINICAL/GENETIC TYPES OF NEUROBLASTOMA[a]

Feature	Type 1	Type 2	Type 3
Age	<12 mo	Any age	Any age
Stage	1, 2, 4S	3,4	Any stage
Ploidy	Hyperdiploid Near triploid	Near diploid Near tetraploid	Near diploid Near tetraploid
Chromosome 1p	Normal	Normal	Deleted
Dmins, HSR	Absent	Absent	Present
MYCN Copy	Normal	Normal	Amplified
Outcome	Good	Intermediate	Bad

[a]Modified from Brodeur (1990a).

The molecular and cytogenetic analysis of human neuroblastomas promises to make available a great deal of information that would be difficult to obtain otherwise. First, these studies may permit the localization of one or more neuroblastoma-predisposition loci. This would make possible the identification of hereditary cases in order to provide family counseling, as well as prenatal diagnosis of affected individuals in informative families. Second, genetic markers provide a more objective means to classify tumors that may appear similar histologically. Third, genetic analysis by karyotype, flow cytometry and/or determination of *MYCN* copy number provides information that has prognostic significance and can direct the most appropriate choice of treatment. A better understanding of these and other genetic abnormalities in human neuroblastomas may allow specific proteins and pathways to be identified, on which future therapeutic approaches could be focused.

Acknowledgments

Some of the material in the chapter was published previously (Brodeur and Fong, 1989; Brodeur, 1990a; Brodeur, 1990b). This work was supported in part by National Institutes of Health Grants RO1-CA-39771, KO4-CA-01027 and U10-CA-05887, the Children's United Research Effort, and the Fern Waldman Memorial Fund for Research in Childhood Cancer.

References

Allen, R. W., Ogden, B., Bentley, F. L., and Jung, A. L. (1980). Fetal hydantoin syndrome, neuroblastoma, and hemorrhagic disease in a neonate. *J.A.M.A.* **244**, 1464–1465.

Amler, L. C., and Schwab, M. (1989). Amplified N-*myc* in human neuroblastoma cells is often arranged as clustered tandem repeats of differently recombined DNA. *Mol. Cell. Biol.* **9**, 4903–4913.

Arenson, E. B. J., Hutter, J. J., Restuccia, R. D., and Holton, C. P. (1976). Neuroblastoma in a father and son. *J.A.M.A.* **235**, 727–729.

Atkin, N. B. (1986). Chromosome 1 aberrations in cancer. *Cancer Genet. Cytogenet.* **21**, 279–285.

Balaban-Malenbaum, G., and Gilbert, F. (1980). Relationship between homogeneously staining regions and double minute chromosomes in human neuroblastoma cell lines. *Prog. Cancer Res. Ther.* **12**, 97–107.

Ballas, K., Lyons, J., Jannsen, J. W. G., and Bartram, C. R. (1988). Incidence of *ras* gene mutations in neuroblastoma. *Eur. J. Pediatr.* **147**, 313–314.

Barr, H. Page, R., and Taylor, W. (1986). Primary small bowel ganglioneuroblastoma and Friedreich's ataxia. *J. R. Soc. Med.* **79**, 612–613.

Bartram, C. R., and Berthold, F. (1987). Amplification and expression of the N-*myc* gene in neuroblastoma. *Eur. J. Pediatr.* **146**, 162–165.

Beckwith, J., and Perrin, E. (1963). *In situ* neuroblastomas: A contribution to the natural history of neural crest tumors. *Am J. Pathol.* **43**, 1089–1104.

Biedler, J. L., and Spengler, B. A. (1976a). Metaphase chromosome anomaly: Association with drug resistance and cell-specific products. *Science* **191**, 185–187.

Biedler, J. L., and Spengler, B. A. (1976b). A novel chromosome abnormality in human neuroblastoma and antifolate-resistant Chinese hamster cell lines in culture. *J. Natl. Cancer Inst.* **57**, 683–695.

Biedler, J. L., Ross, R. A., Shanske, S., and Spengler, B. A. (1980). Human neuroblastoma cytogenetics: Search for significance of homogeneously staining regions and double minute chromosomes. *Prog. Cancer Res. Ther.* **12**, 81–96.

Brodeur, G. M. (1987). The involvement of oncogenes and suppressor genes in human neoplasia. *Adv. Pediatr.* **34**, 1–44.

Brodeur, G. M. (1990a). Neuroblastoma—Clinical applications of molecular parameters. *Brain Pathol.* **1**, in press.

Brodeur, G. M. (1990b). Molecular biology and genetics of human neuroblastoma. In "Neuroblastoma: Tumor Biology and Therapy." (C. Pochedly, ed.), pp. 31–50. CRC Press, Boca Raton, Florida.

Brodeur, G. M., and Fong, C. T. (1989). Molecular biology and genetics of human neuroblastoma. *Cancer Genet. Cytogenet.* **41**, 153–174.

Brodeur, G.M., and Seeger, R. C. (1986). Gene amplification in human neuroblastomas: Basic mechanisms and clinical implications. *Cancer Genet. Cytogenet.* **19**, 101–111.

Brodeur, G. M., Fong, C. T., Morita, M., Griffith, R., Hayes, F. A., and Seeger, R. C. (1988). Molecular analysis and clinical significance of N-*myc* amplification and chromosome 1 abnormalities in human neuroblastomas. *Prog. Clin. Biol. Res.* **271**, 3–15.

Brodeur, G. M., Green, A. A., Hayes, F. A., Williams, K. J., Williams, D. L., and Tsiatis, A. A. (1981). Cytogenetic features of human neuroblastomas and cell lines. *Cancer Res.* **41**, 4678–4686.

Brodeur, G. M., Hayes, F. A., Green, A. A., Casper, J. T., Wasson, J., Wallach, S., and Seeger, R. C. (1987). Consistent N-*myc* copy number in simultaneous or consecutive neuroblastoma samples from sixty individual patients. *Cancer Res.* **47**, 4248–4253.

Brodeur, G. M., Seeger, R. C., Barrett, A. T., *et al.* (1988). International criteria for diagnosis, staging, and response to treatment in patients with neuroblastoma. *J. Clin. Oncol.* **6**, 1874–1881.

Brodeur, G. M., Seeger, R. C., Sather, H., Dalton, A., Siegel, S. E., Wong, K. Y., and Hammond, D. (1986). Clinical implications of oncogene activation in human neuroblastomas. *Cancer* **58**, 541–545.

Brodeur, G. M., Seeger, R. C., Schwab, M., Varmus, H. E., and Bishop, J. M. (1984). Amplification of N-*myc* in untreated human neuroblastomas correlates with advanced disease stage. *Science* **224**, 1121–1124.

Brodeur, G. M., Sekhon, G. S., and Goldstein, M.N. (1977). Chromosomal aberrations in human neuroblastomas. *Cancer* **40**, 2256–2263.

Carroll, S., DeRose, M., Gaudray, P., Moore, C., VanDevanter, D. N., Von Hoff, D., and Wahl, G. (1988). Double minute chromosomes can be produced from percursors derived from a chromosomal deletion. *Mol. Cell. Biol.* **3**, 1525–1533.

Chatten, J., and Voorhess, M. L. (1967). Familial neuroblastoma: Report of a kindred with multiple disorders, including neuroblastomas in four siblings. *N. Engl. J. Med.* **227**, 1230–1236.

Christiansen, H., and Lampert, F. (1988). Tumour karyotype discriminates between good and bad prognostic outcome in neuroblastoma. *Br. J. Cancer* **57**, 121–126.

Comings, D. E. (1973). A general theory of carcinogenesis. *Proc. Natl. Acad. Sci. U.S.A.* **70**, 3324–3328.

Cox, D., Yuncken, C., and Spriggs, A. I. (1965). Minute chromatin bodies in malignant tumours of childhood. *Lancet* **2**, 55–58.

de la Monte, S. M., Hutchins, G. M., and Moore, G. W. (1985). Peripheral neuroblastic tumors and congenital heart disease. Possible role of hypoxic states in tumor induction. *Am. J. Pediatr. Hematol. Oncol.* **7,** 109–116.

Douglass, E. C., Green, A. A., Hayes, F. A., Etcubanas, E., Horowitz, M., and Wilimas, J. A. (1985). Chromosome 1 abnormalities: A common feature of pediatric solid tumors. *J. Natl. Cancer Inst.* **75,** 51–54.

Dracopoli, N. C., Harnett, P., Bale, S. J., Stanger, B. Z., Tucker, M. A., Housman, D. E., and Kefford, R. F. (1989). Loss of alleles from the distal short arm of chromosome 1 occurs late in melanoma tumor progression. *Proc. Natl. Acad. Sci. U.S.A.* **86,** 4614–4618.

Emery, L. G., Shields, M., Shah, N. R., and Garbes, A. (1983). Neuroblastoma associated with Beckwith-Wiedemann syndrome. *Cancer* **52,** 176–179.

Evans, A. E., D'Angio, G. J., Seeger, R. C. (eds.), (1985). In "Advances in Neuroblastoma Research." Alan R. Liss, New York.

Evans, A. E., D'Angio, G. J., Knudson, A. G. J., and Seeger, R. C. (eds.), (1988). In "Advances in Neuroblastoma Research 2." Alan, R. Liss, New York.

Evans, A. E., D'Angio, G. J., Knudson, A. G. J., and Seeger, R. C. (eds.), (1991). In "Advances in Neuroblastoma Research 3." Alan R. Liss, New York.

Fairchild, R. S., Kyner, J. L, Hermreck, A., and Schimke, R. N. (1979). Neuroblastoma, pheochromocytoma, and renal cell carcinoma. Occurrence in a single patient. *J.A.M.A.* **242,** 2210–2211.

Feingold, M., Gheradi, G. J., and Simmons, C. (1971). Familial neuroblastoma and trisomy 13. *Am. J. Dis. Child.* **121,** 451.

Fong, C. T., Dracopoli, N. C., White, P. S., Merrill, P. T., Griffith, R. C., Housman, D. E., and Brodeur, G. M. (1989). Loss of heterozygosity for chromosome 1p in human neuroblastomas: Correlation with N-*myc* amplification. *Proc. Natl. Acad. Sci. U.S.A.* **86,** 3753–3757.

Franke, F., Rudolph, B., Christiansen, H., Harbott, J., and Lampert, F. (1986). Tumour karyotype may be important in the prognosis of human neuroblastoma. *J. Cancer Res. Clin. Oncol.* **111,** 266–272.

Gansler, T., Chatten, J., Varello, M., Bunin, G. R., and Atkinson, B., (1986). Flow cytometric DNA analysis of neuroblastoma. Correlation with histology and clinical outcome. *Cancer* **58,** 2453–2458.

Gilbert, F., Feder, M., Balaban, G., Brangman, D., Lurie, D., Podolsky, R., Rinaldt, V., Vinikoor, N., and Weisband, J. (1984). Human neuroblastomas and abnormalities of chromosome 1 and 17. *Cancer Res.* **44,** 5444–5449.

Grady-Leopardi, E. F., Schwab, M., Ablin, A. R., and Rosenau, W. (1986). Detection of N-*myc* expression in human neuroblastoma by *in situ* hybridization and blot analysis: Relationship to clinical outcome. *Cancer Res.* **46,** 3196–3199.

Grotting, J. C., Kassel, S., and Dehner, L. P. (1979). Nesidioblastosis and congenital neuroblastoma. A histologic and immunocytochemical study of a new complex neurocristopathy. *Arch. Pathol. Lab. Med.* **103,** 642–646.

Hardy, P. C., and Nesbit, M. E. J. (1972). Familial neuroblastoma: Report of a kindred with a high incidence of infantile tumors. *J. Pediatr.* **80,** 74–77.

Hayashi, Y., Hanada, R., Yamamoto, K., and Bessho, F. (1986). Chromosome findings and prognosis in neuroblastoma. *Cancer Genet. Cytogenet.* **29,** 175–177.

Hayashi, Y., Inabada, T., Hanada, R., and Yamamoto, K. (1988). Chromosome findings and prognosis in 15 patients with neuroblastoma found by VMA mass screening. *J. Pediatr.* **112,** 67–71.

Hayashi, Y., Kanda, N., Inaba, T., Hanada, R., Nagahara, N., Muchi, H., and Yamamoto, K. (1989). Cytogenetic findings and prognosis in neuroblastoma with emphasis on marker chromosome 1. *Cancer* **63,** 126–132.

Hecht, F., and Kaiser-McCaw, B. (1981). Chromosomes in familial neuroblastoma *J. Pediatr.* **98,** 334.

Hecht, F., Hecht, B. K., Northrup, J. C., Trachtenberg, N., Wood, S. T., and Cohen, J. D. (1982). Genetics of familial neuroblastoma: Long-range studies. *Cancer Gent. Cytogenet.* **7**, 227–230.

Hunt, J. D., Valentine, M., and Tereba, A. (1990). Excision of N-*myc* from chromosome 2 in human neuroblastoma cells containing amplified N-*myc* sequences. *Mol. Cell. Biol.* **10**, 823–829.

Ikeda, Y., Lister, J., Bouton, J. M., and Buyukpamukcu, M. (1981). Congenital neuroblastoma, neuroblastoma *in situ*, and the normal fetal development of the adrenal. *J. Pediatr. Surg.* **16**, 636–644.

Ireland, C. M. (1989). Activated N-*ras* oncogenes in human neuroblastoma. *Cancer Res.* **49**, 5530–5533.

Kalmanti, M., and Athanasiou, A. (1985). Neuroblastoma occurring in a child with dermatomyositis. *Am. J. Pediatr. Hematol. Oncol.* **7**, 387–388.

Kaneko, Y., Kanda, N., Maseki, N., Sakurai, M., Tsuchida, Y., Takeda, T., Okabe, L., and Sakurai, M. (1987). Different karyotypic patterns in early- and advanced-stage neuroblastomas. *Cancer Res.* **47**, 311–318.

Kinney, H., Faix, R., and Brazy, J. (1980). The fetal alcohol syndrome and neuroblastoma. *Pediatrics* **66**, 130–132.

Kinzler, K. W., Zehnbauer, B. A., Brodeur, G. M., Seeger, R. C., Trent, J. M., Meltzer, P. S., and Vogelstein, B. (1986). Amplification units containing human N-*myc* and c-*myc* genes. *Proc. Natl. Acad. Sci. U.S.A.* **83**, 1031–1035.

Knudson, A. G. (1971). Mutation and cancer: Statistical study of retinoblastoma. *Proc. Natl. Acad. Sci. U.S.A.* **68**, 820–823.

Knudson, A. G. J., and Amromin, G. D. (1966). Neuroblastoma and ganglioneuroma in a child with multiple neurofibromatosis. Implications for the mutational origin of neuroblastoma. *Cancer* **19**, 1032–1037.

Knudson, A. G. J., and Meadows, A. T. (1976). Developmental genetics of neuroblastoma. *J. Natl. Cancer Inst.* **57**, 675–682.

Knudson, A. G. J., and Strong, L. C. (1972). Mutation and cancer: Neuroblastoma and pheochromocytoma. *Am J. Hum. Genet.* **24**, 514–522.

Kohl, N. E., Gee, C. E., and Alt, F. W. (1984). Activated expression of the N-*myc* gene in human neuroblastomas and related tumors. *Science* **226**, 1335–1337.

Kohl, N. E., Kanda, N., Schreck, R. R., Bruns, G., Latt, S. A., Gilbert, F., and Alt, F. W. (1983). Transposition and amplification of oncogene-related sequences in human neuroblastomas. *Cell* **35**, 359–367.

Kushner, B. H., and Helson, L. (1985). Monozygotic siblings discordant for neuroblastoma: Etiologic implications. *J. Pediatr.* **107**, 405–409.

Kushner, B. H., Gilbert, F., and Helson, L., (1986). Familial neublatoma: Case reports, literature review, and etiologic considerations. *Cancer* **57**, 1887–1893.

Kushner, B. H., Hajdu, S. I., and Helson, L. (1985). Synchronous neuroblastoma and von Recklinghausen's disease: A review of the literature. *J. Clin. Oncol.* **3**, 117–120.

Lenarsky, C., Shewmon, A., Shaw, A., and Feig, S. A. (1985). Occurrence of neuroblastoma and asymmetric crying facies: Case report and review of the literature. *J. Pediatr.* **107**, 268–270.

Look, A. T., Hayes, F. A., Nitschke, R., McWilliams, N. B., and Green, A. A. (1984). Cellular DNA content as predictor of response to chemotherapy in infants with unresectable neuroblastoma. *N. Engl. J. Med.* **311**, 231–235.

Look, A. T., Hayes, F. A., Shuster, J. J., Douglass, E. C., Castleberry, R. P., Bowman, L. C., Smith, E. I., and Brodeur, G. M. (1991). Clinical relevance of tumor cell ploidy and N-*myc* gene amplification in childhood neuroblastoma. *J. Clin. Oncol.* **9**, 581–591.

Mathew, C. G. P., Smith, B. A., Thorpe, K., Wong, Z., Royle, N. J., Jeffreys, A. J., and Ponder, B. A. J. (1987). Deletion of genes on chromosome 1 in endocrine neoplasia. *Nature* **328**, 524–526.

Matsunaga, E. (1981). Genetics of Wilms' tumor. *Hum. Genet.* **57**, 231–246.

Meadows, A. T., Baum, E., Fossati-Bellani, F. D. G., Jenkin, R. D. T., Marsden, B., Nesbit, M., Newton, W., Oberlin, O., Sallan, S. G., Siegel, S., Strong, L. C., and Voute, P. A. (1985). Second malignant neoplasms in children: An update from the Late Effects Study Group. *J. Clin. Oncol.* **3**, 532–538.

Miller, D. R., Patel, K., Allen, J. C., and Horten, B. (1983). Neuroblastoma, tuberous sclerosis, and subependymal giant cell astrocytoma. *Am J. Pediatr. Hematol. Oncol.* **5**, 213–218.

Miller, R. W., and Fraumeni, J. F. J. (1968). Neuroblastoma: Epidemiologic approach to its origin. *Am. J. Dis. Child.* **115**, 253–261.

Moley, J. F., Brother, M. B., Wells, S. A., Spengler, B. A., Biedler, J. L., and Brodeur, G. M. (1991). Low Frequency of *ras* Gene Mutations in Neuroblastomas, Pheochromocytomas, and Medullary Thyroid Cancers. *Cancer Res.* **51**, 1596–1599.

Montgomery, K. T., Biedler, J. L., Spengler, B. A., and Melera, P. W. (1983). Specific DNA sequence amplification in human neuroblastoma cells. *Proc Natl. Acad. Sci. U.S.A.* **80**, 5724–5728.

Moorhead, P. S., and Evans, A. E. (1980). Chromosomal findings in patients with neuroblastoma. *In* "Advances in Neuroblastoma Research" (A. E. Evans, ed.), pp. 109–118. Raven Press, New York.

Moss, R. B., Blessing-Moore, J., Bender, S. W., and Weibel, A. (1985). Cystic fibrosis and neuroblastoma. *Pediatrics* **76**, 814–817.

Nagano, H., Kano, Y., Kobuchi, S., and Kajitani, T. (1980). A case of partial 2p trisomy with neuroblastoma. *Jpn. J. Human Genet.* **25**, 39–45.

Nakagawara, A., Ikeda, K., Tsuda, T., Higashi, K., and Okabe, T. (1987). Amplification of N-*myc* oncogene in stage II and IVS neuroblastomas may be a prognostic indicator. *J. Pediatr. Surg.* **22**, 415–418.

Nakissa, N., Constine, L. S., Rubin, P., and Strohl, R. (1985). Birth defects in three common pediatric malignancies: Wilms' tumor, neuroblastoma, and Ewing's sarcoma. *Oncology* **42**, 358–363.

Nevin, N. C., Dodge, J. A., and Allen, I. V. (1972). Two cases of trisomy D associated with adrenal tumors. *J. Med. Genet.* **9**, 199–123.

Nisen, P. D., Waber, P. G., Rich, M. A., Pierce, S., Garvin, J. R. J., Gilbert, F., and Lanskowsky, P. (1988). N-*myc* oncogene RNA expression in neuroblastoma. *J. Natl. Cancer Inst.* **80**, 1633–1637.

Oppedal, B. R., Storm-Mathisen, I., Lie, S. O., and Brandtzaeg, P. (1988). Prognostic factors in neuroblastoma. Clinical, histopathologic, immunohistochemical features and DNA ploidy in relation to prognosis. *Cancer* **62**, 772–780.

Pegelow, C. H., Ebbin, A. J., Powars, D., and Towner, J. W. (1975). Familial neuroblastoma. *J. Pediatr.* **87**, 763–765.

Robinson, M. G., and McCorquodale, M. M. (1981). Trisomy 18 and neurogenic neoplasia. *J. Pediatr.* **99**, 428 429.

Rudolph, B., Harbott, J., and Lampert, F. (1988). Fragile sites and neuroblastoma: Fragile site at 1p13.1 and other points on lymphocyte chromosomes from patients and family members. *Cancer Genet. Cytogenet.* **31**, 83–94.

Sanger, W. G., Howe, J., Fordyce, R., and Purtilo, D. T. (1984). Inherited partial trisomy #15 complicated by neuroblastoma. *Cancer Gent. Cytogenet.* **11**, 153–159.

Schneider, S. S., Zehnbauer, B. A., Vogelstein, B., and Brodeur, G. M., (1991). Yeast artificial chromosome (YAC) vector cloning of the *MYCN*-amplified domain in human neuroblastomas. *Prog. Clin. Biol. Res.* **366**, 71–76.

Schwab, M., Alitalo, K., Klempnauer, K. H., Varmus, H. E., Bishop, J. M., Gilbert, F., Brodeur, G., Goldstein, M., and Trent, J. M. (1983). Amplified DNA with limited homology to *myc* cellular oncogene is shared by human neuroblastoma cell lines and a neuroblastoma tumour. *Nature* **305**, 245–248.

Schwab, M., Varmus, H. E., and Bishop, J. M. (1985). Human N-*myc* gene contributes to neoplastic transformation of mammalian cells in culture. *Nature* **316**, 160–162.

Schwab, M., Varmus, H. E., Bishop, J. M., Grzeschik, K. H., Naylor, S. L., Sakaguchi, A. Y., Brodeur, G., and Trent, J. (1984). Chromosome localization in normal human cells and neuroblastomas of a gene related to c-*myc*. *Nature* **308**, 288–291.

Secker-Walker, L. M., Stewart, E. L., and Todd, A. (1985). Acute lymphoblastic leukaemia with t(4;11) follows neuroblastoma: A late effect of treatment? *Med. Pediatr. Oncol.* **13**, 48–50.

Seeger, R. C., Brodeur, G. M., Sather, H., Dalton, A., Siegel, S. E., Wong, K. Y., and Hammond, D. (1985). Association of multiple copies of the N-*myc* oncogene with rapid progression of neuroblastomas. *N. Engl. J. Med.* **313**, 1111–1116.

Seeger, R. C., Wada, R., Brodeur, G. M., Moss, T. J., Bjork, R. L., Sousa, L., and Slamon, D. J. (1988). Expression of N-*myc* by neuroblastomas with one or multiple copies of the oncogene. *Prog. Clin. Biol. Res.* **271**, 41–49.

Seeler, R. A., Israel, J. N., Royal, J. E., Kaye, C. I., Rao, S., and Abulaban, M. (1979). Ganglioneuroblastoma and fetal hydantoin-alcohol syndromes. *Pediatrics* **63**, 524–527.

Shah, N. R., Miller, D. R., Steinherz, P. G., Garbes, A., and Farber, P. (1983). Acute monoblastic leukemia as a second malignant neoplasm in metastatic neuroblastoma. *Am. J. Pediat. Hematol. Oncol.* **7**, 309–314.

Shiloh, Y., Korf, B., Kohl, N. E., Sakai, K., Brodeur, G. M., Harris, P., Kanda, N., Seeger, R. C., Alt, F., and Latt, S. A. (1986). Amplification and rearrangement of DNA sequences from the chromosomal region 2p24 in human neuroblastomas. *Cancer Res.* **46**, 5297–5301.

Shiloh, Y., Shipley, J., Brodeur, G. M., Bruns, G., Korf, B., Donlon, T., Schreck, R. R., Seeger, R., Sakai, K., and Latt, S. A. (1985). Differential amplification, assembly, and relocation of multiple DNA sequences in human neuroblastomas and neuroblastoma cell lines. *Proc. Natl. Acad. Sci. U.S.A.* **82**, 3761–3765.

Shimizu, K., Goldfarb, M., Perucho, M., and Wigler, M. (1983). Isolation and preliminary characterization of the transforming gene of a human neuroblastoma cell line. *Proc. Natl. Acad. Sci. U.S.A.* **80**, 383–387.

Slavc, I., Ellenbogen, R., Jung, W. H., Vawter, G. F., Kretschmar, C., Grier, H., and Korf, B. R. (1990). *Myc* gene amplification and expression in primary human neuroblastoma. *Cancer Res.* **50**, 1459–1463.

Small, M. B., Hay, N., Schwab, M., and Bishop, J. M. (1987). Neoplastic transformation by the human gene N-*myc*. *Mol. Cell. Biol.* **7**, 1638–1645.

Stark, G. R., Debatisse, M., Giulotto, E., and Wahl, G. M. (1989). Recent progress in understanding mechanisms of mammalian DNA amplification. *Cell* **57**, 901–908.

Suzuki, T., Yokota, J., Mugishima, H., Okabe, I., Ookuni, M., Sugimura, T., and Terada, M. (1989). Frequent loss of heterozygosity on chromosome 14q in neuroblastoma. *Cancer Res.* **49**, 1095–1098.

Sy, W. M., and Edmonson, J. H. (1968). The developmental defects associated with neuroblastoma—Etiologic implications. *Cancer* **22**, 234–238.

Tanaka, T., Slamon, D. J., Shimoda, H., Waki, C., Kawaguchi, Y., Tanaka, Y., and Ida, N. (1988). Expression of Ha-*ras* oncogene products in human neuroblastomas and the significant correlation with a patient's prognosis. *Cancer Res.* **48**, 1030–1034.

Taparowsky, E., Shimizu, K., Goldfarb, M., and Wigler, M. (1983). Structure and activation of the human N-*ras* gene. *Cell* **34**, 581–586.

Taylor, S. R., Blatt, J., Constantino, J. P., Roederer, M., and Murphy, R. F. (1988). Flow-cytometric DNA analysis of neuroblastoma and ganglioneuroma. A 10-year retrospective study. *Cancer* **62**, 749–754.

Thiele, C. J., McKeon, C., Triche, T. J., Ross, R. A., Reynolds, C. P., and Israel, M. A. (1987). Differential protooncogene expression characterizes histopathologically indistinguishable tumors of the peripheral nervous system. *J. Clin. Invest.* **80**, 804–811.

Tsuda, T., Obara, M., Hirano, H., Gotoh, S., Kubomura, S., Higashi, K., Kuroiwa, A., Nakagawara, A., Nagahara, N., and Shimizu, K. (1987). Analysis of N-*myc* amplification in relation to disease stage and histologic types in human neuroblastomas. *Cancer* **60**, 820–826.

Tsutsumi, M., Yokota, J., Kakizoe, T., Koiso, K., Sugimura, T., and Terada, M. (1989). Loss of heterozygosity on chromosomes 1p and 11p in sporadic pheochromocytoma. *J. Natl. Cancer Inst.* **81**, 367–370.

Turkel, S. B., and Itabashi, H. H. (1975). The natural history of neuroblastic cells in the fetal adrenal gland. *Am. J. Pathol.* **76**, 225–243.

Vogel, F. (1979). Genetics of retinoblastoma. *Hum. Genet.* **52**, 1–54.

Wagget, J., Aherne, G., and Aherne, W. (1973). Familial neuroblastoma: Report of two sib pairs. *Arch. Dis. Child.* **48**, 63–66.

Wahl, G. M. (1989). The importance of circular DNA in mammalian gene amplification. *Cancer Res.* **49**, 1333–1340.

Weh, H. J., Kabisch, H., Landbeck, G., and Hossfeld, D. K. (1986). Translocation (9;11)(p21;q23) in a child with acute monoblastic leukemia following 2½ years after successful chemotherapy for neuroblastoma. *J. Clin. Oncol.* **4**, 1518–1520.

Weith, A., Martinsson, T., Cziepluch, C., Bruderlein, S., Amler, L. C., and Berthold, F. (1989). Neuroblastoma consensus deletion maps to 1p36.1-2. *Genes Chrom. Cancer* **1**, 159–166.

Witzleben, C. L., and Landy, R. A. (1974). Disseminated neuroblastoma in a child with von Recklinghausen's disease. *Cancer* **34**, 786–790.

Wong, K. Y., Hanenson, I. B., and Lampkin, B. C. (1971). Familial neuroblastoma. *Am. J. Dis. Child.* **121**, 415–416.

Yancopoulos, G. D., Nisen, P. D., Tesfaye, A., Kohl, N. E., Goldfarb, M. P., and Alt, F. W. (1985). N-*myc* can cooperate with *ras* to transform normal cells in culture. *Proc. Natl. Acad. Sci. U.S.A.* **82**, 5455–5459.

Young, J. L. Jr., Ries, L. G., Silverberg, E., Horm, J. W., and Miller, R. W. (1986). Cancer incidence, survival, and mortality for children younger than 15 years. *Cancer* **58**, 598–602.

Zehnbauer, B. A., Small, D., Brodeur, G. M., Seeger, R., and Vogelstein, B. (1988). Characterization of N-*myc* amplification units in human neuroblastoma cells. *Mol. Cell. Biol.* **8**, 522–530.

Chapter 9

Colonic and Pancreatic Mucin Glycoproteins Expressed in Neoplasia

Young S. Kim and James C. Byrd

*GI Research Lab (151M2), VA Medical Center and Department of Medicine,
University of California, San Francisco, San Francisco, California*

I. Introduction

Many secretory glandular or ductal cells are rich in molecules that contain carbohydrates. These cellular carbohydrate-containing molecules are glycoproteins and glycolipids, which together are called glycoconjugates. Recent studies indicate that many tumor-associated alterations occur in the carbohydrate moieties of these glycoconjugates (Hakomori, 1989; Kim, 1990). In colorectal and pancreatic cancers, which together make up most of the cases of gastrointestinal cancers seen in the United States, both qualitative and quantitative changes in carbohydrate of mucin glycoproteins have been observed. These studies were carried out using histochemical, immunological, and lectin-affinity–staining techniques as well as biochemical analytical methods. Furthermore, using monoclonal antibodies (MAbs), various antigenic epitopes associated with cancers of

BIOCHEMICAL AND MOLECULAR ASPECTS
OF SELECTED CANCERS, VOL. 1

the colorectum and pancreas have recently been demonstrated to be present on mucin glycoprotein molecules.

In this chapter, the biochemical and immunochemical properties of mucin glycoproteins in normal and cancerous cells of colon and pancreas will be discussed.

II. Mucin Glycoproteins

A. GENERAL PROPERTIES

Mucin glycoproteins are the major component of mucus, which forms viscous gels covering the epithelial cell surface (Neutra and Forstner, 1987). Using a variety of histochemical methods, these gel-forming mucin glycoproteins have been shown to be secreted by such specialized epithelial cells as goblet cells, submucosal gland cells, and ductal cells of the respiratory, gastrointestinal, and genitourinary tracts. Goblet cells in the colon and ductal cells in the pancreas are the major epithelial cell types responsible for mucin synthesis and secretion. In addition, mucin-like glycoproteins have also been found to be associated with the plasma membranes of a variety of normal and cancerous cells as integral membrane glycoproteins (e.g., epiglycanin (Coddington *et al.*, 1984), leukosialin (Carlsson and Fukuda, 1986), episialin (Ligtenberg *et al.*, 1990), and epitectin (Bhavanandan, 1988)). These membrane-associated, mucin-like glycoproteins have been suggested to play a biological role in cell–cell, or cell–substratum interaction, invasion, and metastasis. However, the presence of mucin-like membrane glycoproteins has not yet been conclusively demonstrated in the epithelial cells of colon or pancreas.

Models for the structure of mucus gel-forming mucin glycoproteins proposed by several investigators all consist of mucin subunits linked by disulfide bonds, with or without a *link* peptide (Allen, 1983; Mantle *et al.*, 1984; Carlstedt and Sheehan, 1988). These polymeric mucins are thought to contribute to gel formation owing to their large molecular size and high hydrodynamic volume, with the large amount of bound water resulting from heavy glycosylation (Harding, 1989).

This gel-forming property of mucin glycoproteins contributes to some of their protective functions, particularly in parts of the body that must interact in some way with the environment. These functions include lubrication for ingested food or elimination of fecal matter, prevention of dehydration in the various mucous membranes they coat, exclusion of microorganisms and parasites from attacking the gut wall, and protection of the intestinal and pancreatic ductal mucosa from digestive proteases.

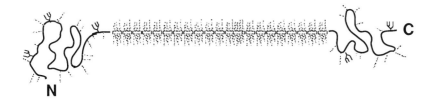

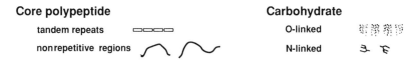

FIG. 1.   Working model of mucin structure.

B. Biochemical Properties

Mucin glycoproteins consist of a protein backbone with many carbohydrate side chains linked to it (Fig. 1). They have the following general biochemical properties: (1) a large molecular weight (4×10^5 to 1×10^7); (2) many "O-glycosidically" linked carbohydrate side chains, which may constitute 50–85% of the total molecular weight; (3) a high content of serine, threonine, and proline in the protein backbone structure; (4) a buoyant density higher than protein (e.g., 1.35–1.50 g/cm³), due to their high carbohydrate content; and (5) a high viscosity and capacity for gel formation, due to their high molecular weight and carbohydrate content.

1. Carbohydrate Moiety

Carbohydrate side chains of mucin glycoproteins are attached to a hydroxyl group of serine or threonine of the protein backbone via N-acetylgalactosamine through O-glycosidic linkages. This is in contrast to most serum and cell-membrane glycoproteins, which have carbohydrate side chains linked to the amide nitrogen molecule of asparagine via N-acetylglucosamine through "N-glycosidic" linkages.

Although it was long thought that mucin glycoproteins contain only O-glycosidically linked oligosaccharides, recent studies indicate that a small number of N-glycosidically linked carbohydrates may also be present in mucin glycoproteins (Denny and Denny, 1982; Hilkens and Buijs, 1988; Linsley et al., 1988; Gum et al., 1989; Gum et al., 1990).

Five different sugars are commonly found in O-glycosidic mucin glycoproteins. These are N-acetylgalactosamine (GalNAc), N-acetylglucosamine (GlcNAc),

N-acetylneuraminic acid (NeuAc), galactose (Gal) and fucose (Fuc). Carbohydrate side chains are often branched, with one to over 20 sugars per chain. They may be negatively changed, owing primarily to NeuAc and ester sulfate. Up to a third of the total amino acid residues may be linked to carbohydrate side chains, making the protein backbone resistant to proteolysis.

O-Linked oligosaccharide side chains may be arbitrarily divided into three regions: inner core, backbone, and periphery (Hounsell and Feizi, 1982), as illustrated in Fig. 2. The sugar or sugars that are attached to the GalNAc that is linked to the protein backbone compose the core-region carbohydrates. Six different types of core-region carbohydrates have been identified (Roussel *et al.,* 1988), but the relative proportions of core sugar structures in normal and cancerous colonic and pancreatic mucins are not known.

In the normal human adult gastrointestinal mucosa in man, the core structures are usually elongated by the major basic backbone structure consisting of type 1 backbone chain (Galβ1-3 GlcNAcβ1-3Galβ-R). This backbone structure may be replaced with a type 2 (lactosamine) chain (Galβ1-4GlcNAcβ1-3Galβ-R), and less frequently with a type 3 chain (Galβ1-3GalNAcα1-3Galβ1-r) or a type 4 chain (Galβ1-3GalNAcβ1-3Galβ1-R) (Hakomori, 1989). The type 2 chain may be repeated in the same oligosaccharide side chain to form a polylactosamine backbone, but the type 1 chain is usually not repeated. The type 1 and type 2 chain backbone structures can also be branched in a β1-6 configuration using Gal as branch point. The backbone chains are terminated or terminally branched by α-linked sugars such as NeuAc, fucose, *N*-acetylgalactosamine or galactose in the peripheral region. All three regions of the oligosaccharide side chains provide specific recognition sites for carbohydrate-specific antibodies,

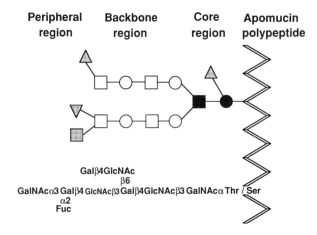

FIG. 2.   Schematic representation of carbohydrate and protein domains in mucins.

and can serve as tumor markers recognized by monoclonal antibodies and lectins.

2. Protein Backbone (Apomucin)

The protein backbones of mucin glycoproteins are rich in serine, threonine, and proline, which can compose over half of the total amino acids. Until recently, relatively little was known about the structure and amino acid sequence of the protein backbones of mucin glycoproteins, because of their heavy glycosylation and the difficulty in removing the sugars without extensive degradation of the protein moiety. The availability of molecular cloning and sequencing techniques has now resulted in the identification of three human mucin gene apomucins (Table I) (Gendler et al., 1987; Siddiqui et al., 1988; Gum et al., 1989, 1990; Ligtenberg et al., 1990).

All three apomucins have a similar structural motif, consisting of central repetitive regions flanked by nonrepetitive unique sequences (Fig. 1). The repetitive segments consist of tandem repeats containing serine and/or threonine, the sites of potential O-glycosylation. In the case of breast cancer apomucin (the MUC1 gene product designated PUM, PEM, or episialin), tandem repeat units consist of 20 amino acids, while the repeat unit of MUC2 and MUC3 type intestinal apomucins have 23 and 17 amino acids respectively. All three types of apomucin have several potential N-glycosylation sites, a finding contrary to long-held views that only O-glycosidically linked oligosaccharide side chains are present in the mucin glycoproteins. All three mucin genes are polymorphic. It has been shown that the variation in the size of breast cancer mucin observed in cell

TABLE I
HUMAN APOMUCINS

Source	Suggested and (published) gene symbol	Tandem repeat (AA res)	mRNA size (kb)	Potential N-glyco-sylation sites	Poly-morphism	Chromosomal location
Intestinal mucin						
Acidic	MUC2 (SMUC)	23	7.6 polydisperse	Yes	Yes	11 p15.5
Neutral	MUC3 (SIB)	17	8 polydisperse	Yes	Yes	7
Mammary mucin	MUC1 (PUM, PEM EPISIALIN)	20	4.1–7.1 discrete	Yes	Yes (length)	1 q21–24

lines derived from different individuals is caused by genetic polymorphism due to variable members of the tandem repeats in each allele (Gendler *et al.*, 1988; Siddiqui *et al.*, 1988). Interestingly, cloning and sequencing of cDNAs obtained by screening a pancreatic cancer cell library with a hybridization probe prepared according to the sequence of breast cancer mucin cDNA (MUC1), yielded a sequence identical to that of breast cancer apomucin (Lan *et al.*, 1990). Though limited data are available on the organ specificities of the expression of different apomucins at this time, all three types of apomucins appear to be expressed in a variety of mucin-synthesizing organs. The available data indicate that MUC1-type apomucin is expressed in normal adult breast, pancreas, and stomach, but not in small intestine and colon, while the reverse is true for MUC2- and MUC3-type intestinal apomucins (Yan *et al.*, 1990; Gum *et al.*, 1990).

C. BIOSYNTHESIS

From immunohistochemical studies at both the light microscopic and electron microscopic level using antibodies to fully deglycosylated intestinal mucins and to synthetic peptides representing the tandem repeat unit of the two intestinal apomucins, the endoplasmic reticulum appears to be the site of biosynthesis of the polypeptide backbone of intestinal mucin glycoproteins (Yan *et al.*, 1990; J. Roth, personal communication, 1990). Similar studies using antibodies to Tn (GalNAc-apomucin) antigen indicate that the site of initial glycosylation of apomucin is in the Golgi apparatus. Although the biosynthesis of O-linked sugars has not been elucidated as well as that of N-linked sugars, it would appear that a stepwise glycosylation of apomucin occurs through the sequential action of a series of specific glycosyltransferases in the Golgi apparatus (Kim *et al.*, 1971; Roth *et al.*, 1986). As shown in Fig. 3, when the first sugar, GalNAc, is attached to the protein backbone apomucin, Tn antigenic activity appears. This reaction is catalyzed by a specific glycosyltransferase, which adds GalNAc to serine and threonine residues of the protein backbone. However, the acceptor specificity of polypeptide GalNAc transferase, which could explain the extensive O-glycosylation of mucins and relative rarity of O-glycosylation of threonine and serine residues in other proteins, is not yet determined. Once formed, the Tn antigen can undergo several biosynthetic pathways, of which the best characterized are indicated. Each pathway is catalyzed by a pathway-specific glycosyltransferase. Synthesis of sialyl Tn by pathway 1 in Fig. 3 is a terminal step, since no further glycosylation occurs once NeuAc is added to Tn antigen (Beyer *et al.*, 1981). In contrast, synthesis along pathways 2 and 3 may proceed to further elongation of carbohydrate side chains with or without branching. The completed carbohydrate side chains will consist of core-region, backbone-region, and peripheral-region carbohydrates. Once fully glycosylated, completed mucin glycoproteins are ei-

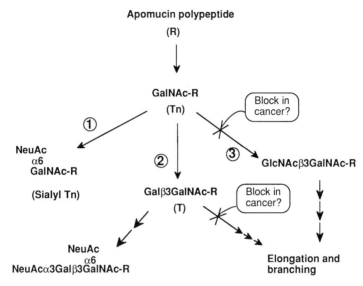

FIG. 3. Synthesis of mucin core structures.

ther stored and secreted or become incorporated into the plasma membrane via membrane vesicles.

D. TISSUE AND CELL DISTRIBUTION OF MUCIN GLYCOPROTEINS IN COLON AND PANCREAS

In studying mucin glycoproteins in the colon, it is important to consider regional and cellular variation in mucin type, since the pattern of their expression may vary considerably depending on these factors. There are a number of regional differences in the mucins present in the proximal versus the distal colon. In normal right colon, histochemical studies have shown that about 70% of the goblet cells stain for neutral mucin, while the rest stained equally for either NeuAc or O-acylated sialic acid (Sugihara and Jass, 1986). In the left colon, the staining intensity for neutral mucin was reduced to 30% of the goblet cells, while staining for NeuAc or O-acylated sialic acid was more intense than in the right colon. Lectin-binding studies also showed that *Ulex europaeus* agglutinin-1 (UEA-1), specific for terminal L-fucosyl residues in mucin glycoproteins, bound to about 65% of the cases in normal right colon, but only to one of 29 cases in the normal left colon, and none of 34 cases in the normal rectum (Bresalier *et al.*, 1985).

Colonic cells in crypt columns vary in degree of differentiation, with immature cells in the lower crypt and mature differentiated cells in the upper colonic crypt. In normal mucosa, lectins that preferentially bind to exposed GalNAc residues (*Dolichos biflorus* agglutinin and soybean agglutinin) bind selectively to the goblet cell mucin of well-differentiated cells in the upper colonic crypt (Boland *et al.*, 1982). In contrast, lectins that require exposed nonreducing galactose residues for binding (*Ricinus communis* agglutinin and *Bauhinia purpurea* agglutinin) preferentially label the mucin of less-differentiated goblet cells located in the lower portion of the colonic crypt. Although the structural bases of these differences in lectin binding have not yet been well established, these results indicate that alterations in the exposed, nonreducing carbohydrate residues occur in human colonic mucin during the process of goblet cell differentiation.

Cell lineage is another factor to consider, since several cell types such as columnar cells, goblet cells, endocrine cells, and Paneth cells reside in the colon (Ho *et al.*, 1989a). Thus far, goblet cells appear to be the main cell type responsible for the synthesis of mucin glycoproteins that can form gels. However, the occurrence of non–gel-forming, mucin-like glycoproteins, such as plasma membrane–associated mucins, in other colonic epithelial cell types cannot be ruled out. Furthermore, additional cell types have recently been described in the intestine (Madara and Trier, 1987; Kim, 1988), and heterogeneity among goblet cells has been demonstrated using human colonic mucin–associated monoclonal antibodies (Podolsky *et al.*, 1986a,b).

Although less is known about pancreatic mucin, one histochemical study on pancreatic biopsy specimens taken at laparotomy indicate that the pancreatic ductal system is responsible for the synthesis and secretion of mucin glycoproteins (Roberts and Burns, 1972). Four different ductal cell types were found to synthesize mucin glycoproteins: cuboidal, low columnar, tall columnar, and goblet. The type of mucin glycoproteins, however, varied in different parts of the ductal system with an inverse relationship between the degree of sulfation and the amount of neutral and sialomucins.

III. Alteration of Mucin Glycoproteins in Premalignant and Malignant Colorectal Cells

From histochemical studies, it has long been observed that both quantitative and qualitative alterations in mucins occur in colorectal cancer. The most consistent observation has been that there is a decrease in total mucin content and a decrease in sulfomucin, but an increase in sialomucin in colon cancer cells (Allen *et al.*, 1988). A reduction in O-acylated sialic acid has also been observed in colon cancer (Sugihara and Jass, 1986).

Although biochemical studies of colon cancer mucins are complicated by the intrinsic heterogeneity and difficulty of purification of mucins from tissues, there do appear to be differences in composition between the mucins of normal colon and colon cancers. One biochemical study on mucins isolated from colon cancer reported an increase in sialic acid (NeuAc) (Gold and Miller, 1978). However, other available biochemical studies on mucin glycoproteins isolated from human normal and cancerous colon indicate that the carbohydrate content of colon cancer mucin glycoproteins is about 50% of that in the normal colon, with significant reductions in Fuc, Gal, GlcNAc, GalNAc and NeuAc (Shimamoto et al., 1989; Boland and Deshmukh, 1990). In addition, oligosaccharide side chains were found to be 20% fewer and the mean oligosaccharide chain length was shorter (4.8 carbohydrate residues per chain versus 10.2 residues in normal colonic mucin glycoprotein) in colon cancer mucin glycoproteins compared to normal colonic mucin. These data are more consistent with previous observations that the activities of glycosyltransferases involved in the synthesis of O-glycosidically linked mucin-type oligosaccharides are reduced significantly in cancerous colonic mucosa compared to normal colon (Kim et al., 1974).

These studies indicate that mucin glycoproteins are abnormally glycosylated in colon cancer both in the number and mean chain length of the oligosaccharides. Several oligosaccharide sequences from normal colonic mucin (lacking the Galβ3GalNAc core) have been reported (Podolsky, 1985), but the structures present in colon cancer mucins have not been elucidated. With the recent availability of monoclonal antibodies of defined specificities, structural alteration in mucin glycoproteins in epithelial cancer cells are beginning to be defined. Three groups of mucin glycoprotein tumor markers with different specificities are shown in Table II. These tumor markers include those whose epitopes are on carbohydrate, those specific for peptide moieties of mucin glycoproteins, and those for which the epitope specificities are, as yet, indeterminate.

A. CARBOHYDRATE ANTIGENS

Cancer-associated changes in carbohydrates in colon and pancreas can be classified into four categories: (1) inappropriate expression of antigenic structures not normally present in a particular location, which may occur owing to reactivation of a fetal gene; (2) deletion of normally expressed antigens, with or without accumulation or exposure of precursors arising as a result of incomplete carbohydrate side-chain elongation; (3) increased level of expression over that found in normal tissues; (4) neosynthesis that occurs as a result of either extension or modification of existing carbohydrate structures or synthesis of new structures (Table III) (Hakomori, 1989). These changes are illustrated by recent data using monoclonal antibodies on the expression of major blood group antigens A, B, H, Le[a], and Le[b] (Yuan et al., 1985a), and of the exposed core-region carbohydrates of mucin glycoproteins, T, Tn, and sialyl Tn (Yuan et al., 1986; Itzkowitz et al., 1989; Samuel et al., 1990), and the modified blood group–related

TABLE II

MUCIN GLYCOPROTEIN TUMOR MARKERS OF
COLORECTAL CANCER

Carbohydrate epitopes

Peripheral and backbone-region carbohydrate changes
A,B,H, Le^a, Le^b
Sialyl Le^a (CA19-9)
Sialyl Le^x, extended Le^x
Extended Le^y
Type 2 polylactosamine (i)
Core-region carbohydrate changes
T, Tn, Sialyl Tn (TAG-72)

Peptide epitopes

Apomucins
MUC1 (PUM, PEM, HMFG, episialyn)
MUC2 (SMUC), MUC3 (SIB)

Indeterminate epitopes

M1 antigen, crypt cell antigens, Cora antigen
NCC-CO-450 antigen

antigens Le^x and Le^y in the normal or cancerous colon (Shı *et al.*, 1984; Itzkow-itz *et al.*, 1986b; Kim *et al.*, 1986). All these antigenic changes, except for mucin core-region carbohydrates, may be found in peripheral regions of carbo-hydrate side chains of either glycolipids or of mucin- or nonmucin–type glyco-proteins. For some antigens, the precise epitope specificities have not been de-termined and for others, both carbohydrate and protein moieties appear to be involved.

TABLE III

COLON CANCER–ASSOCIATED CHANGES IN CARBOHYDRATES

1. Inappropriate expression of antigenic structures not normally present in a particular location in the colon and rectum (e.g., incompatible expression of A, B, H, and Le^b)

2. Deletion of normally expressed antigens, with or without accumulation or exposure of precur-sors (e.g., deletion of A, B, H antigens, expression of T, Tn, and sialyl Tn)

3. Increased level of expression over that found in normal tissues (e.g., short-chain Le^x and Le^y)

4. Neosynthesis
   (a) Modification of existing structures (e.g., CA19-9, extended Le^x, Le^y, or sialyl Le^x)
   (b) New antigenic structure (?)

1. Peripheral and Backbone-Region Carbohydrate Changes

a. A, B, H, Le^a and Le^b Blood Group Antigens.

The antigenic specificities of A, B, H, Le^a and Le^b blood group antigens depend on peripheral carbohydrates at the nonreducing terminus of the oligosaccharide side chains of glycoproteins and glycolipids. The immunodeterminant carbohydrate structures of the ABH, Le^a, and Le^b blood group antigens are shown in simplified form in Fig. 4. When fucose in α-1,2 linkage is added to galactose, blood group H antigen is formed. Addition of either GalNAc or galactose to H antigen converts it to A or B antigen. The ABH antigens can be expressed on both type 1 and type 2 chains, as well as other structures containing β-linked galactose, e.g.,

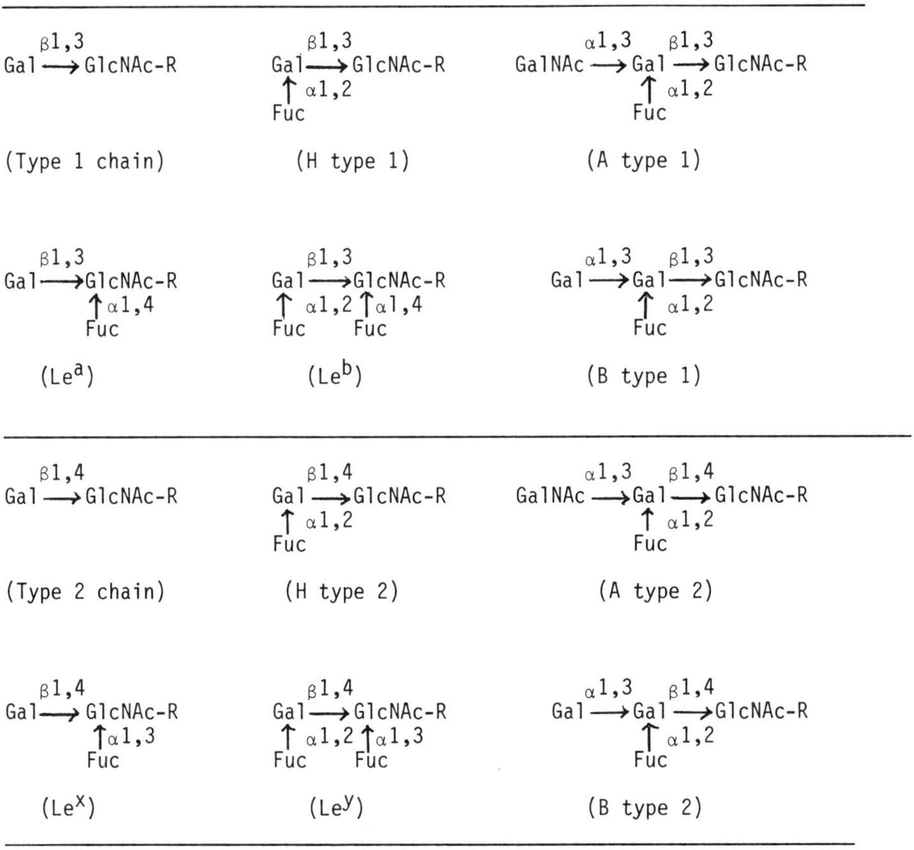

FIG. 4.   Structures of blood group-related carbohydrate antigens. Abbreviations: Gal, galactose; GlcNAc, N-Acetylglucosamine; Fuc, fucose; GalNAc, N-acetylgalactosamine.

the H type 3 antigen Fucα2-Galβ-3GalNAc. In contrast, Le^a and Le^b antigens can be expressed only on type 1 chains, since the fourth carbon position of GlcNAc of the type 2 chain is already occupied, so that fucose cannot be linked to GlcNAc at that position.

When the fucose is added in α1-4 linkage to the penultimate GlcNAc of type 1 chain, Le^a antigen is formed. The addition of a second fucose to H type 1 forms the Le^b antigen. The genes for the glycosyltransferases that add each sugar to its acceptor in a specific anomeric linkage are polymorphic, thereby conferring genetic variation in blood types. The addition or deletion of even one monosaccharide structure can completely alter the antigenicity of the molecule.

In the human embryo and fetus, blood group antigens A, B, H, Le^a, and Le^b are expressed throughout the colon (Szulman *et al.*, 1964, 1973; Yuan *et al.*, 1985a). After birth, however, ABH and Le^b antigens are no longer present in the distal normal colon. There is, however, re-expression of these antigens in 90% of cases of cancer in the distal colon. Furthermore, in 60 to 80% of cases of cancer of both the proximal and the distal colon, there is expression of blood group antigen that is incompatible with the host's blood type. Deletion of the host's blood type in the proximal colon also occurs in nearly half of these cancers (Table IV). Also, adenomatous polyps in 27% of the cases examined re-expressed ABH antigens or expressed incompatible blood group A or B (Itzkowitz *et al.*, 1986a). There was a significant correlation of the reappearance of ABH antigens in distal polyps with increasing grade of dysplasia, though not with polyp size or histologic type. The incompatible expression of blood group A or B antigens may also be a premalignant or malignant phenomenon, since it occurs only in adenomatous polyps and cancer tissues, but not in fetal or adult normal colonic mucosa, or in hyperplastic polyps.

b. Sialyl Le^a-Antigen and Related Antigens (CA50, SPan-1).   An example of modification of existing structure is sialylation of a type 1 backbone chain which leads to CA50-defined antigen (NeuAcα3Galβ3GlcNAc) (Mansson *et al.*, 1985). The addition of fucose in α1,4 linkage to the CA50 antigen leads to another modified structure (sialyl Le^a, NeuAcα3Galβ3[Fucα4]GlcNAc) called gastrointestinal cancer–associated antigen (GICA), or CA19-9, which is recognized by MAb NS19-9 (Atkinson *et al.*, 1982; Magnani *et al.*, 1982). Both antigens occur both as acidic glycolipids and as glycoproteins in the tissues, but in serum and pancreatic juice are found only on mucin glycoproteins (Magnani *et al.*, 1983; Malesci *et al.*, 1987). Because of the similarity in structures, both MAbs show immunological crossreactivity, and the tissue-staining patterns of both antigens are similar, although much more detailed studies are necessary. Most specimens of colon cancer, regardless of degree of differentiation, and also second trimester fetal colon expressed CA19-9 antigen, whereas normal mucosa

TABLE IV

CARBOHYDRATE ANTIGEN EXPRESSION IN COLONIC TISSUES[a]

Antigen alteration	Normal	Adenomatous polyp	Cancer
Reappearance (distal)			
A, B, H	1[b]	73	70–100
Le[b]	5	90	95
Incompatibility			
A, B, H, Le[b]	0	38	61
Deletion (proximal)			
A, Le[b]	0	18	43
Incompletion			
T	0	54	76
Tn	14	100	81
Sialyl Tn (TAG-72)	0	50–63	96
Neosynthesis			
Sialyl-Le[a] (19-9)	0–45	51–81	59–82
Extended Le[x]	0–8	50–55	82–86
Sialyl-extended Le[x]	8–15	45–56	60–67
Difucosyl-(dimeric) Le[x]	0–8	45–48	96
Extended Le[y]	0–38[c]	33–66	79–83
Trifucosyl-Le[y]	0–27	43–67	53–70

[a] Data from Abe et al., 1986; Atkinson et al., 1982; Brown et al., 1984; Fukushima et al., 1984; Itzkowitz et al., 1986a,b, 1988; Kim et al., 1986; Magnani et al., 1982; Sakamoto et al., 1986; Yuan et al., 1985, 1986, 1987; and unpublished observations.

[b] Expressed as the percentage of specimens positive by immunohistochemical methods.

[c] Proximal, 0; distal, 8–38.

rarely expressed it (Table IV) (Itzkowitz et al., 1988). The majority of hyperplastic polyps and practically all adenomatous polyps expressed it independent of polyp size, villous morphology, or degree of dysplasia. Thus, a modification of the type 1 backbone chain by $\alpha 2,3$ sialylation with or without $\alpha 1$-4 fucosylation produces oncodevelopmental antigens in colorectal cancer tissues, but these antigens do not discriminate between the polyps of malignant and nonmalignant potential.

Recently, another MAb, SPan-1, has been produced and was observed to have epitope specificity similar to, but distinct from CA19-9 or CA50 (Chung et al., 1987; Ho et al., 1988). SPan-1 stained Le[a−] Le[b−] colon cancer tissues, while NS19-9 did not. The tissue-staining pattern was similar to that observed with NS19-9.

c. Le^x Related antigens. A number of carbohydrate-specific antigens related to Le^x are examples of modified peripheral and backbone carbohydrate structure. Le^x antigen is a positional isomer of Le^a antigen, with fucose attached to the type 2 (lactosamine) backbone instead of the type 1 backbone (Figs. 4 and 5) backbone. The epitopes for Le^x antigen can be present either on short or extended lactosamine backbones of either glycolipids and glycoproteins, with or without additional internal fucose (Hakomori, 1990).

Recently, several Le^x-related antigens, defined by MAbs, have been described (Fig. 5) (Shi *et al.*, 1984; Itzkowitz *et al.*, 1986b). Among these MAbs, anti-SSEA-1 and AH8-183 MAbs recognize the simple Le^x trisaccharide, whether it is present on short or extended lactosamine backbones. The FH-1, FH-4, and

Antigens (MAb)	Antigenic determinant		Antigens (MAb)
	Le^x(X)	Le^y(Y)	
Le^x (anti-SSEA-1 AH8-183)	$\overset{\beta1,4}{Gal \longrightarrow GlcNAc\text{-}R}$ $\overset{\uparrow \alpha1,3}{Fuc}$	$\overset{\beta1,4}{Gal \longrightarrow GlcNAc\text{-}R}$ $\overset{\uparrow \alpha1,2\ \uparrow\alpha1,3}{Fuc\quad Fuc}$	Le^y (AH6)
Extended Le^x (FH1)	$\overset{\beta1,4\qquad\beta1,3\quad\beta1,4}{Gal \longrightarrow GlcNAc \longrightarrow Gal \longrightarrow GlcNAc\text{-}R}$ $\overset{\uparrow \alpha1,3}{Fuc}$		
		$\overset{\beta1,4\qquad\beta1,3\quad\beta1,4}{Gal \longrightarrow GlcNAc \longrightarrow Gal \longrightarrow GlcNAc\text{-}R}$ $\overset{\uparrow \alpha1,2\ \uparrow\alpha1,3}{Fuc\quad Fuc}$	Extended Le^y (CC-1 CC-2)
Difucosyl or dimeric Le^x (FH4)	$\overset{\beta1,4\qquad\beta1,3\quad\beta1,4}{Gal \longrightarrow GlcNAc \longrightarrow Gal \longrightarrow GlcNAc\text{-}R}$ $\overset{\uparrow\alpha1,3\qquad\qquad\uparrow\alpha1,3}{Fuc\qquad\qquad Fuc}$		
		$\overset{\beta1,4\qquad\beta1,3\quad\beta1,4}{Gal \longrightarrow GlcNAc \longrightarrow Gal \longrightarrow GlcNAc\text{-}R}$ $\overset{\uparrow \alpha1,2\ \uparrow\alpha1,3\qquad\uparrow\alpha1,3}{Fuc\quad Fuc\qquad\qquad Fuc}$	Trifucosyl Le^y (KH-1)
Sialosyl difucosyl Le^x (FH6)	$\overset{\beta1,4\qquad\beta1,3\quad\beta1,4}{Gal \longrightarrow GlcNAc \longrightarrow Gal \longrightarrow GlcNAc\text{-}R}$ $\overset{\uparrow\alpha2,3\ \uparrow\alpha1,3\qquad\uparrow\alpha1,3}{NeuAc\quad Fuc\qquad\qquad Fuc}$		

FIG. 5. Le^x and Le^y antigens recognized by monoclonal antibodies. Abbreviations same as for FIG. 4.

FH-6 MAbs, on the other hand, have greatest affinity for extended Le^x determinants. The epitope for FH-1 MAb is an extended Le^x structure, while FH-4 and FH-6 are specific for an extended Le^x epitope with an additional fucose, linked in α1,3 linkage to GlcNAc of an internal type 2 lactosamine. Thus, the FH-4 determinant can be referred to as difucosyl or dimeric Le^x. The FH-6 MAb also requires the difucosyl Le^x structure, but in addition requires the presence of N-acetylneuraminic acid (NeuAc) linked α2,3 to the terminal galactose of difucosyl Le^x.

Immunohistochemical studies have shown that the short-chain Le^x antigen is present in the normal colon, in cell membranes of the lower colonic crypt (Sakamoto *et al.*, 1986; Itzkowitz *et al.*, 1986b). Short-chain Le^x is also present in fetal colon, colon cancer, and in hyperplastic and adenomatous polyps. All of the extended Le^x antigens, however, were undetectable or present at very low levels in specimens of normal colonic mucosa and hyperplastic polyps, but were present in fetal colon, in colon cancers, and in adenomatous polyps (Table IV) (Itzkowitz *et al.*, 1986b; Yuan *et al.*, 1987). The expression of extended and polyfucosylated Le^x antigen among adenomatous polyps correlated with larger polyp size, villous histology, and severe dysplasia, all of which are measures of malignant potential.

d. Le^y-Related Antigens.   The Le^y antigen, which is a positional isomer of the Le^b antigen, differs from the Le^x antigen by the presence of fucose in α1,2 linkage on the terminal galactose (Figs. 4 and 5). The immunodeterminant tetrasaccharide for Le^y, like Le^x, can be present on either short or extended backbone chains of glycolipids or glycoproteins (Hakomori, 1989). There are also a number of MAbs specific for Le^y determinants. The AH-6 MAb recognizes the Le^y tetrasaccharide whether it is present on short or extended lactosamine backbones. The other three MAbs recognize only extended Le^y determinants. CC-1 and CC-2 MAbs, which have similar epitope specificities, bind best to extended Le^Y structures. KH-1 MAb is specific for an extended Le^y epitope, with an internal fucose linked in α1,3 linkage to GlcNAc, referred to as trifucosyl Le^y (Kim *et al.*, 1986).

The pattern of expression of Le^y antigen in various types of colorectal tissues was, in general, similar to that of Le^x (Table IV) (Brown *et al.*, 1984; Abe *et al.*, 1986; Kim *et al.*, 1986). As markers for premalignant and malignant colorectal tissues, the extended and trifucosylated Le^y antigens were found to be more specific than the short-chain Le^y determinant. Although the level of expression of short-chain Le^y is greatest in the cancerous tissues, this antigen is also often expressed in normal colonic mucosa (lower crypt-cell membrane), as well as in hyperplastic and adenomatous polyps. Extended and trifucosylated Le^y antigens, in contrast, are present in 61 to 80% of colon cancers and are rarely detected in normal colonic mucosa or in hyperplastic polyps. The extended and trifucosyl Le^y antigens are also present in 36 to 51% of adenomas, where there is a positive correlation between increased expression of extended Le^y antigen and histologic criteria of malignant potential. These results indicate that Le^x and Le^y antigens in general are oncodevelopmental antigens in the colon.

e. Polylactosamine Backbone.   The extended type 2 chain polylactosamine backbone structure (i antigen) that is the precursor for Le^x and Le^y antigens (with or without sialylation or fucosylation) appears to be synthesized preferentially by premalignant and malignant colonocytes. A monoclonal antibody (MH21-134) has recently been described that reacts with the repeated unbranched polylacto-samine structure lacking substitution of terminal sugars. The extended polylac-tosamine structures recognized by this antibody were found to be absent or mini-mally present in normal tissues, but preferentially expressed in many cancer tissues, including 59% of colon cancers (Miyake *et al.,* 1989).

2. *Core Region Carbohydrate Changes*

a. T and Tn Antigens.   Many carbohydrate alterations have recently been found to occur in colon cancer mucins. The T and Tn antigens, which are present in the inner-core carbohydrate structures of mucins and are oncodevelopmental anti-gens in the colon and rectum, are examples of this phenomenon. These antigens arise when the biosynthesis of the carbohydrate side chains of mucin glycopro-teins is terminated at an early stage (Fig. 3). When the first sugar GalNAc is attached to the protein backbone apomucin, depicted as R, Tn antigenic activity appears. The Tn antigen can then, by addition of galactose in $\beta 1,3$ linkage, form the Thomsen-Friedenreich (T) antigen (Yuan *et al.,* 1986).

Immunohistochemical studies have indicated that Tn and T antigens are not detectable in the mucosa of normal colon, but are present in colon cancers (Tn 81%, T 71%) (Yuan *et al.,* 1986; Itzkowitz *et al.,* 1989). The T antigen was preferentially expressed by moderately well differentiated and well-differentiated adenocarcinomas. However, Tn antigen was also present in poorly differentiated adenocarcinomas and mucinous carcinomas. Thus, Tn may be useful as a marker for these two histological subsets of colon cancer, which often lack other cancer-associated antigens and which have a particularly poor clinical outcome.

Furthermore, T antigen was present in 54% of adenomatous polyps. Expres-sion of T also correlated with malignant potential as judged by size, histological type, and degree of dysplasia (Yuan *et al.,* 1986). These findings suggest that T antigen could be a useful premalignant and malignant marker.

The appearance of T and Tn antigens provides a clear example of incomplete glycosylation in malignant and premalignant colon cells. Thus, the altered regu-lation of glycosyltransferases in these cells must be responsible for altered expression of core-region carbohydrate antigens. The enzymological basis for alterations in these expressions of mucin core-region carbohydrate antigens is not yet established. However, available data support the hypothesis that in colon cancer cells, the glycosyltransferases responsible for further elongation of T antigen through pathway 2 in Fig. 3 may be blocked, resulting in the accumulation of T antigen as well as its precursor, Tn antigen. Pathway 3, which may be the predominant pathway in the synthesis of mucin carbohydrate side chains in normal colonic mucosa, would also, according to this hypothetical scheme, be decreased in colon cancers, resulting in increased expression of T and Tn antigen.

b. Sialyl Tn Antigen in Colon Cancers. Sialylation of the Tn antigen at the 6-hydroxyl of GalNAc results in the formation of sialyl Tn antigen. Sialyl Tn antigen is recognized by several MAbs, including B72.3 (Gold and Mattes, 1988), TKH2 (Kjeldsen *et al.*, 1988), and MLS 102 (Kurosaka *et al.*, 1988). Sialyl Tn antigen, also designated TAG-72, is present in serum of patients with colonic, pancreatic, and other cancers (Paterson *et al.*, 1986) and has been shown to be very similar to mucin purified from xenografts of LS174T colon cancer cells (Johnson *et al.*, 1986; Byrd *et al.*, 1988).

As for T and Tn, immunohistochemical studies have shown that sialyl Tn is not detectable in normal colon, but is present in most colon cancers (Table 4) (Itzkowitz *et al.*, 1989). Poorly differentiated adenocarcinomas and mucinous carcinomas were stained by antibody to sialyl Tn, in contrast to results for T antigen. The positive staining of adenomatous polyps and the correlation of antigen expression with malignant potential suggests that sialyl Tn could be a premalignant marker.

In a study of 128 primary colorectal carcinoma specimens from 137 patients who underwent curative surgical resection, expression of sialyl Tn antigen was examined and related to clinical outcome (Itzkowitz *et al.*, 1990). Overall, 5-year survival patients with sialosyl Tn–negative versus sialosyl Tn–positive tumor was 100% versus 73% ($P < 0.05$), and the disease-free survival was 94% versus 73% ($P = 0.12$). By multivariate regression analysis, two variances of most importance for predicting survival (disease-free and overall survival) were found to be tumor ploidy ($P < 0.001$) and sialosyl Tn expression ($P < 0.05$). These data indicate that sialosyl Tn expression is an independent prognostic factor in colon cancer.

The enzymatic basis for increased sialyl Tn expression in colon cancers has not yet been established. One possibility is that colon cancer cells could have higher activities of the $\alpha 2,6$ sialyltransferase responsible for its synthesis (pathway 1 in Fig. 3). Alternatively, if there were a decrease in elongation of Tn antigen, for example, pathway 3 in Fig. 3, the accumulation of Tn antigen could result in increased amounts of sialyl Tn endproducts.

B. MUCIN PROTEIN ANTIGENS IN COLON CANCER

Antibodies that react with the protein backbone of MUC1-encoded, mammary-type mucins have been extensively studied because of their potential clinical utility for detection of advanced breast cancer and other malignancies. Immunochemical studies of the pattern of expression of other apomucins in normal and diseased tissues are much more limited.

The mammary-type apomucin is absent from normal colon but can be detected in many colon cancers. In a large-scale immunohistochemical survey of colonic tissues, episialin (MAM-6 antigen), detected by MAbs 115D8, 139H2, and 140C1, was present in 99% of colon cancers but only 7% of non-neoplastic biopsy specimens (Zotter et al., 1987). In another study (Burchell et al., 1987), 10 of 10 colon cancers were stained by SM3, an MAb prepared against mammary apomucin. The results of this study, shown in Table V, agree with the cancer-associated expression of the MUC1-encoded mammary mucin protein in the colon (Byrd et al., 1991). In this study, 89% and 75% of colon cancer specimens were stained by MAbs DF3 and 139H2, respectively, while normal colon was unstained. The staining of colon cancers but not normal colon by antibodies that react with mammary-type apomucin presumably reflects aberrant regulation of the type of mucin polypeptide expressed.

In spite of the staining of colon cancer tissues by MUC1-specific antibodies, none of the colon cancer cell lines studied thus far have high levels of mammary-type apomucin protein or mRNA, and sera of most colon cancer patients do not have elevated levels of these antigens (Hayes et al., 1985; Hilkens et al., 1986; Stahli et al., 1988). Thus, there is still much that is not known about the factors affecting MUC1 gene expression in vitro and about the shedding of the antigen in vivo.

No monoclonal antibodies to the protein backbone of the MUC2-encoded intestinal-type apomucin are yet available. Polyclonal antisera have been prepared

TABLE V
MUCIN PROTEIN ANTIGENS IN COLONIC AND PANCREATIC CANCER[a]

| | | Percentage of cases positive | | | |
| | | Normal colon | Colon cancer | Normal pancreas | Pancreatic cancer |
Antigen	Antibody				
MUC1	DF3	0	89	100	93
	139H2	0	75	100	100
MUC2	Anti-HFB	100	93	90	25
	Anti-MRP	100	81	0	17

[a]Data from Byrd et al., 1991.

against HF deglycosylated colon cancer apomucin (anti-HFB) (Byrd *et al.*, 1989) and also against synthetic mucin repeat peptide (anti-MRP) (Gum *et al.*, 1989). Both antibodies stained all specimens of normal colon, as well as most colon cancers (Table 5) (Yan *et al.*, 1990). In normal colon, goblet cells were stained in the supranuclear area but not in the vacuoles, presumably reflecting apomucin present in the endoplasmic reticulum. In colon cancer cells, however, there was, in most cases, stronger and more diffuse staining, perhaps indicating abnormal processing of apomucin and/or impaired glycosylation. It will be important in the future to survey immunohistochemically the tissue distribution of the MUC3-encoded apomucin, as well as that of other apomucins as they are discovered.

C. ANTIGENS WITH INDETERMINATE EPITOPE SPECIFICITY

The mucin-associated M1 antigens are present in the mucus cells of normal surface gastric epithelium but they are absent from the mucosa of the normal colon. The antigenic epitope of M1 is not well understood but resides in peptide backbone structures. Colon cancers and fetal colonic tissues stain positively, indicating the oncodevelopmental nature of M1 antigens. The expression of M1 antigens is more frequent in proximal colon cancers (55%) than in distal colon cancers (12%). In both proximal and distal colon, on the other hand, over half of colonic adenomas express M1 antigens (Bara *et al.*, 1983, 1984). Thus, M1 antigens appear to be malignant and premalignant markers in colonic mucosa, although they may not be specific enough to be clinically useful.

Several monoclonal antibodies specific for the carbohydrates of high-molecular-weight glycoproteins of intestinal crypt-cell membranes show positive immunohistochemical staining of nearly all the colon cancer tissues but do not stain normal or inflamed colonic mucosa. The epitope specificity seems to reside in O-glycosidically linked oligosaccharides of mucin glycoproteins (Quaroni *et al.*, 1986, 1989). While further studies are necessary, this may be an example of the expression, in colon cancer cells, of developmentally regulated crypt antigens.

A monoclonal antibody (Cora), which recognizes a variably glycosylated membrane glycoprotein (of 75 to 95 kDa in size), has been used in an immunohistochemical study. Cora antigen was present in 100% of colorectal cancer specimens and 70% of the gastric cancer tissues examined, but was undetectable in normal gastrointestinal tissues (Gottlinger *et al.*, 1988). Establishing the clinical utility of Cora antigen will require further studies.

Recently, MAb NCC-CO-450 was produced by using high-molecular-weight mucin glycoproteins isolated from ascitic fluid of a colon cancer patient. This antigen has been characterized as mucin glycoprotein. Immunohistochemical and biochemical analyses have shown that is is present in high concentrations in normal colon, bronchial epithelium, and uterus, but not in other tissues.

However, it is highly expressed in nearly all cases of colon cancer, 70% of pancreatic cancers, and 85% of gastric cancers. Its epitope seems to be present in an O-linked oligosaccharide side chain without terminal NeuAc and is different from those present in other carbohydrate antigens, i.e., sialyl Le^a, Le^x, Le^y and Tn (Sakurai *et al.*, 1988). This antibody may have some clinical utility in serological assays in colon cancer and other epithelial cell cancers.

IV. Alteration of Mucin Glycoproteins in Pancreatic Cancer

Cancer of exocrine pancreas arises most frequently from the pancreatic ducts. The ductal cell adenocarcinomas contain many mucin-synthesizing cells. Because of the difficulty in early diagnosis due to its retroperitoneal location, diagnosis of pancreatic cancer is usually made in an advanced stage. Therefore, it has a high mortality rate and poor prognosis. Furthermore, unlike colorectal cancer, a premalignant lesion is not well defined. It is thought that papillary hyperplasia, involving mucin-containing tall columnar cells, may be a premalignant lesion, but unfortunately this lesion gives no symptoms and is usually diagnosed incidentally or at postmortem (Sindelar *et al.*, 1985).

Histochemical studies of pancreatic tissues do not reveal qualitative cancer-associated differences, but do show an increase in mucin content in pancreatic cancer compared to normal pancreas. Pancreatic cancer mucin glycoproteins have been purified and characterized from ascites fluid of patients with pancreatic tumors (Lan *et al.*, 1985, 1987), from cell lines (Ho *et al.*, 1988), and from nude mouse xenografts produced by subcutaneous injection of human pancreatic cancer cell lines (Nardelli *et al.*, 1988). However, comparison with normal human pancreatic mucin glycoproteins (Gold *et al.*, 1983) is difficult because of the limited availability of normal pancreatic tissues. Pancreatic cancer mucin glycoproteins purified from different sources have the usual properties of mucin glycoproteins (Forstner and Forstner, 1986). They are high in molecular weight, and their amino acid compositions are rich in serine, threonine, and proline. Their carbohydrates consist of five sugars, GalNAc, GlcNAc, NeuAc, Gal, and Fuc, which are O-glycosidically linked to protein backbone.

Recent studies using MAbs have revealed that a number of types of changes in mucin glycoproteins occur in pancreatic cancer (Itzkowitz *et al.*, 1987, 1989; Kim *et al.*, 1988; Pour *et al.*, 1988).

A. CARBOHYDRATE ANTIGENS

1. *Peripheral and Backbone-Region Carbohydrate Changes*

a. A, B, H, Le^a, and Le^b Blood Group Antigens.   Immunohistochemical studies showed that A, B, H, Le^a and Le^b antigens were expressed in pancreatic ducts,

TABLE VI
CANCER-ASSOCIATED ALTERATIONS IN CARBOHYDRATE
ANTIGENS IN PANCREATIC TISSUES[a]

Antigen alteration	Percentage of cases positive	
	Normal pancreas	Pancreatic cancer
Compatible ABH antigens	100	75
Incompatible A or B	0	33
Le^a	100	74–80
Le^b	100	82
19-9	100	84
Short-chain Le^x	0	71
Difucosyl Le^x	0	54
Sialyl extended Le^x	0	63
Short-chain Le^y	77	86
Extended Le^y	55–73	37–49
Trifucosyl Le^y	32	31
Tn	100	100
T	53	44
Sia Tn	0	97

[a]Data from Itzkowitz *et al.*, 1987, 1988; Kim *et al.*, 1988, and unpublished observations.

ductules, and acini of normal pancreas and chronic pancreatitis tissues (Table VI) (Itzkowitz *et al.*, 1987). In pancreatic cancer, two cancer-associated phenomena observed in both the primary and metastatic cancers were (1) deletion of an expected A, B, H, or Le^b antigen (25% of cases), particularly in poorly differentiated cancers, and (2) incompatible expression of unexpected A or B antigens (33% of cases).

b. Sialyl Le^a and Related Antigens.   Although serum sialyl Le^a antigen (CA19-9) has a relatively high degree of specificity for malignancy, tissue staining with MAb NS19-9 is positive in both normal pancreas and pancreatic cancer (Itzkowitz *et al.*, 1988). Staining of pancreatic tissues with NS19-9 is primarily in the ducts and ductules. SPan-1, which has an epitope that is similar but not identical to 19-9, also stains normal pancreas as well as pancreatic cancers (Chung *et al.*, 1987; Ho *et al.*, 1988).

c. Le^x and Le^y-Related Antigens.   Antibodies specific for Le^x-related antigens do not stain normal pancreas, but do stain the majority of pancreatic cancers (Kim *et al.*, 1988). Antibody to short chain Le^x stained 71% of pancreatic cancers, while antibodies specific for extended and/or sialylated Le^x stained 54 to 65%. Thus, expression of the Le^x antigen appears to be a cancer-associated phenomenon in the pancreas. It is not known whether the Le^x is present mainly on glycolipid or on glycoprotein. However, mucin purified from pancreatic cancer xenografts has been shown to have Le^x antigen, detectable immunochemically after removal of sialic acid (Nardelli *et al.*, 1988).

Le^y antigens are expressed in most specimens of normal pancreas, in contrast to results for Le^x. Both single Le^y and extended Le^y antigens were present in 32 to 77% of normal specimens and in 31 to 86% of pancreatic cancer specimens.

2. *Core-region Carbohydrate Changes*

Among the carbohydrate antigens representing the initial steps in mucin glycosylation (T, Tn, and sialyl Tn), the major difference in immunohistochemical staining between normal pancreas and pancreatic cancer is for the sialyl T antigen (Table VI) (Itzkowitz *et al.*, 1991). Normal pancreas was not stained by MAb TKH2, but 97% of the pancreatic cancer specimens examined were positive, with intense staining of cancer cell membranes and secretions. T antigen, as detected by MAb AH9-16, was present in about half of both normal and cancerous pancreatic tissues.

B. MUCIN PROTEIN ANTIGENS IN PANCREATIC CANCERS

Although pancreatic and colonic mucins have several similarities in their reactivity with carbohydrate-specific antibodies, results to date suggest that they differ in their protein core (Lan *et al.*, 1990; Byrd *et al.*, 1991). While monoclonal antibodies against mammary apomucin did not stain normal colon, they stained all specimens of normal pancreas (Table V). Conversely, antibody against the MUC2-encoded, intestinal-type mucin repeat peptide stained all specimens of normal colon, but did not stain normal pancreas (Byrd *et al.*, 1991). The staining of normal pancreas by anti-HFB (fully deglycosylated intestinal mucin) presumably reflects a broader specificity of this polyclonal antibody. The organ specificity of mucin type expressed tends to be looser in cancer specimens, with MUC2 intestinal type apomucin detectable in some pancreatic cancers, and MUC1-encoded mammary type apomucin present in most colon cancers.

The conclusion that pancreatic cancer mucins can have the MUC1-encoded mammary-type mucin core is supported by studies with cultured pancreatic cancer cells. Antibody prepared against deglycosylated pancreatic cancer mucin was found to crossreact with synthetic breast mucin peptide (Lan *et al.*, 1990). The presence of MUC1 mRNA in some pancreatic cancer cell lines was also demonstrated by Northern blotting. In another study (Byrd *et al.*, 1991), the glycosylated mucin prepared from nude mouse xenografts of the SW1990 pancreatic cancer cell line was recognized by MAbs 139H2, DF3, and HMFG2, all of which are directed against the core protein of mammary mucin (Abe and Kufe, 1989; Burchell *et al.*, 1989; Hilkens *et al.*, 1989). However, there was also immunological crossreaction with deglycosylated colon cancer mucin. Thus, pancreatic cancer cells in nude mouse xenografts appear to make both MUC1 and MUC2 encoded mucins, a conclusion also supported by Northern blotting.

Expression of MUC3-encoded mucin in pancreas has not yet been studied. It is also still possible that there could be another, as yet undiscovered, pancreas-specific mucin protein.

C. ANTIGENS OF INDETERMINATE EPITOPES

DuPan-2 antigen, defined by a MAb produced by immunizing with a human pancreatic ductal adenocarcinoma, is a high-molecular-weight mucin glycoprotein (Lan *et al.*, 1985, 1987). Both protein backbone and sialic acid residues may be involved in the antigenic epitopes since its antigenic activity is susceptible to neuraminidase, pepsin, pronase, and papain digestion. The antigen is expressed in both normal and neoplastic cells in the pancreas (Borowitz *et al.*, 1984). Immunohistochemical studies have shown that DuPan-2 antigen is present in nearly all the cancers of pancreas, gallbladder, or bile duct, and in 80% of gastric cancers, whereas it is infrequently expressed in cancers of the colon, breast, and lung (Borowitz *et al.*, 1984). In the normal adult pancreas, the antigen is present on ductal cells but not on acinar or islet cells. DuPan-2 antigen is present in both ductal and acinar cells in fetal pancreas. Although this antigen is present in both normal and cancerous pancreas, its levels in the sera of patients with cancers of pancreas, gallbladder, and bile duct are significantly elevated when compared to the sera from normal subjects (Sawabu *et al.*, 1986).

MAb MUSE 11 was produced by using ascites fluid of a patient with gastric cancer as immunogen. This MAb is thought to react with a peptide epitope of a 300,000 kDa glycoprotein (which may be N-linked), since periodic acid and neuraminidase treatment of the antigen did not affect its immunoreactivity. Immunohistochemical studies showed that MUSE 11 antigen was detectable in virtually all adenocarcinomas (especially pancreatic carcinoma), whereas it was either negative or faintly positive in their normal counterparts (Ban *et al.*, 1989).

MAb YPan-1 was produced using a human pancreatic cancer cell line as immunogen (Yuan *et al.*, 1985). YPan-1 had an 89%, 90%, and 46% positive immunoreactivity with formalin-fixed cancerous pancreas, stomach, and colon, respectively. Although YPan-1 reacts with normal pancreas, it has little or no reaction with normal colon or stomach. Preliminary studies indicate that YPan-1-defined antigen level is increased in the sera of patients with pancreatic cancer (Ho *et al.*, 1988).

V. Clinical Application

A. SEROLOGICAL DIAGNOSIS

As has been discussed, many MAbs directed against mucin glycoproteins have been demonstrated immunohistochemically to show specificity toward premalignant and malignant colorectal and pancreatic tissues. When these MAbs are used in serum assays for the detection of circulating mucin glycoprotein antigens, however, they are not always elevated. Conversely, several mucin glycoprotein–reactive MAbs, which were found to have a high degree of specificity when assayed in serum, show less specificity at the tissue level (Itzkowitz *et al.*, 1988).

Serum assays of CA19-9 (Kuusela *et al.*, 1984; Haglund *et al.*, 1987; Steinberg, 1990), CA-50 (Blind and Dahlgren, 1987; Persson *et al.*, 1988), SPan-1 (Kiriyama *et al.*, 1990), and Le^x- and Le^y-related antigens (Chia *et al.*, 1985; Kawahara *et al.*, 1985; Kannagi *et al.*, 1986; Singhal *et al.*, 1990) have, thus far, had little utility either for the diagnosis of colon cancer or for the management of patients with colorectal cancer (Table VII). Although increased serum levels of CA19-9 are found in 19 to 49% of patients with colorectal cancer, compared with 0.6% in healthy subjects, comparative studies indicate that determinations of carcinoembryonic antigen (CEA) are more sensitive in the prediction of residual disease or recurrence. By combining CEA and CA19-9 determinations, there is only a marginal improvement in sensitivity for the diagnosis and follow-up of colorectal cancer patients (Kuusela *et al.*, 1984). Serum levels of short chain sialyl Le^x antigen (CSLEX 1) were reported to be elevated in 25 to 44% of patients with colorectal cancer, and 33 to 37% of pancreatic cancer patients (Chia *et al.*, 1985; Kawahara *et al.*, 1985). Subsequently, studies on fucosylated type 2–chain polylactosamine antigens in colorectal cancer patients showed that, altogether, 36% of the patients had one or more of these antigens (Le^x, polyfucosyl Le^x, sialyl Le^x, or Le^y) elevated (Kannagi *et al.*, 1986).

Recently, direct determination of Le^x antigen levels in sera was carried out using a double determinant solid phase immunoassay with MAb SH2 (which recognizes difucosyl Le^x antigen) as the capture antibody and MAb SH1 (which recognizes simple Le^x antigens) as the detecting antibody. The levels of serum Le^x correlated well with the Dukes' stages of colorectal cancer; Dukes' A, 20%; Dukes' B, 45%; Dukes' C, 67%; and Dukes' D, 74% (Singhal *et al.*, 1990).

The TAG-72 antigen recognized by MAb B72.3, which depends on sialosyl Tn epitopes on mucin glycoprotein molecules, is reported to be elevated in the serum of patients with colorectal cancer (55%), gastric cancer (52%), pancreatic choledochal cancer (46%), and breast cancer (39%) (Table VII). Those patients with cancers at advanced stages or with recurrent cancers had higher levels of the antigen (71%) than patients with early-stage cancer (12%) (Klug *et al.*, 1986; Ohuchi *et al.*, 1988).

TABLE VII

SERUM LEVELS OF MUCIN GLYCOPROTEIN-ASSOCIATED CARBOHYDRATE AND PEPTIDE ANTIGENS IN COLORECTAL AND PANCREATIC CANCER[a]

Antigen (MAbs)	Normal	Nonneoplastic disease	Colorectal carcinoma	Pancreatic carcinoma	Other carcinoma	
Sialyl Le[a]						
(NS19.9)	0–1[b]	1.5–14	19–49	73–87	35–50	Stomach
					50	Lung
					51	Liver
CA-50	0–2	3–8	37–75	62–80	41	Stomach
SPan-1	0–2	5–23	18–41	81–93	23	Stomach
					63	Liver
DuPan-2	0–4	2–26	6	38–72	24	Stomach
					85	Liver
Le[x]						
(SH1/SH2)	1	13	65	—[c]	60	Lung
					60	Breast
Le[y]						
(AH-6)	3	4	7	41	18	Stomach
					34	Liver
Sialyl Le[x]						
(CSLEX 1)	1–4	1–14	25–44	33–37	19–26	Stomach
Sialyl difucosyl						
Le[x] (FH6)	0–3	2–13	25	32–66	16–23	Stomach
					71	Lung
Sialyl Tn						
(B72.3)	0	0	12–71	46	52	Stomach
					39	Breast
Breast apomucin						
(CA15.3)	1.3	—	44	70	20–80	Breast

[a]Data obtained from Blind and Dahlgren, 1987; Chia et al., 1985; Chung et al., 1987; Haglund et al., 1987; Hayes et al., 1986; Kannagi et al., 1986; Kawahara et al., 1985; Kiriyama et al., 1990; Klug et al., 1986; Kuusela et al., 1984; Ohuchi et al., 1988; Sawabu et al., 1986; Singhal et al., 1990.

[b]Expressed as percentage of patients with serum levels above the normal limits.

[c]Not done.

Serologic determination of CA19-9, CA-50, SPan-1, and DuPan-2 appears to be useful in the diagnosis of pancreatic cancer and also in the monitoring of the patient following surgical resection of the tumor (Sawabu et al., 1986; Chung et al., 1987; Steinberg, 1990; Ho et al., 1989b). The antigenic epitopes for three of these antigens (CA19-9, CA-50, and SPan-1) are all related and represent modified type 1–chain backbone structures. Recent studies indicate that the serum assays of these antigens for the diagnosis of pancreatic cancer are comparable, although the sensitivity was slightly higher for SPan-1 assay than for CA19-9 assay (Kiriyama et al., 1990). DuPan-2 assays showed somewhat lower sensitivity than the assays for the CA19-9 related antigens. Interestingly, serum levels of SPan-1 and DuPan-2 were also elevated significantly in the sera of patients with nonmalignant hepatobiliary diseases (40 and 55%, respectively) and hepatocellular carcinoma (63 and 85%, respectively). The serum assays for CA19-9 (20%), SPan-1 (12%), and DuPan-2 (8%) showed elevated levels of antigens in patients with chronic pancreatitis. When circulating breast cancer apomucin antigen was examined using the CA15-3 assay, serum levels were found to be elevated in advanced breast cancer (80%) and in pancreatic cancer (70%) patients (Hayes et al., 1986).

Although high levels of mucin glycoprotein antigens CA19-9, SPan-1, and DuPan-2 are observed in the serum of patients with pancreatic cancer compared to those of normal subjects, these antigens are present in both the normal and cancerous pancreas. At present, little is known about the mechanisms or factors leading to the high levels of these mucin glycoprotein antigens in the serum. It may be due to increased rates of antigen synthesis and/or release, or to changes in the mode of release, such as direct release into the blood (basolaterally rather than apically into the duct lumen), resulting from loss of polarity of cancer cells. It is also to be noted that both purified pancreatic cancer xenograft mucin glycoproteins and the sera obtained from pancreatic cancer patients carry multiple antigenic epitopes (SPan-1, YPan-1, CA19-9, and DuPan-2) (Lan et al., 1985, 1987; Nardelli et al., 1988; Ho et al., 1988.) However, it is not clear at present how many different types of mucin glycoproteins exist in the sera or tissues.

B. RADIOIMMUNOLOCALIZATION USING RADIOLABELED ANTIBODIES

Radiolabeled MAbs directed against the carbohydrate antigens of mucin glycoproteins have been examined for the detection of primary and metastatic cancers expressing a high concentration and density of the particular antigens on the surface or in the periphery of the cancer cells. The antibodies can be labeled with various radionuclides, e.g., ^{125}I, ^{111}In or [131]Tc. Studies in patients with colon carcinomas using ^{131}I-labeled MAb B72.3 (anti-sialyl Tn) showed a threefold higher localization in tumors compared to normal colon and yielded positive scintigraphic images in 50% of the patients (Tuttle et al., 1988). In addition, a new intraoperative approach to tumor localization is being explored using ^{125}I-labeled MAb B72.3 and a hand-held, gamma-detecting probe. Thirty-one patients with colorectal cancer were administered with radiolabeled MAb and explored surgically 5 to 35 days postinjection. In vivo localization of the labeled MAb, as evaluated by the hand-held, gamma-detecting probe, was confirmed by in vitro analysis of biopsy samples. Using this method, MAb B72.3 localized tumors in 68% of patients. In another study using similar techniques, a positive probe count was obtained in 83% of patients with primary colon cancer and 79% of patients with recurrent colon cancer undergoing second-look procedure (Martin *et al.*, 1988).

C. THERAPY

The biological role of mucin glycoproteins in tumor immunology is not well understood. However, there is some evidence that they may be involved in the host immune response to tumors (Singhal and Hakomori, 1990). Recently, tumor-associated mucin in breast and pancreatic cancer cells has been demonstrated to be recognized by cytotoxic T lymphocytes in a major histocompatibility complex–unrestricted manner (Barnd *et al.*, 1989). This indicates that a patient can mount an immune response against tumor-associated mucin glycoprotein components. In addition, it has been observed that cell-surface carbohydrates containing 2-6 linked NeuAc may be important in a postbinding event in natural killer cell–mediated lysis (Van Rinsum *et al.*, 1986). Recently, two MAbs directed to Le[y]-related, cell-surface antigens of cancer cells (including colon cancer cells) have been studied (Hellstrom *et al.*, 1990). These MAbs were found to have special properties: (1) they have a high tumor specificity for gastrointestinal and other epithelial cancers; (2) both are internalized by antigen-positive cells, and (3) one MAb has a direct cytotoxic effect on antigen-positive tumor cells.

Recently, several purified or synthetic carbohydrate antigens have been used as immunogens in animal studies (Fung *et al.*, 1990). A synthetic tumor-associated conjugate consisting of synthetic T antigen (Galβ1-3GalNAc-R) coupled to bovine serum albumin or keyhole limpet hemocyanin was developed for active specific immunotherapy of a murine mammary carcinoma and was found to be useful in increasing the survival time of the immunized mice compared to untreated ones. Since T antigens are highly expressed by many gastrointestinal cancer cells, this approach needs to be explored further.

VI. Summary and Conclusion

It is now well established that alterations in glycoproteins and glycolipids are among the most common phenomena associated with malignant transformation. In cancers of the gastrointestinal tract, many of the phenotypic markers for malignancy have been found to be mucin glycoproteins. Recent advances in hybridoma technology, molecular biological methods, and sensitive analytical methods for studying small amounts of glycoprotein samples are beginning to have a significant impact on our understanding of the detailed structure of both carbohydrate and protein moieties of mucin glycoproteins in normal and cancerous cells.

Recent molecular cloning and sequencing data on three distinct mucin cDNAs, one encoding breast and pancreatic cancer mucins and two encoding distinct intestinal mucin genes, indicate that the apomucin peptide itself consists of repetitive tandem repeats segment flanked on either side by nonrepetitive unique segments. The repetitive segments are much more heavily glycosylated with O-glycosidically linked oligosaccharides than are the unique segments. In normal mucin glycoproteins, tandem repeat regions of the protein backbone structures are heavily glycosylated, there are more carbohydrate side chains per molecule, and the average chain length is long. With malignant transformation, the tandem repeats are more sparsely glycosylated. Some carbohydrate chains may be much shorter, exposing inner-core sugar structures such as T, Tn, and sialyl Tn antigens. Other oligosaccharides may be modified in the peripheral and backbone regions to form oncodevelopmental antigens such as extended type 2 chain, Le^x, and Le^y, or sialyl Le^x, or polyfucosylated Le^x and Le^y. Altered glycosylation may also lead to exposure of protein-backbone antigens that are normally masked by heavy glycosylation. Thus, the modified sugar structures, or exposed inner sugar-core structures, or the exposed protein backbone may serve as premalignant and malignant markers. In addition, some of these markers have already been found to be useful as prognostic indicators.

Many of these antigens are expressed heterogeneously in cancer tissues exhibiting mosaicism due to tumor cell heterogeneity. At the present time, serological assay methods for the detection of increased levels of these mucin glycoproteins lack sufficient sensitivity and specificity for the early diagnosis of cancers of colorectum and pancreas. The development of more sensitive assay methods and the judicious use of a panel of MAbs may be expected to significantly improve the sensitivity and specificities of serological assays of these tumor antigens. Some of these mucin glycoprotein antigens have been found to be useful in monitoring the patients for recurrence after surgical resection. It is clear that further studies are necessary to elucidate the role of altered mucin glycoproteins in the biological properties of cancer cells, in invasion and metastasis, and in host immune–defense mechanisms.

Thus, further investigation on the structure–function relationship of mucin glycoproteins in normal, premalignant, and malignant lesions of the colorectum and pancreas will undoubtedly lead to further elucidation of the role of mucins in cancer cell biology, and also to development of more effective methods of diagnosis and therapy.

Acknowledgments

Supported by the VA Medical Research Service and by National Cancer Institute Grants CA47551 and CA24321. The authors thank Rita Burns for manuscript preparation.

References

Abe, M., Hakomori, S., and Ohshiba, S. (1986). Differential expression of difucosyl type 2 chain (Le^y) defined by monoclonal antibody AH6 in different locations of colonic epithelia, various histological types of colonic polyps, and adenocarcinomas. *Cancer Res.* **46**, 2639–2644.

Abe, M., and Kufe, D. (1989). Structural analysis of the DF3 human breast carcinoma–associated protein. *Cancer Res.* **49**, 2834–2839.

Allen, A. (1983). The structure of colonic mucus. *In* "Colon: Structure and Function" (M. Bustos-Fernandez, ed.), pp. 45–63. Plenum, New York.

Allen, D. C., Connolly, N. S., and Biggart, J. D. (1988). High iron diamine-alcian blue mucin profiles in benign, premalignant, and malignant colorectal disease. *Histopathology* **13**, 399–411.

Atkinson, B. F., Ernst, C. S., Herlyn, M., Steplewski, Z., Sears, H. F., and Koprowski, H. (1982). Gastrointestinal cancer–associated antigen in immunoperoxidase assay. *Cancer Res.* **42**, 4820–4823.

Ban, T., Imai, K., and Yachi, A. (1989). Immunohistological and immunochemical characterization of a novel pancreatic cancer–associated antigen MUSE 11. *Cancer Res.* **49**, 7141–7146.

Bara, J., Languille, D., Gendron, M. C., Daher, N., Martin, E., and Burtin, P. (1983). Immuno-histological study of precancerous mucus modification in human distal colonic polyps. *Cancer Res.* **43**, 3885–3891.

Bara, J., Nardelli, J., Gadenne, C., Prade, M., and Burtin, P. (1984). Differences in the expression of mucus-associated antigens between proximal and distal colon adenocarcinomas. *Br. J. Cancer* **49**, 495–501.

Barnd, D. L., Lan, M. S., Metzgar, R. S., and Finn, O. J. (1989). Specific, major histocompatibility complex–unrestricted recognition of tumor-associated mucins by human cytotoxic T cells. *Proc. Natl. Acad. Sci. U.S.A.* **86**, 7159–7163.

Beyer, T. A., Sadler, J. E., Rearick, J. I., Paulson, J. C., and Hill, R. L. (1981). Glycosyltransfer-ases and their use in assessing oligosaccharide structure and structure–function relationships. *Adv. Enzymol.* **52**, 23–175.

Bhavanandan, V. P., (1988). Malignancy-related, cell-surface mucin-type glycoproteins. *Indian J. Biochem. Biophys.* **25**, 36–42.

Blind, P. J., and Dahlgren, S. T. (1987). Serum levels of the carbohydrate antigen CA-50 in pancre-atic disease. *Acta Clin. Scand.* **153**, 45–49.

Boland, C. R., Montgomery, C. K., and Kim, Y. S. (1982). Alterations in human colonic mucin occurring with cellular differentiation and malignant transformation. *Proc. Natl. Acad. Sci. U.S.A.* **79**, 2051–2055.

Boland, C. R., and Deshmukh, G. D. (1990). The carbohydrate composition of mucin in colonic cancer. *Gastroenterol* **98**, 1170–1177.

Borowitz, M. J., Tuck, F. L., Sindelar, W. F., Fernsten, P. D., and Metzgar, R. S. (1984). Mono-clonal antibodies against human pancreatic adenocarcinoma: Distribution of DU-PAN-2 antigen on glandular epithelia and adenocarcinomas. *J. Natl. Cancer Inst.* **72**, 999–1005.

Bresalier, R. S., Boland, C. R., and Kim, Y. S. (1985). Regional differences in normal and cancer-associated glycoconjugates of the human colon. *J. Natl. Cancer Inst.* **75**, 249–260.

Brown, A., Ellis, I. O., Embleton, M. J., Baldwin, R. W., Turner, D. R., and Hardcastle, J. D. (1984). Immunohistochemical localization of Y hapten and the structurally related H type-2 blood group antigen on large bowel tumors and normal adult tissues. *Int. J. Cancer* **33**, 727–736.

Burchell, J., Gendler, S., Taylor-Papadimitriou, J., Girling, A., Lewis, A., Millis, R., and Lamport, D. (1987). Development and characterization of breast cancer–reactive monoclonal antibodies directed to the core protein of the human milk mucin. *Cancer Res.* **47**, 5476–5482.

Burchell, J., Taylor-Papadimitriou, J., Boshell, M., Gendler, S., and Duhig, T. (1989). A short sequence, within the amino acid tandem repeat of a cancer-associated mucin, contains immuno-dominant epitopes. *Int. J. Cancer* **44,** 691–696.

Byrd, J. C., Nardelli, J., Siddiqui, B., and Kim, Y. S. (1988). Isolation and characterization of colon cancer mucin from xenografts of LS174T cells. *Cancer Res.* **48,** 6678–6685.

Byrd, J. C., Lamport, D. T. A., Siddiqui, B., Kuan, S.-F., Erickson, R., Itzkowitz, S. H., and Kim, Y. S. (1989). Deglycosylation of mucin from LS174T colon cancer cells by hydrogen fluoride treatment. *Biochem. J.* **261,** 617–625.

Byrd, J. C., Ho, J. J. L., Lamport, D. T. A., Ho, S. B., Siddiqui, B., Huang, J., Yan, P., and Kim, Y. S. (1991). Relationship of pancreatic cancer apomucin to mammary and intestinal apomucins. *Cancer Res.* **51,** 1026–1033.

Carlsson, S. R., and Fukuda, M. (1986). Isolation and characterization of leukosialin, a major sialoglycoprotein on human leukocytes. *J. Biol. Chem.* **261,** 12779–12786.

Carlstedt, I., and Sheehan, J. K. (1988). Structure and macromolecular properties of mucus glyco-proteins. *Monogr. Allergy* **24,** 16–24.

Chia, D., Terasaki, P. I., Suyama, N., Galton, J., Hirota, M., and Katz, D. (1985). Use of mono-clonal antibodies to sialylated Lewis[x] and sialylated Lewis[a] for serological tests of cancer. *Cancer Res.* **45,** 435–437.

Chung, Y. S., Ho, J. J. L., Kim, Y. S., Tanaka, H., Nakata, B., Hiura, A., Motoyoshi, H., Satake, K., and Umeyama, K. (1987). The detection of human pancreatic cancer–associated antigen in the serum of cancer patients. *Cancer* **60,** 1636–1643.

Coddington, J. F., Bhavanandan, V. P., Bloch, J. K., Nikrui, N., Ellard, J. V., Wang, P. S., and Jeanioz, R. W. (1984). Antibody to epiglycanin and radioimmunoassay to detect epiglycanin-related glycoproteins in body fluids of cancer patients. *J. Natl. Cancer Inst.* **73,** 1029–1038.

Denny, P. A., and Denny, P. C. (1982). A mouse submandibular sialomucin containing both N- and O-glycosidic linkages. *Carbohydr. Res.* **110,** 305–314.

Forstner, G., and Forstner, J. (1986). Mucus: biosynthesis and secretion. *In* "The Exocrine Pancreas: Biology, Pathobiology, and Diseases (V. L. W. Go, ed.), pp. 283–286. Raven Press, New York.

Fukushima, K., Hirota, M., Terasaki, P. I., Wakisawa, A., Togashi, H., Chia, D., Suyama, N., Fukushi, Y., Nudelman, E., and Hakomori, S. I. (1984). Characterization of sialylated Lewis[x] as a new tumor-associated antigen. *Cancer Res.* **44,** 5279–5285.

Fung, P. Y. S., Madej, M., Koganty, R. R., and Longenecker, B. M. (1990). Active specific im-munotherapy of a murine mammary adenocarcinoma using a synthetic tumor-associated glycocon-jugate. *Cancer Res.* **50,** 4308–4314.

Gendler, S. J., Burchell, J. M., Duhig, T., Lamport, D., White, R., Parker, M., and Taylor-Papadimitriou, J. (1987). Cloning of partial cDNA-encoding differentiation and tumor-associated mucin glycoproteins expressed by human mammary epithelium. *Proc. Natl. Acad. Sci. U.S.A.* **84,** 6060–6064.

Gendler, S., Taylor-Papadimitriou, J., Duhig, T., Rothbard, J., and Burchell, J. (1988). A highly immunogenic region of a human polymorphic epithelial mucin expressed by carcinomas is made up of tandem repeats. *J. Biol. Chem.* **263,** 12820–12823.

Gold, D. V., and Miller, F. (1978). Comparison of human colonic mucoprotein antigen from normal and neoplastic mucosa. *Cancer Res.* **38,** 3204–3211.

Gold, D. V., Hollingsworth, P., Kreimer, T., and Nelson, D. (1983). Identification of a human pancreatic duct tissue-specific antigen. *Cancer Res.* **43,** 235–238.

Gold, D. V., and Mattes, M. J. (1988). Monoclonal antibody B72.3 reacts with a core region struc-ture of O-linked carbohydrates. *Tumour Biol.* **9,** 137–144.

Gottlinger, H. G., Lobo, F. M., Grimm, T. W., Reithmuller, G., and Johnson, J. P. (1988). Bio-chemical characterization and tissue distribution of the Cora antigen, a cell surface glycoprotein differentially expressed on malignant and benign gastrointestinal epithelia. *Cancer Res.* **48,** 2198–2203.

Gum, J. R., Byrd, J. C., Hicks, J. W., Toribara, N. W., Lamport, D. T. A., and Kim, Y. S. (1989). Molecular cloning of human intestinal mucin cDNAs: Sequence analysis and evidence for genetic polymorphism. *J. Biol. Chem.* **264,** 6480–6487.

Gum, J. R., Hicks, J. W., Swallow, D. M., Lagace, R. L., Byrd, J. C., Siddiqui, B., and Kim, Y. S. (1990). Molecular cloning of cDNAs derived from a novel human intestinal mucin gene. *Biochem. Biophys. Res. Commun.* **171,** 405–415.

Haglund, C., Kuusela, P., Jalanko, H., and Roberts, P. J. (1987). Serum CA 50 as a tumor marker in pancreatic cancer: A comparison with CA19-9. *Int. J. Cancer* **39,** 477–481.

Hakomori, S. I. (1989). Aberrant glycosylation in tumors and tumor-associated carbohydrate antigens. *Adv. Cancer Res.* **52,** 257–331.

Harding, S. E. (1989). The macrostructure of mucus glycoproteins in solution. *Adv.Carbohydr. Chem. Biochem.* **47,** 345–381.

Hayes, D. F., Sekine, H., Ohno, T., Abe, M., Keefe, K., and Kufe, D. W. (1985). Use of a murine monoclonal antibody for detection of circulating plasma DF3 antigen levels in breast cancer patients. *J. Clin. Invest.* **75,** 1671–1678.

Hayes, D. F., Zurawski, V. R., and Kufe, D. W. (1986). Comparison of circulating CA 15-3 and carcinoembryonic antigen level in patients with breast cancer. *J. Clin. Oncol.* **4,** 1542–1550.

Hellstrom, I., Garrigues, J. H., Garrigues, V. and Hellstrom, K. E. (1990). Highly tumor-reactive, internalizing, mouse monoclonal antibodies to Le^y-related cell surface antigens. *Cancer Res.* **50,** 2183–2190.

Herlyn, M., Sears, H. F., Steplewski, Z., and Koprowski, H. (1982). Monoclonal antibody detection of a circulating tumor associated antigen: I. Presence of antigen in sera of patients with colorectal, gastric, and pancreatic carcinoma. *J. Clin. Immunol.* **2,** 135–140.

Hilkens, J., Kroezen, V., Bonfrer, J. M. G., DeJong-Bakker, M., and Bruning, P. F. (1986). MAM-6 antigen, a new serum marker for breast cancer monitoring. *Cancer Res.* **46,** 2582–2587.

Hilkens, J., and Buijs, F. (1988). Biosynthesis of MAM-6, an epithelial sialomucin: Evidence for involvement of a rare proteolytic cleavage step in the endoplasmic reticulum. *J. Biol. Chem.* **263,** 4215–4222.

Hilkens, J., Buijs, F., and Ligtenberg, M., (1989). Complexity of MAM-6, an epithelial sialomucin associated with carcinomas. *Cancer Res.* **49,** 786–793.

Ho, J. J. L., Chung, Y., Fujimoto, Y., Bi, N., Ryan, W., Yuan, S., Byrd, J. C., and Kim, Y. S. (1988). Mucin-like antigens in a human pancreatic cancer cell line identified by murine monoclonal antibodies SPan-1 and YPan-1. *Cancer Res.* **48,** 3924–3931.

Ho, S. B., Itzkowitz, S. H., Friera, A. M., Jiang, S., and Kim, Y. S. (1989a). Cell lineage markers in premalignant and malignant colonic mucosa. *Gastroenterol.* **97,** 392–404.

Ho, J. J. L., Chung, Y., Ryan, W., Henslee, J. G., and Kim, Y. S. (1989b). Evaluation of factors affecting the performance of enzymatic SPan-1 immunoassays for pancreatic cancer. *J. Immunol. Methods* **125,** 97–104.

Hounsell, E. G., and Feizi, T. (1982). Gastrointestinal mucins: Structures and antigenicities of their carbohydrate chains in health and disease. *Med. Biol.* **60,** 227–236.

Itzkowitz, S. H., Yuan, M., Ferrell, L. D., Palekar, A., and Kim, Y. S. (1986a). Cancer-associated alterations of blood group antigen expression in human colorectal polyps. *Cancer Res.* **46,** 5976–5984.

Itzkowitz, S. H., Yuan, M., Fukushi, Y., Palekar, A., Phelps, P. C., Shamsuddin, A. M., Trump, B. F., Hakomori, S., and Kim, T. S. (1986b). Lewis^x- and sialylated Lewis^x-related antigen expression in human malignant and nonmalignant colonic tissues. *Cancer Res.* **46,** 2627–2632.

Itzkowitz, S. H., Yuan, M., Ferrell, L. D., Ratcliffe, R. M., Chung, Y.-S., Satake, K., Umeyama, K., Jones, R. T., and Kim, Y. S. (1987). Cancer-associated alterations of blood group antigen expression in the human pancreas. *J. Natl. Cancer Inst.* **79,** 425–434.

Itzkowitz, S. H., Yuan, M., Fukushi, Y., Lee, H., Shi, Z., Zurawski, V., Hakomori, S., and Kim,

Y. S. (1988). Immunohistochemical comparison of Le[a], monosialosyl Le[a] (CA19-9), and disialosyl Le[a] antigens in human colorectal and pancreatic tissues. *Cancer Res.* **48**, 3834–3842.

Itzkowitz, S. H., Yuan, M., Montgomery, C. K., Kjeldsen, T., Takahashi, H. K., Bigbee, W. L., and Kim, Y. S. (1989). Expression of Tn, sialosyl Tn, and T antigens in human colon cancer. *Cancer Res.* **49**, 197–204.

Itzkowitz, S. H., Bloom, E. J., Kokal, W. A., Modin, G., Hakomori. S., and Kim, Y. S. (1990). Sialosyl Tn: A novel mucin antigen associated with poor prognosis in colorectal cancer patients. *Cancer* **66**, 1960–1966.

Itzkowitz, S. H., Kjeldsen, T., Friera, A., Hakomori, S., Yang, U. S., and Kim, Y. S. (1991). Expression of Tn, Sialosyl Tn, and T antigens in human pancreas. *Gastroenterol.* **100**, 1691–1700.

Johnson, V. G., Schlom, J., Paterson, A. J., Bennett, J., Magnani, J. L., and Colcher, D. (1986). Analysis of a human tumor-associated glycoprotein (TAG-72) identified by monoclonal antibody B72.3. *Cancer Res.* **46**, 850–857.

Kannagi, R., Fukushi, Y., Tachikama, T., Noda, A., Shigeta, K., Hiraiwa, N., Fukuda, Y., Inamoto, T., Hakomori, S. I., and Imura, H. (1986). Quantitative and qualitative characterization of human cancer–associated serum glycoprotein antigen expressing fucosyl or sialyl-fucosyl type 2 chain polylactosamine. *Cancer Res.* **46**, 2619–2626.

Kawahara, M., Chia, D., and Terasaki, P. I. (1985). Detection of sialylated Lewis[x] antigen in cancer sera using a sandwich radioimmunoassay. *Int. J. Cancer* **36**, 421–424.

Kim, Y. S., Perdomo, J., and Nordberg, J. (1971). Glycoprotein biosynthesis in small intestinal mucosa. I. A study of glycosyltransferases in microsomal subfractions. *J. Biol. Chem.* **246**, 5466–5476.

Kim, Y. S., Isaacs, R., and Perdomo, J. M. (1974). Alterations of membrane glycopeptides in human colonic adenocarcinoma. *Proc. Natl. Acad. Sci. U.S.A.* **71**, 4869–4873.

Kim, Y. S., Yuan, M., Itzkowitz, S. H., Sun, Q., Kaizu, T., Palekar, A., Trump, B. F., and Hakomori, S. (1986). Expression of Le[y] and extended Le[y] blood group–related antigens in human malignant, premalignant, and nonmalignant colonic tissues. *Cancer Res.* **46**, 5985–5992.

Kim, Y. S., Itzkowitz, S. H., Yuan, M., Chung, Y.-S., Satake, K., Umeyama, K., and Hakomori, S. (1988). Le[x] and Le[y] antigen expression in human pancreatic cancer. *Cancer Res.* **48**, 475–482.

Kim, Y. S. (1988). Differentiation of normal and cancerous colon cells. *In* "The Status of Differentiation Therapy of Cancer" (S. Waxman, G. B. Rossi, F. Takaku, eds.), pp. 29–44. Raven Press, New York.

Kim, Y. S. (1990). Carbohydrate antigen expression in colorectal cancer. *Sem. Cancer Biol.* **1**, 189–197.

Kiriyama, S., Kayakawa, T., Kondo, T., Shibata, T., Kitagawa, M., Ono, H., and Sakai, Y. (1990). Usefulness of a new tumor marker, SPan-1, for the diagnosis of pancreatic cancer. *Cancer* **65**, 1557–1561.

Kjeldsen, T., Clausen, H., Hirohashi, S., Ogawa, T., Iijima, H., and Hakomori, S. (1988). Preparation and characterization of monoclonal antibodies directed to the tumor-associated O-linked sialosyl-2,6-α-N-acetylgalactosaminyl (Sialosyl-Tn) epitope. *Cancer Res.* **48**, 2214–2220.

Klug, T. L., Sattler, M. A., Colcher, D., and Schlom, J. (1986). Monoclonal antibody immunoradiometric assay for an antigenic determinant (CA72) on a novel pancarcinoma antigen (TAG-72). *Int. J. Cancer* **38**, 661–669.

Kurosaka, A., Kitagawa, H., Fukui, S., Numata, Y., Nakada, H., Funakoshi, I., Kawasaki, T., Ogawa, T., Iijima, H., and Yamashina, I. (1988). A monoclonal antibody that recognizes a cluster of a dissacharide, NeuAcα2-6GalNAc, in mucin-type glycoproteins. *J. Biol. Chem.* **263**, 8724–8726.

Kuusela, P., Jalanko, H., Roberts, P. J., Sipponen, P., Mecklin, J. P., Patkanen, R., and Makela,

D., (1984). Comparison of CA19-9 and CEA levels in the serum of patients with colorectal diseases. *Br. J. Cancer* **49**, 135–139.

Lan, M. S., Finn, O. J., Fernsten, P. D., and Metzgar, R. S. (1985). Isolation and properties of a human pancreatic adenocarcinoma–associated antigen, DU-PAN-2. *Cancer Res.* **45**, 305–310.

Lan, M. S., Khorrami, A., Kaufman, B., and Metzgar, R. S. (1987). Molecular characterization of a mucin-type antigen associated with human pancreatic cancer: The DU-PAN-2 antigen. *J. Biol. Chem.* **262**, 12863–12870.

Lan, M. S., Hollingsworth, M. A., and Metzgar, R. S. (1990). Polypeptide core of a human pancreatic tumor mucin antigen. *Cancer Res.* **50**, 2997–3001.

Ligtenberg, M. J. L., Vos, H. L., Gennissen, A. M. C., and Hilkens, J. (1990). Episialin, a carcinoma-associated mucin, is generated by a polymorphic gene encoding splice variants with alternative amino termini. *J. Biol. Chem.* **265**, 5573–5578.

Linsley, P. S., Kallestad, J. C., and Horn, D. (1988). Biosynthesis of high-molecular-weight breast carcinoma–associated mucin glycoproteins. *J. Biol. Chem.* **263**, 8390–8397.

Madara, J. L., and Trier, J. S. (1987). Functional morphology of the mucosa of the small intestine. *In* "Physiology of the Gastrointestinal Tract" (L. R. Johnson, ed.), pp. 1209–1249. Raven Press, New York.

Magnani, J. L., Nilsson, B., Brockhaus, M., Sopf, D., Steplewski, Z., Koprowski, H., and Ginsburg, V. (1982). A monoclonal antibody–defined antigen associated with gastrointestinal cancer is a ganglioside containing sialylated lacto-N-fucopentaose II. *J. Biol. Chem.* **257**, 14365–14369.

Magnani, J. L., Steplewski, Z., Koprowski, H., and Ginsburg, V. (1983). Identification of the gastrointestinal and pancreatic cancer–associated antigen detected by monoclonal antibody 19-9 in the sera of patients as a mucin. *Cancer Res.* **43**, 5489–5492.

Malesci, A., Tommasini, M. A., Bonato, C., Bocchia, P., Bersani, M., Zerbi, A., Beretta, E., and DiCarlo, V. (1987). Determination of CA19-9 antigen in serum and pancreatic juice for differential diagnosis of pancreatic adenocarcinoma from chronic pancreatitis. *Gastroenterol* **92**, 60–67.

Mansson, J. E., Fredman, P., Nilsson, O., Lindholm, L., Holmgren, J., and Svennerholm, L. (1985). Chemical structure of carcinoma ganglioside antigens defined by monoclonal antibody C-50 and some allied gangliosides of human pancreatic adenocarcinoma. *Biochim. Biophys. Acta* **834**, 110–117.

Mantle, M., Forstner, G. G., and Forstner, J. F. (1984). Antigenic and structural features of goblet-cell mucin of human small intestine. *Biochem. J.* **217**, 159–167.

Martin, E. W., Mojzisik, C. M., Hinkle, G. H., Sampsel, J., Siddiqui, M. A., Tuttle, S. E., Sickle-Santanello, B., Colcher, D., Thurston, M. O., Bell, J. G., Farrar, W. B., and Schlom, J. (1988). Radioimmunoguided surgery using monoclonal antibody. *Am. J. Surg.* **156**, 386–392.

Miyake, M., Kohno, N., Nudelman, E. D., and Hakomori, S. (1989). Human IgG$_3$ monoclonal antibody directed to unbranched type 2 chain (Galβ1-4GlcNAcβ1-3 Galβ1-GlcNAcβ1-3Gal 1-R), which is highly expressed in colonic and hepatocellular carcinoma. *Cancer Res.* **49**, 5689–5695.

Nardelli, J., Byrd, J. C., Ho, J., Fearney, F. J., Tasman-Jones, C., and Kim, Y. S. (1988). Pancreatic cancer mucin from xenografts of SW1990 cells: Isolation, characterization, and comparison to colon cancer mucin. *Pancreas* **3**, 631–641.

Neutra, M. R., and Forstner, J. F. (1987). Gastrointestinal mucus: Synthesis, secretion, and function. *In* "Physiology of the Gastrointestinal Tract," 2nd Ed. (L. R. Johnson, ed.), pp. 975–1009. Raven Press, New York.

Ohuchi, N., Matoba, N., Taira, Y., Takahashi, K., Sakai, N., Sato, K., Fujita, N., Mochizubi, F., Nishihira, T., and Mori, S. (1988). Levels of circulating tumor–associated glycoprotein (TAG-72) in patients with carcinoma using a novel tumor marker CA72.4. *Jpn. J. Cancer Chemother.* **15**, 2767–2772.

Paterson, A. J., Schlom, J., Sears, H. F., Bennett, J., and Colcher, D. (1986). A radioimmunoassay for the detection of a human tumor–associated glycoprotein (TAG-72) using monoclonal antibody B72.3. *Int. J. Cancer* **37,** 659–666.

Persson, B. E., Stahle, E., Pahlman, L., Glimelius, B., Nilsson, O., Lindholm, L., Norrgand-Pedersen, B., and Holmgren, J. (1988). A clinical study of CA-50 as a tumour marker for monitoring of colorectal cancer. *Med. Oncol. Tumor Pharmacother.* **5,** 165–171.

Podolsky, D. K. (1985). Oligosaccharide structures of isolated human colonic mucin species. *J. Biol. Chem.* **260,** 15510–15515.

Podolsky, D. K., Fournier, D. A., and Lynch, K. E. (1986a). Development of anti–human colonic mucin monoclonal antibodies: Characterization of multiple colonic mucin species. *J. Clin. Invest.* **77,** 1251–1262.

Podolsky, D. K., Fournier, D. A., and Lynch, K. E. (1986b). Human colonic goblet cells: Demonstration of distinct subpopulations defined by mucin-specific monoclonal antibodies. *J. Clin. Invest.* **77,** 1263–1271.

Pour, P. M., Tempero, M. M., Takasaki, H., Uchida, E., Takiyama, Y., Burnett, D. A., and Steplewski, Z. (1988). Expression of blood group–related antigens ABH, Lewis A, Lewis B, Lewis X, Lewis Y, and CA19-9 in pancreatic cancer cells in comparison with the patient's blood group type. *Cancer Res.* **48,** 5422–5426.

Quaroni, A., Weiser, M., Lee, S., and Amodeo, D. (1986). Expression of developmentally regulated crypt cell antigens in human and rat intestinal tumors. *J. Natl. Cancer Inst.* **77,** 405–411.

Quaroni, A., Weiser, M. M., Herrera, L., and Fay, D. (1989). Crypt-cell antigens (CCA): New carbohydrate markers for human colon cancer cells. *Immunol. Invest.* **18,** 391–404.

Roberts, P. F., and Burns, J. (1972). A histochemical study of mucins in normal and neoplastic human pancreatic tissue. *J. Path.* **107,** 87–94.

Roth, J., Taatyes, D. J., Weinstein, J., Paulson, J. C., Greenwell, P., and Watkins, W. M. (1986). Differential subcompartmentation of terminal glycosylation in the Golgi apparatus of intestinal absorptive and goblet cells. *J. Biol. Chem.* **261,** 14307–14312.

Roussel, P., Lamblin, G., Lhermitte, M., Houdret, N., Lafitte, J., Perini, J., Klein, A., and Scharfman, A. (1988). The complexity of mucins. *Biochimie* **70,** 1471–1482.

Sakamoto, J., Furukawa, K., Cordon-Cardo, C., Yin, B. M. T., Rettig, W., Oettgen, H. F., Old, J., and Lloyd, K. O. (1986). Expression of Lewis[a], Lewis[b], X, and Y blood group antigens in human colonic tumors and normal tissue and in human tumor–derived cell lines. *Cancer Res.* **46,** 1553–1561.

Sakurai, Y., Hirohashi, S., Shimosato, Y., Kodaira, S., and Abe, O. (1988). Selection of a monoclonal antibody reactive with a high-molecular-weight glycoprotein circulating in the body fluid of gastrointestinal cancer patients. *Cancer Res.* **48,** 4053–4058.

Samuel, J., Noujaim, A. A., MacLean, G. D., Suresh, M. R., and Longenecker, B. M. (1990). Analysis of human tumor–associated Thomsen-Friedenreich antigen. *Cancer Res.* **50,** 4801–4808.

Sawabu, N., Toya, D., Takemori, Y., Hattori, N., and Fukui, M. (1986). Measurement of a pancreatic cancer–associated antigen (DU PAN 2) detected by a monoclonal antibody in sera of patients with digestive cancers. *Int. J. Cancer* **37,** 693–696.

Shi, Z. R., McIntyre, L. J., Kowles, B. B., Solter, D., and Kim, Y. S. (1984). Expression of a carbohydrate differentiation antigen, SSEA-1, in human colonic adenocarcinoma. *Cancer Res.* **44,** 1142–1147.

Shimamoto, C., Deshmukh, G. D., Rigot, W. L., and Boland, C. R. (1989). Analysis of cancer-associated colonic mucin by ion-exchange chromatography: Evidence for a mucin species of lower molecular charge and weight in cancer. *Biochim. Biophys. Acta* **991,** 284–295.

Siddiqui, J., Abe, M., Hayes, D., Shani, E., Yunis, E., and Kufe, D. (1988). Isolation and sequencing of a cDNA coding for the human DF3 breast carcinoma–associated antigen. *Proc. Natl. Acad. Sci. U.S.A.* **85,** 2320–2323.

Sindelar, W. F., Kinsella, T. J., and Mayer, R. J. (1985). Cancer of the pancreas. *In* "Cancer:

Principles and Practice of Oncology," Vol. 1 (V. T. DeVita, S. Hellman, S. A. Rosenberg, eds.), pp. 691–739. J. B. Lippincott, Philadelphia.

Singhal, A. K., Orntoft, T. F., Nudelman, E., Nance, S., Schibig, L., Stroud, M. R., Clausen, H., and Hakomori, S. (1990). Profiles of Lewis[x]-containing glycoproteins and glycolipids in sera of patients with adenocarcinoma. *Cancer Res.* **50**, 1375–1380.

Singhal, A., and Hakomori, S. (1990). Molecular changes in carbohydrate antigens associated with cancer. *Bioessays* **12**, 223–230.

Stahli, C., Caravatti, M., Aeschbacher, M., Kocyba, C., Takacs, B., and Carmann, H. (1988). Mucin-like carcinoma-associated antigen defined by three monoclonal antibodies against different epitopes. *Cancer Res.* **48**, 6799–6802.

Steinberg, W. (1990). The clinical utility of CA19-9 tumor-associated antigen. *Am. J. Gastroenterol.* **85**, 350–355.

Sugihara, K., and Jass, J. R. (1986). Colorectal goblet cell sialomucin heterogeneity: Its relation to malignant disease. *J. Clin. Pathol.* **39**, 1088–1095.

Szulman, A. E. (1964). The histological distribution of the blood group substances in man as disclosed by immunofluorescence IV. The ABO and H antigens in embryos and fetuses from 18 mm in length. *J. Exp. Med.* **119**, 503–515.

Szulman, A. E., and Marcus, D. M. (1973). The histological distribution of the blood group substances in man as disclosed by immunofluorescence, VI. The Le[a] and Le[b] antigens during fetal development. *Lab. Invest.* **28**, 565–574.

Tuttle, S. E., Jewell, S. D., Mojzisik, C. M., Hinkle, G. H., Colcher, D., Schlom, J., and Martin, E. W. (1988). Intraoperative radioimmunolocalization of colorectal carcinoma with a hand-held gamma probe and MAb B72.3: Comparison of *in vivo* gamma probe counts with *in vitro* MAb radiolocalization. *Int. J. Cancer* **42**, 352–358.

Van Rinsum, J., Smets, L. A., VanRooy, H., and Van den Eijnden, D. H. (1986). Specific inhibition of human natural killer cell–mediated cytotoxicity by sialic acid and sialo-oligosaccharides. *Int. J. Cancer* **38**, 915–922.

Yan, P.-S., Ho, S. B., Itzkowitz, S. H., Byrd, J. C., Siddiqui, B., and Kim, Y. S. (1990). Expression of native and deglycosylated colon cancer mucin antigens in normal and malignant epithelial tissues. *Lab. Invest.* **62**, 698–706.

Yuan, M., Itzkowitz, S. H., Palekar, A., Shamsuddin, A. M., Phelps, P. C., Trump, B. F., and Kim, Y. S. (1985a). Distribution of blood group antigens A, B, H, Lewis[a], and Lewis[b] in human normal, fetal, and malignant colonic tissue. *Cancer Res.* **45**, 4499–4511.

Yuan, M., Itzkowitz, S. H., Boland, C. R., Kim, Y. D., Tomita, J. T., Palekar, A., Bennington, J. L., Trump, B. F., and Kim, Y. S. (1986). Comparison of T antigen expression in normal, premalignant, and malignant human colonic tissue using lectin and antibody immunohistochemistry. *Cancer Res.* **46**, 4841–4847.

Yuan, M., Itzkowitz, S. H., Ferrell, L. D., Fukushi, Y., Palekar, A., Hakomori, S., and Kim, Y. S. (1987). Expression of Lewis[x] and sialylated Lewis[x] antigens in human colorectal polyps. *J. Natl. Cancer Inst.* **78**, 479–488.

Yuan, S., Ho, J.J.L., Yuan, M., and Kim, Y. S. (1985b). Human pancreatic cancer–associated antigens detected by murine monoclonal antibodies. *Cancer Res.* **45**, 6179–6187.

Zotter, S., Lossnitzer, A., Hageman, P. C., Delemarre, J. F. M., Hilkens, J., and Hilgers, J. (1987). Immunohistochemical localization of the epithelial marker MAM-6 in invasive malignancies and highly dysplastic adenomas of the large intestine. *Lab. Invest.* **57**, 193.

Chapter 10

Pyruvate Kinase in Selected Human Tumors

G. E. J. STAAL AND G. RIJKSEN

Department of Haematology, Laboratory of Medical Enzymology,
University Hospital Utrecht
3508 GA Utrecht,
The Netherlands

I. Introduction

Control of gene expression is of fundamental importance in metabolic regulation. Since many manifestations of cancer appear to originate from an abnormal pattern of gene expression, studies on its regulation should provide important information for the understanding of cancer. After the discovery by Markert and Möller in 1959 that enzymes can exist in multimolecular forms, it became evident that alteration in gene expression in neoplasia may be manifested (among other things) by a change in isozyme distribution. This observation is important because changes in the expression of isozymes with altered regulatory properties

BIOCHEMICAL AND MOLECULAR ASPECTS
OF SELECTED CANCERS, VOL. 1

may affect the metabolic pathways of the tumor cell. Various studies with malignant hepatoma cell lines have shown that isozymes of regulatory enzymes appear that are also present in fetal or regenerating liver (Ibsen and Fishman, 1979; Schapira, 1981). In addition, it was shown that the extent of the appearance of some of these isozymes correlated well with the proliferative capacity of the cell (Weinhouse, 1973).

It has been recognized for many years that glucose is one of the most important metabolic fuels for malignant tumors. Glucose catabolism not only represents the principal source of energy production but also supplies the tumor cell with metabolites that are used in various biosynthetic pathways. Therefore, the glycolytic pathway takes a central position in the metabolism of the tumor cell. Pyruvate kinase (ATP:pyruvate O^2-phosphotransferase, EC 2.7.1.40), which catalyzes the conversion of phosphoenolpyruvate to pyruvate with generation of ATP, is a key enzyme of the glycolytic pathway, and different isozymes of pyruvate kinase are known. The pyruvate kinase isozyme system appears to be a good model system for studying the alteration of gene expression by the determination of the isozyme pattern in neoplasia. In this chapter we describe the expression and characteristics of pyruvate kinase isozymes in human tumors after presenting a short overview of the genetic system of pyruvate kinase and the structural and kinetical differences between the various isozymes.

II. Genetic System of Pyruvate Kinase

Pyruvate kinase is a tetramer consisting of identical or nearly identical subunits of about 60 kDa of which four forms, the M (or M_1), K (or M_2), L and R types, exist in mammals (reviewed in Imamura et al, 1986; Staal and Rijksen, 1985).

M (or M_1) is the main type in skeletal muscle, heart, and brain. K type is predominant in fetal tissues, neoplasias, and proliferating tissue but may also be expressed in adult tissues. L type is mainly found in liver and, to a lesser extent, in kidney and intestines. R type is present in erythrocytes.

A. L- and R-type Pyruvate Kinase

Comparing the L type found in liver with the R type present in erythrocytes, differences are found with respect to molecular weight (Kahn et al., 1978), kinetics (Sprengers and Staal, 1979), ability to be phosphorylated (Marie and Kahn, 1080), and electrophoretic properties (Kahn et al., 1978). However, important similarities are also observed. First, an antiserum raised in rabbits against pure human L-type pyruvate kinase does not discriminate between the liver and the erythrocyte enzymes (Imamura et al., 1972). This indicates a large structural similarity between the enzymes from these two sources. Second, a deficiency of the human erythrocyte pyruvate kinase is also expressed in the liver (Kahn *et al.*, 1976; Staal *et al.* 1982). This is an argument for the statement that the enzymes from liver tissue and erythrocytes are derived from one and the same gene. In order to test this hypothesis, mRNA fractions from liver and erythrocytes have been isolated and translated in a cell-free reticulocyte system (Marie *et al.*, 1981). The results demonstrated that two different mRNAs encode for the L- and R-type pyruvate kinase. The two types of mRNAs are transcribed from a single gene, presumably involving gene rearrangement or differential processing of a common nuclear RNA precursor (Marie *et al.*, 1981; Saheki *et al.*, 1982). In more recent studies, it was shown that the L-type pyruvate kinase gene possesses two tissue–specific promoters generating heterogeneous mRNAs (Cognet *et al.*, 1987; Noguchi *et al.*, 1987; Tremp *et al.*, 1989). Also, additional heterogeneity is created by an alternative use of polyadenylation sites of the mRNAs (Marie *et al.*, 1986).

B. M- AND K-TYPE PYRUVATE KINASE

Both M and K isozymes consist of four identical subunits. The K subunit has been reported to be 1000 to 2000 daltons larger than the M subunit, and the two isozymes have different isoelectric points (Muroya *et al.*, 1976). The question of whether the M- and K-type isozymes of pyruvate kinase are synthesized by a common mRNA has been examined by isolating total RNA from rat skeletal muscle and AH-130 Yoshida ascites hepatoma cells, which express the M- and K-type isozymes, respectively, and translating the preparations in a rabbit reticulocyte lysate system (Noguchi and Tanaka, 1982). The pyruvate kinase subunit synthesized from hepatoma RNA has a slightly larger molecular weight and higher pI value than the subunit from muscle RNA. This indicates that one gene but two mRNAs may be involved in the synthesis of M- and K-type isozymes. This hypothesis was further supported by the results obtained by Saheki *et al.* (1982) and Levin *et al.* (1982). A definitive answer was given by the determination of the complete nucleotide sequences for both M- and K-type pyruvate kinase from the rat by sequencing the cDNAs (Noguchi *et al.*, 1986). The derived amino acid sequences turned out to be identical except for one region of 45 residues.

In summary, two structural genes, L-type gene (for L and R isozymes) and M-type gene (M and K isozymes) and four different mRNAs control the synthesis of pyruvate kinase isozymes (Imamura *et al.*, 1986).

III. Kinetics: Phosphorylation

Pyruvate kinase belongs to the group of allosteric enzymes. Tanaka *et al.* (1967) were the first to demonstrate that the L type is under allosteric control.

The enzyme exhibits cooperativity with respect to phosphoenolpyruvate and is activated by fructose 1,6-diphosphate, which shifts the kinetics from sigmoidal to hyperbolic (Carminatti *et al.*, 1968; Rozengurt *et al.*, 1969). The enzymatic activity of the L type can be modulated to a great extent. The enzyme is allosterically inhibited by ATP and alanine, the inhibitory effects of which can be counteracted by the addition of fructose 1,6-diphosphate (Tanaka *et al.*, 1967).

Fructose 2,6-diphosphate is a potent allosteric activator of 6-phosphofructo-1-kinase (Hers and Van Schaftingen, 1982). The activating effect of fructose 2,6-diphosphate will result in an increase of fructose 1,6-diphosphate which, in turn, activates pyruvate kinase. In this way fructose 2,6-diphosphate influences indirectly the activity of pyruvate kinase.

Jimenez de Asua *et al.* (1971) showed that the K type from rat liver is inhibited by a series of amino acids while the M type from muscle is inhibited only by phenylalanine (Rozengurt *et al.*, 1970). Pyruvate kinase, type K from leukocytes, shows cooperative interaction between the binding sites for phosphoenolpyruvate (Van Berkel and Koster, 1973). Activity curves obtained in the presence of the allosteric inhibitor alanine are sigmoidal and very similar to the normal activity curves obtained with the L type (Staal *et al.*, 1971, Rozengurt *et al.*, 1970). Alanine and phenylalanine act as allosteric inhibitors. These properties are in agreement with the two-state R ⇌ T model. In this model fructose 1,6-diphosphate and phosphoenolpyruvate should favor the R state, whereas alanine and other inhibitory amino acids possess a higher affinity for the T state. The affinity constant for phosphoenolpyruvate is different for the M and K types, being higher for the latter (Imamura *et al.*, 1986; Consler *et al.*, 1989). This is probably due to a different allosteric constant, that is, a difference in the position of the equilibrium between the R and T states (Van Berkel *et al.*, 1973). In agreement with this assumption is that the M type exhibits Michaelis–Menten kinetics with regard to its substrate phosphoenolpyruvate, whereas the K type shows allosteric properties and can be activated by fructose 1,6-diphosphate. In conclusion, both isoenyzmes are subjected to similar modes of allosteric regulation. However, the distribution between the R and T forms is different owing to structural differences. As mentioned before, M- and K-type isozymes differ only in a region of 45 amino acids, of which only 21 are different. The remaining parts of the molecule, including the active sites, are identical. The region of difference was shown to be the structural region responsible for intersubunit contact (Stuart *et al.*, 1979; Muirhead *et al.*, 1986), which supports the idea of different cooperativity between the subunits, leading to a different allosteric constant. However, structural information provided by Consler *et al.* (1989) showed that, in addition, long-range conformational differences exist along the enzyme molecule resulting in different affinity constants.

Regulation of liver L-type pyruvate kinase by a phosphorylation mechanism has been intensively studied. Ljungström *et al.* (1974) were the first to report that rat liver pyruvate kinase can be phosphorylated by a cyclic AMP–dependent protein kinase. The effect of cyclic AMP–dependent phosphorylation can be reversed by a phosphoprotein phosphatase (Titanji et al., 1976). The phosphorylation of L-type pyruvate kinase causes important changes in the kinetics of the enzyme: decreased affinity for phospho-enol-pyruvate and increased inhibition by the allosteric inhibitors ATP and alanine (Ekman et al., 1976; Pilkis et al., 1978). These kinetic modifications are expected to play an important physiological role in the dynamic balance between glycolysis and gluconeogenesis. Much less is known about the possible contribution of phosphorylation to the regulation of the M- and K-type kinase. Phosphorylation of pyruvate kinase type K by a cAMP-independent protein kinase has been demonstrated in isolated chicken hepatocytes (Fister et al., 1983), in rat pancreatic islet cells (MacDonald and Kowluru, 1985), in rat medullary thyroid carcinomas (Rijksen et al., 1988) and in human gliomas (Oude Weernink et al., 1990). Furthermore, transformation of chicken embryo cells by Rous sarcoma virus resulted in phosphorylation of type K pyruvate kinase on a tyrosine residue, which was accompanied by inactivation of the enzyme activity (Presek et al., 1980; Glossmann et al., 1981; Presek et al, 1988). However, phosphorylation on tyrosine residues seems to be restricted to cells transformed by the Rous sarcoma virus, as in all other cases, phosphorylation on only serine and threonine residues could be detected. The effects of the latter phosphorylation on the kinetic properties of the enzyme are unknown to date. Although both K- and L-type pyruvate kinase can be phosphorylated on serine and threonine residues, there are some fundamental differences: (1) The stoichiometry of the incorporation of phosphate is much lower for the K type; (2) the phosphorylation of the K type is independent of the presence of cAMP, in contrast to the L type; and (3) the phosphorylation site of the L type (Ser 12 at the N-terminal end of the molecule) is not present in the K type (Hjelmquist et al., 1974; Noguchi et al., 1987), so the latter must be phosphorylated at an entirely other—yet undefined—phosphorylation site. Therefore, it must be anticipated that the effects on the properties of both enzymes are not comparable either. In that respect, however, it is remarkable that fructose 1,6-diphosphate has a similar inhibitory effect on the phosphorylation of both the L type and the K type, suggesting a potential similar physiological meaning. To our knowledge, no phosphorylation of the M type has ever been reported.

IV. Antibodies Specific for Type K Pyruvate Kinase. Application in Immunohistochemical Studies

As already mentioned, the M- and K-type isozymes are structurally and immunologically closely related. Noguchi et al. (1986) determined the complete nucleotide sequences for both M- and K-type pyruvate kinase from rat by sequencing the cDNAs. The derived amino acid sequences turned out to be identical except for one region of 45 residues. In order to obtain antibodies specific for the K type, a synthetic tetradecapeptide was constructed (Oude Weernink *et al.*, 1988). The sequence of this peptide was chosen from the K-type specific region of rat pyruvate kinase (Noguchi *et al.*, 1986). Immunization of rabbits with this peptide, coupled to keyhole limpet hemocyanin as a carrier protein, resulted in antibodies reacting not only with this peptide, but also with the K type and not crossreacting with the M type (Oude Weernink *et al.*, 1988). This was established by immunoblot analysis under both dissociating and nondissociating conditions.

Van Erp *et al.* (1988) obtained monoclonal antibodies against K-type pyruvate kinase purified from human kidney not crossreacting with the other pyruvate kinase isoenzymes (M, L, and R types). The specificity of the monoclonal antibodies was proven by enzyme-linked immunosorbent assay, immunoprecipitation, and immunoblotting experiments. The monoclonal antibodies could be successfully used in immunohistochemical studies (Van Erp *et al.*, 1988). Neurons and astrocytes in the brain, Kupffer's cells in liver, connective tissue cells, and vascular smooth muscle cells showed immunoreactivity. However, striated muscle cells in skeletal muscle, heart, and hepatocytes were not immunoreactive. Other types of glial cells, e.g., oligodendrocytes and microglia, showed no reaction either.

V. Isozyme Distribution in Neoplasia

The similarity of some isozyme patterns to those of fetal organs is probably one of the most remarkable features of malignant tumors (Weinhouse, 1982; Schapira, 1981). However, many isozymes (e.g., adult liver) undergo substantial changes in activity in response to normal dietary and hormone alterations. Furthermore, in many cases it is still a question of whether isozyme alterations are due to true changes in isozyme composition of a homogeneous cell population or to differences in the cell populations comprising the tumor.

It has been hypothesized that type K pyruvate kinase is the prototype or undifferentiated type of the pyruvate kinase isozymes, while the L and M types are differentiated types (Imamura *et al.*, 1986). This hypothesis is supported by the predominance of the K type in many tumors.

A. Brain Tumors

Pyruvate kinase type M_4 is predominant in adult brain, whereas type K_4 is present in minor amounts. In the fetal brain, five forms are found (K_4, K_3M, K_2M_2, KM_3, and M_4), indicating that both K and M subunits are synthesized simultaneously (Van Veelen *et al.*, 1978). In the newborn, both type M_4 and K_4 are present but M_4 is predominant, whereas in the adult, type M_4 is mainly present with little K_4. It seems likely that during development, the synthesis of M subunits is favored. As already mentioned, the K type is strongly inhibited by the amino acid alanine, but the M type shows no sensitivity to alanine. Based on these properties an alanine-inhibition assay was developed (Van Veelen *et al.*, 1981). With this assay it is possible to determine the proportion of K and M subunits in normal brain and brain tumors. It should be noted that the alanine-inhibition assay can be performed within 10 min after a biopsy is taken and fits well within the scope of a surgical procedure (Van Veelen *et al.*, 1988). The activity of pyruvate kinase in a biopsy specimen in the presence of alanine can be expressed as the residual percentage of the activity in the absence of alanine. Thus high residual activity correlates with the predominance of M type; low residual activity indicates the prevalence of K type.

1. *Astrocytomas and Glioblastomas*

A switch toward the K type in human brain tumors was first observed by Bennett *et al.* (1975). Pyruvate kinase of grade IV astrocytomas is characterized by a marked, increased inhibition by alanine, which indicates the presence of mainly type K_4 (Van Veelen *et al.*, 1979). The electrophoretic pattern is in agreement with the observed alanine inhibition: only K_4 and little K_3M are present, and no M_4 isozyme can be detected (Van Veelen *et al.*, 1979). A correlation also exists between histological grading of gliomas and pyruvate kinase activity in the presence of alanine: well-differentiated grade I and II astrocytomas are characterized by relatively high residual activities. The reverse is found for the anaplastic astrocytoma III and IV and also for the poorly differentiated glioblastomas (Van Veelen *et al.*, 1979; Van Veelen *et al.*, 1982). Electrophoresis of pyruvate kinase from the tumors of the different groups is in agreement with the alanine inhibition. Figure 1 shows the electrophoretic pattern of examples of tumors representative for the respective histological classification. From this figure, it can be concluded that the presence of both M_4 and K_4 and the hybrid K_3M is a specific property of well-differentiated astrocytomas, but in highly malignant glioblastomas, the synthesis of K subunits is favored; therefore, more K_4 and K_3M are observed, in agreement with the alanine inhibition (Van Veelen *et al.*, 1979; Van Veelen *et al.*, 1982).

2. *Oligodendrogliomas*

The degree of inhibition of pyruvate kinase by alanine was investigated in well-differentiated (grade II) and anaplastic oligodendrogliomas (Van Veelen *et al.*, 1979). In this variety of glioma, high residual activity of the enzyme corresponds with low grading of cancer. Relatively low residual activity is seen in

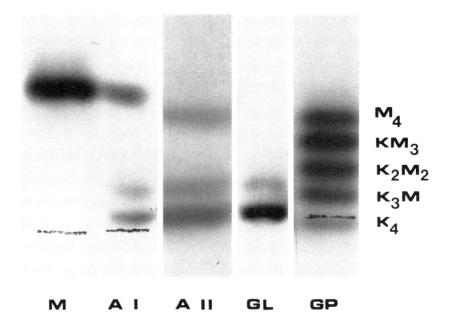

M_4
KM_3
K_2M_2
K_3M
K_4

M   A I   A II   GL   GP

Fig. 1.   Electrophoretic pattern of pyruvate kinase from tumors representative of the respective histological classification and grades. AI, astrocytoma grade I; AII astrocytoma grade II; GL, glioblastoma. M (muscle) and GP (glandula pinealis) served as references.

tumors that were classified as more malignant, so in well-differentiated tumors, relatively more M subunits are present, while in less-differentiated tumors, the synthesis of K subunits is favored (Van Veelen *et al.*, 1986).

3. *Ependymomas*

In this kind of tumor, a shift from the M to the K type is also observed (Van Veelen *et al.*, 1986). Ependymomas appear to have lower residual activities than astro- and oligodendrogliomas, and so far no correlation has been found between histological differentiation and residual activity.

4. *Gliomas in Children*

Van Veelen *et al.* (1986) studied 27 gliomas in patients under 20 years of age. No correlation could be found between residual activity and histological grading. This group of tumors was in fact characterized by low residual activities irrespective of their histological grading.

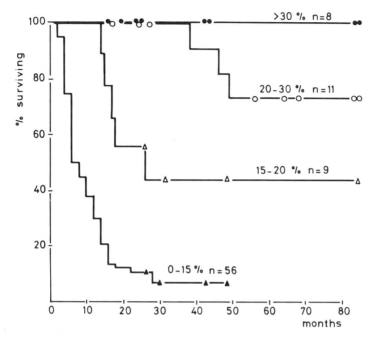

Fɪɢ. 2. Postoperative survival of adult patients with glioma (n = 84) in relation to residual activity of pyruvate kinase in the presence of alanine. The symbols (●, ○, △, ▲) represent patients in the different groups who are still alive.

a. Correlation between alanine inhibition and survival of the total or subtotal resections of gliomas. The correlation between alanine inhibition of pyruvate kinase and post-operative survival in 84 adult patients with gliomas was studied (Van Veelen *et al.*, 1986). Figure 2 shows the survival after the resection of these tumors, subdivided into four groups according to the residual activity. In the group of tumors in which 15% or less residual activity was found, the majority of the patients did not survive 18 months. In the group with over 15% residual activity, all patients survived the first year after surgery. Those who died in this group and had tumors with less than 20% residual activity had a shorter survival than those who died of tumors that had residual activities between 20 and 30%. Finally, all patients who had tumors in which residual activity over 30% was found were still alive after 6 years.

b. Correlation between alanine inhibition and presence or absence of tumor at histological examination. Maximal alanine inhibition of pyruvate kinase is found in the center of a poorly differentiated glioma. The alanine inhibition decreases going toward the periphery of the tumor. Therefore, in biopsies away

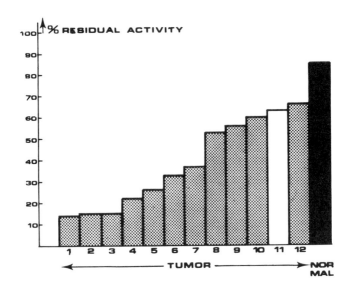

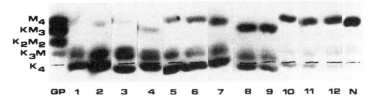

FIG. 3.   Residual pyruvate kinase activity in the presence of alanine of different parts (1 to 12) of an anaplastic oligodendroglioma developing into a glioblastoma. The electrophoretic pattern of pyruvate kinase is shown in the photograph below. Glandula pinealis (GP) and normal brain tissue (N) were used as references.

from the center of such tumors, one may expect a correlation quite different from that already mentioned. This is illustrated in Fig. 3 for an anaplastic oligodendroglioma (Van Veelen *et al.*, 1979). Samples from 12 different locations were taken, and all but one (specimen 11) were diagnosed as tumor by pathological examination. In the same figure, the electrophoretic pattern of pyruvate kinase from the 12 different specimens is given. At the time of surgery, only specimens one to six were considered suspect for tumor growth, whereas at microscopic examination of the paraffin slides, five other specimens appeared to contain tumor as well. Therefore, the result of an alanine inhibition assay of an individual tumor can only be appreciated as a diagnostic parameter, if the biopsy is taken from the center of the tumor.

B. RETINOBLASTOMA, NEUROBLASTOMA, AND MEDULLOBLASTOMA

Normal fetal retina is characterized by the presence of five forms of pyruvate kinase, representing the M_4 and K_4 type and the hybrids KM_3, K_2M_2 and K_3M (Beemer et al., 1982). Normal adult retina contains the same set of isozymes but only a small amount of K_4. By contrast, in retinoblastoma the M_4 type is almost absent. The alanine inhibition was found to be in good agreement with the observed electrophoretic pattern (Beemer et al., 1982).

Neuroblastomas are characterized by the presence of all five forms (Beemer et al., 1986). By contrast, childhood gliomas are characterized by the presence of mainly K_4 and only a little K_3M. In neuroblastoma the residual activity of pyruvate kinase in the presence of alanine is $74 \pm 11\%$ as compared with $7 \pm 4\%$ in childhood gliomas.

Like retino- and neuroblastomas, medulloblastomas belong to the so-called embryonal neuroectodermal tumors (Palmer et al., 1981). Electrophoretically, medulloblastomas show all five forms of pyruvate kinase (Beemer et al., 1984). Like neuroblastomas, medulloblastomas show a relatively high pyruvate kinase activity in the presence of alanine ($53 \pm 7\%$). Cottreau et al. (1982) studied thirteen neuroblastomas. Different forms were detected, with K_4 as the predominate type. Retinoblastoma, neuroblastoma, and medulloblastoma resemble one another with respect to the expression of pyruvate kinase isozymes.

C. BREAST CANCER

Hilf et al. (1973) studied pyruvate kinase activity in samples of normal breast tissue, fibrocystic disease, fibroadenomas, and infiltrating ductal carcinomas. Compared with normal breast tissue, the pyruvate kinase activity was found to be significantly elevated in carcinomas. Furthermore, the activity of pyruvate kinase was significantly higher in carcinomas compared with samples of fibrocystic disease and fibroadenoma (Hilf et al., 1973).

The levels of multimolecular forms of pyruvate kinase present in four normal human breast specimens, nine benign tumors, and thirteen malignant breast carcinomas were studied by Ibsen et al. (1982). A correlation between specific activity and malignancy was found. The mean specific activities of the normal, benign, and malignant tissue were 0.078 ± 0.006, 0.36 ± 0.072, and 3.50 ± 0.696 units/mg protein, respectively. Both K and M types were expressed in all tissues, but the K type predominated. Lopez-Alarcon et al. (1981) measured the sensitivity to ATP of the pyruvate kinase activity of homogenates of human mammary carcinomas of different degrees of histological differentiation. The inhibition by ATP was found to be significantly lower ($p < 0.001$) in well-differentiated carcinomas than in poorly differentiated carcinomas. The pyruvate kinase activity of normal mammary tissue had, in turn, a significantly lower sensitivity to ATP than that of well-differentiated carcinomas. The results were explained on the basis of the isoenzyme shift from M to K type (Lopez-Alarcon *et al.*, 1981).

Balinsky *et al.* (1983) reported that the K_4 isozyme of pyruvate kinase was the major form in most malignant breast tissue, but accounted for only 41% in normal tissue, 30% in fibrocystic disease specimens, and 46% in fibroadenomas. Balinsky *et al.* (1984b) also determined the pyruvate kinase activity in normal, dysplastic, and cancerous human breast tissues. Benign lesions generally showed enzyme activities similar to those of normal breast tissue. Malignant tumors had significantly increased pyruvate kinase activity. Pyruvate kinase activity in the malignant tumors was always higher than that in apparently normal or fibrocystic tissue from the same patients. Hennipman *et al.* (1987) determined pyruvate kinase activity in normal human breast tissue, fibrocystic disease, fibroadenomas, and carcinomas of the breast. The enzyme activity was significantly higher in carcinomas than in normal breast tissue. The pyruvate kinase activity in benign tumors was intermediate between normal tissue and carcinomas. In normal breast tissue, the larger part of pyruvate kinase consisted of K subunits, distributed mainly between K_4 and K_3M hybrids. The total amount of K subunits appeared to be increased in benign tumors compared to normal breast tissues. This increase, however, was found to be insignificant. In carcinomas, a significant shift in isozyme composition was observed, favoring the expression of K subunits. Furthermore, it was shown (Hennipman *et al.*, 1988) that pyruvate kinase activities were significantly higher in breast cancer metastases than in primary tumors. However, no changes in the isozyme patterns were observed when the metastases were compared with primary breast cancers. In conclusion, all reports mentioned showed that pyruvate kinase activity and the expression of the K subunit in breast cancer are increased.

D. THYROID NEOPLASMS

Verhagen *et al.* (1985) studied pyruvate kinase expression in human thyroid carcinomas, follicular adenomas, and normal thyroid tissue. The specific activity in carcinomas (0.94 ± 0.44) was found to be significantly increased in comparison with pyruvate kinase in normal tissue (0.14 ± 0.05). Specific activities of follicular adenomas were rather heterogeneous. When these tumors were divided into three groups of increasing proliferative activity, as judged by histopathological criteria, the highest specific activities of pyruvate kinase were found in the group with the highest proliferative activity. On the other hand, specific activities of the least active tissues (colloid-containing follicular adenomas) were comparable to normal. The isozyme composition of pyruvate kinase was also studied. Normal thyroid tissue was characterized by the presence of K_4, K_3M, and K_2M_2. In carcinomas, mainly K_4 and K_3M were found. Undifferentiated tumors expressed more K_4 compared with follicular and papillary carcinomas. The alanine inhibition was in agreement with the observed electrophoretic pattern.

E. Chronic Lymphocytic Leukemia

Kraayenhagen *et al.* (1982 and 1985) studied the isozyme distribution of pyruvate kinase in lymphocytes from patients with chronic lymphocytic leukemia (CLL). The CLL lymphocytes were different from normal non–T lymphocytes with respect to the pyruvate kinase residual activity in the presence of alanine. The same authors also compared the pyruvate kinase in two T-cell lines and two B-cell lines with the enzyme of normal T and non–T lymphocytes from peripheral blood. All cell types studied contained K_4-type pyruvate kinase and the hybrid K_3M. In addition, in the two T-cell lines and the T lymphocytes from peripheral blood, the K_2M_2 hybrid was also present.

F. Soft-Tissue Tumors

1. Fibroblastic Proliferations

Pyruvate kinase was studied in 57 fibroblastic and fibrohistiocytic proliferations and 10 normal fibrous tissues (Elbers *et al.*, 1990b). The specific activity was significantly increased in malignant tumors (1.67 ± 0.25) compared with normal tissue (0.26 ± 0.04) and benign proliferations (0.52 ± 0.05). A strong overlap was found between aggressive fibromatosis and the benign group. In all groups studied, the expression of K subunits was predominant. In malignant tumors, there was a statistically significant shift toward greater expression of K subunits compare to that in normal fibrous tissue and benign fibrous proliferation. However, the difference in mean activity of pyruvate kinase between metastasizing and nonmetastasizing tumors was not associated with an isozyme shift from M toward K isozyme (Elbers *et al.*, 1990b).

2. Smooth Muscle Proliferations

Elbers *et al.* (1990a) determined the specific activity of pyruvate kinase in normal smooth muscle, leiomyomas, and leiomyosarcomas. The enzyme activity was found to be slightly higher in leiomyomas and leiomyosarcomas as compared to that of normal smooth muscle tissue. No difference in pyruvate kinase activity was found between leiomyomas and leiomyosarcomas. In normal smooth muscle tissue, the larger part of pyruvate kinase consisted of K subunits distributed mainly between K_4 isozyme and the K_3M hybrid that were present in nearly equivalent proportions (Elbers *et al.*, 1990a). The total amount of K_4 as well as the total percentage of K subunits appeared to be decreased in leiomyomas as compared to normal smooth muscle tissue. These differences were found to be statistically significant. In leiomyosarcomas a significant shift in isozyme composition was observed, as compared to leiomyomas, favoring the expression of K subunits.

3. Rhabdomyosarcomas

Normal adult muscle expresses the M_4 type. In poorly differentiated rhabdomyosarcomas, no M_4 type can be detected, and K_4 mainly is found. In more differentiated rhabdomyosarcomas, both K_4 and M_4 with their hybrids are expressed (Cottreau et al., 1982). Staal et al. (1989) compared the pyruvate kinase isoenzyme pattern of three rhabdomyosarcomas with fetal skeletal muscle tissue of 19 and 23 weeks of gestation and with adult muscle. Two of the three neoplasms were poorly differentiated. The third one was more differentiated in microscopic characteristics. In the fetal tissues, five forms of pyruvate kinase isozymes were present with K_2M_2 as the predominant form. In adult muscle tissue, only M_4 was present. The tumors were characterized by a profound shift to the K type, whereas the M_4 type was not expressed at all. A difference in isozyme composition of pyruvate kinase was found between the morphologically less-differentiated tumors and the more-differentiated tumors; in the latter, more M subunits were expressed.

G. HEPATOMAS

The levels of pyruvate kinase were assayed in the cancerous and morphologically normal portions of livers from nine primary malignant hepatoma cases obtained at autopsy as well as in two normal human adult and two fetal livers (Balinsky et al., 1973). Pyruvate kinase activity was found to be statistically raised in hepatoma relative to the corresponding host tissue. In normal liver, type L pyruvate kinase predominates with only traces of type K. In hepatoma tissue, type K predominates, with type L faint or absent. In the host tissue both types L and K appeared to be present in approximately equal amounts (Balinsky et al., 1973; Hammond and Balinsky, 1978).

H. LUNG TUMORS

The isozyme patterns and activities of pyruvate kinase were examined in surgical samples of lung tumors and nonneoplastic pulmonary areas (Balinsky et al., 1984a). Electrophoretic analysis of lung tumors showed K_4 to be the major isozyme in all but 1 of 14 tumors examined. However, two thirds of the adult lung tissues also had K_4 as the major band. Tumors showed a threefold to fivefold increase in pyruvate kinase activity. Fetal lung tissue had lesser increases.

VI. Discussion

It is well established that malignant cells usually exhibit a high rate of glycolysis and an increased amino acid uptake, dependent on their growth rate. This may be favorable for tumor cells in terms of increased energy production and the supply of precursors for biosynthetic processes, although they also show increased lactate production when oxygen is adequately supplied. Increased glycolytic fluxes and the channeling of intermediates into metabolic-related pathways occur only if enzymes catalyzing individual steps through these routes are either increased in activity or altered in their regulatory properties. In this chapter we focused on pyruvate kinase as a key enzyme in glycolysis.

A. Pyruvate Kinase Activity

In Table I we summarize data obtained in our laboratory on the pyruvate kinase activity of several normal human tissues and derived human tumors. In most, but not all, tumors an increase in enzyme activity is observed, which tends to be correlated with progressively increasing malignancy. This observation is most obvious in tumors from breast and thyroid and in fibroblastic and lipoblastic proliferations, and is in line with the concept of increasing lactate production in cancer. However, tumors residing in tissues that are known to be glycolytically very active, such as brain, muscle, and retina, show decreased pyruvate kinase activities. Apparently in these tumors, glycolytic activity might be decreased. Remarkably, in these cases an isozyme shift occurs as well. In muscle and brain, the M type is the predominant form of pyruvate kinase, whereas in retina both K and M types are present in approximately equal proportions (Beemer *et al.*, 1982). In the corresponding tumors, a shift occurs toward the K type, which is the predominant isozyme in all tumors mentioned in Table I. The extent of this shift correlates with the degree of malignancy in brain tumors (van Veelen *et al.*, 1979); this observation has been exploited for diagnostic purposes (van Veelen *et al.*, 1988).

These findings raise the question of why the presence of K type could be favorable for the metabolism of a tumor, even when its specific activity is decreased with respect to the M type in the corresponding host tissue. Apparently, alterations in the regulation of enzyme activity are more important than the amount of enzyme present.

B. Biological Significance of the M-to-K Isozyme Shift

As mentioned earlier, type K pyruvate kinase has a lower affinity for its substrate phosphoenolpyruvate and is more strongly inhibited by amino acids such as alanine. At first glance this seems in conflict with the proposition of a high

TABLE I
MEAN ACTIVITY OF PYRUVATE KINASE IN NORMAL HUMAN TISSUES AND DERIVED NEOPLASIAS[a]

Normal tissue	Neoplasia	Pyruvate kinase activity (U/mg protein ± SEM)	Reference
Breast (13)		0.042 ± 0.006	Hennipman et al., 1987
	Fibrocystic breast disease (8)	0.17 ± 0.031	Hennipman et al., 1987
	Primary breast cancer (79)	0.98 ± 0.18	Hennipman et al., 1987
	Metastatic breast cancer (24)	1.28 ± 0.18	Hennipman et al., 1988
Thyroid (12)		0.14 ± 0.050	Verhagen et al., 1985
	Follicular thyroid adenoma (32)	0.29 ± 0.29	Verhagen et al., 1985
	Thyroid carcinoma (9)	0.94 ± 0.44	Verhagen et al., 1985
Brain, gray matter (2)		7.0	Van Veelen et al., 1978
Brain, white matter (2)		7.6	Van Veelen et al., 1978
Brain, fetal (2)		2.0	Van Veelen et al., 1978
	Neuroblastoma (9)	1.26 ± 0.84	Beemer et al., 1984
	Glioma (5)	1.90 ± 0.70	Van Veelen et al., 1978
	Meningioma (12)	1.94 ± 0.87	Van Veelen et al., 1978
	Glioma, child (8)	3.02 ± 1.41	Beemer et al., 1984

Retina (11)		4.2	Beemer et al., 1982
	Retinoblastoma (3)	1.86	Beemer et al., 1982
Muscle, striated (11)		6.6 ± 3.0	Own observations, unpublished
	Rhabdomyosarcoma (2)	2.50	Staal et al., 1982
Fibrous tissue (10)		0.26 ± 0.04	Elbers et al., 1990b
	Fibroma (3)	0.50 ± 0.09	Elbers et al., 1990b
	Fibromatosis (18)	0.53 ± 0.05	Elbers et al., 1990b
	Aggressive fibromatosis (10)	0.55 ± 0.06	Elbers et al., 1990b
	Fibrosarcoma (9)	1.60 ± 0.40	Elbers et al., 1990b
	Malignant fibrous histiocytoma (17)	2.37 ± 0.42	Elbers et al., 1990b
Smooth muscle (12)		0.81 ± 0.06	Elbers et al., 1990a
	Leiomyoma (20)	1.06 ± 0.28	Elbers et al., 1990a
	Leiomyosarcoma (21)	1.05 ± 0.19	Elbers et al., 1990a
Fatty tissue (14)		0.22 ± 0.02	Elbers et al., 1990c
	Lipoma (14)	0.32 ± 0.08	Elbers et al., 1990c
	Liposarcoma (12)	0.79 ± 0.23	Elbers et al., 1990c

[a]The number of samples is shown in parentheses.

glycolytic flux in tumor cells. However, it only means that the enzyme need higher levels of substrate to support the same flux. As a result, the presence of K-type pyruvate kinase assures higher steady-state levels of phosphoenolpyruvate and other glycolytic metabolites upstream of phosphoenolpyruvate, while at the same time the net lactate production is not necessarily different from a situation in which M type is present. This damming up of glycolytic metabolites enables increased channeling into three synthetic pathways: serine synthesis from glycerate 3-phosphate; phospholipid, triglyceride, and sphingomyelin synthesis from glycerol 3-phosphate; and ribose 5-phosphate for phosphoribosylpyrophosphate synthesis, ultimately leading to increased purine and pyrimidine synthesis (Eigenbrodt et al., 1985).

A second property in which K type distinguishes itself from M-type pyruvate kinase is its ability to become phosphorylated. As mentioned before, the difference in the primary structure of M- and K-type isozymes resides in a region of only 45 amino acids. This region has been shown to be important for subunit interaction and does not contain sequences belonging to either catalytic sites or a phosphorylation site. Probably the same reasoning explaining kinetic differences between K and M types can be used to explain the difference in the ability to become phosphorylated: a loss of cooperativity between the subunits together with conformational changes along the enzyme molecule abolish the ability of the M type to become phosphorylated. Recent experiments in our laboratory (Oude Weernink et al., unpublished) have shown that in the absence of fructose 1,6-diphosphate, the K-type enzyme from the lung is present as a dimer and is readily phosphorylated. In the same sample and under the same condition, the M type is present as a tetramer and is not phosphorylated. This finding again argues for the importance of subunit interaction in the regulation of phosphorylation. At the same time this experiment shows that the presence or absence of the protein kinase involved is not a determining factor.

It is attractive to hypothesize on the effects of phosphorylation on the properties of the enzyme. It has been suggested that in analogy to the L-type pyruvate kinase, the K type becomes inactivated on phosphorylation in terms of decreased substrate affinity and increased inhibition by allosteric inhibitors (Eigenbrodt et al., 1985). Such a change of kinetic parameters would nicely fit into a hypothesis as proposed above, resulting in the damming up of glycolytic intermediates to be used as precursors for various biosynthetic pathways. Indeed, transformation of chicken embryo cells by Rous sarcoma virus results in phosphorylation of pyruvate kinase type K on a tyrosine residue, accompanied by inactivation of the enzyme (Presek et al., 1980; Glossmann et al., 1981; Presek et al., 1988). However, the sites of phosphorylation of pyruvate kinase in human and rat tumors appear to be serine and threonine (Rijksen et al., 1988; Oude Weernink et al., 1990), which precludes comparison with the studies on Rous sarcoma virus–transformed cells. Consequently, the effects of phosphorylation on K-type pyruvate kinase from mammalian tissues remain to be demonstrated. However, similar to the L-type pyruvate kinase, the phosphorylation of the K type could be completely inhibited by fructose 1,6-diphosphate (Oude Weernink *et al.*, 1990), suggesting a potentially similar physiological meaning of the phosphorylation reaction. An argument against a role for phosphorylation in regulating enzyme activity by altering the kinetic properties is governed by the very low stoichiometry of the incorporation of phosphate. In *in vitro* experiments less than 1% of the enzyme molecules become phosphorylated. Although one has to realize that in such studies only a turnover of phosphorylated residues is measured, it has to be expected that *in vivo* only a small amount of enzyme molecules are phosphorylated as well. Kinetic differences induced in such a small proportion of the enzyme are not expected to cause large metabolic changes unless that proportion has a special spatial organization within the cytoplasm. In that respect, it is interesting to note that in rat glioma cells, 8% of the pyruvate kinase activity was found to be loosely associated with the plasma membrane (Daum *et al.*, 1988).

Alternatively, phosphorylation or dephosphorylation of K-type pyruvate kinase may be hypothesized to function as a flag to mark the enzyme for proteolytic degradation. Using a model peptide representing the phosphorylation site of pyruvate kinase, Benore-Parsons *et al.* (1989) showed that phosphorylation of the peptide rendered it far less susceptible to proteolytic attack by trypsin-like enzymes at sequences adjacent to the phosphorylation site. In contrast, in earlier studies Bergström *et al.* (1978) showed that L-type pyruvate kinase was 10-fold more sensitive *in vitro* to proteolytic attack in the phosphorylated form than in the unphosphorylated form. It may be concluded from these studies that phosphorylation–dephosphorylation may play a role in the long-term regulation of enzyme activity by selectively influencing protein processing and turnover. Phosphorylation is implicated as a regulator of turnover of several other proteins and may either decrease or increase the susceptibility to proteolysis (Benore-Parsons *et al.*, 1989). To date, however, experimental evidence supporting the involvement of such a mechanism in the regulation of K-type pyruvate kinase activity *in vivo* is still lacking.

C. K-type Pyruvate Kinase in Normal and Malignant Tissues

The K type is the prototype isozyme in both normal and malignant proliferating cells. Since the K type is also expressed in some adult normal tissues, no tumor-specific pyruvate kinase exists, although K type is expressed in all tumors. However, one may wonder whether different properties can be ascribed to tumor-derived and normal K type. Most reports on the enzyme from both sources do not provide any evidence for fundamental differences. Some authors claim the presence of a tumor-specific isozyme with a higher electrophoretic mobility than the normal K-type isozyme (Marchut *et al.*, 1988; Guminska *et al.*, 1989). This tumor-specific pyruvate kinase is selectively inhibited by L-cysteine. However, these authors use their own nomenclature to describe the various isozymic forms of pyruvate kinase and fail to connect it with more commonly used nomenclatures. They especially neglect the presence of tetrameric hybrids of M and K subunits. Moreover, it is not shown that K_4 isozyme purified from normal tissue and freed from other homotetrameric and heterotetrameric isozymes is not inhibited by L-cysteine under the conditions used in their studies. Although K-type pyruvate kinase is present in both normal and malignant tissues, the isoenzyme shift found in some kinds of tumors is nevertheless of diagnostic importance: (1) the isozyme shift in hemispheric gliomas of adults is well correlated with the histological differentiation and postoperative survival after macroscopic, total, or subtotal resection; (2) the shift can be rapidly demonstrated with the alanine-inhibition assay and fits well within the scope of a surgical procedure, and (3) since macroscopic normal brain surrounding a tumor may still harbor tumor cells, this assay may also be helpful in detecting tumor tissue in apparently normal brain tissue.

It should be noted that the alanine-inhibition assay is done on whole cytosolic extracts and obviously does not provide information about the expression of pyruvate kinase in individual cells. Consequently, it is unable to identify cell types for which expression of K-type pyruvate kinase serves as an oncodevelopmental marker. By immunohistochemical studies using a monoclonal antibody specific for the K type (van Erp *et al.*, 1988), it is possible to discriminate between the proliferation of tumors derived from cells that already contain the K type and cells with an altered gene expression of pyruvate kinase. Recent immunohistochemical studies in our laboratory (van Erp *et al.*, unpublished) have shown that both normal astrocytes and astrocytomas express the K type. Consequently, the gene expression in astrocytomas is not really altered. In contrast, the isozyme shift observed in rhabdomyosarcomas really represent altered gene expression, since cross-striated muscle cells predominantly contain the M type.

VII. Concluding Remarks

In this chapter we showed that the K-type isozyme of pyruvate kinase is the predominant form in all types of malignancies regardless of the isozyme composition of the cells from which these malignancies are derived. The presence of this particular isozyme provides the cell with metabolic advantages most probably aimed at supplying the cell with sufficient precursors for several metabolic pathways. In tumors residing in tissues that predominantly express the M type, the extent of the appearance of the K type can be exploited for diagnostic purposes.

In some tumors, the enzyme activity is increased dependent on the grade of malignancy. In others, most notably those derived from tissues expression the M-type isozyme, enzyme activity is decreased, indicating that alterations in enzyme properties are more important than the enzyme activity as measured *in vitro*.

References

Balinsky, D., Cayanis, E., Geddes, E. W., and Bersoku, O. (1973). Activities and isoenzyme patterns of some enzymes of glucose metabolism in human primary malignant hepatoma. *Cancer Res.* **33**, 249–255.

Balinsky, D., Platz, C. E., and Lewis, J. W. (1983). Isozyme patterns of normal, benign, and malignant human breast tissues. *Cancer Res.* **43**, 5895–5901.

Balinsky, D., Greengard, D., Cayanis, E., and Head, J. F. (1984a). Enzyme activities and isozyme patterns in human lung tumors. *Cancer Res.* **44**, 1058–1062.

Balinsky, D., Platz, C. E., and Lewis, J. W. (1984b). Enzyme activities in normal, dysplastic, and cancerous human breast tissues. *J. Natl. Cancer Inst.* **72**, 217–224.

Beemer, F.A., Vlug, A. M. C., Rijksen, G., Hamburg, A., and Staal, G. E. J. (1982). Characterization of some glycolytic enzymes from human retina and retinoblastoma. *Cancer Res.* **42**, 4228–4232.

Beemer, F. A., Vlug, A. M. C., Rousseau-Merck, M. F., Van Veelen, C. W. M., Rijksen, G., and Staal, G. E. J. (1984). Glycolytic enzymes from human neuroectodermal tumors of childhood. *Eur. J. Cancer Clin. Oncol.* **20**, 253–259.

Beemer, F. (1986). Characterization of some glycolytic enzymes from human retina, retinoblastoma, neuroblastoma, and medulloblastoma. In "Markers of Human Neuroectodermal Tumors" (G. E. J. Staal and C. W. M. van Veelen, eds.), pp. 85–96, CRC Press, Boca Raton, Florida.

Bennett, M. J., Timperley, W. R., Taylor, C. B. and Hill, A. S. (1975). Fetal forms of pyruvate kinase isozymes in tumors of the human nervous system. *Neuropathol. Appl. Neurobiol.* **1**, 347–356.

Benore-Parsons, M., Seidah, N. G., and Wennogle, L. P. (1989). Substrate phosphorylation can inhibit proteolysis by trypsin-like enzymes. *Arch. Biochem. Biophys.* **272**, 274–280.

Bergström, G., Ekman, P., Humble, E., and Engström, L. (1978). Proteolytic modification of pig and rat liver pyruvate kinase type L including phosphorylatable site. *Biochim. Biophys. Acta* **532**, 259–267.

Carminatti, H., Jimenez de Asua, L., Recondo, E., Passeron, S., and Rozengurt, F. (1968). Some kinetic properties of liver pyruvate kinase (type L). *J. Biol. Chem.* **243**, 3051–3056.

Cognet, M., Lone, Y.C., Vaulont, S., Kahn, A., and Marie, J. (1987). Structure of the rat L-type pyruvate kinase gene. *J. Mol. Biol.* **196**, 11–25.

Consler, T. G., Woodard, S. H., and Lee, J. C. (1989). Effects of primary sequence differences on the global structure and function of an enzyme: A study of pyruvate kinase isozymes. *Biochemistry* **28**, 8756–8764.

Cottreau, B., Rousseau-Merck, M. F., Nezelof, C., and Kahn, A. (1982). Pyruvate kinase and phosphofructokinase isozymes in childhood cancer. *Pediatr. Res.* **16**, 199–202.

Daum, G., Keller, K., and Lange, K. (1988). Association of glycolytic enzymes with the cytoplasmic side of the plasma membrane of glioma cell. *Biochim. Biophys. Acta* **939**, 277–281.

Eigenbrodt, E., Fister, P., Reinacher, M. (1985). New perspectives on carbohydrate metabolism in tumor cells. *In* "Regulation of Carbohydrate Metabolism" (R. Beitner, ed.) Vol. II., pp. 141–180, CRC Press, Boca Raton, Florida.

Ekman, P., Dahlquist, U., Humble, E., and Engström, L. (1976). Comparative kinetic studies on the L-type pyruvate kinase from rat liver and the enzyme phosphorylated by cyclic 3′,5′-AMP–stimulated protein kinase. *Biochim. Biophys. Acta* **429**, 374–382.

Elbers, J. R. J., Rijksen, G., Staal, G. E. J., Van Unnik, J. A. M., Roholl, P. J. M., Van Oirschot, B. A., and Oosting, J. (1990a). Activity of glycolytic enzymes and glucose-6-phosphate dehydrogenase in smooth muscle proliferations. *Tumour Biol.* **11**, 210–219.

Elbers, J. R. J., Van Unnik, J. A. M., Rijksen, G., Van Oirschot, B. A., Roholl, P. J. M., Oosting, J., and Staal, G. E. J. (1990b). Pyruvate kinase activity and isozyme composition in normal fibrous tissue and fibroblastic proliferations. *Cancer,* in press.

Elbers, J. R. J., Van Unnik, J. A. M., Rijksen, G., Roholl, P. J. M., Van Oirschot, B. A., and Staal, G. E. J. (1990c). Activity of glycolytic enzymes and glucose-6-phosphate dehydrogenase in lipoblastic and neurogenic proliferations. *Tumour Biol.* **11**, 262–273.

Fister, P., Eigenbrodt, E., Presek, P., Reinacher, M., and Schoner, W. (1983). Pyruvate kinase type M_2 is phosphorylated in the intact chicken liver cell. *Biochem. Biophys. Res. Commun.* **115**, 409–414.

Glossmann, H., Presek, P., and Eigenbrodt, E. (1981) Association of the src-gene product of Rous sarcoma virus with a pyruvate kinase inactivating factor. *Mol. Cell. Endocrinol.* **23**, 49–63.

Guminska, M., Stachurska, M. B., and Ignacak, J. (1988). Pyruvate kinase isoenzymes in chromatin extracts of Ehrlich ascites tumour, Morris hepatoma 7777, and normal mouse and rat livers. *Biochim. Biophys. Acta* **966**, 207–213.

Guminska, M., Stachurska, M. B., Christensen, B., Tromholt, V., Kieler, J., Radzikowski, C., and Dus, D. (1989). Pyruvate kinase inhibited by L-cysteine as a marker of tumorigenic human urothelial cell lines. *Experientia* **45**, 571–574.

Hammond, K. D., and Balinsky, D. (1978). Isozyme studies of several enzymes of carbohydrate metabolism and cell cultures. *Cancer Res.* **38**, 1323–1328.

Hennipman, A., Smits, J., Van Oirschot, B., Van Houwelingen, J. C., Rijksen, G., Neyt, J. P., Van Unnik, J. A. M., and Staal, G. E. J. (1987). Glycolytic enzymes in breast cancer, benign breast disease, and normal breast tissue. *Tumour Biol.* **8**, 251–263.

Hennipman, A., Van Oirschot, B. A., Smits, J., Rijksen, G., and Staal, G. E. J. (1988). Glycolytic enzyme activities in breast cancer metastases. *Tumour Biol.* **9**, 241–248.

Hers, H. G., and Van Schaftingen, E. (1982). Fructose 2,6-biphosphate 2 years after discovery. *Biochem. J.* **206**, 1–12.

Hilf, R., Witliff, J. L, Rector, W. D., Savlov, E. C., Hall, T. C., Orlando, R. A. (1973). Studies on certain cytoplasmic enzymes and specific estrogen receptors in human breast cancer and in nonmalignant tissues of the breast. *Cancer Res.* **33**, 2054–2062.

Hjelmquist, G. Andersson, J., Edlund, B., and Engström, L. (1974). Amino acid sequence of a (32p) phosphopeptide from pig liver pyruvate kinase phosphorylated by cyclic 3′,5′,-AMP–stimulated protein kinase and gamma-(32P)ATP. *Biochem. Biophys. Res. Commun.* **61**, 559–563.

Ibsen, H. I., and Fishman, W. H. (1979). Developmental gene expression in cancer. *Biochim. Biophys. Acta* **560**, 243–280.

Ibsen, K. H., Orlando, R. A., Garratt, K. N., Hernandez, A. M., Giorlando, S., Nungaray, G. (1982). Expression of multimolecular forms of pyruvate kinase in normal, benign, and malignant human breast tissue. *Cancer Res.* **42**, 888–892.

Imamura, K., Taniuchi, K., and Tanaka, T. (1972). Multimolecular forms of pyruvate kinase II. Purification of M_2-type pyruvate kinase from Yoshida ascites hepatoma 130 cells and comparative studies on the enzymological and immunological properties of the three types of pyruvate kinase, L, M, and M_2. *J. Biochem.* **71**, 1001–1015.

Imamura, K., Noguchi, T., and Tanaka, T. (1986). Regulation of isozyme patterns of pyruvate kinase in normal and neoplastic tissues. In "Markers of Human Neuroectodermal Tumors" (G. E. J. Staal and C. W. M. van Veelen, eds.), pp. 191–222, CRC Press, Boca Raton, Florida.

Jimenez de Asua, L., Rozengurt, E., De Valle, J. J., and Carminatti, H. (1971). Some kinetic differences between the M isoenzymes of pyruvate kinase from liver and muscle. *Biochim. Biophys. Acta* **235**, 326–334.

Kahn, A., Marie, J., Galand, C., and Boivin, P. (1976). Chronic haemolytic anemia in two patients heterozygous for erythrocyte pyruvate kinase deficiency. Electrofocusing and immunological studies of erythrocyte and liver pyruvate kinase. *Scand. J. Haematol.* **16**, 250–257.

Kahn, A., Marie, J., Garreau, H., and Sprengers, E. D. (1978). The genetic system of the L-type pyruvate kinase forms in man. *Biochim. Biophys. Acta* **523**, 59–74.

Kraayenhagen, R. J., Van der Heijden, M. C. M., Streefkerk, M., Rijksen, G., De Gast, G. C., and Staal, G. E. J. (1982). Isozyme patterns of glycolytic regulator enzymes in T- and B-lymphoblastic cell lines, compared with T- and non-T-lymphocytes from peripheral blood. *Hum. Lymphocyte Diff.* **1**, 241–250.

Kraayenhagen, R. J., De Gast, G. C., Van der Heijden, M. C. M., Streefkerk, M., Gmelig-Meijling, F. H. J., Rijksen, G., and Staal, G. E. J. (1985). Isozyme distribution of hexokinase, phosphofructokinase, and pyruvate kinase in lymphocytes from patients with chronic lymphocytic leukemia. *Clin. Chim. Acta* **124**, 91–101.

Levin, M. J., Daegelen, V. D., Meienhofer, M. C. Dreyfus, J. L., and Kahn, A. (1982). Two different species of messenger RNAs specify synthesis of M_1 and M_2 pyruvate kinase subunits. *Biochim. Biophys. Acta* **699**, 77–83.

Ljungström, O., Hjelmquist, G., and Engström, L. (1974). Phosphorylation of purified rat liver pyruvate kinase by cyclic 3',5'-AMP–stimulated protein kinase. *Biochim. Biophys. Acta* **358**, 280–298.

Lopez-Alarcon, L., Ruiz, P., and Gosalvez, M. (1981). Quantitative determination of the degree of differentiation of mammary tumors by pyruvate kinase kinetic analysis. *Cancer Res.* **41**, 2019–2020.

MacDonald, M. J., and Kowluru, A. (1985). Evidence for calcium-enhanced phosphorylation of pyruvate kinase by pancreatic islets. *Mol. Cell. Biochem.* **68**, 107–114.

Marchut, E., Guminkska, M., Kedryna, T., Radzikowski, C., and Kusnierczyk, H. (1988). A pyruvate kinase variant in different mouse transplanted tumors. *Experientia* **44**, 25–27.

Marie, J., and Kahn, A. (1980). Proteolytic processing of human L-type pyruvate kinase increases its ability to be phosphorylated. *Biochem. Biophys. Res. Commun.* **94**, 1387–1391.

Marie, J., Simon, M. P., Dreyfus, J. C., and Kahn, A. (1981). One gene, but two messenger RNAs encode liver L and red cell L pyruvate kinase subunits. *Nature* **292**, 70–73.

Marie, J., Simon, M. P., Lone, Y. C., Cognet, M., and Kahn, A. (1986). Tissue-specific heterogeneity of the 3'-untranslated region of L-type pyruvate kinase mRNAs. *Eur. J. Biochem.* **158**, 33–41.

Market, C., and Möller, G. (1959). Multiple forms of enzymes: Ontogenic and species specific patterns. *Proc. Natl. Acad. Sci. U.S.A.* **45**, 753–763.

Muirhead, H., Clayden, D. A., Barford, D., Lorimer, C. G., Fothergill-Gilmore, L. A., Schiltz, E., and Schmitt, W. (1986). The structure of cat muscle pyruvate kinase. *EMBO J.* **5**, 475–481.

Muroya, N., Nago, Y., Miyasaki, K., Nishikawa, K., and Horio, T. (1976). Pyruvate kinase isozymes in various tissues of rat and increase in spleen type pyruvate kinase in liver by injecting chromatins from spleen and tumor. *J. Biochem.* **79**, 203–215.

Noguchi, T., and Tanaka, T. (1982). The M_1 and M_2 subunits of rat pyruvate kinase are encoded by different messenger RNAs. *J. Biol. Chem.* **257**, 1110–1113.

Noguchi, T., Inoue, H., and Tanaka, T. (1986). The M_1- and M_2-types isozymes of rat pyruvate kinase are produced from the same gene by alternative RNA splicing. *J. Biol. Chem.* **261**, 13807–13812.

Noguchi, T., (1987). The L- and R-type isozymes of rat pyruvate kinase are produced from a single gene by use of different promoters. *J. Biol. Chem.* **262**, 14366–14371.

Oude Weernink, P. A., Rijksen, G., and Staal, G. E. J. (1988). Production of a specific antibody against pyruvate kinase type M_2 using a synthetic peptide. *FEBS Lett.* **236**, 391–395.

Oude Weernink, P. A., Rijksen, G., Van der Heijden, M. C. M., and Staal, G. E. J. (1990). Phosphorylation of pyruvate kinase type K in human gliomas by a cyclic AMP-independent protein kinase, *Cancer Res.* **50**, 4604–4610.

Palmer, J. O., Kasselber, A. G., and Netsky, M. G. (1981). Differentiation of medulloblastoma. Studies including immunohistochemical localization of glial fibrillary acidic protein. *J. Neurosurg.* **55**, 161–169.

Pilkis, W. J., Pilkis, J., and Claus, T. H. (1978). The effect of fructose diphosphate and phosphoenol-pyruvate on cyclic AMP–mediated inactivation on rat hepatic pyruvate kinase. *Biochem. Biophys. Res. Commun.* **81**, 139–146.

Presek, P., Glossmann, H., Eigenbrodt, E., Schoner, W., Rübsamen, H., Fris, R. R., and Bauer, H. (1980). Similarities between a phosphoprotein (pp60^src)-associated protein kinase of Rous sarcoma virus and a cyclic AMP–independent protein kinase that phosphorylates pyruvate kinase type M_2. *Cancer Res.* **40**, 1733–1741.

Presek, P., Reinacker, M., and Eigenbrodt, E. (1988). Pyruvate kinase type M_2 is phosphorylated at tyrosine residues in cells transformed by Rous sarcoma virus. *FEBS Lett.* **242**, 194–198.

Rijksen, G., Van der Heijden, M. C. M., Oskam, R., and Staal, G. E. J. (1988). Subunit-specific phosphorylation of pyruvate kinase medullary thyroid carcinomas of the rat. *FEBS Lett.* **233**, 69–73.

Rozengurt, E., Jimenez de Asua, L., and Carminatti, H. (1969). Some kinetic properties of liver pyruvate kinase (type-L) II. Effect of pH on its allosteric behaviour. *J. Biol. Chem.* **244**, 3142–3247.

Rozengurt, E., Jimenez de Asua, L., and Carminatti, H. (1970). Allosteric inhibition of muscle pyruvate kinase by phenylalanine. *REBS Lett.* **11**, 284–286.

Saheki, S., Saheki, K., and Tanaka, T. (1982). Peptide structures of pyruvate kinase isozymes. I. Comparison of the four pyruvate kinase isozymes of the rat. *Biochim. Biophys. Acta* **704**, 484–493.

Schapira, F. (1981). Resurgence of fetal isozymes in cancer: Study of aldolase, pyruvate kinase, lactic dehydrogenase, and hexosaminidase. *Curr. Top. Biol. Med. Res.* **5**, 27–75.

Sprengers, E. D., and Staal, G. E. J. (1979). Functional changes associated with the sequential transformation of L_4^i into L_4 pyruvate kinase. *Biochim. Biophys. Acta* **570**, 259–270.

Staal, G. E. J., and Rijksen, G. (1985). Regulation of pyruvate kinase in normal and pathological condition. In "Regulation of Carbohydrate Metabolism" (R. Beitner, ed.), Vol. I, pp. 143–160, CRC Press, Boca Raton, Florida.

Staal, G. E. J., Koster, J. F., Kamp, H., Van Milligen-Boersma, L., and Veeger, C. (1971). Human erythrocyte pyruvate kinase, its purification, and some properties. *Biochim. Biophys. Acta* **227**, 86–96.

Staal, G. E. J., Rijksen, G., Vlug, A. M. C., Vromen-Van den Bos, B., Akkerman, J. W. N., Gorter, G., Dierick, J., and Petermans, M. (1982). Extreme deficiency of L-type pyruvate kinase with moderate clinical expression. *Clin. Chim. Acta* **118**, 241–253.

Staal, G. E. J., Rijksen, G., Van Oirschot, B. A., and Roholl, P. J. M. (1989). Characterization of pyruvate kinase from human rhabdomyosarcoma in relation to immunohistochemical and morphological criteria. *Cancer* **63**, 479–483.

Stuart, D. I., Levine, M., Muirhead, H., and Stammers, D. K. (1979). Crystal structure of cat muscle pyruvate kinase at a resolution of 2.6 A. *J. Mol. Biol.* **134**, 109–142.

Tanaka, T., Harano, Y., Sue, F., and Morimura, H. (1967). Crystallization, characterization, and metabolic regulation of two types of pyruvate kinase isolated from rat tissues. *J. Biochem.* **62**, 71–91.

Titanji, V. P. K., Zetterquist, D., and Engström, L. (1976). Regulation *in vitro* of rat liver pyruvate kinase by phosphorylation-dephosphorylation reaction, catalyzed by cyclic-AMP-dependent protein kinases and a histone phosphatase. *Biochim. Biophys. Acta* **422**, 98–108.

Tremp, G. L., Boquet, J., Kahn, A., and Doegelen, D. (1989). Expression of the rat L-type pyruvate kinase gene from its dual erythroid- and liver-specific promoter in transgenic mice. *J. Biol. Chem.* **264**, 19904–19910.

Van Berkel, Th. J. C., and Koster, J. F. (1973). M-type pyruvate kinase of leukocytes: An allosteric enzyme. *Biochem. Biophys. Acta* **293**, 134–139.

Van Erp, H. E., Roholl, P. J. M., Rijksen, G., Sprengers, E. D., Van Veelen, C. W. M. and Staal, G. E. J. (1988). Production and characterization of monoclonal antibodies against human type K pyruvate kinase. *Eur. J. Cell Bio.* **47**, 388–394.

Van Veelen, C. W. M., and Staal, G. E, J. (1986). Pyruvate kinase and human brain tumors. *In* "Markers of Human Neuroectodermal Tumors" (G. E. J. Staal and C. W. M. van Veelen, eds.), pp. 63–84, CRC Press, Boca Raton, Florida.

Van Veelen, C. W. M., Verbiest, H., Vlug, A. M. C., Rijksen, G., and Staal, G. E. J. (1978). Isozymes of pyruvate kinase from human brain, meningiomas, and malignant gliomas. *Cancer Res.* **38**, 4681–4687.

Van Veelen, C. W. M., Verbiest, H., Zülch, K. J., Van Ketel, B. A., Van der Vlist, M. J. M., Vlug, A. M. C., Rijksen, G., and Staal, G. E. J. (1979). L-α-alanine inhibition of pyruvate kinase from tumors of the human central nervous system. *Cancer Res.* **39**, 4263–4269.

Van Veelen, C. W. M., Rijksen, G., Vlug, A. M. C., and Staal, G. E. J. (1981). Correlation between alanine inhibition of pyruvate kinase and composition of K-M hybrids. *Clin. Chim. Acta* **110**, 113–120.

Van Veelen, C. W. M., Verbiest, H., Zülch, K. J., van Ketel, B., Van der Vlist, M. J. M., Vlug, A. M. C., Rijksen, G., and Staal, G. E. J. (1982). Pyruvate kinase in human brain tumours. Its significance in the treatment of gliomas. *Acta Neurochir. (Wien)* **61**, 145–159.

Van Veelen, C. W. M., Rijksen, G., Van Ketel B. A., and Staal, G. E. J. (1988). The pyruvate isoenzyme shift in human gliomas: A potential marker in treatment of gliomas. *Br. J. Neurosurg.* **2**, 257–263.

Verhagen, J. N., van der Heijden, M. C. M., De Jong-van Dijken, J., Rijksen, G., Der Kinderen, P. J., Van Unnik, J. A. M., and Staal, G. E. J. (1985). Pyruvate kinase in normal human thyroid tissue and thyroid neoplasms. *Cancer* **55**, 142–148.

Weinhouse, S. (1973). Metabolism and isozyme alterations in experimental hepatomas. *Fed. Proc.* **32**, 2162–2167.

Weinhouse, S. (1982). What are isozymes telling us about gene regulation in cancer. *J. Natl. Cancer Inst.* **68**, 343–349.

Chapter 11

Biochemical Basis for Multidrug Resistance in Cancer

MICHAEL M. GOTTESMAN,* PATRICIA V. SCHOENLEIN,* STEPHEN J. CURRIER,*
EDWARD P. BRUGGEMANN,† AND IRA PASTAN†

*Laboratory of Cell Biology and †Laboratory of Molecular Biology, National Cancer
Institute, National Institutes of Health, Bethesda, Maryland 20892

I. Introduction

The strategy of treating human cancers with many different cytotoxic drugs
with diverse mechanisms of action was predicated on the assumption that development of resistance to any one class of drugs would not result in resistance to
other classes of chemotherapeutic agents. Thus, it should be possible to cure
human cancers by combining anticancer agents, each of which would kill a substantial fraction of surviving cancer cells until there were either no cancer cells
remaining in the body, or so few that they could be handled by normal host
defenses. This strategy has been successful in the cure of several human cancers
including childhood acute lymphocytic leukemia, Hodgkin's disease, and testicular cancer.

Unfortunately, it appears that it is possible for many human cancers to express intrinsically or develop simultaneous resistance to several classes of anticancer drugs, each with different mechanisms of action. This phenomenon, which can be mimicked in tissue culture cells selected for resistance to anticancer drugs, is known as multidrug resistance (Gottesman and Pastan, 1988; Endicott and Ling, 1989; Pastan and Gottesman, 1990). Recent evidence indicates that there are many kinds of multidrug resistance, each of which results in crossresistance to several different anticancer drugs.

How is it possible to develop crossresistance in a single step to drugs that have different mechanisms of action? In theory, there are several ways in which this can occur including (1) decreased permeability to drugs with similar transport mechanisms; (2) increased metabolism or altered covalent modification such as by the cytochrome P450 system or glutathione S-transferase; (3) alterations in cellular physiology, such as changes in pH or ionic environment that affect the activity of different classes of drugs; and (4) increased active extrusion of drugs. This latter mechanism, the energy-dependent efflux of many different classes of natural product drugs, is a common means by which cancer cells become resistant to chemotherapy. This mechanism for crossresistance to anticancer agents is the topic of this chapter.

A. Multidrug Transporter

Cells selected in tissue culture for resistance to one anticancer drug such as an anthracycline (daunomycin, doxorubicin), *Vinca* alkaloid (vinblastine, vincristine), epipodophyllotoxin (etoposide, teniposide), actinomycin D, or taxol, are frequently crossresistant to all these drugs, as well as to other cytotoxic natural products, such as colchicine, puromycin, emetine, and gramicidin D. Although the chemistry of these agents is very different, they are all relatively hydrophobic natural products, with planar ring structures and a positive charge at neutral pH. When mutant cell lines exhibiting this pattern of multidrug resistance are isolated (see Section II for details), they express an energy-dependent mechanism that keeps the intracellular accumulation of the drug low. This mechanism is an active extrusion of the drug, which had originally entered through the plasma membrane (Fojo *et al.*, 1985a; Willingham *et al.*, 1986).

The gene encoding this pump system, or multidrug transporter, has been cloned from tissue culture cells in which it is expressed at high levels (Chen *et al.*, 1986; Gros *et al.*, 1986b; Scotto *et al.*, 1987; Gerlach *et al.*, 1986). The protein product of the gene, generally known as P-glycoprotein, is a 170,000 dalton plasma membrane glycoprotein. As described in Section III, the primary structure of the transporter encoded by the *MDR1* gene in the human, and the *mdr1a* and *mdr1b* genes in the mouse, has been deduced from their nucleotide sequence, and a model of their structure in the plasma membrane has been proposed (Chen *et al.*, 1986; Gros *et al.*, 1986b). Either the human or mouse transporter is sufficient to confer the complete phenotype of multidrug resistance on drug-sensitive cells, as indicated by studies involving transfection or retroviral infection of full-length cDNAs (Gros *et al.*, 1986a; Ueda *et al.*, 1987; Guild *et al.*, 1988; Pastan *et al.*, 1988). Plasma membrane vesicles from multidrug-resistant cells are able to transport drugs in an energy-dependent manner (Horio *et al.*, 1988).

B. Expression of Multidrug Transporter in Normal Tissues

The existence in cancer cells of a multidrug transporter for anticancer drugs was at first rather perplexing. It was necessary to determine where this transport system was normally expressed in order to gain insight into its normal function. Studies in which *MDR1* mRNA expression was detected by nucleic acid hybridization techniques (Fojo *et al.*, 1987), or P-glycoprotein was localized by immunohistochemistry (Thiebaut *et al.*, 1987), indicate a consistent pattern of expression in human tissues. The bulk of P-glycoprotein in the human is found on the apical surfaces of epithelial cells lining the small and large intestine, on the biliary face of hepatocytes, and on the brush border of kidney proximal tubules. This localization is consistent with a normal transport function for the multidrug transporter in moving hydrophobic natural products into the bile, urine, and lumen of the gastrointestinal tract. The origin of such compounds could be endogenous metabolism or contaminants in a normal human diet, which includes many toxic plant and fungal products. The idea that P-glycoprotein found on the apical surface of epithelial cells can facilitate transepithelial transport of hydrophobic drugs is supported by an experimental study in which P-glycoprotein introduced by retroviral infection into canine kidney (MDCK) cells is expressed on the apical surface of these cells, resulting in transepithelial transport of drugs across MDCK monolayers (Horio *et al.*, 1989).

Several other tissues also express P-glycoprotein, including capillary endothelial cells of the brain and testes (Cordon-Cardo *et al.*, 1989; Thiebaut *et al.*, 1989), and adrenal cortex (Thiebaut *et al.*, 1987). The capillary endothelial localizations are also consistent with a transport function, perhaps to protect the brain and testes from toxic natural products. The expression in the adrenal cortex suggests possible involvement in handling steroids or steroid metabolites.

The tissue-specific expression of the *MDR1* gene indicates that levels of *MDR1* RNA may be regulated in mammals. Although very little is known about the factors that determine basal expression in different tissues, a few studies have demonstrated increases in RNA levels for P-glycoprotein after cytotoxic stress such as heat shock (Chin *et al.*, 1990), treatment with chemotherapeutic drugs

(Chin *et al.*, 1990), and partial hepatectomy (Thorgeirrson *et al.*, 1987; Marino *et al.*, 1990). These RNA increases are not associated with proportionate increases in transcription as measured by nuclear run-off, suggesting that mRNA turnover may control *mdr* RNA levels in many cases. These studies demonstrating increased P-glycoprotein mRNA levels in response to cell injury support a role for P-glycoprotein in protecting cells against damage by toxic natural products.

C. Expression of Multidrug Transporter in Human Cancer

The demonstration of an efflux pump system for anticancer drugs in selected, cultured cancer cells does not prove its expression or function in human cancers. Many recent studies have demonstrated expression of *MDR1* RNA in drug-resistant human cancer. Cancers of the colon, kidney, liver, adrenal, and pancreas, which are generally drug-resistant, express levels of *MDR1* RNA equivalent to levels found in fourfold to sixfold multidrug-resistant tissue culture cells (Goldstein *et al.*, 1989). Similar levels of expression are found in a minority of human leukemias and lymphomas before chemotherapy, and in higher percentages of treated leukemias, lymphomas, neuroblastomas, and cancers of the ovary and breast from patients who have received chemotherapy. Thus, expression of the *MDR1* gene is found at high levels in cancers derived from tissues that normally express this gene (e.g., kidney, intestine, liver, pancreas, and adrenal). *MDR1* RNA is found less frequently in cancers derived from cells that do not normally express the *MDR1* gene, either as a sporadic event, perhaps related to the process of malignant transformation, or following selection *in vivo* with anticancer drugs. Since the bone marrow of transgenic mice that express the human *MDR1* cDNA at similar levels to the *MDR1* positive tumors is drug-resistant (Galski *et al.*, 1989), it seems reasonable to conclude that expression of the *MDR1* gene in a large variety of human cancers does contribute to their clinical drug-resistance. Therefore, a complete understanding of the biochemistry and molecular biology of the multidrug transporter is an important priority for the design of new anticancer drugs and the development of agents that can circumvent the multidrug transport system in human cancers.

II. Derivation of Multidrug-Resistant Cell Lines

A. Genetic Selection of Multidrug-Resistant Cell Lines

Our current understanding of the biochemical basis of multidrug resistance in cancer cells has resulted from the analysis of drug-resistant cell lines selected *in vitro*. A variety of multidrug-resistant cell lines have been established in tissue culture, e.g., multidrug-resistant rodent cells (Biedler and Riehm, 1970; Riehm and Biedler, 1971; Danø, 1972; Ling and Thompson, 1973; Bech-Hansen *et al.*, 1976; Ling and Baker, 1978; Meyers and Biedler, 1981); human leukemia and sarcoma cells (Beck *et al.*, 1979; Siegfried *et al.*, 1983) and human KB epidermoid carcinoma cell lines, a Hela variant (Akiyama *et al.*, 1985; Shen *et al.*, 1986b). For purposes of this review, we will limit discussion to multidrug-resistant cell lines with the following properties: (1) The cells are crossresistant to many well-defined chemotherapeutic agents (see Section I,A) that are structurally and functionally unrelated to the specific therapeutic agent used in the initial selection. (2) Multidrug-resistant cell lines consistently show increased expression of an *mdr* gene that encodes the 170 kDa membrane glycoprotein, P-glycoprotein (Juliano and Ling, 1976; Biedler and Peterson, 1981; reviewed in Riordan and Ling, 1985). Other patterns of crossresistance not mediated by P-glycoprotein expression are beginning to be defined in tissue culture studies, but the biochemical basis of these forms of multidrug resistance is as yet poorly defined.

To isolate multidrug-resistant cell lines, cells are subjected to a series of single-step selections in which the concentration of the selecting drug is gradually increased. After multiple step selections, the resulting population of cells will express high-level resistance to the selecting agent as well as crossresistance to many other drugs. This sequential single-step selection protocol was employed in all cell systems that generated highly resistant lines expressing the multidrug-resistant phenotype. In some of the derived cell lines, spontaneous drug-resistant clones could not be easily obtained in the initial step(s) of selection. In these cases, exponentially growing cells were treated with the mutagen, ethyl methanesulfonate (EMS) (Biedler and Riehm, 1970; Ling and Thompson, 1973; Akiyama *et al.*, 1985; and Shen *et al.*, 1986a). Later steps in the selection occurred readily, and cells rapidly adapted to relatively high levels of the selecting drug. It should be noted that the step-wise selection of populations of cells in increasing drug concentrations favors the introduction of multiple independent mutations; therefore, many of the existing multidrug-resistant cells may also express other mechanisms of resistance unrelated to P-glycoprotein.

The multidrug-resistant human carcinoma KB cells have served as a model system in which to study the molecular basis of drug resistance in human cancer. These lines were selected independently in colchicine, doxorubicin, or vinblastine (Akiyama *et al.*, 1985; Shen *et al.*, 1986b). To avoid the introduction of extraneous drug-resistance mutations into the KB cells, they were initially cloned at each selection step, and only clones that exhibited a classic pattern of multidrug resistance were carried through further steps of selection. However, after several steps of selection, some of the KB multidrug-resistant cell lines were significantly more resistant to the drug used as the selecting agent (Akiyama *et al.*, 1985; Shen *et al.*, 1986a). This preferential resistance to the selecting agent has been observed in other multidrug-resistant cell lines of different origin (reviewed in Bradley *et al.*, 1988). This could result from the introduction of mutations either affecting P-glycoprotein or unrelated to P-glycoprotein, which specifically confer resistance to the selecting drug. In the case of the KB cells, a mutation altering P-glycoprotein itself has been discovered (see Section III, B,3 for details).

Genetic analysis of the multidrug-resistant KB cell lines demonstrated that the multidrug-resistance genotype was dominant in somatic cell hybrids, and all drug resistances co-segregated when chromosomes were lost in these hybrids (Akiyama *et al.*, 1985). These results were similar to genetic studies of the multidrug-resistant CHO cell lines (Ling and Thompson, 1973) and indicated that either a single gene or a small cluster of linked genes was affected by mutation(s) incurred by the cell lines during the step-wise selection protocol. In the multidrug-resistant KB cell lines, short-term growth in nonselective medium generated *partial* revertants that had coordinately lost some of their resistance to colchicine, vinblastine, and actinomycin D. Prolonged growth in nonselective medium resulted in the isolation of drug-sensitive revertants from which the simultaneous loss of all drug resistances (co-reversion) had occurred. This unstable genotype suggested that a gene-amplification event contributed to the multidrug-resistant phenotype in cultured cells.

B. GENE AMPLIFICATION IN MULTIDRUG-RESISTANT CELLS

Cytogenetic analysis of the human multidrug-resistant KB cells provided additional genetic evidence that the multidrug-resistance phenotype of most cell lines resulted from gene amplification (Fojo *et al.*, 1985b), a common mechanism employed by cells to express higher levels of genes encoding drug resistances, e.g., methotrexate resistance (reviewed in Schimke, 1988; Stark *et al.*, 1989). Karyotypic analysis of the highly multidrug-resistant KB cell lines and several other multidrug-resistant cell lines showed the presence of minute and double-minute chromosomes (DMs), homogeneously staining regions (HSRs), or abnormally banding regions (ABRs) (reviewed in Bradley and Ling, 1988). These types of chromosomal aberrations are often associated with an increase in the copy number of specific genes conferring a selective growth advantage to these cells. In several cell lines, the degree of drug resistance correlated with the number of DMs or the length of the HSR. Further, as cell lines were cultured in the absence of drug, loss of drug resistance paralleled a loss in either the number of DMs or the length of the HSR (Dahllof *et al.*, 1984; Meyers *et al.*, 1985; Roy and Horwitz, 1985; Lothstein and Horwitz, 1986). In the human KB cells, drug-sensitive revertants of the multidrug-resistant phenotype showed the complete absence of the multiple-minute and double-minute chromosomes that had been observed in the highly resistant lines (Fojo *et al.*, 1985b).

The amplification of the genes responsible for multidrug resistance in KB cells was exploited to clone the human *MDR1* gene. By using a novel in-gel renaturation technique, an amplified genomic fragment from multidrug-resistant hamster cell lines was cloned (Roninson *et al.*, 1984) and subsequently used to detect and isolate homologous amplified DNA sequences in the multidrug-resistant human KB cells (Roninson *et al.*, 1986). Although two homologous human genes were detected, designated *MDR1* and *MDR2*, only the *MDR1* gene was consistently amplified and overexpressed in the human multidrug-resistant cell lines (Roninson *et al.*, 1986). Northern and Southern blot analysis using the human *MDR1* DNA probe, pMDR1, demonstrated that the stepwise selection of cultured KB cells in colchicine (Akiyama *et al.*, 1985) resulted initially in increased expression of the *MDR1* gene, followed by its amplification (Shen *et al.*, 1986a). The pMDR1 probe hybridized to a 4.5–5 kb mRNA species whose levels correlated with the level of drug resistance in the KB sublines. An *mdr* mRNA of similar size is overexpressed in mouse (Gros *et al.*, 1986a,b) and hamster multidrug-resistant cell lines (Gros *et al.*, 1986c; Teeter *et al.*, 1986).

The human *MDR1* genomic probe was also used to isolate complementary DNAs from the highly drug-resistant KB cell line (KB-C2.5), which encoded a functional *MDR1* gene product (Ueda *et al.*, 1987). Complementary DNAs that encode the rodent P-glycoprotein have also been cloned (Kartner *et al.*, 1985; Riordan *et al.*, 1985; Van der Bliek *et al.*, 1986; Scotto *et al.*, 1987) and sequence analysis has been performed on all these cDNAs (Section III,A). Substantial progress also has been made in mapping and sequencing the endogenous *MDR1* amplicon in human cells. Both the mouse (Raymond and Gros, 1989) and human *MDR1* (Chin *et al.*, 1989) genes have been cloned, and the DNA sequences at their exon–intron junctions have been determined. The human *MDR1* gene encompasses greater than 100 kb of DNA and contains 27 introns in the coding region (Chin *et al.*, 1989).

C. STRUCTURAL ANALYSIS OF THE *MDR1* AMPLICON

The region of amplification in multidrug-resistant mammalian cell lines has been analyzed using probes derived from *mdr* genes and from cDNAs of other co-amplified genes whose RNAs increase in amount during the amplification process. These studies employed conventional Southern blot analysis and pulsed-field gel electrophoresis of high-molecular-weight DNAs restricted with infrequently cutting restriction enzymes (Smith *et al.*, 1987a,b). In multidrug-resistant CHO cells selected in colchicine, the amplified region includes several hundred kb of functional DNA encoding at least five genes in addition to the *mdr* gene (Van der Bliek *et al.*, 1986). Recent studies of mouse multidrug-resistant cell lines demonstrate that all three *mdr* genes are co-amplified in an amplicon of minimum size 625 kb (Raymond *et al.*, 1990). However, some multidrug-resistant mouse (DeBruijn *et al.*, 1986) and hamster (Hsu *et al.*, 1989) cell lines show differential amplification of the *mdr* genes.

In human KB-C4 cells, selected in 4 μg/ml colchicine, the amplified region carries the *MDR1* gene, its homolog *MDR2*, which does not confer drug-resistance, and several hundred kb of adjacent DNA. The *MDR1* and *MDR2* genes are linked within 330 kilobases and are contained within a 600 kb *Nru*I fragment (Chin *et al.*, 1989) on chromosome 7, band q21.1 (Fojo *et al.*, 1986; Callen *et al.*, 1987) (Fig. 1). Analysis of KB-C4 DNA using field-inversion gel electrophoresis did not reveal any detectable rearrangements in the *MDR* amplicon. Similar analysis of the vinblastine (KB-V1) and adriamycin (KB-A1)-derived cell lines demonstrated that the *MDR1* amplicon did not contain the *MDR2* gene. In this amplicon, several novel DNA fragments, presumably resulting from DNA rearrangements, were generated during drug selection. In all of the multidrug-resistant cell lines harboring complex amplicons, amplification of a particular *mdr* gene does not necessarily correlate with its level of expression. For example, the amplification of the *MDR2* gene parallels that of *MDR1* in KB-C4; however, expression of *MDR2* is much less than that of *MDR1* (Chin *et al.*, 1989).

To further characterize the *MDR1* amplicon in multidrug-resistant human KB cell lines, genomic DNA, deproteinized *in situ,* has been analyzed by high-voltage gel electrophoresis and pulsed-field gel electrophoresis following γ-irradiation to linearize circular DNA molecules. These techniques allow the detection of episomes, extrachromosomal elements smaller than 1000 kb, the approximate limit of resolution of circular DNA molecules, such as DMs, by light microscopy (Barker, 1979). Episomes contain amplified genes and replicate

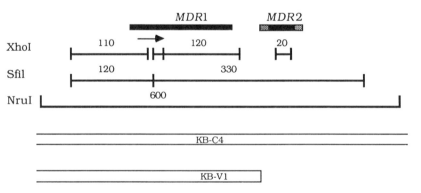

FIG. 1. Map of the human *MDR1* locus (adapted from Chin *et al.*, 1989). The restriction fragments are shown in kilobase (kb) pairs. The known amplified sequences in KB-C4 and KB-V1 are boxed. The arrow denotes the direction of transcription of the *MDR1* gene.

autonomously, approximately once per cell cycle (Carroll *et al.,* 1987; Maurer *et al.,* 1987; von Hoff *et al.,* 1988; Wahl, 1989). In the colchicine-selected murine cell line, J774.2, small extrachromosomal elements (approximately 400 kb and 800 kb) have been detected using these methods (Meese *et al.,* 1990). In the highly multidrug-resistant human KB-V1 cell line (selected in 1.0 μg/ml vinblastine), there are two episomal species of approximately 600 kb and 750 kb (Ruiz *et al.,* 1989). However, this study did not determine whether these episomes contain one or multiple copies of the *MDR1* gene. Preliminary results demonstrate that the 750-kb episome is present in the KB-V.05 cell line (selected in 50 ng/ml vinblastine), which represents one of the early stages in the vinblastine selection, and that the copy number of this episome and its multimers increase during increased drug selection (P. V. Schoenlein, I. Pastan, and M. M. Gottesman, unpublished data). Since the earliest stages of selection have not been studied, the 750-kb episome may represent an initial excision event or other circular extrachromosomal DNAs may have preceded its formation.

High-molecular-weight episomes have also been identified in most of the other multidrug-resistant human KB cell lines in which the endogenous *MDR1* gene is amplified (Schoenlein *et al.,* 1990). Episomes containing the *MDR1* and/or *MDR2* gene, ranging in size from approximately 750 kb to 890 kb are present at very early steps in drug-selected KB cells. For example, KB-Ch^R-8-5-11, selected in colchicine at 100 ng/ml, harbors an approximately 890-kb episome. This episome is formed immediately following a mutagenesis step, the same step in the selection protocol in which amplification of *MDR1* DNA was initially detected by conventional Southern blot analysis (Shen *et al.,* 1986a). This would indicate that amplification was mediated via episome formation. Further, the KB-C1.5, C2.5, C4.5, and C6.0 cell lines, which were selected from the KB-Ch^R-8-5-11 cell line by increasing the colchicine concentration in a stepwise fashion, no longer harbor the 890-kb episome but contain DMs ($\sim$1780 kb). This observation is consistent with Wahl's hypothesis that episomes are precursors to DMs (Wahl, 1989). The episomal structures in these cell lines are very stable and appear to be unchanged in structure after continuous passaging for 1 year. Since chromosomally integrated structures such as HSRs and ABRs are typically more stable than extrachromosomal elements that lack centromeres, one might speculate that the maintenance of the extrachromosomal amplicon provides some selective growth advantage to the cells.

These studies on episome formation during selection of multidrug-resistant cells raise several questions: (1) Do the unidentified genes, as well as the *MDR2* gene present on the episome in colchicine-derived cell lines, contribute to the overall drug-resistance phenotype of these cells (Shen *et al.,* 1986a,b)? (2) Are extrachromosomal structures such as episomes subject to a higher mutation rate than native chromosomes? Several point mutations have been identified in the KB-C1.5 cell line that result in an altered amino acid in the *MDR1* cDNA at position 185 of the P-glycoprotein. This change alters the crossresistance profile of this cell line (see Section III,C,3 for details). (3) Do the amplicon structures derived in tissue culture lines have any clinical relevance? Although amplification of *MDR1* DNA has not been reported in tumor samples, if only 10% of the cells in a tumor harbor extrachromosomal elements, the amplification phenotype may not be detected. Studies to evaluate the role of extrachromosomal elements in conferring drug resistance in human cancers are in progress.

III. Molecular Biology of Multidrug Transporter

A. OVERALL STRUCTURE: SUPERFAMILY OF ATP-DEPENDENT TRANSPORTERS

As previously noted, drug-sensitive cells grown *in vitro* can be made multidrug resistant by introduction of a full-length cDNA for the *MDR1* gene (Gros *et al.*, 1986a; Ueda *et al.*, 1987). There is a second human gene, known as *MDR2* or *MDR3*, which apparently does not confer drug resistance in simple transfection experiments (Van der Bliek *et al.*, 1988). In the mouse, there are a total of three *mdr* genes of which two can confer drug resistance: *mdr1a* (also called *mdr3*) and *mdr1b* (also called *mdr1*) (Gros *et al.*, 1986a; 1990). The two human genes encode proteins that are 80% homologous at the amino acid level. In general, *mdr* genes code for P-glycoproteins of approximately 1280 amino acid residues. The primary amino acid sequence predicts a protein with 12 transmembrane domains and two large cytoplasmic loops whose primary sequence suggests that they are ATP-binding sites. A simple model of the human P-glycoprotein based on its predicted amino acid sequence is shown in Fig. 2. P-glycoprotein consists of two homologous halves, with 43% amino acid–sequence identity between the amino- and carboxy-terminal halves (reviewed in Kane *et al.*, 1990).

Numerous other prokaryotic and eukaryotic proteins have been identified with similar ATP-binding sites and multiple transmembrane regions, suggesting that there is a superfamily of genes encoding ATP-binding proteins involved in membrane traffic (Hyde *et al.*, 1990). Some examples of members of this family are the extensively characterized multisubunit ATP-dependent nutrient transport systems of *Escherichia coli*, which include the ATP-binding peptides encoded by the *hisP*, *malK* and *oppD* genes. These are involved in histidine, maltose–maltodextran, and oligopeptide transport, respectively (Higgins *et al.*, 1986). Several members of this family are involved in export of proteins and carbohydrates including the hemolysin export protein *hlyB* (Felmlee *et al.*, 1985); the β-(1→2) glucan transporter of *Rhizobium meliloti*, *ndvA* (Stanfield *et al.*, 1988); a leukotoxin transporter of *Pasteurella haemolytica*, *lktB* (Strathdee *et al.*, 1989); and *cyaB*, a factor involved in the movement of adenylate cyclase in

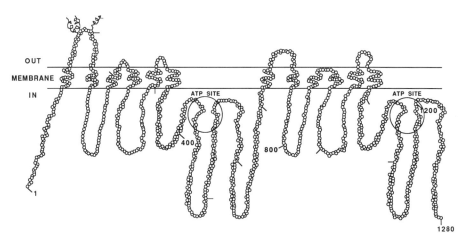

Fig. 2. Schematic model of the human multidrug transporter based on its predicted amino acid sequence. The wiggly lines are potential glycoprotein sites. This figure is adapted from Gottesman and Pastan (1988).

Bordetella pertussis (Glaser *et al.*, 1988). Examples of ATP-utilizing transporters in eukaryotic cells are increasing rapidly and include a transporter of eye pigment encoded by the white and brown locus of *Drosophila melanogaster* (O'Hare *et al.*, 1984; Dreesen *et al.*, 1988); the drug efflux pump that mediates chloroquine resistance of *Plasmodium falciparum* (pfmdr) (Wilson *et al.*, 1989; Foote *et al.*, 1989); the STE6 protein of yeast (McGrath and Varsharsky, 1989; Kuchler *et al.*, 1989), which is involved in the secretion of mating-type factor a; a major liver peroxisomal membrane protein of rats (Kamijo *et al.*, 1990); and CFTR, the product of the cystic fibrosis locus (Riordan *et al.*, 1989). The common unifying feature of members of this family is the presence of one or two short ATP-binding motifs, frequently referred to as Walker motifs (Walker *et al.*, 1982; Higgins *et al.*, 1985), associated with multiple transmembrane domains. Figure 3 shows the most homologous sequences in a comparison of several of these ATP binding–utilization domains and indicates the near identity among the prokaryotic and eukaryotic members of this family.

Recent studies on the structure of the human *MDR1* gene have provided some insight into the evolution of these ATP-dependent transporters. The location of each of the introns in the >100kb *MDR1* gene in the human and the *mdr3* (*mdr 1a*) gene in the mouse has been determined (Chen *et al.*, 1990; Raymond and Gros, 1989). The two halves of the molecule have similar amino acid sequences, which can be aligned. When the 27 introns that interrupt the coding sequences are located in these alignments of the amino- and carboxy-terminal halves of P-glycoprotein, it is obvious that they do not occur in homologous regions in both

HisP	G S G K S T	——	Q Q R	-	-	-	A R A	-	-	-	-	P D V L L F D E
MalK	G C G K S T	——	R Q R	-	-	-	G R T	-	-	-	-	P S V F L L D E
OppD	G S G K S Q	——	R Q R	-	-	-	A M A	-	-	-	-	P K L L I A D E
HMDR1(N)	G C G K S T	——	K Q R	-	-	-	A R A	-	-	-	-	P K I L L L D E
HMDR1(C)	G C G K S T	——	K Q R	-	-	-	A R A	-	-	-	-	P H I L L L D E
MMDR1(N)	G C G K S T	——	K Q R	-	-	-	A R A	-	-	-	-	P K I L L L D E
MMDR1(C)	G C G K S T	——	K Q R	-	-	-	A R A	-	-	-	-	P H I L L L D E
MMDR2(N)	G C G K S T	——	K Q R	-	-	-	A R A	-	-	-	-	P K I L L L D E
MMDR2(C)	G C G K S T	——	K Q R	-	-	-	A R A	-	-	-	-	P R V L L L D E
PMP70	G C G K S S	——	K Q R	-	-	-	A R A	-	-	-	-	P Q F A I L D E
CFTR(N)	G A G K S T	——	R A R	-	-	-	A R A	-	-	-	-	A D L Y L L D S
CFTR(C)	G S G K S T	——	K Q L	-	-	-	A R S	-	-	-	-	A K I L L L D E
STE6(N)	G S G K S T	——	Q Q R	-	-	-	A R A	-	-	-	-	T P I L F L D E
STE6(C)	G T G K S T	——	A Q R	-	-	-	A R A	-	-	-	S K I L I L D E

FIG. 3.   Amino acid identity in highly conserved regions of several members of the superfamily of ATP-dependent transporters, which are involved in ATP binding and utilization. The core of the A domain is on the left, and B domain is on the right with nonconserved amino acids indicated by a dashed line. The letters in parentheses indicate whether the sequence of the amino- (N) or carboxyl-(C) terminal ATP site is shown. The continuous line indicates a gap introduced for the alignment, and the dashes represent nonconserved amino acid residues. His, Mal, and Opp are genes involved in histidine, maltose, and peptide transport in *E. coli;* HMDR and MMDR are human and mouse MDR genes, respectively; CTFR is the cystic fibrosis transmembrane regulator, and STE6 is the transporter for the sex factor a of *Saccharomyces cerevisiae.*

halves. The only exceptions to this observation are the two introns within the two ATP-binding folds. This result suggests that the transmembrane regions in the amino- and carboxy-terminal halves of P-glycoprotein evolved independently, whereas the ATP-binding domains in both halves were of similar origin.

B. Molecular Manipulation of Multidrug Transporter

1. *Deletions*

To determine the essential structural components of the multidrug transporter, the *MDR1* gene was altered *in vitro* by deletion and insertional mutagenesis (Currier *et al.*, 1989). Many of these deletions and insertions are summarized in Fig. 4. A four–amino acid insertion in either the fourth transmembrane segment or preceding the Walker motif of the amino half of the second ATP-binding domain did not alter the ability of P-glycoprotein to confer colchicine resistance

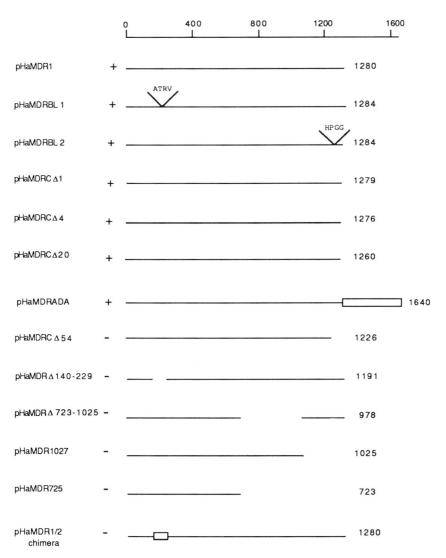

FIG. 4. Summary of deletions, point mutations, and chimeras affecting P-glycoprotein. The (+) or (−) sign to the right of the name of the mutant denotes whether the transfected mutant transporter is active (+) or inactive (−).

to transfected cells. Carboxyl-terminal deletions of one to three amino acids had no effect on activity of the transporter, while a deletion of 23 amino acids reduced the activity of the transporter. In pHaMDR725, an insertion of a nonsense mutation near the center of the *MDR1* cDNA results in translation of only the amino terminal half of the transporter. This molecule is interesting because it tests whether the internal duplication in P-glycoprotein results in redundancy of function. RNAs of transfectants with this construction showed that pHaMDR725 transcripts were present even though no protein was ever identified. This finding suggests that both halves of the molecule are necessary to form an active transporter, because either half of the molecule is unstable or it is insufficient to confer drug resistance.

Internal deletions of the *MDR1* cDNA were designed to modify either the amino or carboxyl-terminal halves of the transporter. None of these mutants resulted in the formation of an active transporter, emphasizing the need for an intact molecule with two functional halves.

2. *Chimeras*

Since the *MDR2* cDNA is unable to confer drug resistance after transfection, but is highly homologous to the *MDR1* cDNA, the construction of chimeras between *MDR1* and *MDR2* was undertaken to study which amino acids may be critical in the formation of an active transporter. DNA sequence analysis of cDNAs isolated from KB cells more resistant to either colchicine or vinblastine revealed that amino acid residue 185 might be involved in this differential relative resistance (see Section III,B,3). Using these two observations, a molecule was constructed using the "functional" *MDR1* gene as a backbone to introduce potentially "nonfunctional" *MDR2* nucleotide sequences corresponding to the amino acid residues 140 through 229. This chimeric P-glycoprotein differs at 17 residues between amino acids 140 and 229 from the *MDR1*-encoded product. Transfection of this chimeric cDNA did not confer drug resistance on drug-sensitive cells (S. Currier, I. Pastan, M. M. Gottesman, unpublished data). After several rounds of site-directed mutagenesis, it has been possible to restore transport activity to the chimera by introducing *MDR1* specific amino acids. We are currently determining which residue or residues are critical for restoration of a functional transporter. This detailed analysis should make it possible to pinpoint important functional residues in P-glycoprotein.

Based on the observation that small carboxyl-terminal deletions of P-glycoprotein are possible, chimeras have been formed between P-glycoprotein and adenosine deaminase (ADA). These experiments show clearly that both P-glycoprotein and ADA are still functional when ADA is attached to the carboxyl-terminus of P-glycoprotein (Germann *et al.,* 1989). These results suggest that a free carboxyl-terminus of P-glycoprotein is not essential for function, and support the structural model of P-glycoprotein (Fig. 2) in which the carboxyl-terminus is free in the cytoplasm. Results with these chimeras are also summarized in Fig. 4.

3. Point Mutations

Three point mutations in P-glycoprotein have been identified in *MDR1* cDNAs from KB cells selected in high levels of colchicine when compared to cDNAs derived from KB cells selected stepwise in vinblastine (Choi *et al.*, 1988). These mutations resulted in the introduction of a diagnostic *DdeI* restriction site (a silent mutation), and a change from the wild-type glycine to valine at residue 185. Detection of the new *DdeI* restriction site was used to determine at what step during colchicine selection these mutations occurred. It was discovered that the relative colchicine resistance of the KB cells increased substantially at the selection step corresponding to the introduction of the mutations at position 185. To verify the significance of the gly→val change at residue 185, expression vectors were made *in vitro* with interchanges at this position. A vector, with the valine at position 185, resulted in cells able to grow in threefold to sixfold higher concentrations of colchicine than a vector with glycine at this position. A difference in relative resistance for these two drugs, as mediated by residue 185, has been verified when comparing nucleotide sequences of cDNA isolated from human adrenal cells (wild-type) and that of the highly colchicine-resistant cell line, KB-C2.5, which carries the mutant valine at position 185 (Kioka *et al.*, 1989). The cDNA isolated from the adrenal cells has glycine at 185 and confers higher relative resistance to vinblastine than colchicine, when transfected into NIH3T3 cells.

It is also possible to ascertain the role of specific amino acid residues in determining relative drug resistance by comparing the patterns of drug resistance obtained with the two functional mouse *mdr* genes. The two mouse *mdr* genes that confer drug resistance when transfected into drug-sensitive cells also give somewhat different resistance patterns in these cells (Devault and Gros, 1990). For example, *mdr1b* (*mdr1*) shows sevenfold to tenfold preferential resistance to colchicine and Adriamycin; while *mdr1a* (*mdr3*) shows a twofold to threefold higher resistance to actinomycin D. These differences occur even though the two genes share 84% identical residues. A more detailed analysis will be needed to determine which specific residues affect the pattern of drug resistance.

To ascertain the necessity for two nucleotide-binding domains in a functional transporter, amino acid substitutions were made in the core of the Walker motif, GXGKST (Azzaria *et al.*, 1989). Mutants of the mouse *mdr1b* (*mdr1*) gene with either GXAKST or GXGRST at either domain, or one with duplicate GXGRST sequences were nonfunctional. The mutants were able to bind 8-azido ATP, but were unable to reduce intracellular accumulation of [^{3}H]vinblastine.

This would suggest that the two nucleotide-binding domains must both be active in a functional transporter, and that ATP binding alone does not define an active ATPase site.

C. VECTORS BASED ON MULTIDRUG TRANSPORTER

Three approaches have been reported for the use of the human *MDR1* gene as a dominant and amplifiable selective marker. In every case, the *MDR1* cDNA was under control of a Harvey murine sarcoma virus LTR promoter, which gives high levels of *MDR1* cDNA (Pastan *et al.*, 1988).

The first system used the *MDR1* gene to coamplify another cointroduced unselectable gene, cathepsin L (Kane *et al.*, 1988). In this experiment the level of expression of cathepsin L, encoded either by a small cDNA or a larger genomic fragment, increased as the concentration of the selective drug, colchicine, was increased. This coamplification was probably due to the co-integration of the two DNAs into the host genome. Therefore, the *MDR1* gene can be used for coamplification of cotransfected DNAs and represents a good system to produce large amounts of a second, otherwise nonselectable, gene product. More recently, the HIV receptor CD4 has been overexpressed in CHO cells after cotransfection with a vector encoding the *MDR1* gene (Konig *et al.*, 1989).

Another approach involved making a fusion molecule between the carboxyl-terminus of the *MDR1* gene and the amino-terminus of a second gene, the ADA gene (see Section III,B,2). The feasibility of this construction was based on the knowledge that small perturbations of the carboxyl-terminus of the *MDR1* gene could be tolerated. As before, increased selective pressure resulted in more drug-resistant cells having increased coexpressed functional protein product, the ADA enzyme (Germann *et al.*, 1989). Such an approach could prove useful for introducing unselectable cytoplasmic proteins into cells, as in human gene therapy.

Recently, a third vector for expressing nonselectable genes was reported (Kane *et al.*, 1990). In this vector, the *MDR1* gene is under the control of the Harvey murine sarcoma promoter, while the second gene is controlled by the SV40 promoter. In a pilot experiment, a cDNA for the IL2 receptor was introduced via this vector into NIH 3T3 cells, which normally do not express the IL2 receptor. Drug-resistant cells were readily isolated, and the membrane expression of the IL2 receptor could be increased by selection of cells in higher concentrations of colchicine. Thus, high-level expression of currently nonselectable genes can be achieved with this type of plasmid construction.

The use of vectors with retroviral LTRs also allows packaging of the *MDR1* cDNA as a defective retrovirus. Such viruses have been used to infect a variety of eukaryotic cells, which become multidrug resistant at high frequency (Pastan *et al.*, 1988; Germann *et al.*, 1990). Recently, high-efficiency infection of mouse bone marrow with such a vector has been shown (McLachlin *et al.*, 1990), demonstrating the feasibility of using the *MDR1* cDNA for gene therapy into bone marrow, or simply for conferring multidrug resistance on bone marrow to protect it during cancer chemotherapy.

IV. Drug Interaction Sites on Multidrug Transporter

A. PHOTOAFFINITY LABELS

Photoaffinity labels were used initially to test the general hypothesis that P-glycoprotein is responsible for multidrug resistance. If P-glycoprotein protects multidrug-resistant cells by pumping cytotoxic drugs through the plasma membrane and out of the cell, then P-glycoprotein should contain specific binding sites for these drugs, and the sites would be labeled by photoaffinity drug analogs. Cornwell *et al.* (1986a), demonstrated that plasma membrane vesicles prepared from multidrug-resistant human KB cells contained specific binding sites for ³H-vinblastine, but plasma membrane vesicles prepared from the drug-sensitive parent cell line did not contain these sites (Cornwell *et al.*, 1986a). Because the plasma membrane from multidrug-resistant cells contains P-glycoprotein, this protein was assumed to be responsible for the specific binding of vinblastine. However, it was not possible to demonstrate this directly without the use of photoaffinity drug analogs.

Cornwell *et al.* (1986b) then prepared two different photoaffinity vinblastine analogs and showed that these compounds specifically labeled P-glycoprotein. The specificity of labeling was defined by three criteria: (1) The photoaffinity vinblastine analogs labeled a 170-kDa protein in the plasma membrane of multidrug-resistant cells, but it did not label any such protein in the plasma membrane vesicles prepared from the drug-sensitive parent cells. (2) It was possible to inhibit the labeling by adding excess vinblastine to the reaction. (3) The 170-kDa–labeled protein was immunoprecipitated by antibodies raised against P-glycoprotein (Safa *et al.*, 1986). These results demonstrated that P-glycoprotein contains specific binding sites for vinblastine and thus supported the hypothesis that P-glycoprotein pumps this drug out of multidrug-resistant cells.

An essential aspect of these experiments was that excess vinblastine prevented the photoaffinity analogs from labeling P-glycoprotein. Excess vinblastine also competed successfully to prevent ³H-vinblastine from binding to plasma membrane vesicles prepared from multidrug-resistant cells. These results show that vinblastine binding and labeling is a saturable process, and from this one may infer that vinblastine binds to a specific site on P-glycoprotein. Other drugs, which are also presumed to be substrates for P-glycoprotein transport, did not necessarily inhibit vinblastine binding and labeling. For instance, daunomycin inhibited vinblastine binding to P-glycoprotein, but colchicine and actinomycin

D did not, even though the multidrug-resistant cells are crossresistant to all of these drugs. This pattern of inhibition is very similar to that found when vinblastine transport into plasma membrane vesicles prepared from multidrug-resistant cells was studied (Horio *et al.*, 1988).

Many different drugs are able to interfere with the activity of the multidrug transporter and also reverse the multidrug-resistance phenotype of cultured cells. These include the calcium channel blocker verapamil, the antiarrhythmic quinidine, the antihypertensive reserpine, and the immune suppressant cyclosporin A (reviewed in Tsuruo, 1988). Verapamil is one of the most potent of these agents, but its mechanism of action was somewhat mysterious until it was shown to block photoaffinity-labeling of P-glycoprotein (Cornwell *et al.*, 1986b; Akiyama *et al.*, 1988). Since it is also a substrate for P-glycoprotein (Cano-Gauci and Riordan, 1987), and inhibits ATP-dependent transport of vinblastine into vesicles containing P-glycoprotein (Horio *et al.*, 1988), it is likely that verapamil works as a competitive inhibitor of the multidrug transporter.

The results from the competition experiments with vinblastine, daunomycin, and verapamil suggested that daunomycin and verapamil bind to P-glycoprotein, although the situation with colchicine and actinomycin D is not clear. Photoaffinity anologs of verapamil (Safa, 1988; Qian and Beck, 1990), colchicine (Safa *et al.*, 1989), and daunomycin (Busche *et al.*, 1989a,b) have since been prepared and used to specifically label P-glycoprotein. These results demonstrate that these drugs have binding sites on P-glycoprotein and support the hypothesis that P-glycoprotein is responsible for pumping these drugs out of the multidrug-resistant cells. In addition, a prazosin analog (Greenberger *et al.*, 1990; Safa *et al.*, 1990), which is a α_1-adrenergic receptor probe, and some isoprenoid derivatives (Akiyama *et al.*, 1989) label P-glycoprotein; the significance of these drugs and their interaction with P-glycoprotein remains unknown.

Because it is commercially available, inexpensive, and easy to use, the photoaffinity label azidopine has become the standard for many different labeling experiments of P-glycoprotein. Azidopine is an arylazide dihydropyridine calcium channel blocker (Ferry *et al.*, 1984), which has been shown to label P-glycoprotein specifically (Safa *et al.*, 1987). Many other calcium channel blockers, including the dihydropyridines, reverse multidrug resistance, and bind to membrane vesicles prepared from multidrug-resistant cells (Cornwell *et al.*, 1987). The pattern by which other anticancer agents competed with and inhibited azidopine labeling of P-glycoprotein was similar, but not identical, to that with vinblastine. For instance, vinblastine competed, but colchicine and verapamil did not. Actinomycin D was an intermediate inhibitor, but Adriamycin was a poor inhibitor. Azidopine has also been used to screen potential multidrug-resistance reversing agents (Kamiwatari *et al.*, 1989). The logic behind this strategy is the assumption that dihydropyridines must first bind to P-glycoprotein before they can reverse multidrug resistance. Newly synthesized dihydropyridines may be quickly tested for their ability to bind to P-glycoprotein by measuring how successfully they compete with azidopine labeling. A photoaffinity vinblastine analog has also been used to screen potential multidrug-reversing agents (Nogae *et al.*, 1989).

B. Strategies for Identifying Labeled Sites

The pattern by which other drugs inhibit the binding of vinblastine and the photoaffinity labels to P-glycoprotein should reveal something about binding sites on P-glycoprotein for these compounds. Several hypotheses that might account for the data are possible. (1) All drugs bind to the same site or sites of P-glycoprotein, and different affinities account for the different levels of competition. It is not known how all of the substrates for P-glycoprotein, which bear no obvious structural or functional similarity, can bind to a single site. (2) There is a different binding site for each drug or class of drugs. In this case only drugs that bind to the same site would show binding competition. No information is currently available to infer the number and other characteristics of such putative binding sites. (3) It is possible that other proteins or factors are somehow involved in multidrug transport and that the presence or absence of these other functional factors may lead to the patterns of competition detected in the *in vitro* assays. The common working hypothesis, based on gene-transfer experiments, is that P-glycoprotein alone is sufficient for multidrug transport. In principle, several features of these hypotheses should be distinguishable by their transport kinetics, but so far this approach has not been definitive (Horio *et al.*, 1990).

Several groups have taken a more direct approach by using the photoaffinity labels to identify drug-binding sites on P-glycoprotein. In this strategy, P-glycoprotein is first labeled with a photoaffinity drug analog and then digested into fragments with proteolytic enzymes. The labeled fragments are recovered, identified, and assumed to contain the binding site for the drug. Bruggemann *et al.* (1989) and Yoshimura *et al.* (1989) independently labeled human P-glycoprotein with azidopine and digested the labeled protein with trypsin or V8 protease. By using specific antibodies, labeled fragments from both the amino- and carboxyl-terminus were identified. The smallest amino-terminal fragment was a 38-kDa trypsin fragment comprising transmembrane domains 1–6. The smallest carboxyl-terminus fragment was a 30-kDa V8 fragment comprising transmembrane domains 7–12 (Fig. 5). These results, summarized in Fig. 6, may be explained by either of two possibilities: (1) There are two binding sites on P-glycoprotein for azidopine, one in each of the homologous halves of the protein. Azidopine binds to each site independently and labels it. (2) There is one binding site on P-glycoprotein that is formed by the two homologous halves of the protein. After azidopine binds to this site, it labels both halves of the protein. Azidopine can label some of the proteolytic fragments of P-glycoprotein

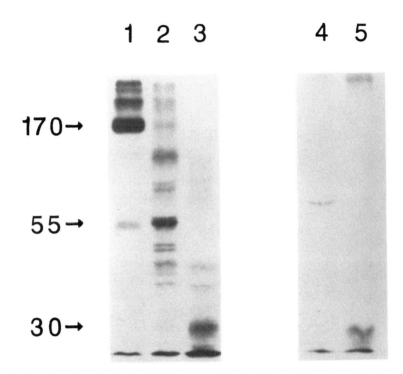

FIG. 5.   Examples of azidopine labeling, proteolytic digestion, and immunoprecipitation of P-glycoprotein. Results were analyzed by SDS-PAGE. Lane 1: P-glycoprotein, labeled with azidopine and immunoprecipitated with anti–P-glycoprotein antiserum 4007 (Tanaka *et al.*, 1990) runs at 170 kDa. The higher molecular-weight bands above P-glycoprotein are aggregates of P-glycoprotein. Lane 2: Azidopine-labeled P-glycoprotein was digested with 1 mg/ml V8 protease. A 55-kDa–labeled fragment is the major product. Lane 3: After digestion with 10 mg/ml V8 protease, the 55-kDa fragment is reduced to 30 kDa. Lane 4: The azidopine-labeled 30-kDa V8 fragment was incubated with the antipeptide antiserum anti-P4. The peptide used to raise this antiserum comprised amino acid residues 100–112 of human P-glycoprotein (Richert *et al.*, 1988). Lane 5: Immunoprecipitation of the 30-kDa fragment with anti-P0. This antipeptide antiserum was raised against amino acid residues 740–749 of human P-glycoprotein (Richert *et al.*, 1988).

(Yoshimura *et al.*, 1989), which shows that these fragments contain a binding site, but this result does not eliminate either possibility.

Although small fragments allow a more precise definition of the binding site, the small fragments are usually much more difficult to identify. Mouse P-glycoprotein was labeled with azidopine, digested with trypsin, and one small labeled fragment was obtained by high-performance liquid chromatography (HPLC) (Yang *et al.*, 1988). Unfortunately, the position of this fragment within P-glycoprotein has not yet been determined, and it is also possible that other

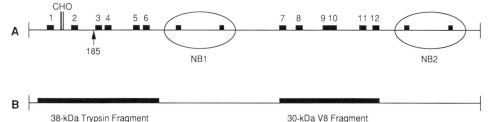

FIG. 6. Regions of P-glycoprotein labeled by azidopine. A: A linear map of P-glycoprotein is shown; the amino terminus is on the left. The twelve transmembrane domains of P-glycoprotein are numbered 1–12, and the two nucleotide-binding sites are circled (NB). The predicted sites of glycosylation (CHO) and the location of amino acid residue 185 are shown. B: The two smallest azidopine-labeled fragments obtained by proteolytic digestion of P-glycoprotein are shown.

labeled fragments were missed. Greenberger *et al.* (1990) labeled mouse P-glycoprotein either with azidopine or with a prazosin photoaffinity analog. They obtained several small fragments of about 6 kDa, but were not able to identify their location in P-glycoprotein. They did show by V8 mapping, however, that azidopine and the prazosin analog labeled identical fragments of P-glycoprotein. This suggests that these two drugs bind to the same site, or that they bind to closely related sites. This 6-kDa fragment labeled with prazosin has also been obtained with hamster P-glycoprotein (Safa *et al.*, 1990).

These experiments with photoaffinity labels have failed to identify the putative binding sites with any degree of precision. Ideally, one would like to obtain very small labeled fragments, then purify and sequence them. This would not only identify the fragment, but also might reveal the exact amino acid residues labeled by the photoaffinity labels. Unfortunately, it has simply not been possible to recover enough labeled fragment to pursue this approach. Even if this approach were successful, the labeled site might not be coincident with the binding site. For example, it is possible that the tertiary structure of P-glycoprotein is such that the binding site is at some distance in the primary structure from the labeled site. So, unfortunately, the location and nature of the drug-binding site remain elusive.

Another approach to identifying drug-binding sites is to examine the sequence of different *mdr* alleles and the drug-binding characteristics of the proteins they encode. For instance, Choi *et al.* (1988) demonstrated that KB cells selected for multidrug resistance with vinblastine retain a wild-type glycine at position 185 of P-glycoprotein, but KB cells selected with colchicine contain a valine at this position (see also Section III,B,3). These two cell lines also showed different patterns of resistance to vinblastine and colchicine, and this pattern was retained when the cDNAs were transfected into another cell line. These results suggest that amino acid residue 185 is an important residue for drug binding or transport. Others have examined the crossresistance of mouse cell lines that express the different mouse *mdr* alleles (Lothstein *et al.*, 1989; Devault and Gros, 1990). They have shown that the differences in crossresistance between these lines depend on the specific allele expressed. Although the putative drug binding site(s) may be responsible, there are many differences between the alleles, and it is not possible to draw any firm conclusions from these data.

Chloroquine resistance in *Plasmodium falciparum* is associated with a P-glycoprotein–like molecule. Specific point mutations have been identified in the structural gene that may be important to drug resistance (Foote *et al.*, 1990). These amino acid residues correspond in the human sequence to amino acid residues 106, 204, 945, 953, and 1108. Obviously, from comparing the primary sequence, none is close to amino acid 185, but one is not far away and some or all may be close in the folded molecule. Although these results are suggestive, it is not yet possible to infer from these data anything about the drug-binding sites on P-glycoprotein. Azidopine can label P-glycoprotein from *P. falciparum* (Ye *et al.*, 1989), but in these experiments the identity of the allele was not known, nor were different strains of the parasite compared. Rather than look for alleles with interesting patterns of drug resistance, the most fruitful approach in the long run will be to introduce specific point mutations into P-glycoprotein and examine their effects on drug binding. Such studies are underway in several laboratories.

V. Mechanism of Action of Drug Transport

A. GENERAL CONSIDERATIONS IN DRUG TRANSPORT

Despite the accumulation of data defining the important structural components of P-glycoprotein, the means by which a single transporter identifies and translocates so many chemically different drugs across the plasma membrane remains mysterious. We do know that the net effect of the action of the transporter is to reduce accumulation of drugs within the cells, and the bulk of physiological evidence suggests that this results from increased efflux (Fojo *et al.*, 1985a). Energy is required for this process, as indicated by increased turnover of ATP in drug-resistant cells (Broxterman *et al.*, 1988), the inhibitory effects of azide and 2-deoxyglucose (Willingham *et al.*, 1986), and the direct demonstration of an ATP requirement for ^{3}H-vinblastine transport into P-glycoprotein–containing vesicles (Horio *et al.*, 1988). The binding of 8-N_3-ATP to P-glycoprotein (Cornwell *et al.*, 1987), and the presence of two canonical ATP-utilization sites in the primary sequence of the protein, indicating its obvious relationship to the superfamily of ATP-dependent transporters (see Section III,A), provide further circumstantial evidence for a critical role of ATP in its mechanism of action.

How is the hydrolysis of ATP harnessed to the movement of drugs through the plasma membrane? How are so many different drugs recognized by the transporter? These are questions on which we can only speculate.

There are several epiphenomena associated with overexpression of P-glycoprotein that are worthy of comment, since they may shed some light on these questions. First, in cells selected in multiple steps in tissue culture, where the *MDR1* gene is amplified (see Section II,B), there is frequently overexpression of other co-amplified genes (see Section II,C). It is at present unclear whether the proteins encoded by these co-amplified genes play a significant role in the transport process. However, no other neighboring protein is known to be overexpressed in all multidrug-resistant cell lines (Van der Bliek *et al.*, 1986; De Bruijn *et al.*, 1986), and transfection of a full-length *MDR1* cDNA is sufficient to confer multidrug resistance, suggesting that overexpression of P-glycoprotein alone is sufficient to confer drug resistance. It must be kept in mind, however, that these transfection experiments do not rule out a cellular co-factor or constitutively expressed protein present in very high amounts, which is involved in transport but is never limiting in drug-sensitive cells.

Numerous studies have shown that P-glycoprotein is phosphorylated (reviewed in Endicott and Ling, 1989) by both cAMP-dependent protein kinase (Mellado and Horwitz, 1987) and C-kinase (Chambers *et al.*, 1990). The functional effect of this direct phosphorylation of P-glycoprotein is not yet known, but it could affect the pumping efficiency or specificity of the transporter. In addition, reduced levels of cAMP-dependent protein kinase result in reduced amounts of mRNA for P-glycoprotein, suggesting a role for this kinase in regulating synthesis or turnover of *mdr* RNA (Abraham *et al.*, 1987, 1990).

Another phenomenon associated with drug resistance is a rise in intracellular pH in many (but not all) multidrug-resistant cell lines (Keizer and Joenje, 1989; Thiebaut *et al.*, 1990; Boscoboinik *et al.*, 1990). Some multidrug-resistant cells will quickly acidify medium in the presence or absence of substrate drugs (Thiebaut *et al.*, 1990). Our preferred current interpretation of these data is that there are cationic endogenous substrates for the multidrug transporter whose transport results in the net efflux of a proton. Another interpretation of this result is that the multidrug transporter is primarily a proton pump. The alkalinization of the cytoplasm resulting from this activity could increase the pH gradient across the plasma membrane and promote efflux of cationic drugs. However, the small pH gradients so far observed do not seem sufficient to explain the much greater gradient of drugs, and this hypothesis certainly does not account for the direct interaction of drugs with the transporter (see Section IV,A).

Another hypothesis is that the drugs are covalently modified, perhaps by glutathione (West, 1990) or some other covalent addition, which is recognized by the transporter as a common feature in all drugs so modified. Although superficially this is an attractive hypothesis, it fails to take into account three kinds of data: (1) no one has demonstrated such a covalent modification of any of the drugs in question; (2) unmodified drugs interact directly with the transporter as shown by photoaffinity-labeling experiments and vesicle-transport studies; and (3) this explanation does not solve the problem of specificity in the least, since it does not account for how the putative modifying system can recognize the diverse chemical structures in the first place!

B. POSSIBLE MECHANISM OF ACTION BASED ON HYDROPHOBIC NATURE OF SUBSTRATES

One striking feature of virtually all of the substrates for P-glycoprotein is that they consist of both hydrophobic and positively charged moieties. These structural features suggest that the drugs, most of which are not very water-soluble, will partition between nonaqueous and aqueous milieus. In cells, in the absence of specific binding sites, or shortly after exposure to the drugs, they would be expected to be embedded in cellular membranes with hydrophobic domains in the lipid bilayer and charged moieties in the aqueous phase. Thus, what the transporter might see could be the hydrophobic portion embedded in or associated with lipid, or the interface between lipid and aqueous phase. Current models do not allow us to predict what these structures would look like, but it is possible that all of the drugs present a common appearance to the transporter.

Two kinds of evidence suggest that the transporter recognizes drugs in the lipid bilayer and functions primarily to exclude such drugs from the plasma membrane. The photoaffinity label ^{125}I-INA (iodonaphthalene azide) is highly insoluble in water and will nonspecifically label many transmembrane proteins, including P-glycoprotein (Raviv et al., 1990). Specificity of labeling can be conferred by photoactivating INA by energy transfer from the chromophores daunorubicin or rhodamine 123, which are substrates for P-glycoprotein. In drug-sensitive cells, such an experiment can be utilized to localize the drugs in cells. The complex pattern of labeling of transmembrane proteins obtained in such an experiment indicates that the drug is diffusely dissolved in the lipid bilayer, in contact with most transmembrane proteins. In multidrug-resistant cells, however, this diffuse pattern of labeling is lost in favor of relatively specific labeling of P-glycoprotein. Such an experiment suggests that in the presence of P-glycoprotein, the drugs have been removed by the transporter from the plasma membrane. Hence, the pump may act as a hydrophobic vacuum cleaner to identify, bind, and expel harmful hydrophobic substances from the plasma membrane.

Spectral evidence also supports this model. Kessel (1989) has shown that the environment of rhodamine 123, as indicated by its diagnostic fluorescence-excitation spectrum, is primarily hydrophobic in drug-sensitive cells. In multi-

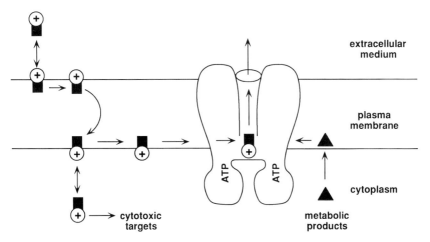

FIG. 7. Hypothetical model for action of the multidrug transporter. A theoretical anticancer drug with a hydrophobic domain (filled-in region) and a positively charged domain (+) is shown diffusing into and across the plasma membrane where it encounters the multidrug transporter by lateral diffusion. Whether the positively charged or neutral form of the drug diffuses across the plasma membrane has not been determined. The transporter uses energy transduced from two essential ATP sites to pump the drug out of the membrane. To the right, a hypothetical hydrophobic metabolic product, produced in the cytoplasm or in the membrane, is shown as a potential substrate for the transporter (solid triangle). One pathway of drug or metabolite efflux within the transporter is shown for simplicity's sake, but there may be more than one.

drug-resistant cells, however, rhodamine 123 appears to be in a primarily aqueous environment, consistent with exclusion from the lipid bilayer.

A model for the action of P-glycoprotein, which incorporates these ideas, is shown in Fig. 7. The drugs, containing both hydrophobic and cationic components, are believed to diffuse across and through the plasma membrane where they encounter the multidrug transporter. Hydrophobic metabolites produced in the cytoplasm, or the membrane itself, may also be substrates for the transporter. As shown in this model, the transporter uses the energy provided by two ATP sites to remove drugs or endogenous metabolites from the membrane.

VI. Conclusions

The application of somatic cell genetics and molecular biology has made possible the isolation and initial characterization of a multidrug efflux pump, which contributes to the multidrug resistance of many human cancers. Although the precise mechanism of action of this transporter is not yet known, approaches combining molecular genetics and biochemistry are yielding valuable clues as to how it functions, and how this function can be inhibited. This system promises to reveal important new information about the energetics of membrane transporters, and the interaction of hydrophobic and amphipathic compounds with proteins. The reward for a true biochemical understanding of the multidrug transporter may be improved therapy of human cancer.

References

Abraham, I., Hunter, R. J., Sampson, K. E., Smith, S., Gottesman, M. M., and Mayo, J. K. (1987). Cyclic AMP–dependent protein kinase regulates sensitivity of cells to multiple drugs. *Mol. Cell. Biol.* **7**, 3098–3106.

Abraham, I., Chin, K.-V., Gottesman, M. M., Mayo, J., and Sampson, K. E. (1990). Transfection of a mutant regulatory subunit of cAMP-dependent protein kinase causes increased drug sensitivity and decreased expression of P-glycoprotein. *Exp. Cell Res.* **189**, 133–141.

Akiyama, S.-i., Fojo, A., Hanover, J. A., Pastan, I., Gottesman, M. M. (1985). Isolation and genetic characterization of human KB cell lines resistant to multiple drugs. *Somat. Cell Mol. Genet.* **11**, 117–126.

Akiyama, S.-i., Cornwell, M. M., Kuwano, M., Pastan, I., and Gottesman, M. M. (1988). Most drugs that reverse multidrug resistance also inhibit photoaffinity labeling of P-glycoprotein by a vinblastine analog. *Mol. Pharmacol.* **33**, 144–147.

Akiyama, S.-i., Yoshimura, A., Kikuchi, H., Sumizawa, T., Kuwano, M., and Tahara, Y. (1989). Synthetic isoprenoid photoaffinity labeling of P-glycoprotein specific to multidrug-resistant cells. *Mol. Pharmacol.* **36**, 730–735.

Azzaria, M., Schurr, E., and Gros, P. (1989). Discrete mutations introduced in the predicted nucleotide-binding sites of the *mdr1* gene abolish its ability to confer multidrug resistance. *Mol. Cell. Biol.* **9**, 5289–5297.

Barker, P. E., and Stubblefield, E. (1979). Ultrastructure of double minutes from a human tumor cell line. *J. Cell Biol.* **83**, 663–666.

Bech-Hansen, N. T., Till, J. E., and Ling, V. (1976). Pleiotropic phenotype of colchicine-resistant CHO cells: Crossresistance and collateral sensitivity. *J. Cell. Physiol.* **88**, 23–32.

Beck, W. T., Mueller, T. J., and Tanzer, L. R. (1979). Altered surface membrane glycoproteins in *Vinca* alkaloid–resistant human leukemic lymphoblasts. *Cancer Res.* **39**, 2070–2076.

Biedler, J. L., and Riehm, H. (1970). Cellular resistance to actinomycin D in Chinese hamster cells *in vitro:* Crossresistance, radioautographic, and cytogenetic studies. *Cancer Res.* **30**, 1174–1184.

Biedler, J. L., and Peterson, R. H. F. (1981). Altered plasma membrane glycoconjugates of Chinese hamster cells with acquired resistance to actinomycin D, daunorubicin, and vincristine. *In* "Molecular Actions and Targets for Cancer Chemotherapeutic Agents" (A. C. Sartorelli, J. S. Lazo, and J. R. Bertino, eds.), pp. 453–482. Academic Press, New York.

Boscoboinik, D., Gupta, R. S., and Epand, R. M. (1990). Investigation of the relationship between altered intracellular pH and multidrug resistance in mammalian cells. *Br. J. Canc.* **61**, 568–572.

Bradley, G., Juranda, P. F., and Ling, V. (1988). Mechanism of multidrug resistance. *Biochim. Biophy. Acta* **948**, 87–128.

Broxterman, H. J., Pinedo, H. M., Kuiper, C. M., Kaptein, L. C. M., Schuurhuis, G. J., and Lankelma, J. (1988). Induction of a rapid decrease in ATP consumption by verapamil in multidrug resistant tumor cells. *FASEB J.* **2**, 2278–2282.

Bruggemann, E. P., Germann, U. A., Gottesman, M. M., and Pastan, I. (1989). Two different regions of P-glycoprotein are photoaffinity labeled by azidopine. *J. Biol. Chem.* **264,** 15483–15488.

Busche, R., Tümmler, B., Cano-Gauci, D. F., and Riordan, J. R. (1989a). Equilibrium, kinetic, and photoaffinity-labeling studies of daunomycin binding to P-glycoprotein-containing membranes of multidrug-resistant Chinese hamster ovary cells. *Eur. J. Biochem.* **183,** 189–197.

Busche, R., Tümmler, B., Riordan, J. R., and Cano-Gauci, D. F. (1989b). Preparation and utility of a radioiodinated analogue of daunomycin in the study of multidrug resistance. *Mol. Pharmacol.* **35,** 414–421.

Callen, D. F., Baker, E., Simmers, R. N., Seshadri, R., and Roninson, I. B. (1987). Localization of the human multiple drug resistance gene, *MDR1,* to 7q21.1. *Hum. Genet.* **77,** 142–144.

Cano-Gauci, D. F., and Riordan, J. R. (1987). Action of calcium antagonists on multidrug-resistant cells. Specific cytotoxicity independent of increased cancer drug accumulation. *Biochem. Pharmacol.* **13,** 2115–2123.

Carroll, S. M., Gaudray, P., DeRose, M. L., Emery, J. F., Meinkoth, J. L., Nakkim, E., Subler, M., Von Hoff, D. D., and Wahl, G. M. (1987). Characterization of an episome produced in hamster cells that amplify a transfected CAD gene at high frequency; functional evidence for a mammalian replication origin. *Mol. Cell. Biol.* **7,** 1740–1750.

Chambers, T. C., McAvoy, E. M., Jacobs, J. W., and Eilon, G. (1990). Protein kinase C phosphorylates P-glycoprotein in multidrug-resistant human KB carcinoma cells. *J. Biol. Chem.* **265,** 7679–7686.

Chen, C.-J., Chin, J. E., Ueda, K., Clark, D., Pastan, I., Gottesman, M. M., and Roninson, I. B. (1986). Internal duplication and homology with bacterial transport proteins in the *mdr1* (P-glycoprotein) gene from multidrug-resistant human cells. *Cell* **47,** 381–389.

Chen, C.-J., Clark, D., Ueda, K., Pastan, I., Gottesman, M. M., and Roninson, I. B. (1990). Genomic organization of the human multidrug resistance (*MDR1*) gene and origin of P-glycoproteins. *J. Biol. Chem.* **265,** 506–514.

Chin, K.-V., Tanaka, S., Darlington, G., Pastan, I., and Gottesman, M. M. (1990). Heat shock and arsenite increase expression of the multidrug-resistance (*MDR1*) gene in human carcinoma cells. *J. Biol. Chem.* **265,** 221–226.

Chin, K.-V., Chauhan, S., Pastan, I., and Gottesman, M. M. (1990). Regulation of *mdr* gene expression in acute response to cytotoxic insults in rodent cells. *Cell Growth and Differentiation* **1,** 361–365.

Chin, J. E., Soffir, R., Noonan, K. E., Choi, K., and Roninson, I. B. (1989). Structure and expression of the human MDR (P-glycoprotein) gene family. *Mol. Cell. Biol.* **9,** 3808–3820.

Choi, K., Chen, C., Kriegler, M., and Roninson, I. B. (1988). An altered pattern of crossresistance in multidrug-resistant human cells results from spontaneous mutations in the *mdr1* (P-glycoprotein) gene. *Cell* **53,** 519–529.

Cordon-Cardo, C., O'Brien, J. P., Casals, D., Rittman-Grauer, L., Biedler, J. L., Melamed, M. R., and Bertino, J. R. (1989). Multidrug-resistance gene (P-glycoprotein) is expressed by endothelial cells at blood–brain barrier sites. *Proc. Natl. Acad. Sci. U.S.A.* **86,** 695–698.

Cornwell, M. M., Gottesman, M. M., and Pastan, I. H. (1986a). Increased vinblastine binding to membrane vesicles from multidrug-resistant KB cells. *J. Biol. Chem.* **261,** 7921–7928.

Cornwell, M. M., Safa, A. R., Felsted, R. L., Gottesman, M. M., and Pastan, I. (1986b). Membrane vesicles from multidrug-resistant human cancer cells contain a specific 150- to 170-kDa protein detected by photoaffinity labeling. *Proc. Natl. Acad. Sci. U.S.A.* **83,** 3827–3830.

Cornwell, M. M., Pastan, I., and Gottesman, M. M. (1987). Certain calcium channel blockers bind specifically to multidrug-resistant human KB carcinoma membrane vesicles and inhibit drug binding to P-glycoprotein. *J. Biol. Chem.* **262,** 2166–2170.

Croop, J. M., Grow, P., and Housman, D. E. (1988). Genetics of multidrug resistance. *J. Clin. Invest.* **81,** 1303–1309.

Currier, S. J., Ueda, K., Willingham, M. C., Pastan, I., and Gottesman, M. M. (1989). Deletion and insertion mutants of the multidrug transporter. *J. Biol. Chem.* **264,** 14376–14381.

Dahllof, B., Martinsson, T., and Levan, G. (1984). Resistance to actinomycin D and to vincristine induced in a SEWA mouse tumor cell line with concomitant appearance of double minutes and a low-molecular-weight protein. *Exp. Cell Res.* **152,** 415–426.

Danø, K. (1972). Crossresistance between vinca alkaloids and anthracyclines in Ehrlich ascites tumor *in vivo. Cancer Chemother. Rep.* **56,** 701–708.

De Bruijn, M. H. L., Van der Bliek, A. M., Biedler, J. L., and Borst, P. (1986). Differential amplification and disproportionate expression of five genes in three multidrug-resistant Chinese hamster lung cell lines. *Mol. Cell. Biol.* **6,** 4717–4722.

Devault, A., and Gros, P. (1990). Two members of the mouse *mdr* gene family confer multidrug resistance with overlapping but distinct drug specificities. *Mol. Cell. Biol.* **10,** 1652-1663.

Dreesen, T. D., Johnson, D. H., and Henikott, S. (1988). The brown protein of *Drosophila melanogaster* is similar to the white protein and to components of active transport complex. *Mol. Cell. Biol.* **8,** 5206–5215.

Endicott, J. A., and Ling, V. (1989). The biochemistry of P-glycoprotein–mediated multidrug resistance. *Annu. Rev. Biochem.* **58,** 137–171.

Ferry, D. R., Rombusch, M., Goll, A., and Glossmann, H. (1984). Photoaffinity labelling of Ca^{2+} channels with [^{3}H]azidopine. *FEBS Lett.* **169,** 112–118.

Felmlee, T., Pelleh, S., and Welch, R. A. (1985). Nucleotide sequence of an *Escherichia coli* chromosomal hemolysin. *J. Bacteriol.* **163,** 94–105.

Fojo, A. T., Akiyama, S.-i., Gottesman, M. M., and Pastan, I. (1985a). Reduced drug accumulation in multiply drug-resistant human KB carcinoma cell lines. *Cancer Res.* **45,** 3002–3007.

Fojo, A. T., Whang-Peng, J., Gottesman, M. M., and Pastan, I. (1985b). Amplification of DNA sequences in human multidrug-resistant KB carcinoma cells. *Proc. Natl. Acad. Sci. U.S.A.* **82,** 7661–7665.

Fojo, A. T., Lebo, R., Simizu, N., Chin, J. E., Roninson, I. B., Merlino, G. T., Gottesman, M. M., and Pastan, I. (1986). Localization of multidrug resistance–associated DNA sequences to human chromosome 7. *Somatic Cell. Mol. Genet.* **12,** 415–420.

Fojo, A. T., Ueda, K., Slamon, D. J., Poplack, D. G., Gottesman, M. M., and Pastan, I. (1987). Expression of a multidrug-resistance gene in human tumors and tissues. *Proc. Natl. Acad. Sci. U.S.A.* **84,** 265–269.

Foote, S. J., Thompson, J. K., Cowman, A. F., and Kemp, D. J. (1989). Amplification of the multidrug resistance gene in some chloroquine-resistant isolates of *P. falciparum. Cell* **57,** 921–930.

Foote, S. J., Kyle, D. E., Martin, R. K., Oduola, A. M. J., Forsyth, K., Kemp, D. J., and Cowman, A. F. (1990). Several alleles of the multidrug-resistance gene are closely linked to chloroquine resistance in *Plasmodium falciparum. Nature* **345,** 255–258.

Galski, H., Sullivan, M., Willingham, M. C., Chin, K.-V., Gottesman, M. M., Pastan, I., and Merlino, G. T. (1989). Expression of a human multidrug-resistance cDNA (*MDR1*) in the bone marrow of transgenic mice: Resistance to daunomycin-induced leukopenia. *Mol. Cell. Biol.* **9,** 4357–4363.

Gerlach, J. H., Endicott, J. A., Juranka, P. F., Henderson, G., Sarangi, F., Deuchars, K. L., and Ling, V. (1986). Homology between P-glycoprotein and a bacterial haemolysin transport protein suggests a model for multidrug resistance. *Nature* **324,** 485–489.

Germann, U., Gottesman, M. M., and Pastan, I. (1989). Expression of a multidrug resistance–adenosine deaminase fusion gene. *J. Biol. Chem.* **264,** 7418–7424.

Germann, U., Chin, K.-v., Pastan, I., and Gottesman, M. M. (1990). Retroviral transfer of a chimeric multidrug resistance–adenosine deaminase gene. *FASEB J.* **4,** 1501–1507.

Glaser, P., Sakamoto, H., Bellalou, J., Ulmann, A., and Danchin, A. (1988). Secretion of cyclolysin, the calmodulin-sensitive adenylate cyclase-haemolysin bifunctional protein of *Bordetella pertussis. EMBO J.* **7**, 3997–4004.

Goldstein, L. J., Galski, H., Fojo, A. T., Willingham, M. C., Lai, S.-L., Gazdar, A., Pirker, R., Green, A., Crist, W., Brodeur, G. M., Lieber, M., Cossman, J., Gottesman, M. M., and Pastan, I. (1989). Expression of a multidrug-resistance gene in human cancers. *J. Natl. Cancer Inst.* **81**, 116–124.

Gottesman, M. M., and Pastan, I. (1988). The multidrug transporter, a double-edged sword. *J. Biol. Chem.* **263**, 12163–12166.

Greenberger, L. M., Yang, C. H., Gindin, E., and Horwitz, S. B. (1990). Photoaffinity probes for the α_1-adrenergic receptor and the calcium channel bind to a common domain in P-glycoprotein. *J. Biol. Chem.* **265**, 4394–4401.

Gros, P., Ben-Neriah, Y. U., Croop, J., and Housman, D. E. (1986a). Isolation and expression of a complementary DNA that confers multidrug resistance. *Nature* **323**, 728–731.

Gros, P., Croop, J., and Housman, D. E. (1986b). Mammalian multidrug-resistance gene: Complete cDNA sequence indicates strong homology to bacterial transport proteins. *Cell* **47**, 371–380.

Gros, P., Croop, J., Roninson, I., Varshavsky, A., and Housman, D. E. (1986c). Isolation and characterization of DNA sequences amplified in multidrug-resistant hamster cells. *Proc. Natl. Acad. Sci. U.S.A.* **83**, 337–341.

Guild, B. C., Mulligan, R. C., Gros, P., and Housman, D. E. (1988). Retroviral transfer of a murine cDNA for multidrug resistance confers pleiotropic drug resistance to cells without prior drug selection. *Proc. Natl. Acad. Sci. U.S.A.* **85**, 1595–1599.

Higgins, C. F., Hiles, I. D., Salmonel, G. P. C., Gill, D. R., Downie, J. A., Evans, I. J., Holland, I. B., Gray, L., Buckel, S. D., Bell, A. W., and Hermodson, M. A. (1986). A family of related ATP-binding subunits coupled to many distinct biological processes in bacteria. *Nature* **323**, 448–450.

Higgins, C. F., Hiles, I. D., Whalley, K., and Jamieson, D. J. (1985). Nucleotide binding by membrane components of bacterial periplasmic binding protein-dependent transport systems. *EMBO J.* **4**, 1033–1039.

Horio, M., Gottesman, M. M., and Pastan, I. (1988). ATP-dependent transport of vinblastine in vesicles from human multidrug-resistant cells. *Proc. Natl. Acad. Sci. U.S.A.* **85**, 3580–3584.

Horio, M., Chin, K.-V., Currier, S. J., Goldenberg, S., Williams, C., Pastan, I., Gottesman, M. M., and Handler, J. (1989). Transepithelial transport of drugs by the multidrug transporter in cultured Madin-Darby canine kidney cell epithelia. *J. Biol. Chem.* **264**, 14880–14884.

Horio, M., Lovelace, E., Pastan, I., and Gottesman, M. M. (1990). Agents which reverse multidrug resistance are inhibitors of ³H-vinblastine transport by isolated vesicles. *Biochim. Biophys. Acta,* in press.

Howell, N., Belli, T. A., Zaczkiewics, L. T., and Belli, J. A. (1984). High-level, unstable adriamycin resistance in a Chinese hamster mutant cell line with double-minute chromosomes. *Cancer Res.* **44**, 4023–4030.

Hsu, S. I. H., Lothstein, L., and Horwitz, S. B. (1989). Differential overexpression of three *mdr* gene family members in multidrug resistant J774-2 mouse cells. Evidence that distinct P-glycoprotein precursors are encoded by unique *mdr* genes. *J. Biol. Chem.* **264**, 12053–12062.

Hyde, S. C., Emsley, P., Hartshorn, M. J., Mimmack, M. M., Gileadi, U., Pearce, S. R., Gullagher, M. P., Gill, D. R., Hubbard, R. E., and Higgins, C. F. (1990). Structural and functional relationships of ATP-binding proteins associated with cystic fibrosis, multidrug resistance, and bacterial transport. *Nature* **346**, 362–365.

Juliano, R. L., and Ling, V. (1976). A surface glycoprotein-modulating drug permeability in Chinese hamster ovary cell mutants. *Biochim. Biophys. Acta* **455**, 152–162.

Kamijo, K., Taketani, S., Yokota, S., Osumi, T., and Hashimoto, T. (1990). The 70-kDa peroxisomal membrane protein is member of the MDR (P-glycoprotein)-related ATP-binding protein superfamily. *J. Biol. Chem.* **265,** 4534–4540.

Kamiwatari, M., Nagata, Y., Kikuchi, H., Yoshimura, A., Sumizawa, T., Shudo, N., Sakoda, R., Seto, K., and Akiyama, S. (1989). Correlation between reversing of multidrug resistance and inhibiting of [³H]azidopine photolabeling of P-glycoprotein by newly synthesized dihydropyridine analogues in a human cell line. *Cancer Res.* **49,** 3190–3195.

Kane, S. E., Pastan, I., and Gottesman, M. M. (1990). Genetic basis of multidrug resistance of tumor cells. Review. *J. Bioenerg. Biomembr.* **22,** 593–618.

Kane, S. E., Reinhard, D. H., Fordis, C. M., Pastan, I., and Gottesman, M. M. (1990). A new vector using the human multidrug-resistance gene as a selectable marker enables overexpression of foreign genes in eukaryotic cells. *Gene* **84,** 439–446.

Kane, S. E., Troen, B. R., Gal, S., Ueda, K., Pastan, I., and Gottesman, M. M. (1988). Use of a cloned multidrug-resistance gene for coamplification and overproduction of a major excreted protein, a tranformation-regulated secreted acid protease. *Mol. Cell. Biol.* **8,** 3316–3321.

Kartner, N., Evernden-Porelle, D., Bradley, G., and Ling, V. (1985). Detection of P-glycoprotein in multidrug-resistant cell lines by monoclonal antibodies. *Nature* **316,** 820–823.

Kessel, D. (1989). Exploring multidrug resistance using rhodamine 123. *Cancer Commun.* **1,** 145–149.

Keizer, H. G., and Joenje, H. (1989). Increased cytosolic pH in multidrug-resistant human lung tumor cells: Effect of verapamil. *J. Natl. Cancer Inst.* **81,** 706–709.

Kioka, N., Tsubota, J., Kakehi, Y., Komano, T., Gottesman, M. M., Pastan, I., and Ueda, K. (1989). P-glycoprotein gene (*mdr1*) cDNA from human adrenal: Normal P-glycoprotein carries gly185 with an altered pattern of multidrug resistance. *Biochem. Biophys. Res. Commun.* **162,** 224–231.

Konig, R., Ashwell, G., and Hanover, J. A. (1989). Overexpression and biosynthesis of CD4 in Chinese hamster ovary cells: Coamplification using the multidrug-resistance gene. *Proc. Natl. Acad. Sci. U.S.A.* **86,** 9188–9192.

Kuchler, K., Sterne, R. E., and Thorner, J. (1989). *Saccharomyces cerevisiae* STE6 gene product: A novel pathway for protein export in eukaryotic cells. *EMBO J.* **8,** 3973–3984.

Ling, V., and Baker, R. M. (1978). Dominance of colchicine resistance in hybrid CHO cells. *Somat. Cell. Genet.* **4:** 193–200.

Ling, V., and Thompson, L. H. (1973). Reduced permeability in CHO cells as a mechanism of resistance to colchicine. *J. Cell. Physiol.* **83:** 103–116.

Lothstein, L., Hsu, S. I., Horwitz, S. B., and Greenberger, L. M. (1989). Alternate overexpression of two P-glycoprotein genes is associated with changes in multidrug resistance in a J774.2 cell line. *J. Biol. Chem.* **264,** 16054–16058.

Lothstein, L., and Horwitz, S. B. (1986). Expression of phenotype traits following modulation of colchicine resistance in J774.2 cells. *J. Cell. Physiol.* **127,** 253–260.

Marino, P., Gottesman, M. M., and Pastan, I. (1990). Regulation of the multidrug-resistance gene in regenerating rat liver. *Cell Growth and Differentiation* **1,** 57–62.

Maurer, B. J., Lai, E., Hamkalo, B. A., Hood, L., and Attardi, G. (1987). Novel submicroscopic extrachromosomal elements containing amplified genes in human cells. *Nature* **327,** 434–437.

McGrath, J. P., and Varsharsky, A. (1989). The yeast STE6 gene encodes a homologue of the mammalian multidrug-resistance P-glycoprotein. *Nature* **340,** 400–404.

McLachlin, J. R., Eglitis, M. A., Ueda, K., Kantoff, P. W., Pastan, I., Anderson, W. F., and Gottesman, M. M. (1990). Expression of a human complementing DNA for the multidrug-resistance gene in murine hematopoietic precursor cells with the use of retroviral gene transfer. *J. Natl. Cancer Inst.* **82,** 1260–1263.

Mellado, W., and Horwitz, S. B. (1987). Phosphorylation of the multidrug-resistance-associated glycoprotein. *Biochemistry* **26,** 6900–6904.

Meese, E., Olson, S., Horwitz, S., and Trent, J. (1990). Gene amplification is mediated by extra-chromosomal elements in the multidrug resistant J774.2 murine cell line. *Proc. A.A.C.R.* **31,** 380.

Meyers, M. B., and Biedler, J. L. (1981). Increased synthesis of a low-molecular-weight protein in vincristine-resistant cells. *Biochem. Biophys. Res. Commun.* **99,** 228–235.

Meyers, M. B., Spengler, B. A., Chang, T. D., Melera, P. W., and Biedler, J. L. (1985). Gene amplification–associated cytogenetic aberrations and protein changes in vincristine-resistant Chinese hamster, mouse, and human cells. *J. Cell Biol.* **100,** 588–597.

Nogae, I., Kohno, K., Kikuchi, J., Kuwano, M., Akiyama, S., Kiue, A., Suzuki, K., Yoshida, Y., Cornwell, M. M., Pastan, I., and Gottesman, M. M. (1989). Analysis of structural features of dihydropyridine analogs needed to reverse multidrug resistance and to inhibit photoaffinity labeling of P-glycoprotein. *Biochem. Pharmacol.* **38,** 519–527.

O'Hare, K., Murphy, C., Levis, R., and Rubin, G. M. (1984). DNA sequence of the *white* locus of *Drosophila melanogaster*. *J. Mol. Biol.* **180,** 437–455.

Pastan, I., Gottesman, M. M., Ueda, K., Lovelace, E., Rutherford, A. V., and Willingham, M. C. (1988). A retrovirus carrying an *MDR1* cDNA confers multidrug resistance and polarized expression of P-glycoprotein in MDCK cells. *Proc. Natl. Acad. Sci. U.S.A.* **85,** 4486–4490.

Pastan, I., and Gottesman, M. M. (1990). Drug resistance: Biological warfare at the cellular level. *In* "Molecular Foundations of Oncology" (Samuel Broder, ed.), Williams and Wilkins, pp. 83–93.

Qian, X., and Beck, W. T. (1990). Binding of an optically pure photoaffinity analogue of verapamil, LU-49888, to P-glycoprotein from multidrug-resistant human leukemic cell lines. *Cancer Res.* **50,** 1132–1137.

Raviv, Y., Pollard, H. B., Bruggemann, E. P., Pastan, I., and Gottesman, M. M. (1990). Photosensitized labeling of a functional multidrug transporter in living drug-resistant tumor cells. *J. Biol. Chem.* **265,** 3975–3980.

Raymond, M., and Gros, P. (1989). Mammalian multidrug-resistance gene: Correlation of exon organization with structural domains and duplication of an ancestral gene. *Proc. Natl. Acad. Sci. U.S.A.* **86,** 6488–6492.

Raymond, M., Rose, E., Housman, D. E., and Gros, P. (1990). Physical mapping, amplification, and overexpression of the mouse *mdr* gene family in multidrug-resistant cells. *Mol. Cell. Biol.* **10,** 1642–1651.

Richert, N. D., Aldwin, L., Nitecki, D., Gottesman, M. M., and Pastan, I. (1988). Stability and covalent modification of P-glycoprotein in multidrug-resistant KB cells. *Biochemistry* **27,** 7607–7613.

Riehm, H., and Biedler, J. L. (1971). Cellular resistance to daunomycin in Chinese hamster cells *in vitro*. *Cancer Res.* **31,** 409–412.

Riordan, J. R., and Ling, V. (1985). Genetic and biochemical characterization of multidrug resistance. *Pharmacol. Ther.* **28,** 51–75.

Riordan, J. R., Denchars, K., Kartner, N., Alon, M., Trent, J., and Ling, V. (1985). Amplification of P-glycoprotein genes in multidrug-resistant mammalian cell lines. *Nature (London)* **316,** 817–819.

Riordan, J. R., Rommens, J. M., Kerem, B.-s., Alon, N., Rozmahel, R., Grzelczak, Z., Zielenski, J., Lok, S., Plavsic, N., Chou, J-l., Drumm, M. L., Iannuzzi, M. C., Collins, F. S., and Tsui, L.-c. (1989). Identification of the cystic fibrosis gene: Cloning and characterization of complementary DNA. *Science* **245,** 1066–1073.

Roninson, I. B., Abelson, H. T., Housman, D. E., Howell, N., and Varshavsky, A. (1984). Amplification of specific DNA sequences correlates with multidrug resistance in Chinese hamster cells. *Nature (London)* **309,** 626–638.

Roninson, I. B., Chin, J. E., Choi, K., Gros, P., Housman, D. E., Fojo, A., Shen, D.-w., Gottesman, M. M., and Pastan, I. (1986). Isolation of the human *mdr* DNA sequences amplified in multidrug-resistant KB carcinoma cells. *Proc. Natl. Acad. Sci. U.S.A.* **83,** 4538–4542.

Roy, S. M., and Horwitz, S. B. (1985). A phosphoglycoprotein associated with taxol resistance in J774.2 cells. *Cancer Res.* **45,** 3856–3863.

Ruiz, J. C., Choi, K., Von Hoff, D. D., Roninson, I. B., and Wahl, G. M. (1989). Autonomously replicating episomes contain *mdr1* genes in a multidrug-resistant human cell line. *Mol. Cell. Biol.* **9,** 109–115.

Safa, A. R., Glover, C. J., Meyers, M. B., Biedler, J. L., and Felsted, R. L. (1986). Vinblastine photoaffinity labeling of a high-molecular-weight surface membrane glycoprotein specific for multidrug-resistant cells. *J. Biol. Chem.* **261,** 6137–6140.

Safa, A. R. (1988). Photoaffinity labeling of the multidrug-resistance-related P-glycoprotein with photoactive analogs of verapamil. *Proc. Natl. Acad. Sci. U.S.A.* **85,** 7187–7191.

Safa, A. R., Glover, C. J., Sewell, J. L., Meyers, M. B., Biedler, J. L., and Felsted, R. L. (1987). Identification of the multidrug resistance–related membrane glycoprotein as an acceptor for calcium channel blockers. *J. Biol. Chem.* **262,** 7884–7888.

Safa, A. R., Mehta, N. D., and Agresti, M. (1989). Photoaffinity labeling of P-glycoprotein in multidrug-resistant cells with photoactive analogs of colchicine. *Biochem. Biophys. Res. Commun.* **162,** 1402–1408.

Schimke, R. T. (1988). Gene amplification in cultured cells. *J. Biol. Chem.* **263,** 5989–5992.

Schoenlein, P. V., Shen, D.-w., Johnson, B. P., Pastan, I., and Gottesman, M. M. (1990). The amplification of the human *MDR1* gene occurs via episome formation in KB carcinoma cells. *Proc. A.A.C.R.* **31,** 356.

Scotto, K. W., Biedler, J. L., and Melera, P. W. (1987). Amplification and expression of genes associated with multidrug resistance in mammalian cells. *Science* **232,** 751–755.

Shen, D.-w., Fojo, A., Chin, J. E., Roninson, I. B., Richert, N., Pastan, I., and Gottesman, M. M. (1986a). Human multidrug-resistant cell lines: Increased *mdr1* expression can proceed gene amplification. *Science* **232,** 643–645.

Shen, D.-w., Cardarelli, C., Hwang, J., Cornwell, M., Richert, N., Ishii, S., Pastan, I., and Gottesman, M. M. (1986b). Multiple drug-resistant human KB carcinoma cells independently selected for high-level resistance to colchicine, adriamycin, or vinblastine show changes in expression of specific proteins. *J. Biol. Chem.* **261:** 7762–7770.

Siegfried, J. A., Tritton, T. R., and Sartorelli, A. C. (1983). Comparison of anthracycline concentrations in S180 cell lines of varying sensitivity. *Eur. J. Cancer Clin. Oncol.* **19,** 1133–1141.

Smith, C. L., Econome, J., Schutt, A., Kico, A., and Cantor, C. R. (1987a). A physical map of the *Escherichia coli* K-12 genome. *Science* **236,** 1448–1453.

Smith, C. L., Lawrence, S. K., Gillespie, G. A., Cantor, C. R., Weissman, S. M., and Collins, F. S. (1987b). Strategies for mapping and cloning macroregions of mammalian genomes. *Methods Enzymol.* **151,** 461–489.

Stanfield, S. W., Ielpi, L., O'Brochta, D., Helinski, D. R., and Ditta, G. S. (1988). The ndvA gene product of *Rhizobium meliloti* is required for β-(1→2) glucan production and has homology to the ATP-binding export protein Hly B. *J. Bacteriol.* **170,** 3523–3530.

Stark, G. R., Debatisse, M., Giulotto, E., and Wahl, G. M. (1989). Recent progress in understanding mechanisms of mammalian DNA amplification. *Cell* **57,** 901–908.

Strathdee, C. A., and Lo, R. Y. (1989). Cloning, nucleotide sequence, and characterization of genes encoding the secretion function of the *Pasteurella haemolytica* leukotoxin determinant. *J. Bacteriol.* **171,** 916–928.

Tanaka, S., Currier, S. J., Bruggemann, E. P., Germann, U. A., Pastan, I., and Gottesman, M. M. (1990). Use of recombinant P-glycoprotein fragments to produce antibodies to the multidrug transporter. *Biochem. Biophys. Res. Commun.* **166,** 180–186.

Teeter, L. D., Atsumi, S.-i., Sen, S., and Kuo, T. (1986). DNA amplification in multidrug, cross-resistant Chinese hamster ovary cells: Molecular characterization and cytogenetic localization of amplified DNA. *J. Cell Biol.* **103,** 1159–1166.

Thiebaut, F., Tsuruo, T., Hamada, H., Gottesman, M. M., Pastan, I., and Willingham, M. C. (1987). Cellular localization of the multidrug-resistance gene product P-glycoprotein in normal human tissues. *Proc. Natl. Acad. Sci. U.S.A.* **84,** 7735–7738.

Thiebaut, F., Tsuruo, T., Hamada, H., Gottesman, M. M., Pastan, I., and Willingham, M. C. (1989). Immunohistochemical localization in normal tissues of different epitopes in the multidrug transport protein P170: Evidence for localization in brain capillaries and crossreactivity of one antibody with a muscle protein. *J. Histochem. Cytochem.* **37,** 159–164.

Thiebaut, F., Currier, S. J., Whitaker, J., Haugland, R. P., Gottesman, M. M., Pastan, I., and Willingham, M. C. (1990). Activity of the multidrug transporter results in alkalinization of the cytosol: Measurement of cytosolic pH by microinjection of a pH-sensitive dye. *J. Histochem. Cytochem.* **38,** 685–690.

Thorgeirrson, S., Huber, B., Sorrell, S., Fojo, A. T., Pastan, I., and Gottesman, M. M. (1987). Expression of the multidrug-resistance gene in hepatocarcinogenesis and regenerating rat liver. *Science* **236,** 1120–1122.

Tsuruo, T. (1988). Mechanisms of multidrug resistance and implications for therapy. *Jpn. J. Cancer Res.* **79:** 285–296.

Ueda, K., Cardarelli, C., Gottesman, M. M., and Pastan, I. (1987). Expression of a full-length cDNA for the human "*MDR1*" (P-glycoprotein) gene confers multidrug resistance to colchicine, doxorubicin, and vinblastine. *Proc. Natl. Acad. Sci. U.S.A.* **84,** 3004–3008.

Van der Bliek, A. M., Van der Velde-Koerts, T., Ling, V., and Borst, P. (1986). Overexpression and amplification of five genes in a multidrug-resistant Chinese hamster ovary cell line. *Mol. Cell. Biol.* **6,** 1671–1678.

Van der Bliek, A. M., Kooiman, P. M., Schneider, C., and Borst, P. (1988). Sequence of *mdr3* cDNA encoding a human P-glycoprotein. *Gene* **71,** 401–411.

Von Hoff, D. D., Needham-Van Devanter, D. R., Yucel, J., Windle, B. E., and Wahl, G. M. (1988). Amplified human MYC oncogenes localized to replicating submicroscopic circular DNA molecules. *Proc. Natl. Acad. Sci. U.S.A.* **85,** 4804–4808.

Wahl, G. M. (1989). The importance of circular DNA in mammalian gene amplification. *Cancer Res.* **49,** 1333–1340.

Walker, J. E., Saraste, M., Runswick, M. J., and Gay, N. J. (1982). Distantly related sequences in the α- and β-subunits of ATP synthase, myosin, kinases, and other ATP-requiring enzymes and a common nucleotide binding fold. *EMBO J.* **1,** 945–951.

West, I. (1990). What determines the substrate specificity of the multidrug-resistance pump? *Trends Biochem. Sci.* **15,** 42–46.

Willingham, M. C., Cornwell, M. M., Cardarelli, C. O., Gottesman, M. M., and Pastan, I. (1986). Single-cell analysis of daunomycin uptake and efflux in multidrug-resistant and sensitive KB cells: Effect of verapamil and other drugs. *Cancer Res.* **46,** 5941–5946.

Wilson, C. M., Serrano, A. E., Wasley, A., Bogenshutz, M. P., Shankar, A. H., and Wirth, D. F. (1989). Amplification of a gene related to mammalian *mdr* genes in drug-resistant *Plasmodium falciparum*. *Science* **244,** 1184–1186.

Yang, C. H., Mellado, W., and Horwitz, S. B. (1988). Azidopine photoaffinity labeling of multidrug resistance–associated glycoproteins. *Biochem. Pharmacol.* **37,** 1417–1424.

Ye, Z., Dyke, K. V., Spearman, T., and Safa, A. R. (1989). ^{3}H-azidopine photoaffinity labeling of high-molecular-weight proteins in chloroquine-resistant falciparum malaria. *Biochem. Biophys. Res. Commun.* **162,** 809–813.

Yoshimura, A., Kuwazuru, Y., Sumizawa, T., Ichikawa, M., Ikeda, S., Uda, T., and Akiyama, S. (1989). Cytoplasmic orientation and two-domain structure of the multidrug transporter, P-glyco-protein, demonstrated with sequence-specific antibodies. *J. Biol. Chem.* **264,** 16282–16291.

Chapter 12

Role of p53 in Neoplasia

MOSHE OREN

Department of Chemical Immunology,
The Weizmann Institute of Science,
Rehovot 76100, Israel

I. Introduction

The cellular phosphoprotein p53 was initially discovered by virtue of its presence, at elevated levels, in a variety of *in vitro* transformed and tumor-derived cell lines (DeLeo *et al.*, 1979), as well as owing to its ability to form specific complexes with large T antigen, the major oncogenic protein of the DNA tumor virus SV40 (Lane and Crawford, 1979; Linzer and Levine, 1979; Melero *et al.*, 1980). The augmented levels of p53 in transformed cells raised the possibility that this protein possesses some growth-stimulatory activity, an excess of which could promote neoplastic transformation. This proposal was in line with the finding that inhibition of p53 function, mediated by the microinjection of anti-p53 antibodies into cell nuclei, prevented quiescent cells from resuming proliferation on exposure to serum (Mercer *et al.*, 1982, 1984). In addition, p53 levels were shown to increase severalfold in serum-stimulated mouse fibroblasts (Reich and Levine, 1984).

The contention that p53 was an oncogene whose augmented activity could be conducive to neoplasia was seemingly supported by the demonstration that p53 expression plasmids could make cells more transformed (for reviews see Crawford, 1983; Rotter and Wolf, 1984; Oren, 1985; O'Reilly, 1986; Jenkins and Sturzbecher, 1988). However, more recent work established that only mutant forms of p53 were capable of exerting such transforming effects. On the other

BIOCHEMICAL AND MOLECULAR ASPECTS
OF SELECTED CANCERS, VOL. 1

hand, wild-type (wt) p53, did not exhibit any transforming activity. Not only that, but overexpression of wt p53 could suppress oncogene-mediated transformation. It now appears very likely that wt p53 is, in fact, a tumor suppressor. Tumor-suppressor genes are presumed to interfere with neoplasia, either by possessing a direct antiproliferative activity or by imposing a restriction on the progression of a transformed cell toward a more malignant phenotype (for recent reviews see Bock and March, 1989; Sager, 1989; Weinberg, 1989; Mikkelsen and Cavenee, 1990; Levine, 1990). The presence of excess p53 in tumor cells, previously believed to represent an enhanced activity of wt p53, now appears to reflect, in fact, the accumulation of mutationally inactivated forms of the protein. The pattern of p53-related abnormalities, which is now emerging from the study of many types of human and rodent tumors, indicates that the p53 gene is a very frequent target for mutational alterations in cancer cells. Whether all these events simply cause the loss of the suppressor activity associated with wt p53, or whether some of them actually generate a *bona fide* oncogenic protein, is still an unresolved issue.

II. Historical Perspective

A. MUTANT P53 IS ONCOGENIC

p53 was first described in cells transformed by the DNA tumor virus SV40 as well as in a variety of other tumor-derived and *in vitro* transformed cell types. In all these systems, the protein was present at levels greatly above those found in normal cells. Based on the simple assumption that more protein implies more activity, it was inferred that the activity of p53 might play a positive role in promoting neoplastic processes. In other words, the possibility arose that p53 might be an oncogene product.

The molecular cloning of murine p53 cDNA and genomic DNA (Oren and Levine, 1983; Zakut-Houri *et al.*, 1983; Jenkins *et al.*, 1984b; Pennica *et al.*, 1984; Wolf and Rotter, 1984) made it possible to test directly the oncogenic potential of p53. When plasmids encoding p53 were introduced into primary rat embryo fibroblasts (REF) together with an activated human Ha-*ras* oncogene, morphologically transformed foci were induced (Eliyahu *et al.*, 1984; Parada *et al.*, 1984). The cells had a typical refractile, spindle-shaped morphology. All cell lines derived from such foci expressed high levels of the transfected mouse p53, in large excess over the endogenous rat p53, and usually much higher than seen in lines originating in non–virally induced mouse tumors (Fig. 1). On injection into syngeneic rats, such cell lines induced rapidly growing fibrosarcomas visible within less than 2 weeks after the subcutaneous injection of 10^6 cells. A similar assay had previously been described for *myc*. The results therefore indi-

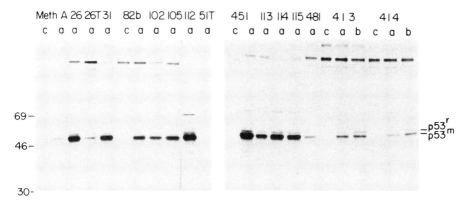

FIG. 1. Detection of p53 in various tumor-derived cell lines. Foci derived by the cotransfection of REF with plasmids encoding mutant p53 and *ras* were expanded into cell lines. Proteins were radiolabeled, extracted, and subjected to analysis by immunoprecipitation with an anti-p53 monoclonal antibody, followed by SDS-polyacrylamide gel electrophoresis. Depicted, in addition to the p53 + *ras* transformants, are also lines Meth A, derived from a chemically induced mouse fibrosarcoma, and 51T, originating in REF transformed by *myc* + *ras*. Reactions in a and b were done with two different p53-specific monoclonal antibodies; c, Control hybridoma supernatant. $p53^r$ and $p53^m$ identify the positions of endogenous rat p53 and transfected mouse p53, respectively.

cated that p53 could mimic the *in vitro* effects of deregulated *myc* expression, supporting the idea that the p53 gene was indeed an oncogene of a *myc*-like type. Quantitatively, the number of foci induced by p53 + *ras* was severalfold lower than seen in parallel dishes transfected by *myc* + *ras*, suggesting that p53 was somewhat less efficient than *myc* as an oncogene (Eliyahu *et al.*, 1984; Parada *et al.*, 1984). An interesting property of p53 + *ras* transformants was revealed when foci were trypsinized and transferred into new dishes, in an attempt to generate stable cell lines. Foci induced by a combination of *ras* with either *myc* or adenovirus E1A could be easily expanded into cell lines. On the other hand, p53 + *ras* foci often proved harder to expand. In many cases, only a fraction of such foci eventually gave rise to stable cell lines. This was particularly manifest with p53 plasmids possessing moderate, rather than very high, transforming activity (Eliyahu *et al.*, 1984; Finlay *et al.*, 1988; Hinds *et al.*, 1989). One likely interpretation was that the cells in such foci, although displaying a typical transformed morphology, were often still not immortalized. Furthermore, the data were consistent with the possibility that an additional genetic events had to occur in such cells before they could become a stable, immortal cell line.

The oncogenic activity of p53 was also revealed in a number of other systems, most of which had previously been shown to serve as good model systems for the oncogenic effects of overproduced *myc*. Introduction of p53 plasmids into adult rat chondrocytes (Jenkins *et al.*, 1984a, 1985) or into REF (Rovinski and

Benchimol, 1988) caused their conversion into immortal cell lines, still possessing a nontransformed cell morphology. In the former case, transfection of such p53-immortalized lines with activated Ha-*ras* led to their neoplastic transformation, giving rise to highly tumorigenic lines (Jenkins *et al.*, 1984a).

Growth-deregulating effects of p53 plasmids could also be observed in established cell lines. Accordingly, p53-expression plasmids relieved mouse Swiss 3T3 cells of their dependence on platelet-derived growth factor (PDGF) for proliferation (Kaczmarek *et al.*, 1986; Gai *et al.*, 1988). *In vivo*, transfection of p53 could give rise to a more malignant phenotype in a number of systems. Introduction of p53 plasmids into Rat-1 fibroblasts, possessing a low tumorigenic potential in nude mice, made such cells highly tumorigenic (Eliyahu *et al.*, 1985). A striking example was seen in the case of the L12 mouse lymphoid cell line. These cells, transformed by Abelson MuLV, are devoid of any detectable p53 protein expression, owing to insertional inactivation by a Moloney leukemia provirus (Wolf and Rotter, 1984). Unlike similar lines that express p53, these p53-negative cells cannot elicit lethal tumors in syngeneic mice (Rotter *et al.*, 1983b). However, following the introduction of a p53 plasmid, L12 cells now became capable of causing lethal tumors (Wolf *et al.*, 1984). Finally, an expression plasmid containing mouse genomic p53 DNA was transfected into a murine bladder carcinoma line of low metastatic capacity. The resultant lines exhibited elevated p53 protein levels, and a significantly increased metastatic potential in syngeneic mice (Pohl *et al.*, 1988).

All the above findings seemingly suggested that, like *myc*, p53 was a typical nuclear oncogene whose overproduction contributed positively to neoplastic processes. Further work, however, clearly established that none of the p53 plasmids employed in these studies represented the true wt version of the gene. In fact, all these plasmids carried mutations in the protein-coding region, although different mutations were present in different clones (Eliyahu *et al.*, 1988; Finlay *et al.*, 1988; Hinds *et al.*, 1989). When tested for the cotransformation of REF in cooperation with *ras*, plasmids encoding wt p53 had no detectable transforming activity; only certain mutant forms of the gene could exhibit such cooperation (Eliyahu *et al.*, 1988; Finaly *et al.*, 1988; Hinds *et al.*, 1989). An apparent activating effect of p53 mutations had previously also been reported by Jenkins *et al.* (1985), studying the immortalization of rat chondrocytes. All these findings demonstrated that wt mouse p53 is actually not oncogenic, and mutations are needed in order to endow it with oncogenic activity *in vitro*. This was very different from the case of *myc*, where the mere deregulated overexpression of the otherwise wt protein rendered it highly oncogenic in the REF assay (Lee *et al.*, 1985). Thus, wt p53 was not an oncogene, and at best could be considered a protooncogene, whose activation was contingent upon the acquisition of mutations in the protein-coding region. As detailed in the next section, subsequent work revealed that the differences between p53 and *myc* were far more extensive.

In fact, it is now clear that not only is wt p53 nononcogenic, but also it is actually capable of interfering with neoplastic processes.

B. WILD-TYPE p53 IS A POTENTIAL TUMOR SUPPRESSOR

Results which were not easy to reconcile with the notion that p53 is a dominant oncogene were reported as early as 1985. Benchimol and co-workers studied the induction of murine erythroleukemia by the Friend virus. Clonal erythroleukemic cell lines were established from spleens of Friend virus–infected mice. Analysis of such lines revealed that while many had elevated p53 levels, a significant proportion (over 20%) of the lines either had no detectable p53 at all, or made only a truncated form of the protein (Mowat *et al.*, 1985). The molecular basis for this aberrant p53 expression was found to vary among the independent lines. While in some cases there were deletions in the p53 gene (Munroe *et al.*, 1988; Ben David *et al.*, 1988), in other cases the loss of expression was due to the integration of retroviral DNA within the gene (Ben David *et al.*, 1988). Most significantly, analysis of cells isolated at late stages of the disease demonstrated that transformed cell lines, defective in p53 expression, were always clonal (Chow *et al.*, 1987). The data indicated that the responsible p53 gene rearrangements must have occurred very early in the process of Friend virus–induced tumorigenesis. It was therefore proposed that such rearrangements, abolishing normal p53 expression, might have conferred a strong selective advantage on these transformed cells (Chow *et a.*, 1987). Cases of loss of p53 expression were also reported in human tumor cells, albeit more sporadically (see Section II).

The evidence in favor of a selection against p53 expression in certain types of malignant cells, along with the realization that wt p53 was not oncogenic, prompted a reevaluation of the normal role of p53. One could now speculate that, whereas p53 mutants could exhibit a transforming capacity, the wt gene was, in fact, even capable of interfering with certain types of neoplastic processes. In that case, abrogation of its expression could have a positive contribution to malignant transformation. In other words, p53 could now be considered a potential tumor-suppressor gene. This idea was tested by studying the effects of wt p53–encoding plasmids on oncogene-mediated transformation of REF (Finlay *et al.*, 1989; Eliyahu *et al.*, 1989). REF can become neoplastically transformed through the combined action of plasmids overproducing mutant p53 and activated Ha-*ras* (see Section I, A). If wt p53 was indeed a tumor suppressor, it was now conceivable that the oncogenic activity of mutant p53 could be due, at least in part, to the ability of the mutant protein to block the function of the endogenous wt p53 in the transfected cells. In that case, mutant p53 could be acting in a dominant negative fashion (Herskowitz, 1987).

If this model is correct, then one should, potentially, be able to antagonize transforming p53 mutants by increasing the amount of wt p53 in the cell. Therefore, the effects of various p53 plasmids were tested on the transformation of REF by a combination of *ras* and pLTRcGval135; the latter plasmid directs the abundant synthesis of mutant p53 (Eliyahu *et al.*, 1985, 1988; Finlay *et al.*, 1988). Experiments done by Finlay *et al.* (1989) and by Eliyahu *et al.* (1989), indeed proved that inclusion of wt p53 plasmids in the assay led to a major reduction in the number of transformed foci. The results of one such series of experiments are portrayed in Fig. 2. The bottom line of the figure lists the various oncogene combinations employed to transform the REF. The cotransfected plasmids were pSPCMV (vector only), pCMVp53dl (containing a highly deleted version of the p53 coding region), pCMVc5 (encoding a tumor-derived mutant mouse p53), and pCMVNc9 (encoding wt murine p53). The "p53 + *ras*" columns display the number of foci elicited by p53val135 + *ras* in presence of each cotransfected DNA. Clearly, addition of wt p53-expression plasmid greatly reduced the ability of an oncogenic p53 mutant to elicit foci in concert with *ras*. This apparent suppression of transformation was dependent on the production of wt p53 protein, and was abolished by the mutations present in pCMVc5.

The ability of wt p53 to act *in vitro* as a tumor suppressor is not restricted to cases in which transformation is driven by mutant p53. Actually a similar, though somewhat less complete, inhibitory effect is exerted by wt p53 plasmids on the transformation of REF by a variety of oncogene combinations. These include *myc* + *ras*, adenovirus E1A + *ras*, and adenovirus E1A + E1B (Fig. 2). In all these cases, tumor-derived p53 mutants proved utterly devoid of any suppressor activity (Finlay *et al.*, 1989; Eliyahu *et al.*, 1989; Halevy *et al.*, 1990). The latter fact is highly significant, as it supports the contention that the

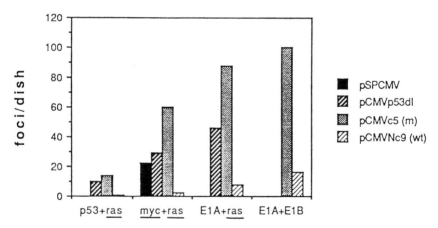

FIG. 2.   Transformation of REF by different oncogene combinations in presence of mouse p53 plasmids. Oncogene pairs used for transfection are indicated at the bottom. See text for details of p53 plasmids. Adapted, with permission, from Eliyahu *et al.*, 1990.

apparent suppressor activity, revealed in this *in vitro* assay, is indeed selected against in the course of actual tumorigenesis.

Interestingly, plasmids encoding mutant p53 were often found to enhance the ability of various oncogene combinations to transform REF (Finaly *et al.*, 1989; Eliyahu *et al.*, 1989; Halevy *et al.*, 1990; Michalovitz *et al.*, 1990). Such enhancement is consistent with the possibility that these mutants may contribute a distinct positive oncogenic activity, resulting in an additive effect. However, it could equally imply that the activity of the endogenous wt rat p53 in REF restricts the ability of oncogenes such as *myc* and/or *ras* to promote stable cell transformation. In such cases, the cotransfected mutant p53 could be acting dominant-negatively to extinguish the function of the endogenous protein, thereby increasing transformation efficiencies.

The proposal that wt p53 may be a tumor suppressor, as suggested by these *in vitro* studies, gained strong independent support from the analysis of p53-related alterations in human cancer, detailed in the next section.

III. p53-Related Alterations in Human Cancer

A. Solid Tumors

1. *Osteosarcoma*

Aberrations related to p53 are rapidly emerging as some of the most frequent genetic alterations in human solid tumors. One of the first pertinent reports involved a study of human osteosarcoma lines and tumors (Masuda *et al.*, 1987). Rearrangements of the p53 gene were found in three of six osteogenic sarcoma specimens, whereas no rearrangement was seen when normal tissue from one of these patients was examined. Rearranged p53 genes were also identified in human osteosarcoma cell lines. In most of the latter cases, no p53 mRNA or protein was detectable. A seemingly contradictory observation was that in another osteosarcoma line, HOS, p53 was very abundant, rather than absent (Masuda *et al.*, 1987). Subsequently, however, these cells were shown to harbor a mutant p53 gene (Romano *et al.*, 1989). Unlike wt p53, the mutant protein encoded by this gene forms stable complexes with heat-shock proteins (Ehrhart *et al.*, 1988), and fails to interact with the SV40 large T antigen (Van Roy *et al.*, 1990).

2. *Colorectal Cancer*

The study of 58 human colorectal carcinoma tumors (Vogelstein *et al.*, 1989), indicated that more than 75% of them carried deletions in the short arm of one chromosome 17. The p53 gene is located in this region (McBride *et al.*, 1986; Isobe *et al.*, 1986; Miller *et al.*, 1986). Careful restriction fragment–length polymorphism (RFLP) analysis revealed that in all cases, the deleted region also included the p53 gene itself, suggesting that p53 may be the target of these deletions. In several such cases, the remaining p53 allele was subjected to fine structural analysis. It was found that, in tumors exhibiting a loss of heterozygosity for p53, the remaining p53 allele was usually not wt. In different tumors, different mutations were present in the p53 protein coding region (Baker *et al.*, 1989; Nigro *et al.*, 1989). On the assumption that these were primarily loss-of-function mutations, Vogelstein and coworkers concluded that the elimination of wt p53 expression may be an essential step in the development of colorectal carcinoma. They therefore proposed that the wt p53 gene has a tumor-suppressor function, which serves as a target for mutational inactivation during colorectal tumor progression (Baker *et al.*, 1989).

Of note, a minor fraction of colorectal carcinomas seem to progress without the loss of wt p53 expression. Of two cases still retaining both p53 alleles, one apparently expressed both wt and mutant p53, whereas the other failed to provide any evidence for the presence of mutant p53 (Nigro *et al.*, 1989). While the first case is compatible with a dominant negative model for wt p53 inactivation, the other is not. In the latter case, p53-related events may not be involved at all. Alternatively, however, the protein made in such cells could nevertheless end up being inactive, due to some unique posttranslational modification, or to the elimination of a molecular target needed for its suppressor activity.

3. *Lung Cancer*

A similar situation was subsequently reported in human lung cancer (Takahaski *et al.*, 1989; Nigro *et al.*, 1989; Iggo *et al.*, 1990). Here, too, it was discovered that the p53 gene is frequently mutated or inactivated in all types of lung cancer. The changes include gross rearrangements, homozygous deletions, and a high frequency of point or minor mutations, all of which change the amino acid sequence of this protein. On the basis of their findings, Minna and coworkers (Takahashi *et al.*, 1989) also proposed that p53 is an antioncogene, whose disruption is involved in the pathogenesis of human lung cancer. A role for abnormal p53 expression in lung carcinogenesis was also suggested by immunohistological studies on primary lung cancer samples (Iggo *et al.*, 1990). Employing a new p53-specific monoclonal antibody, PAb240, it was found that more than 50% of the tumors displayed a gross overexpression of p53, whereas no such case was observed among normal lung biopsies, or in seven low-malignancy carcinoid tumors. While this antibody can react with wt p53 under the conditions of immunohistological staining (Gannon *et al.*, 1990), previous studies on mouse cells indicate that stabilization of p53 is highly diagnostic of the presence of structural alterations (Jenkins *et al.*, 1985; Rovinski *et al.*, 1988; Finaly *et al.*, 1988; Halevy *et al.*, 1989). This was directly confirmed for several representative human lung carcinomas by sequencing PCR-amplified cDNA. In all the tested cases, strong staining with PAb240 correlated with the homozygous expression of mutant p53 (Iggo *et al.*, 1990). Finally, it is noteworthy that transgenic mice, overexpressing mutant p53 alleles, display a very high incidence of lung tumors; the latter constitute the most frequent malignancy in such mice (Lavigeur *et al.*, 1989).

4. *Breast Cancer*

While consistent deletions in 17p were earlier reported for colon and lung cancer, they were not considered a typical aberration in breast cancer. More recently, however, a refined RFLP analysis revealed a high frequency of marker loss on 17p in breast tumors (Mackay *et al.*, 1988; Devilee *et al.*, 1989). Here, too, the suggestion was made that a suppressor gene may reside in that region. While still compatible with the presence of more than a single suppressor gene on 17p, it appeared very reasonable that p53 might be implicated in breast cancer, too. Circumstantial evidence supporting this notion was provided by a number of studies. Crawford and co-workers reported the presence of circulating anti-p53 antibodies in the blood of 11.5% of breast cancer patients (Crawford *et al.*, 1984; Crawford, 1985). One interesting possibility is that those patients possessed an altered, more immunogenic form of p53 generated by point mutations or other gene alterations. Similarly, elevated p53 levels were observed by the same investigators, using a radioimmunoassay, in 24% of breast cancer tumors (Crawford *et al.*, 1984; Crawford, 1985). Another group, using immunohistochemistry on frozen sections, found elevated p53 levels in about 15% of the patients; a higher frequency was found when high-grade tumors were grouped separately (Catoretti *et al.*, 1988a,b). As in lung cancer (Section II, A, 3), an enhanced staining pattern most probably indicates the presence of p53 mutations in these tumors.

More recent data seem to confirm this prediction. Nigro *et al.* (1989) and Bartek *et al.* (1990) found p53 mutations in six of six breast cancer lines analyzed. In all cases, no wt p53 was expressed in these cells. So far, published information about actual tumors (rather than cell lines) is practically nonexistent. The only case described to date of a primary human biopsy was homozygous for p53, but no mutation was detected (Nigro *et al.*, 1989). It is therefore too early to decide whether the cell-line data reflect a prominent role for p53 mutations in breast cancer, or whether such mutations are merely advantageous for establishing stable breast cancer lines *in vitro*.

5. *Other Solid Tumors*

Information about p53-related aberrations in other human solid tumors is relatively sparse, although this situation is likely to change rapidly. Nigro *et al.*

(1989) found p53 mutations in four of four brain tumors (glioblastoma multiforme), all of which were homozygous for p53 expression. No mutations were detected in a single cell line of a similar origin. Additionally, they identified a p53 mutation in a neurofibrosarcoma tumor. The relevance of the latter finding is underscored by recent work of Menon *et al.* (1990), involving cases of von Recklinghausen's neurofibromatosis. These investigators studied genetic alterations associated with the progression of benign neurofibromas to malignant neurofibrosarcomas. Whereas no loss of markers on 17p was seen in any of 30 benign tumors, the majority of malignant tumors displayed such a loss. In some of these cases, the remaining p53 allele was mutant. This may, therefore, be another type of cancer in which p53 aberrations play a role in malignant progression.

Aberrant p53 expression may also play a role in the pathogenesis of hepatocellular carcinoma. This was suggested by the work of Bressac *et al.* (1990). In a survey of seven human hepatocellular carcinoma–derived cell lines, they found that six of those exhibited p53-related abnormalities. These ranged from accumulation of a long-lived, presumably mutant protein, to a partial deletion of the gene, coupled with the lack of any detectable p53 mRNA.

More work is obviously needed before one can tell with certainty whether p53 alterations are prevalent in all types of solid tumors, or whether they occur in a nonrandom way in only a subset of tumors. In any event, such alterations appear to be very frequent, at least in the most common types of human solid tumors.

An interesting observation was made with the HeLa cell line derived from cervical carcinoma. In these cells, the p53 gene appears intact, and the cells contain normal-size p53 mRNA, which can be translated *in vitro* to yield full-size p53. Nevertheless, no p53 protein can be detected in these cells, owing to either an exceptionally fast rate of degradation or a unique translational selectivity operating in HeLa cells (Matlashewski *et al.*, 1986). This observation stands to illustrate that even the analysis of tumor mRNA, let alone genomic DNA, probably provides an underestimate of the actual prevalence of p53 lesions in tumors.

B. Hematopoietic Malignancies

Leukemias were the first type of human malignancy in which losses of p53 expression were unequivocally documented. For instance, in line HL60, originating in a case of acute promyelocytic leukemia (APL), there is absolutely no p53 expression, due to deletion of a major part of the human p53 gene (Wolf and Rotter, 1985). A rearrangement in the p53 gene was also found in fresh material from an APL patient (Prokocimer *et al.*, 1986). In addition, Prokocimer *et al.* (1986) detected no p53 protein in any of the 17 acute myelocytic leukemia

(AML), 11 chronic myelocytic leukemia, 10 myelofibrosis, and 4 polycythemia vera fresh samples tested.

Evidence for a possible role of p53 aberrations in human CML is particularly compelling. This disease is characterized by a slow chronic phase, which is usually followed by an accelerated phase and eventually by a lethal acute blast crisis. In addition to the finding of Prokocimer *et al.* (1986), Lubbert *et al.* (1988) also reported a complete lack of p53 protein in a number of myeloid CML lines, including some that expressed easily detectable p53 mRNA. More recent work (Ahuja *et al.*, 1989; Kelman *et al.*, 1989), revealed that p53-related changes were frequently seen in the blast crisis, but not in the chronic phase. In total, 12 of 48 blast crisis patients had gross structural alteration in the p53 gene. Ten of 16 cases, with and without such structural alteration, had no detectable p53 mRNA. On the other hand, only 2 of 77 chronic-phase samples displayed p53 gene rearrangements. It was suggested that disruption of normal p53 expression is a common event in blast crisis, and may therefore by a key inactivation step, causing the transition from the chronic phase to the more malignant acute phase.

Less is known about p53 aberrations in other hematopoietic malignancies. It is of note, though, that minor deletions in chromosome 17p, in the vicinity of the p53 gene locus, are frequently observed in myelodysplastic syndrome patients (Kerndrup *et al.*, 1987). A role for wt p53 inactivation is therefore also conceivable in this group of disorders.

C. MUTATIONAL HOT SPOTS

The rapidly expanding body of information about p53 mutations in human and rodent tumors clearly shows that such mutations can occur at any of a large number of residues within the protein-coding region. This feature is consistent with the proposal that wt p53 acts as a tumor suppressor gene. This proposal predicts that any mutation that interferes with the ability of the protein to function properly, will be selected for in the course of tumor progression (Green, 1989). On the other hand, the distribution of the mutations is not random. As evident from Fig. 3, containing a compendium of most p53 mutations detected so far in tumors, the vast majority cluster within a number of defined regions. These regions display a striking degree of overlap with previously defined *homology boxes,* whose sequence has been highly conserved in evolution (Soussi *et al.*, 1987). Such a high degree of conservation strongly suggests that the integrity of these domains is essential for the ability of p53 to carry out its normal functions. It is thus not surprising that such structural elements serve as primary targets for the presumptive mutational inactivation. In addition, in most cases in which mutations were found outside the homology boxes, they nevertheless still hit

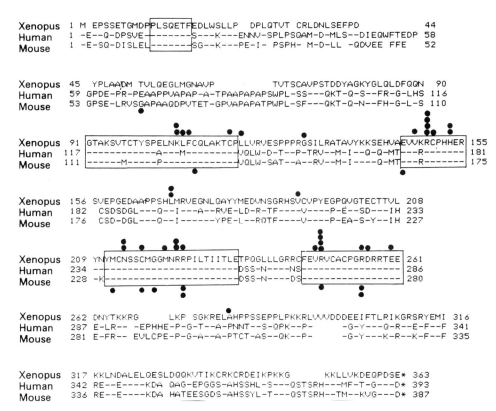

FIG. 3. Positions of p53 mutations in tumors relative to those of the conserved homology boxes. The sequence data are reproduced, with permission, from Soussi *et al.*, 1987. Homology boxes are identified by roman numerals. Each dot indicates a mutation in an individual tumor. Dots above and below each line represent mutations in human and mouse tumors, respectively. Compiled from Baker *et al.* (1989), Eliyahu *et al.* (1988), Takahaski *et al.* (1989), Nigro *et al.* (1989), Bartek, *et al.* (1990), Iggo *et al.* (1990), Halevy *et al.* (1990), and O. Halevy and M. Oren (unpublished data.) A cDNA clone derived from a vulvar carcinoma line (Harlow *et al.* 1985), now known to be mutant, was also included.

individual residues, which remained invariant throughout vertebrate evolution. The nonrandom distribution of the mutations also argues against the possibility that, during tumor formation, the p53 gene becomes an accidental target for indiscriminate alterations that have no relevance to the progression of the disease. On the contrary, it supports the contention that these mutations are indeed selected for, because they endow the cell with some new properties.

Within the conserved domains, many different residues appear to serve as appropriate targets. Nevertheless, there do appear to be a few preferred individual hot spots. In human p53, these are most notably arginine 175 and arginine 273. Whether this reflects a qualitative difference in the resultant mutant proteins, or merely some structural feature of the DNA in that region, is still an open issue.

IV. Molecular Properties of the p53 Protein

A major limitation for properly evaluating the consequences of p53 mutations, as well as the mechanism underlying its tumor-suppressor capacity, is the fundamental lack of understanding about the biochemical functions of the protein. Yet, from what has been learned thus far, one can glean clues for the types of activities that p53 may be involved in.

The p53 protein is predominantly localized in the nucleus (Dippold *et al.*, 1981; Rotter *et al.*, 1983a; Zantema *et al.*, 1985). This is especially true for molecules that carry the wt sequence (Gannon *et al.*, 1990). On the other hand, a variety of mutations, including some of those originating in tumors, result in a much higher fraction of the protein's being present in the cytoplasm (Sturzbecher *et al.*, 1987; Gannon *et al.*, 1990; Ginsberg *et al.*, 1991). Furthermore, cells harboring a temperature-sensitive (ts) p53 mutant proliferate at 37.5° C, but arrest at 32.5° C (Michalovitz *et al.*, 1990). This growth arrest correlates with the induction of a wt protein conformation, presumably coupled with a biochemical activity responsible for this "suppression" (Michalovitz *et al.*, 1990). Interestingly, while the ts protein is present in large amounts in the cytoplasm at 37.5° C, it exhibits an almost exclusively nuclear staining pattern at 32.5° C (Ginsberg *et al.*, 1991). It is therefore most likely that the suppressor activity of wt p53 requires interaction with certain nuclear targets. One is therefore inclined to suspect that p53 may play a role in processes related to regulation of gene expression or DNA replication.

The overall organization of the p53 protein is compatible with its acting as a transcription factor (see Levine, 1990). This possibility is supported by recent evidence (Fields and Jang, 1990; Raycroft *et al.*, 1990). Alternatively, there are some clues that seem to implicate p53 in the control of DNA synthesis. Iguchi-Ariga *et al.* (1988) reported the molecular cloning of a mammalian genomic DNA fragment, specifically recognized by p53, which was capable of autonomous replication. They therefore suggested that this DNA may represent a p53-dependent origin of cellular DNA replication. While these results are very provocative, their relevance is hard to assess owing to the lack of a proper definition for an authentic mammalian replication origin. A link between p53 and DNA replication is perhaps also provided by studies on SV40 DNA replication. The DNA of this tumor virus is replicated from a well-defined origin, and requires the presence of the SV40 large T antigen. This process can be inhibited both *in vitro* and *in vivo* by wt p53 (Braithwaite *et al.*, 1987; Sturzbecher *et al.*, 1988; Wang *et al.*, 1989). On the other hand, many p53 mutants fail to exert such an inhibitory effect. Interestingly, all tumor-derived p53 mutants examined to date, as well as a number of *in vitro*–generated p53 mutants exhibiting comparable biological properties, have a markedly reduced affinity for T antigen (Tan *et al.*, 1986; Jenkins *et al.*, 1988; Halevy *et al.*, 1990). Finally, the regions of p53 implicated in its interaction with T antigen correspond very closely to two of the conserved homology boxes in which mutations are often found in tumors (Jenkins *et al.*, 1988). One can therefore entertain the idea that under normal circumstances in which no T antigen is present, wt p53 engages in interactions with some cellular protein(s), through these same conserved domains. These proteins may, in this case, be cellular counterparts of the viral protein, also intimately involved in the control of DNA replication (Gannon and Lane, 1987). So far, however, this model is sheerly speculative.

Whichever biochemical activities of p53 are eventually uncovered, a basic prerequisite for their being related to tumor suppression is their abrogation or attenuation in tumor-derived mutants. In addition, one can not rule out the possibility that certain p53 mutants are overtly oncogenic, rather than simply capable of eliminating the tumor-suppressor function of wt p53. Such mutants, if indeed present in tumors, may well turn out to have certain augmented biochemical activities, or even carry new activities not normally present in wt p53.

V. Conclusion

In recent years, our understanding of the role of p53 in neoplasia has undergone fundamental changes. The conceptual switch, from an oncogene to a tumor-suppressor gene, also calls for a change of methodologies for studying the relevance of p53 to a given type of cancer. Previously, inspired by impressive progress in the study of *myc* and other oncogenes, investigators tried repeatedly to identify cases of p53 gene amplification. In addition, attempts were made to detect consistent gene rearrangements expected to lead to a deregulated overexpression of the protein. The realization that the ongoing presence of wt p53 interferes with tumorigenesis, rather than promoting it, now dictates different experimental strategies. Not surprisingly, the common type of p53-related gene rearrangement involves chromosomal deletions, entailing a complete loss of one allele along with many flanking genes. Such events will usually not be scored by the type of Southern hybridization assays that worked so well for *myc* in plasmacytoma and Burkitt's lymphoma. Rather, they call for analysis of tumor material by RFLP. Ideally, one would want to have informative probes derived from within or the close vicinity of the p53 gene. Additionally, it is now obvious that the most frequent aberration in p53 expression is manifested as point mutations. Whether the resultant mutant protein is simply an inactive version of its wt counterpart, or whether certain mutants are overtly oncogenic, owing to a gain of function, will be a matter for future research. In addition, it would be of great interest to determine whether tumors of a given type, which retain the ability to produce apparently wt p53, differ in any relevant way from similar tumors in which wt p53 expression has been ablated. Finally, one would wish to find out whether the malignant properties of tumor cells, defective in wt p53 expression, can be reversed on reconstitution of the latter. This issue is not only of scientific interest, but may also potentially have practical implications. It is therefore very likely to be at the focus of numerous studies in a multitude of systems.

References

Ahuja, H., Bar-Eli, M., Advani, S. H., Benchimol, S., and Cline, M. J. (1989). Alteration in the p53 gene and the clonal evolution of the blast crisis of chronic myelocytic leukemia. *Proc. Natl. Acad. Sci. U.S.A.* **86**, 6783–6787.

Baker, S. J., Fearon, E. R., Nigro, J. M., Hamilton, S. R., Preisinger, A. C., Jessup, J. M., van-Tuinen, P., Ledbetter, D. H., Barker, D. F., Nakamura, Y., White, R., and Vogelstein, B. (1989). Chromosome 17 deletions and p53 gene mutations in colorectal carcinomas. *Science* **244**, 217–221.

Bartek, J., Iggo, R., Gannon, J., and Lane, D. P. (1990). Genetic and immunochemical analysis of mutant p53 in human breast cancer cell lines. *Oncogene* **5**, 893–899.

Ben David, Y., Prideaux, V. R., Chow, V., Benchimol, S., and Bernstein, A. (1988). Inactivation of the p53 oncogene by the internal deletion or retroviral integration in erythroleukemic cell lines induced by Friend leukemia virus. *Oncogene* **3**, 179–185.

Bock, G., and Marsh, J., eds. (1989). "Genetic Analysis of Tumor Suppression." Wiley-Interscience, New York.

Braithwaite, A. W., Sturzbecher, H. - W., Addison, C., Palmer, C., Rudge, K., and Jenkins, J. R. (1987). Mouse p53 inhibits SV40 origin-dependent DNA replication. *Nature* **329**, 458–460.

Bressac, B., Galvin, K. M., Liang, T. J., Isselbacher, K. J., Wands, J. R., and Ozturk, M. (1990). Abnormal structure and expression of p53 gene in human hepatocellular carcinoma. *Proc. Natl. Acad. Sci. U. S. A.* **87**, 1973–1977.

Cattoretti, G., Andreola, S., Clements, C., D'Amato, L., and Rilke, F. (1988a). Vimentin and p53 expression on epidermal growth factor receptor–positive, oestrogen receptor–negative breast carcinomas. *Br. J. Cancer* **57**, 353–357.

Cattoretti, G., Rilke, F., Andreola, S., D'Amato, L. D., and Della, D. (1988a). p53 expression in breast cancer. *Int. J. Cancer* **41**, 178–183.

Chow, V., Ben-David, Y., Bernstein, A., Benshimol, S., and Mowat, M. (1987). Multistage Friend erythroleukemia: Independent origin of tumor clones with normal or rearranged p53 cellular oncogenes. *J. Virol.* **61**, 2771–2781.

Crawford, L. V. (1983). The 53,000-dalton cellular protein and its role in transformation. *Int. Rev. Exp. Pathol.* **25**, 1–50.

Crawford, L. (1985). Human p53 and human tumours. *Bio Essays* **3**, 117–120.

Crawford, L. V., Pim, D., and Lamb, P. (1984). The cellular protein p53 in human tumors. *Mol. Biol. Med.* **2**, 261–272.

DeLeo, A. B., Jay, G., Appella, E., Dubois, G. C., Law, L. W., and Old, L. J. (1979). Detection of a transformation-related antigen in chemically induced sarcomas and other transformed cells of the mouse. *Proc. Natl. Acad. Sci. U.S.A.* **78,** 1695–1699.

Devilee, P., Pearson, P. L., and Cornelisse, C. J. (1989). Allele losses in breast cancer. *Lancet* **i,** 154.

Dippold, W. D., Jay, G., Deleo, A. B., Khoury, G., and Old, L. J. (1981). p53-Transformation-related protein. Detection by monoclonal antibody in mouse and human cells. *Proc. Natl. Acad. Sci. U.S.A.* **78,** 1695–1699.

Ehrhart, J. C., Duthu, A., Ullrich, S., Appella, E., and May, P. (1988). Specific interaction between a subset of the p53 protein family and heat-shock proteins hsp72/hsc73 in a human osteosarcoma cell line. *Oncogene* **3,** 595–603.

Eliyahu, D., Raz, A., Gruss, P., Givol, P., Givol, D., and Oren, M. (1984). Participation of p53 cellular tumor antigen in transformation of normal embryonic cells. *Nature (London)* **312,** 646–649.

Eliyahu, D., Michalovitz, D., and Oren, M. (1985). Overproduction of p53 antigen makes established cells highly tumorigenic. *Nature (London)* **316,** 158–160.

Eliyahu, D., Goldfinger, N., Pinhasi-Kimhi, O., Shaulsky, G., Skurnik, Y., Arai, N., Rotter, V., and Oren, M. (1988). Meth A fibrosarcoma cells express two transforming mutant p53 species. *Oncogene* **3,** 313–321.

Eliyahu, D., Michalovitz, D., Eliyahu, S., Pinhasi-Kimhi, O., and Oren, M. (1989). Wild-type p53 can inhibit oncogene-mediated focus formation. *Proc. Natl. Acad. Sci. U. S. A.* **86,** 8763–8767.

Eliyahu, D., Michalovitz, D., Eliyahu, S., Pinhasi-Kimhi, O., Oren, M. (1990). p53—Oncogene or antioncogene? *In* "Oncogenes in Cancer Diagnostics" (Munk, ed.), Vol 39, pp. 125–134, Karger, Basel, Switzerland.

Fields, S. and Jang, S. K. (1990). Presence of a potent transcription activating sequence in the p53 protein. *Science* **249,** 1046–1049.

Finlay, C. A., Hinds, P. W., Tan, T.-H., Eliyahu, D., Oren, M., and Levine, A. J. (1988). Activating mutations for transformation by p53 produce a gene product that forms an hsc70-p53 complix with an altered half-life. *Mol. Cell. Biol.* **8,** 531–539.

Finlay, C. A., Hinds, P. W., and Levine, A. L. (1989). The p53 protooncogene can act as a suppressor of transformation. *Cell* **57,** 1083–1093.

Gai, X., Rizzo, M. G., Lee, J., Ullrich, A., and Baserga, R. (1988). Abrogation of the requirements for added growth factors in 3T3 cells constitutively expressing the p53 and IGF-1 genes. *Oncogene Res.* **3,** 377–386.

Gannon, J. V., and Lane, D. P. (1987). p53 and DNA polymerase compete for binding to SV40 T antigen. *Nature* **329,** 456–458.

Gannon, J. V., Greaves, R., Iggo, R., and Lane, D. P. (1990). Activating mutations in p53 produce a common conformational effect. A monoclonal antibody specific for the mutant form. *EMBO J.* **9,** 1595–1602.

Ginsberg, D., Michalovitz, D., Ginsberg, D., and Oren, M. (1991). Induction of growth arrest by a temperature-sensitive p53 mutant is correlated with increased nuclear localization and decreased stability of the protein. *Mol. Cell Biol.* **11,** 582–585.

Green, M. R. (1989). When the products of oncogenes and antioncogenes meet. *Cell* **56,** 1–3.

Halevy, O., Hall. A., and Oren, M. (1989). Stabilization of the p53 transformation-related protein in mouse fibrosarcoma cell lines: effects of protein sequence and intracellular environment. *Mol. Cell Biol.* **9,** 3385–3392.

Halevy, O., Michalovitz, D., and Oren, M. (1990). Different tumor-derived p53 mutants exhibit distinct biological activities. *Science* **250,** 113–116.

Harlow, E., Williamson, N. M., Ralston, R., Helfman, D. M., and Adams, T. E. (1985). Molecular cloning and *in vitro* expression of a cDNA clone for human cellular tumor antigen p53. *Mol. Cell. Biol.* **5,** 1601–1610.

Herskowitz, I. (1987). Functional inactivation of genes by dominant negative mutations. *Nature* **329**, 219–222.

Hinds, P., Finlay, C., and Levine, A. J. (1989). Mutation is required to activate the p53 gene for cooperation with the *ras* oncogene and transformation. *J. Virol* **63**, 739–746.

Iggo, R., Gatter, K., Bartek, J., Lane, D., Harris, A. (1990). Increased expression of mutant forms of p53 oncogene in primary lung cancer. *Lancet* **335**, 675–679.

Iguchi-Ariga, S. M. M., Okazaki, T., Itani, T., and Ariga, H. (1988). Cloning of the p53-dependent origin of cellular DNA replication. *Oncogene* **3**, 509–515.

Isobe, M., Emanuel, B. S., Givol, D., Oren, M., and Croce, C. M. (1986). Localization of gene for human p53 tumour antigen to band 17p13. *Nature* **320**, 84–85.

Jenkins, J. R. and Struzbecher, H.-W. (1988). The p53 oncogene. *In* "The Oncogene Handbook" (E. P. Reddy, A. M. Skalka, and T. Curran, eds.). pp. 403–423. Elsevier Science Publishers, New York.

Jenkins, J. R., Rudge, K., and Currie, G. A. (1984a). Cellular immortalization by a cDNA clone encoding the transformation-associated phosphoprotein p53. *Nature (London)* **312**, 651–654.

Jenkins, J. R., Rudge, K., Redmond, S., and Wade-Evans, A. (1984b). Cloning and expression of full-length mouse cDNA sequences encoding the transformation-associated protein p53. *Nucleic Acids Res.* **12**, 5609–5626.

Jenkins, J. R., Rudge, K., Chumakov, P., and Currie, G. A. (1985). The cellular oncogene p53 can be activated by mutagenesis. *Nature (London)* **317**, 816–818.

Jenkins, J. R., Chumakov, P., Addison, C., Sturzbecher, H. - W., and Wade-Evans, A. (1988). Two distinct regions of the murine p53 primary amino acid sequence are implicated in stable complex formation with simian virus 40 T antigen. *J. Virol.* **62**, 3903–3906.

Kaczmarek, L., Oren, M., and Baserga, R. (1986). Cooperation between the p53 protein tumor antigen and platelet-poor plasma in the induction of cellular DNA synthesis. *Exp. Cell Res.* **152**, 268–272.

Kelman, Z., Prokocimer, M., Peller, S., Kahn, Y., Rechavi, G., Manor, Y., Cohen, A., and Rotter, V. (1989). Rearrangements in the p53 gene in Philadelphia chromosome–positive chronic myelogenous leukemia. *Blood* **74**, 2318–2324.

Kerndrup, G., Pedersen, B., and Bendix-Hansen, K. (1987). Specific minor chromosome deletions in myelodysplastic syndromes: Clinical and morphological correlation. *Cancer Genet. Cytogenet.* **26**, 227–234.

Lane, D. P., and Crawford, L. V. (1979). T antigen is bound to a host protein in SV40-transformed cells. *Nature (London)* **278**, 261–263.

Lavigueur, A., Maltby, V., Mock, D., Rossant, J., Pawson, T., and Bernstein, A. (1989). High incidence of lung, bone, and lymphoid tumors in transgenic mice overexpressing mutant alleles of the p53 oncogene. *Mol. Cell Biol.* **9**, 3982–3991.

Lee, W. M. F., Schwab, M., Westaway, D., and Varmus, H. E. (1985). Augmented expression of normal c-*myc* is sufficient for cotransformation of rat embryo cells with a mutant *ras* gene. *Mol. Cell. Biol.* **5**, 3345–3356.

Levine, A. J. (1990). Tumor-suppressor genes. *Bioessays* **12**, 60–66.

Linzer, D. I. H., and Levine, A. J. (1979). Characterization of a 54K dalton cellular SV40 tumor antigen present in SV40-transformed cells and uninfected embryonal carcinoma cells. *Cell* **17**, 43–52.

Lubbert, M., Miller, C. W., Crawford, L., and Koeffler, H. P. (1988). p53 in chronic myclogcnous leukemia. *J. Exp. Med.* **167**, 873–886.

Mackay, J., Steel, M., Elder, P. A., Forrest, A. P. M., and Evans, H. J. (1988). Allele loss on short arm of chromosome 17 in breast cancer. *Lancet* **ii**, 1384–1385.

Masuda, H., Miller, C., Koeffler, H. P., Battifora, H., and Cline, M. J. (1987). Rearrangement of the p53 gene in human osteogenic sarcoma. *Proc. Natl. Acad. Sci. U.S.A.* **84**, 7716–7719.

Matlashewski, G., Banks, L., Pim. D., and Crawford, L. V. (1986). Analysis of human p53 proteins and mRNA levels in normal and transformed cells. *Eur. J. Biochem.* **154,** 665–672.

McBride, O. W., Merry, D., and Givol, D. (1986). The gene for human p53 cellular tumor antigen is located on chromosome 17 short arm (17p13). *Proc. Natl. Acad. Sci. U.S.A.* **83,** 130–134.

Melero, J. A., Tur, S., and Carrol, R. B. (1980). Host nuclear proteins expressed in simian virus 40–transformed and –infected cells. *Proc. Natl. Acad. Sci. U.S.A.* **77,** 97–101.

Menon, A. G., Anderson, K. M., Riccardi, V. M., Chung, R. Y., Whaley, J. M., Yandell, D. W., Farmer, G. E., Freiman, R. N., Lee, J. K. Li, F. P., Barker, D. F., Ledbetter, D. H., Kleider, A., Martuza, R. L., Gusella, J. F., and Seizinger, B. R. (1990). Chromosome 17p deletions and p53 gene mutations associated with the formation of malignant neurofibrosarcomas in von Recklinghausen neurofibromatosis. *Proc. Natl. Acad. Sci. U.S.A.* **87,** 5435–5439.

Mercer, W. E., Nelson, D., De Leo, A. B., Old, L. J., and Baserga, R. (1982). Microinjection of monoclonal antibody to protein p53 inhibits serum-induced DNA synthesis in 3T3 cells. *Proc. Natl. Acad. Sci. U.S.A.* **79,** 6309–6312.

Mercer, W. E., Avignollo, C., and Baserga, R. (1984). Role of the p53 protein in cell proliferation as studied by microinjection of monoclonal antibodies. *Mol. Cell. Biol.* **4,** 276–281.

Michalovitz, D., Halevy, O., and Oren, M. (1990). Conditional inhibition of transformation and of cell proliferation by a temperature-sensitive mutant of p53. *Cell* **62,** 671–680.

Mikkelsen, T., and Cavenee, W. K. (1990). Suppressors of the malignant phenotype. *Cell Growth Diff.* **1,** 201–207.

Miller, C., Mohandas, T., Wolf, D., Prokocimer, M., Rotter, V., and Koeffler, H. P. (1986). Human p53 gene localized to short arm of chromosome 17. *Nature (London)* **319,** 783–784.

Mowat, M., Cheng, A., Kimura, N., Berntein, A., and Benchimol, S. (1985). Rearrangements of the cellular p53 gene in erythroleukaemic cells transformed by Friend virus. *Nature (London)* **314,** 633–636.

Munroe, D. G., Rovinski, B., Bernstein, A., and Benchimol, S. (1988). Loss of a highly conserved domain on p53 as a result of gene deletion during Friend virus–induced erythroleukemia. *Oncogene,* **2,** 621–624.

Nigro, J., Baker, S. J., Preisinger, A. C., Jessup, J. M., Hostetter, R., Cleary, K., Bigner, S. H., Davidson, N., Baylin, S., Devilee, P., Glover, T., Collins, F. S., Weston, A., Modali, R., Harris, C. C., and Vogelstein, B. (1989). Mutations in the p53 gene occur in diverse human tumour types. *Nature (London)* **342,** 705–708.

O'Reilly, D. R. (1986). p53 and transformation by SV40. *Biol. Cell* **57,** 187–196.

Oren, M. (1985). The p53 cellular tumor antigen: Gene structure, expression, and protein properties. *Biochim. Biophys. Acta* **823,** 67–78.

Oren, M., and Levine, A. J. (1983). Molecular cloning of a cDNA specific for the murine p53 cellular tumor antigen. *Proc. Natl. Acad. Sci. U.S.A.* **80,** 56–59.

Parada, L. F., Land, H., Weinberg, R. A., Wolf, D., and Rotter, V. (1984). Cooperation between the gene encoding p53 tumor antigen and *ras* in cellular transformation. *Nature (London)* **312,** 649–651.

Pennica, D., Goeddel, D. V., Hayflick, J. S., Reich, N. C., Anderson, C. W., and Levine, A. J. (1984). The amino acids sequence of murine p53 determined from a cDNA clone. *Virology* **134,** 477–482.

Pohl, J., Goldfinger, N., Radler-Pohl, A., Rotter, V., and Schirrmacher, V. (1988). p53 increases experimental metastatic capacity of murine carcinoma cells. *Mol. Cell. Biol.* **8,** 2078–2081.

Prokocimer, M., Shaklai, M., Ben Bassat, H., Wolf, D., Goldfinger, N., and Rotter, V. (1986). Expression of p53 in human leukemia and lymphoma. *Blood* **68,** 113–118.

Raycroft, L., Wu, H., and Lozano, G. (1990). Transcriptional activation by wild-type but not transforming mutants of the p53 anti-oncogene. *Science* **249,** 1049–1051.

Reich, N. C., and Levine, A. J. (1984). Growth regulation of a cellular tumor antigen, p53, in nontransformed cells. *Nature (London)* **308,** 199–201.

Romano, J. W., Ehrhart, J. C., Duthu, A., Kim, C. M., Appella, E., and May, P. (1989). Identification and characterization of a p53 gene mutation in a human osteosarcoma cell line. *Oncogene* **4**, 1483–1488.

Rotter, V., and Wolf, D. (1984). Biological and molecular analysis of p53 cellular encoded tumor antigen. *Adv. Cancer Res.* **43**, 113–141.

Rotter, V. Abutbul, H., and Ben-Zeev, A. (1983a). p53 transformation–related protein accumulates in the nucleus of transformed fibroblasts in association with the chromatin and is found in the cytoplasm in non-transformed fibroblasts. *EMBO J.* **2**, 1041–1047.

Rotter, V., Abutbul, H., and Wolf, D. (1983b). The presence of p53 transformation–related protein in Ab-MuLV transformed cells is required for their development into lethal tumors in mice. *Int. J. Cancer* **31**, 315–320.

Rovinski, B., and Benchimol, S. (1988). Immortalization of rat embryo fibroblasts by the cellular p53 oncogene. *Oncogene* **2**, 445–451.

Sager, R. (1989). Tumor-suppressor genes: The puzzle and the promise. *Science* **246**, 1406–1412.

Soussi, T., Caron de Fromentel, C., Mechali, M., May, P., and Kress, M. (1987). Cloning and characterization of a cDNA from *Xenopus laevis* coding for a protein homologous to human and murine p53. *Oncogene* **1**, 71–78.

Sturzbecher, H. - W., Chumakov, P., Welch, W. J., and Jenkins, J. R. (1987). Mutant p53 proteins bind hsp72/73 cellular heat shock–related proteins in SV40-transformed monkey cells. *Oncogene*, **1**, 201–211.

Sturzbecher, H.-W., Brain, R., Maimets, T., Addison, C., Rudge, K., and Jenkins, J. R. (1988). Mouse p53 blocks SV40 DNA replication *in vitro* and down-regulates T antigen DNA helicase activity. *Oncogene* **3**, 405–412.

Takahashi, T., Nau, M. M., Chiba, I., Birrer, M. J., Rosenberg, R. K., Vinocour, M., Levitt, M., Pass, H., Gazdar, A. F., and Minna, J. D. (1989). p53: A frequent target for genetic abnormalities in lung cancer. *Science* **246**, 491–494.

Tan, T. H., Wallis, J., and Levine, A. J. (1986). Identification of the p53 protein domain involved in formation of the simian virus 40 large T-antigen-p53 protein complex. *J. Virol.* **59**, 574–583.

Van Roy, F., Leibaut, G., Mareel, M., and Fiers, W. (1990). Partial transformation of human cell lines showing defective interaction between unusual p53 gene product and SV40 large T antigen. *Oncogene* **5**, 207–218.

Vogelstein, B., Fearon, E. R., Kern, S. E., Hamilton, S. R., Preisinger, A. C., Nakamura, Y., and White, R. (1989). Allelotypes of colorectal carcinomas. *Science* **244**, 207–211.

Wang, E. H., Friedman, P. N., and Prives, C. (1989). The murine p53 protein blocks replication of SV40 DNA *in vitro* by inhibiting the initiation functions of SV40 large T antigen. *Cell* **57**, 379–392.

Weinberg, R. A. (1989) Oncogenes, antioncogenes, and the molecular bases of multistep carcinogenesis. *Cancer Res.* **49**, 3713–3721.

Wolf, D., and Rotter, V. (1984). Inactivation of p53 gene expression by an insertion of Moloney murine leukemia virus–like DNA sequences. *Mol. Cell. Biol.* **4**, 1402–1410.

Wolf, D., Harris, N., and Rotter, V. (1984). Reconstitution of p53 expression in a nonproducer Ab-MuLV-transformed cell line by transfection of a functional p53 gene. *Cell* **38**, 119–126.

Wolf, D., and Rotter, V. (1985). Major deletions in the gene encoding the p53 antigen cause lack of p53 expression in HL60 cells. *Proc. Natl. Acad. Sci. U.S.A.* **82**, 790–794.

Zakut-Houri, R., Oren, M., Bienz, B., Lavie, V., Hazum, S., and Givol, D. (1983). A single gene and a psuedogene for the cellular tumor antigen p53. *Nature (London)* **306**, 594–597.

Zantema, A., Schrier, P. I., Davis-Olivier, A., van Laar, T., Vaessen, R. T. M. J., and van der Eb, A. J. (1985). Adenovirus serotype determines association and localization of the large E1B tumor antigen with cellular tumor antigen p53 in transformed cells. *Mol. Cell. Biol.* **5**, 3084–3091.

Chapter 13

Chromosomal Markers of Cancer

SANDRA R. WOLMAN* AND ANWAR N. MOHAMED*

*Program in Cancer Genetics, Michigan Cancer Foundation,
Detroit, Michigan 48201

I. Introduction[1]

The chromosomal aberrations found in tumors are visibly different from the normal diploid pattern that is expected in somatic cells. As such, they can serve as markers to identify tumor cells. To the degree that they can be correlated with specific tumor types or grades, morphologic or behavioral, chromosomal markers can contribute to diagnosis and staging. Furthermore, the finding of chromosome changes in individuals who are predisposed to tumor development or who have been exposed to environmental agents that are associated with tumorigenesis, constitutes evidence that chromosome alterations may play a causal role in tumor formation, in addition to providing documentation of the exposure or underlying condition.

[1] Cytogenetic nomenclature is based on An International System for Human Cytogenetic Nomenclature (1985) published in collaboration with the March of Dimes Birth Defects Foundation and Cytogenetics and Cell Genetics by S. Karger, Basel, Switzerland.

393

BIOCHEMICAL AND MOLECULAR ASPECTS
OF SELECTED CANCERS, VOL. 1

A. VALUE OF CYTOGENETICS TO DIAGNOSIS, PROGNOSIS, AND DEFINITION OF TUMOR PROGRESSION

Metaphase cells derived from human cancers usually show structural and numerical aberrations of chromosomes. When a set of particular aberrations marks one cell of the tumor, and the same or similar and related aberrations are present in many cells from the same tumor, the aberrations are described as clonal. Clonality indicates either that a single cell with those aberrations propagated to give rise to the tumor or that the aberrations conferred a growth advantage that resulted in repopulation of the tumor. Appreciation that chromosome aberrations, gross depictions of mutation, represent and can be responsible for major alterations in biological behavior of the cells is widely prevalent. When a single type or set of aberrations is found in many examples of tumors of similar or identical morphology, then the aberration(s) are considered *specific,* have diagnostic value, and may point to genetic loci that are causally altered in the formation of the particular tumors. Certain chromosome changes common to many tumor types are explicitly assumed to confer properties necessary for tumor growth.

The first and best-known illustration of tumor cell cytogenetic aberration is the Philadelphia chromosome (Ph), which marks the cells of chronic myelogenous leukemia (CML). It is a translocation (exchange of segments between two or more chromosomes) involving chromosomes 9 and 22 and designated t(9;22). It is specific to CML, is present in most or all cells of the tumor and, therefore, is clonal in the population. It is observed in a high frequency of cases of the disorder. The Ph chromosome is not found in constitutional cells of patients with CML but is confined to the tumor cell population. Individuals without the Ph chromosome may have a different clinical form of CML from those patients with this particular chromosome aberration. Moreover, with progression to a blastic phase of the disease, additional chromosome alterations in the leukemic cells are superimposed on the t(9;22) characteristic of the chronic phase.

B. HISTORICAL HIGHLIGHTS

The association of genetic and chromosomal aberrations with malignancy was first highlighted by Boveri in his promulgation of a somatic mutational basis for the origin of tumors (1914). Muller (1928) showed that chromosome damage was one of the immediate biological results of exposure to ionizing radiation. Animal experimentation indicated that a later consequence of radiation exposure was tumor formation (Furth and Furth, 1936). If further proof were necessary, many years later the atomic bomb explosions resulted, among other grim sequelae, in ample evidence of dose-related induction of tumors in humans by radiation (National Research Council, Advisory Committee on the Biological Effects of Ionizing Radiation, 1980). Effects similar to those of radiation on chromosomes (breakage, rearrangements) could be induced by a variety of chemicals that were also implicated in tumor induction. These observations eventually led to the conviction that agents capable of inducing chromosome damage were potentially tumorigenic and therefore that the chromosome aberrations could have an etiologic role in tumor formation.

Direct observations of aberrant and recombinant chromosomes in human tumors began in 1960 with the Ph chromosome (Nowell and Hungerford, 1960). Since that time an increasing body of information characterizing chromosome changes in the leukemias and, more recently, in solid tumors has been accumulating. Description and evaluation of some chromosomal tumor markers form the major topic of this chapter. Chromosomal aberrations associated with gene amplification provided the first direct link between cytogenetic and molecular genetic events in cancer (Biedler and Spengler, 1976). Additionally, gene amplification was recognized as contributing prognostic information in specific tumors (Brodeur et al., 1987). In some instances the amplified gene has been selected for drug resistance and results in failure of response to therapy (Stark et al., 1989); in others, amplification of an oncogene may reflect a biological propensity for poor prognosis (Wolman and Henderson, 1989). The degree to which these events occur in human tumors is uncertain, but the chromosomal representations of gene amplification are common in certain tumor types.

Observation of a common translocation, t(8;14), in Burkitt's lymphoma was the basis for the next major step in understanding how changes relevant to tumor could be effected by chromosome rearrangement (Dalla Favera et al., 1982; Taub et al., 1982; Kirsch et al., 1982; Croce et al., 1982). The location of the breaks resulted in transposition of the c-myc oncogene from 8q24 to a region of immunoglobulin production (14q), which is presumed to function actively in cells of B-lymphoid lineage. The result of the rearrangement then should be overproduction of the c-myc product (Klein and Klein, 1985). In contrast, the t(9;22) of CML juxtaposes the c-abl oncogene with the bcr locus on chromosome 22 to form a hybrid gene that generates a functionally altered protein with strikingly increased tyrosine kinase activity (Kurzrock et al., 1988).

At present, tumor-specific sites of chromosome rearrangements are expected to serve as pointers to genes that are critical either to specific tissue differentiation or to tumor behavioral determinants. The landmark example is the single case of familial adenomatous polyposis in which a chromosomal deletion in 5q led to localization of the gene by linkage studies (Herrera et al., 1986; Bodmer et al., 1987; Leppert et al., 1987). That, in turn, led to an explosion of work at the molecular level that influences current understanding of the relationship between rare, heritable colon cancer and the common sporadic form of the disease and to a better understanding of the sequence of gene changes involved (Vogelstein et al., 1988).

C. Overview

We assume that tumors are genetically abnormal, that they are often chromosomally abnormal, and that three important properties characterize tumor cell chromosome patterns. The first is clonality, evidence that the cells within a tumor are derived from a single parent cell by virtue of the uniformity or relative uniformity of the chromosome aberrations contained within many or all cells of the progeny. The second is specificity, the concordance between a particular chromosome pattern and a particular disease state. If specificity is related to the tissue of tumor origin, we might expect the genes altered by the aberration to be important in normal differentiation of that tissue. Alternatively, the chromosome aberrations could involve genes that are specific to tumor properties in a more general sense, such as oncogenes or repressor genes. The third common property is chromosome instability, a potential for variability in number or structure— an important property that permits tumor cell populations to evolve to new and altered biological states.

Approximately 20 years has elapsed since the advent of chromosome banding techniques and their application to the analysis of human tumors. Much of the accumulated data on chromosome studies in human cancer has been catalogued by Mitelman, most recently in 1988. Of the over 9,000 tumors included, more than 7,600 were disorders of hemopoietic cells (see Table I), leaving only approximately 15% of the entire listing to represent the cumulative data on human solid tumors. Both neural tumors and soft-tissue sarcomas were represented greatly in excess of their true frequency among human tumors. The most common tumors, namely lung, colon, breast, and prostate, were substantially underrepresented. The listing is neither entirely representative nor comprehensive in the following respects: It does not include cases of CML in which the only cy-

TABLE I
CHROMOSOME ABERRATIONS IN HUMAN TUMORS[a]

9069 tumors[b]
5211 nonlymphocytic leukemias
2460 hematologic or lymphomatous neoplastic proliferations
1398 solid tumors, including
354 neural (130 benign)
140 soft-tissue sarcomas
110 breast tumors (primary, metastatic, and effusions)

[a]From Mitelman (1988).

[b]This compilation did not include tumors that were cytogenetically normal or cases of CML that were marked only by t(9;22).

togenetic aberration was the typical t(9;22). It does not include any tumors whose cytogenetic characterization revealed only normal diploid cells, either by direct analysis or after growth in culture. In fact, relatively few tumors from which cytogenetic data were derived after prolonged periods in culture were included, because of the known propensity for spontaneous chromosome evolution in cultured cells. Thus, although this catalog comprises a valuable compilation of karyotypic information on human tumors, the lymphoid and myeloid tumors are disproportionately well represented, and some of the commonest solid tumors are very underrepresented.

II. Myeloid and Lymphoid Tumors

A. PREVALENCE AND SPECIFICITY OF ABERRATIONS

1. Acute Myeloid Leukemias

Although the presence of acquired cytogenetic abnormalities in hematopoietic cells is an indicator that the patient has some type of bone marrow neoplasia, the distribution of these aberrations is nonrandom; some changes show remarkable specificity to distinctive morphologic subtypes that are also associated with disease presentation and response to chemotherapy. Discussions at the Fourth International Workshop on Chromosomes in Leukemia (1984) demonstrated convincingly that the karyotypic picture at diagnosis is an important independent prognostic factor, conveying information about the probability of attainment of complete remission and duration of remission.

The classic example of chromosome changes in CML has been described. When the disease progresses to a more acute or blastic phase, it is characterized by the acquisition of additional aberrations. The most common chromosomal changes in blastic crisis are an extra Ph, trisomy 8, or formation of an isochromosome of 17q; less common are $+19$, $+17$, and rearrangement of 7. These secondary aberrations usually precede the hematologic and clinical manifestations of blastic crisis by several months and thus may serve as valuable prognostic indicators.

The tissue site of origin for clonal evolution in CML has been studied by a number of investigators. It was found that in some cases the karyotypic evolution appeared to be generated in an extramedullary site (spleen, lymph node, or soft tissue) rather than in the bone marrow that is infiltrated secondarily. An illustration of these chromosomal event in CML was found in an individual with two cell populations in the bone marrow at initial presentation, one population with the t(9;22) and the second with t(9;22) and $-7, +8q$. After treatment, the patient had the presumably original pattern of 46,XX,t(9;22) for over a year, but complained of intermittent and worsening back pain. Aspiration of a lesion in

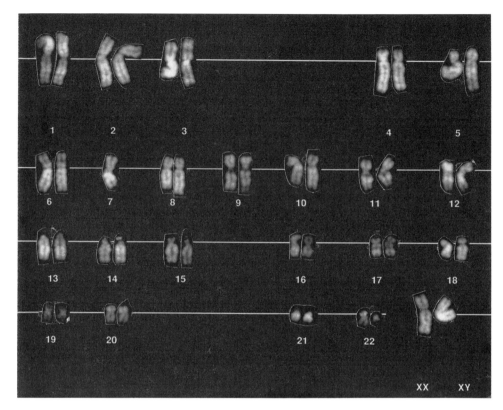

FIG. 1.   A Q-banded karyotype from a solid-tumor mass in the deep pelvic muscle of a 34-year-old woman with a 1-year history of CML. The pattern seen in the tumor, 46,XX,t(9;22), − 7, + 8q, was identical to that observed in marrow cells at the time of her initial presentation.

the pelvic muscles revealed cells with 46,XX,t(9;22), − 7, + 8q in the tumor mass (see Fig. 1). Thus, this patient demonstrated an unusual clinical course with the classical chromosome pattern of clonality, specificity, and karyotypic evolution with tumor progression.

Some of the common chromosome aberrations associated with subtypes in the FAB (French, American, British) classification of acute myeloid leukemias are shown in Table II. The specific morphologic subtypes of leukemia have been associated with relatively specific and different chromosome aberrations. They are, therefore, helpful in differential diagnosis. In addition, because of their known clinical correlates, they may also convey information relevant to prognosis for the individual patient who has been studied. Clonal visible abnormalities including gains, losses, translocations, and rearrangements have been seen in

TABLE II

CHROMOSOME ABERRATIONS OF ACUTE
MYELOID LEUKEMIAS

Leukemic subtype	Associated chromosomal aberrations
M1	t(9;22)(q34;q11)
Stem cell	inv(3)(q21q26)—thrombocytotic
M2	t(8;21)(q22;q22)
Myeloblastic	t(6;9)(p21-22;q34)
	del(12)(p11-13)—basophilic
M3	t(15;17)(q22;q12)
Promyelocytic	
M4	inv/del(16)(p13q22)—eosinophilic
Myelomonocytic	+4
M5	del(11)(q23)
Monoblastic	t(9;11)(p13;q23)
	t(8;16)(p11;p13)—phagocytic
M6	variable
Erythroleukemia	
M7	variable;
Megakaryoblastic	? rearrangement (21)
All	+8, −7,

more than half of newly diagnosed cases of acute nonlymphocytic leukemia (ANLL) by conventional analyses and in well over 85% of cases when extended or prophase banding is achieved. These abnormalities disappear when remission is obtained, and the original aberrations reappear with disease relapse. The superposition of additional rearrangements often presages evolution to a more malignant clinical phase, as it does in CML.

Within a given leukemia subtype, specific aberrations are associated with different clinical courses and responses to therapy. The 8;21 translocation is the most common structural rearrangement reported in ANLL. It is found mainly in the ANLL-M2 subtype. The typical t(8;21) marrow displays a certain degree of eosinophilia, and the leukemic cells contain substantial numbers of Auer rods. The t(8;21) is seen more frequently in young patients and is rare past the age of 50. Men develop t(8;21) more often than women. This group of patients, although showing a high remission rate with survival durations varying from 5 to 49 months, is associated with a clinical course marked by multiple relapses and remissions. Translocation of chromosomes 15 and 17 in ANLL-M3 has proved to be the most specific leukemic aberration. This translocation has never been seen in any other type of tumor nor has it been observed as a constitutional abnormality. Patients with t(15;17) have low remission rates and very short survival with conventional chemotherapy, but intensive chemotherapeutic treatment in these patients has improved prognosis. Thus, cytogenetic subgrouping of ANLL patients may provide guidelines to optimize therapeutic regimens.

Cytogenetic distinctions may lead to better definition of morphologic subgroups; for example, the abnormality of chromosome 16 in ANLL is usually associated with bone-marrow eosinophilia. The specificity of hematologic–cytogenetic association has led the FAB study group to single out ANLL-M4 with eosinophilia as a separate subgroup. This leukemic category has been associated with high remission rate and long survival.

The picture, however, is not simple and straightforward. The same breakpoint at chromosome 9q34 is noted in both the M1 and M2 forms of leukemia, although the molecular breakpoints may differ. The inv(3) is not restricted to any subtype of acute myelogenous leukemia *de novo*. Usually aberrations of 3 are associated with megakaryocytic and platelet abnormality, but they have also been reported in secondary leukemia and myelodysplastic syndromes (see Fig. 2). The del(11) recorded for M5 is also seen in some cases of M4— not surprising, since both are leukemias in which there is some degree of monocytic differentiation. More important, however, a number of chromosome aberrations, i.e., $+8$, -7, del(5q), del(7q), $-Y$, and $+21$ are common to essentially all forms of the myeloid leukemias, regardless of their differentiation. Aberrations of chromosomes 5 and 7 appear associated with poor response to chemotherapy (Arthur *et al.*, 1989). These aberrations are not restricted to particular FAB subgroups, even though they are relatively specific for myeloid disorders and relatively rare in lymphatic leukemia. A typical problem of interpretation is exemplified (in Fig. 3) by a karyotype prepared from an individual with M7, the megakaryoblastic variant of acute myelogenous leukemia. A clonal aberration was found in all cells examined from the marrow of this patient, resulting from a translocation between chromosomes 16 and 21. In addition, a few cells had additional chromosome aberrations superimposed on the t(16;21) depicted. Our laboratory has found structural aberrations involving chromosome 21 in a number of cases of M7 leukemia (Mohamed *et al.*, 1990). Does this represent a new and specific association for which we should expect to find clinical correlates that will define a subgroup in this form of leukemia? Or should these observation be lumped with involvement of chromosome 21 in M2 and trisomy for 21 that is common in other acute myeloid leukemias as a nonspecific change? Certainly, the existence of chromosome aberrations in the leukemic cell population helps to make the diagnosis. What is unclear is whether it will help to predict the patient's clinical course.

Information summarized recently on the relation of chromosome aberrations to clinical outcome indicates that, in general, those leukemic individuals with only normal diploid metaphases in the marrow have the best survival (Arthur *et*

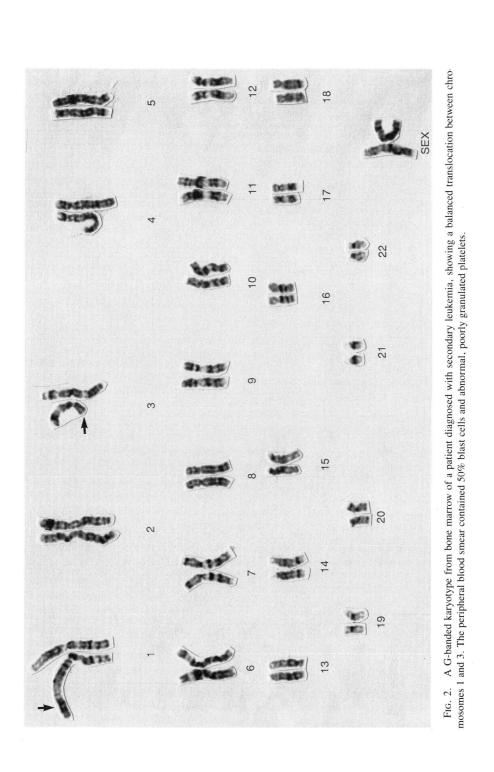

FIG. 2. A G-banded karyotype from bone marrow of a patient diagnosed with secondary leukemia, showing a balanced translocation between chromosomes 1 and 3. The peripheral blood smear contained 50% blast cells and abnormal, poorly granulated platelets.

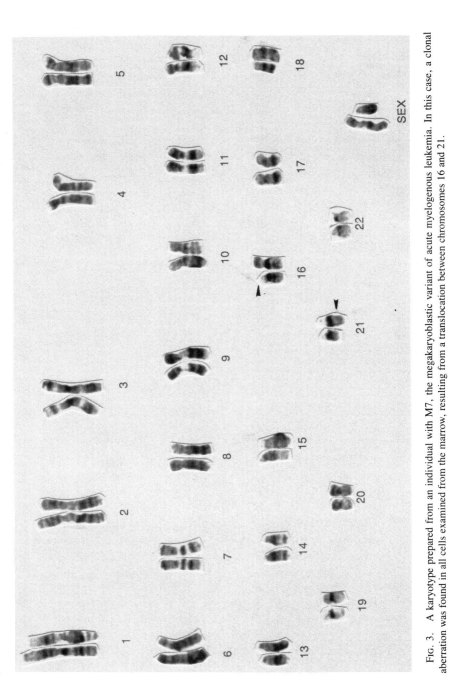

Fig. 3. A karyotype prepared from an individual with M7, the megakaryoblastic variant of acute myelogenous leukemia. In this case, a clonal aberration was found in all cells examined from the marrow, resulting from a translocation between chromosomes 16 and 21.

al., 1989) and are more likely to achieve prolonged remission after therapy. A few abnormal karyotypes, such as the inv(16) associated with M4 leukemia, appear to confer an almost equally good prognosis. Patients with both normal and abnormal karyotypes have done as well as the diploid cases in some studies, and have shown intermediate or poor prognoses in others. In a further refinement, the proportion of diploid cells in the marrow was correlated with duration of survival (Keating *et al.*, 1986). It is generally agreed that the more complex aberrations, those involving five or more different chromosomes, are associated with the poorest overall patient survival (Arthur *et al.*, 1989). Thus, there appears to be a quantitative component in chromosome aberrations so that, as a general rule, tumors with the least aberration appear to be those associated with the best patient survival.

The general principles that have emerged from chromosome studies in leukemia are that chromosome aberrations have great value in identification of tumor cell populations, and the corollary, that they can be important adjuncts to the identification of remission and relapse states in individual patients. In addition, they contribute useful information to the classification of tumor subtypes and to prediction of prognosis within those subtypes. Although these lessons are clear from study of leukemic disorders, it remains to be seen whether the same rules will apply to human solid tumors.

2. Lymphoid Neoplasias

Cytogenetic studies of acute lymphoblastic leukemia (ALL) are technically more difficult to obtain than for ANLL. The chromosome preparations are usually fuzzy, sticky, and difficult to band. Approximately two thirds of all ALL patients have recognizable chromosomal aberrations. The aberrations, both structural and numerical, are quite varied, but show a distinctly nonrandom distribution. Some rearrangements are closely associated with certain hematologic and immunologic subtypes. In addition, the karyotypic pattern has been shown to be important in predicting the rate and duration of remission, independent of other factors. At the Third International Workshop on Chromosomes in Leukemia (1981), 10 major cytogenetic subgroups were recognized. The clonal abnormalities were characterized by one of the following structural abnormalities (t(4;11), t(8;14), 14q +, Ph, 6q −) or were divided, in the remaining cases, also clonal, and categorized according to aberrant chromosome number. Patients with high remission rates usually showed normal karyotypes or chromosome numbers greater than 50. Patients with t(4;11), t(8;14), and 14q + showed low remission rates and poor survival. These patients clearly should be considered high-risk patients and treated accordingly.

Cytogenetic studies in non–Hodgkin's lymphoma show clearly that nonrandom chromosomal changes characterize each of the histologic subtypes

(Bloomfield *et al.*, 1983; Fifth International Workshop on Chromosomes in Leukemia–Lymphoma, 1987). The 14q+ abnormality is seen in 65% of malignant non–Hodgkin's lymphoma. The distal end of the long arm of chromosome 8(q24-qter), chromosome 11(q13-qter), or chromosome 18(q21-qter) translocates to 14q32 and contributes to form the 14q+ abnormality. The translocations t(14;18) and t(8;14) can be correlated with the histologic grade of lymphoma, with the former strongly associated with low-grade lymphoma of nodular histology, whereas the t(8;14) is associated with lymphomas of high grade, such as Burkitt's lymphoma. Recent studies on the genes located at the breakpoints in the specific translocations have shown that the three recurrent translocations defined above bring about the juxtaposition of the cellular oncogenes c-myc (8q24), bcl-1 (11q13), or bcl-2 (18q21) with the immunoglobulin-bearing determinant at 14q32 (Bakhshi *et al.*, 1985; Klein and Klein, 1985; Tsujimoto *et al.*, 1985). Translocation-mediated deregulation of c-myc has been demonstrated, and it is highly likely that the other two genes are similarly deregulated by the respective translocations. Further, the bcl-2 gene seems to be interrupted in most cases of follicular lymphomas carrying the 14;18 translocation (Croce, 1987). These observations indicate possible involvement of oncogenes other than c-myc in the genesis of lymphomas.

B. METHODS AND LIMITATIONS

In patient with leukemic disorders, chromosome analysis of the bone marrow for diagnostic purposes is sometimes hampered by a low yield of mitoses with poor morphology. Marrow aspiration may be difficult or nonproductive, so that studies are limited to peripheral blood cells.

The simplest and most rapid method of chromosome analysis is the direct preparation, by which cells are harvested immediately upon removal from the patient. Only cells that are dividing at the time of sample collection can be studied; this method is, therefore, of value only in tissues that have high mitotic indices, such as bone marrows. Direct preparation has been the standard method for diagnosis of hematologic disorders in many cytogenetic laboratories. Direct harvest procedures give more rapid results than tissue culture growth before harvest, and avoid the possibility of culture artifacts. However, most cytogenetic laboratories now use short-term (24–72 h) cultures routinely, believing that better quality and more plentiful mitoses are obtained and that culture artifacts are not a significant problem. Neither method is optimal for detection of tumor metaphases in all cases and, when feasible, application of several approaches will yield the greatest diagnostic information. The choice of procedures should be determined by the preference of each laboratory, based on experience and expertise, and the timing, volume, and quality of the clinical samples received for diagnosis.

A methotrexate(MTX)-synchronization technique was reported by Yunis (1981) to achieve high-quality preparations that permit improved identification of leukemic chromosomes. In our experience, this technique is reliable in CML and acute nonlymphocytic leukemias, but in ALL it sometimes interferes with growth in culture of the leukemic cells, resulting in a low mitotic index or in growth of normal cells. In addition, MTX-synchronization techniques are labor-intensive and require great precision in timing (especially in the duration of thymidine incubations). Therefore, use of these methods may not always be practical in a busy clinical laboratory. However, for those who acquire experience and are prepared to take the trouble, the results are often rewarding in certain cases.

To improve mitotic activity and to permit cytogenetic analysis from hypocellular bone marrow samples or peripheral blood analysis when white blood cell counts (WBC) are low in patients with myeloid leukemia, we routinely perform short-term cultures (48–72 hr) in the presence of 20% conditioned medium (CM), in parallel with conventional 24- and 48-hour unsupplemented harvests. The CM we use is derived from a human bladder carcinoma cell line (5637) that generates colony-stimulating factors supporting the growth of myeloid stem cells. Other reliable sources of myeloid colony-stimulating factors are commercially available, and factors that stimulate growth of other cell lineages could be applied to appropriate cases. We have observed a pronounced enhancement of mitotic activity even in samples in which the conventional 24-hour cultures fail to yield mitoses, and especially when the peripheral blood WBC is 5×10^{-3} or below. These cultures often demonstrate improved quality of chromosome morphology, with enhanced chromosome banding enabling better identification of rearranged chromosomes. Moreover, in some cases, minor chromosomally aberrant subclones, which are not found in the conventional cultures, are detected in cultures supplemented with CM. Therefore, we believe that CM culture is a reliable and valuable adjunct to cytogenetic studies in myeloid leukemia.

In general, bone marrow is a poor source of cells for definition of lymphoma cytogenetics, because the percentage of lymphoma cells may be low, as is their mitotic activity. As with other human malignancies, cytogenetic abnormalities in lymphomas are best established from the tumor-affected tissues, i.e., lymph node, spleen, or pleural or ascitic fluids. The main problem in achieving cytogenetic analysis is the rapid death of lymphoma cells *in vitro*. Direct preparations are preferred, but may yield insufficient numbers of dividing tumor cells. In those cases, a brief period of culture (6–24 hr) is usually helpful. Longer-term cultures, particularly when supplemented with T- or B-cell mitogens or growth factors, e.g., PHA-LPS, B-cell growth factor, or various interleukins, provide an alternative method. In using such stimulants, the possibility that normal lymphoid cells also will be stimulated to divide must be recognized.

III. Solid Tumors

Can the conclusions from leukemia studies be applied to chromosome studies in solid tumors? As should be clear from the paucity of accumulated data noted earlier, one of the problems is that for many solid tumors there is not an adequate base of information from which to draw conclusions. Some groups of solid tumors have been comparatively well studied; for example, tumors of the central nervous system that appear to adapt well to growth in tissue culture have yielded much cytogenetic data but little specificity other than a high frequency of trisomy 7 (Bigner *et al.*, 1990). Although infrequent and usually highly lethal, the soft-tissue sarcomas have been particularly amenable to chromosome analysis because the tumor cells often show clonal balanced translocations and are near-diploid; for examples of specificity, see Table III. Another comparatively well-studied group includes the developmental tumors of childhood: retinoblastoma, Wilms' tumor, and neuroblastoma. Overall, however, the number of solid tumors that have been reported to show consistent changes, without major discrepancies, by two or more laboratories are few (Teyssier, 1989), and even for these, there are many well-documented exceptions.

TABLE III

SOME CONSISTENT CHROMOSOME ABERRATIONS IN SOLID TUMORS

Solid tumors	Chromosome aberration
Sarcomas	
Rhabdomyosarcoma	t(2;13)
Synovial sarcoma	t(X;18)
Ewing's sarcoma	t(11;22)
Myxoid liposarcoma	t(12;16)
Fibrous histiocytoma	? 19p +
Other solid tumors	
Transitional-cell carcinoma of bladder	? 11p −
Renal carcinoma	del(3p)
Small-cell carcinoma of lung	del(3p)
Ovarian adenocarcinoma	t(6;14) or del(6)
Male germ–cell tumors (seminoma)	i(12p)
Melanomas	rearr(1);(6);(7)
Developmental tumors	
Retinoblastoma	del(13)(q14)
Wilms' tumor	del(11)(p13)
Neuroblastoma	1p −
PNET	i(17q)
Nephroblastoma	del(11)(p13)

A. Tumor Specificity

The level of specificity and frequency of aberration that prevails in the leukemias does not appear in chromosome-specific associations with solid tumors. For example, in a recent, fairly large series of Wilms' tumors, only 10% of cases showed the characteristic deletion in 11p13 (Solis *et al.*, 1988). Similarly, the chromosomal deletion of 13q14 that is sometimes constitutional in patients with hereditary retinoblastoma is found in approximately 21% of the tumors (Potluri *et al.*, 1986). A typical retinoblastoma (see Fig. 4) did not demonstrate 13q deletion, although numerous other chromosome aberrations were evident; high-resolution banding of lymphocytes was similarly uninformative with respect to 13q14, even though this patient had a sibling similarly afflicted with retinoblastoma. By a variety of molecular approaches, evidence of alteration at that chromosomal locus can be demonstrated in far higher frequency (Cavanee *et al.*, 1983).

The constitutional deletions sometimes found in association with retinoblastoma or Wilms' tumor have led to important hypotheses about genetic events in tumorigenesis. When a visible chromosomal aberration can not be detected, it is often assumed that the lesion will be detectable with molecular tools. However, in some cases, such as the retinoblastoma described above, molecular investigation fails to reveal a genomic lesion and, therefore, does not show the expected *specificity*. Similarly, in a Wilms' tumor, examination of loci on 11p flanking the critical 11p13 region showed neither loss of heterozygosity nor quantitative gene loss (Wolman *et al.*, 1990). Further, the specificity of the chromosomal lesion in Wilms' tumor is in doubt because of reported involvement of another locus (11p15) (Reeve *et al.*, 1989), and linkage studies do not support 11p13 as the locus for familial predisposition to Wilms' tumor (Henry *et al.*, 1989).

Specific chromosome aberrations have been described in association with several of the less-common solid tumors. These include the i(12p) in germ cell tumors of the testes, the del(3p) reported in small cell carcinoma of the lung and renal carcinomas, and a few others. These chromosomal lesions are not uniformly prevalent in the associated tumors for reasons that depend, at least in part, on the technical difficulties of performing solid-tumor analysis. Further, they are often obscured by the presence of extensive chromosome aberrations in the tumor cells, with considerable variability from cell to cell. Some of the aberrations may be common to many tumor types and could represent specificity of oncogene or tumor-suppressor gene involvement that might be expected in many tumors without regard to tissue of origin. Trisomy 7, for example, has been reported in renal tumors, glial tumors, bladder tumors, and melanomas. Multiple copies of 1q have been reported in breast cancers, myeloid leukemias, testicular tumors, and others. Thus, certain chromosome aberrations are more remarkable for their ubiquity rather than their specificity.

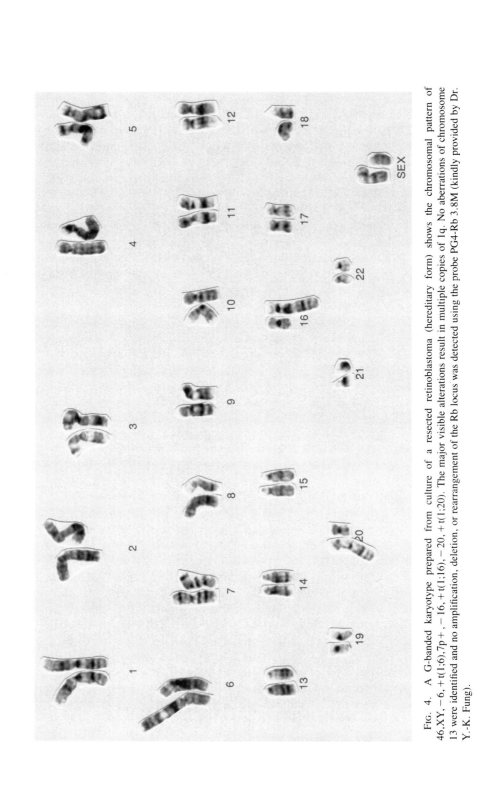

FIG. 4. A G-banded karyotype prepared from culture of a resected retinoblastoma (hereditary form) shows the chromosomal pattern of 46,XY, −6, +t(1:6),7p+, −16, +t(1:16), −20, +t(1:20). The major visible alterations result in multiple copies of 1q. No aberrations of chromosome 13 were identified and no amplification, deletion, or rearrangement of the Rb locus was detected using the probe PG4-Rb 3.8M (kindly provided by Dr. Y.-K. Fung).

Identification of a new specific aberration is exciting because of potential for new biological insights, and can seem remarkably convincing even from examination of small numbers of cases. We recently examined two examples of dedifferentiated chondrosarcoma, a cartilaginous tumor, which was first defined as a new entity by Dahlin and Beaubaut (1971), and which is an aggressive variant of chondrosarcoma clinically. The most surprising observation, although somewhat obscured in one of the tumors by multiplicity of aberrations, was that both cases showed deletion or rearrangement of the same locus on chromosome 1 (1p36) in both homologs (Zalupski *et al.*, 1990). The cytogenetic similarities strongly suggest that genes relevant to cartilaginous development or function are associated with the specific chromosome locus.

Specificity that depends on observations in limited numbers of cases leads to problems in interpretation of results. The t(2;13) was originally described as specific for the alveolar morphologic subtype of rhabdomyosarcoma, but additional cases have confirmed the presence of the same translocation in embryonal and undifferentiated rhabdomyomatous tumors as well (Nilbert and Heim, 1990). The t(X;18) characteristic of synovial sarcoma occasionally is not found in the cultured synovial tumors and has also been reported in association with other soft-tissue tumors (Limon *et al.*, 1989; Bridge *et al.*, 1988). Should we question the specificity of the association or the techniques used to derive the information?

B. CLONALITY

The assumption of clonality in tumors may not sufficiently take into account the prolonged periods of growth and powerful selective influences that could result in dominance of a single pattern despite multiple cells of origin. Arguments favoring a single cell of origin depend on the identification of markers that are relatively uniform within a tumor cell population and differ from the host (cytogenetic aberrations, uniformity of X chromosome inactivation) or, more powerful, the identification of a presumptive *causal* relation between the marker and altered behavior in the tumor cell population. Prime examples, described earlier, are the t(8;14) of Burkitt's and the t(9;22) of CML that result in quantitative or qualitative changes in important cellular proteins.

Multiclonality appears to be the norm for some of the most ordinary of human tumors: the squamous and basal tumors of the skin (Heim *et al.*, 1989b), and squamous and other tumors of the respiratory tract, as well as some leukemias (Kobayashi *et al.*, 1990; Heim and Mitelman, 1989c), gliomas (Shapiro *et al.*, 1981), and possibly some AIDS-related tumors. It may prove to be common in other solid tumors as our ability to study them improves. The appearance of clonality is potentially misleading. Many cells could respond to the initiating event(s) at the time of onset to form a tumor; however, a subpopulation within the mass that is more resistant to local host conditions, e.g., low oxygen supply, or is dividing more rapidly, could easily become the dominant and apparently sole population of the tumor. Clonal evolution has been studied in the course of tumor growth by incorporating cells with different genetic markers into experimental tumors (Kerbel *et al.*, 1988). Clonal selection rapidly resulted in homogeneous populations that appeared as if they had originated from single cells. Conversely, the term *multiclonal* may be descriptive but not necessarily reflective of tumor origin. If the cell of origin were diploid but genetically unstable, then one would expect not only multiple aberrant clones but also an array of nonclonal aberrations (which are frequently seen and usually ignored in tumor-cell analysis). A few recent studies have emphasized that frequent nonclonal numerical and structural aberrations served to distinguish tumor-derived from non-tumor-derived cultures (Geleick *et al.*, 1990; Wurster-Hill *et al.*, 1990).

C. Diploid Tumors

The next major issue concerns the observations of apparently normal diploid cells in cultures or direct preparations of malignant tumors and how they are interpreted. Information is available from divergent sources. For example, several cases of Wilms' Tumor that, when cultured, revealed only cytogenetically diploid cells, did show the expected loss of information at 11p13 when examined genomically (Dao *et al.*, 1987). Another cogent example is that of a cell line originally established from a uterine leiomyosarcoma that was diploid cytogenetically but tumorigenic when inoculated into nude mice (Chen, 1988). Indirect evidence that also supports the existence of diploid tumor cells is based on data from direct studies of chromosome aberrations in breast cancer. A recent report presented evidence of cytogenetic aberrations in the primary tumor and in a metastasis from the same individual (Gerbault-Seureau *et al.*, 1987). However, the aberrations in the two lesions were nonoverlapping and independent, and the interpretation of the authors was that the early stages in evolution of the primary tumor were likely to have been diploid cytogenetically. The same interpretation has been invoked to explain the coexistence of cytogenetically unrelated clones in leukemia (Kobayashi *et al.*, 1990).

We (1985) and others (Zhang *et al.*, 1989; Geleick *et al.*, 1990) have presented evidence based on cell-culture studies that a large proportion of primary breast cancers give rise in culture to cytogenetically diploid cell populations. Culture systems devised by Dr. Helene Smith and colleagues permit limited growth in culture of material from approximately two thirds of the primary breast cancers received. Similar techniques permit the growth of cells from normal breast as well; however, when cultures of normal breasts were examined, aneuploid or structurally rearranged cells were not seen. In primary cultures derived from breast cancer, it was rare to see either structural or numerical aberrations; when such aberrations were found, they were nonclonal. However, the frequency of aberration in cells that were able to grow in culture changed markedly in the metastatic lesions, and clonal chromosomal rearrangements were more common. When metastatic breast cancer effusions were examined, they consisted almost uniformly of cells with both structural and numerical rearrangements, sometimes extensive and invariably clonal. Thus in this system, karyotypic aberration was concordant with increasing malignancy or biologic progression of the lesions. In addition to cytologic markers of breast specificity, evidence in support of the malignant nature of the diploid cells was their growth and invasion of amniotic cell membranes, a functional property strongly resembling that of tumor cells *in vivo* (Smith *et al.*, 1985). The ultimate proof, i.e., retrieval of cells after invasion of the membrane and demonstration of maintenance of diploidy, was not possible because of the limited life span of these cells in culture. These examples emphasize the importance of concurrent marker studies to define the cultured cells, not only for specificity of tissue origin, but also to distinguish malignant from nonmalignant cells of the same tissue type.

Other sets of experiments emphasize the same problems of diploidy, heterogeneity in culture, and cell identity. Cells cultured from renal tumors contained few aberrations and were often cytogenetically normal (Wolman *et al.*, 1988a). Concurrent flow cytometry in several cases indicated that the fresh tumors had populations that were aneuploid by DNA content that were never identified in culture. Loss of aneuploid populations may result from disaggregation procedures, particularly with enzymatic digestion (Costa *et al.*, 1987). Electron microscopy furnished evidence of morphological similarities between the cells growing in culture and those of the original surgical specimen. The renal tumors, unlike breast tumors that may interdigitate with normal tissue, tend to grow as mass lesions easily separable from the normal kidney tissues by dissection before culture. Cultures of prostatic tumors yield results remarkably similar to those from breast, with a preponderance of normal diploid tumors and occasional clonally aberrant cultures (Brothman *et al.*, 1990). The data from these tumors (breast, kidney, prostate) are clouded by questions of interpretation that derive from dependence on tissue culture for tumor analysis. Work in progress, utilizing *in situ* hybridization with centromere-specific chromosome probes (Waldman *et al.*, 1990), supports our original cytogenetic observations on renal tumors in tissue culture by demonstrating similarity of type and extent of aneuploidy in disaggregated cells from the original tumor masses.

Overall, when we look at the collected data on direct and culture analysis of human tumors, particularly in solid tumors, we can conclude that some tumors show specificity of chromosomal aberration, but that not all tumors show the same defects, even among tumors of the same histotype. It is also probable that some changes common to many different tumor types relate to progression of the disease. Further, it seems clear that some malignant tumor cells do not show any detectable karyotypic alterations at the level of the light microscope, and that some of the karyotypic aberrations identified are not specific to the tumors in which they are found.

D. Benign Tumors

A new and different kind of challenge to the presumed association between cytogenetic aberration and malignancy is the accumulating evidence of aberrations in benign proliferations. It should not be surprising in light of the first solid tumor in which consistent chromosome aberrations were identified, the loss of 22 in meningiomas, which is reported in approximately 50% of cases examined cytogenetically. The assumption that cytogenetic clonal aberration should be associated with malignancy can lead to problems in diagnosis. A soft-tissue lesion that we studied had been characterized as a desmoid tumor, a benign but locally invasive proliferation, but revealed extensive clonal karyotypic rearrangements in the cultured tumor cells. The lesion was reclassified as a fibrosarcoma, a malignant tumor, and the reclassification may have been influenced by the reported chromosome aberrations. Other examples of reclassification and reinterpretation have appeared recently in the cytogenetic and cancer literature. In the case of fibrous-tissue proliferations, caution in such interpretations is especially important, because clonal cytogenetic aberrations appear common in benign neoplasias, such as Dupuytren's contractures (Wurster-Hill et al., 1988) as well as desmoid tumors (Karlsson et al., 1988).

Several benign tumor-specific aberrations and some reported associations of clonal changes with other proliferative lesions that are less well defined as neoplastic are listed in Table IV. The presence of chromosome change in parotid adenomas or colonic adenomatous polyps could indicate risk of malignant progression, since these tumors frequently recur and have some probability of evolving to frank malignancy. Similarly, trisomy 12 in ovarian tumors that are considered benign or of low-grade malignancy (Pejovic et al., 1990; Leung et al., 1990) may be predictive of biologic potential for further growth. In follicular thyroid tumors, the interpretation is more complex, owing to the difficulty of establishing a diagnosis on the basis of histopathology: the attribution of diagnostic value to cytogenetic aberrations, whether specific or not, remains to be determined. A large proportion of lipomas show chromosome aberration, usually involving rearrangement at chromosome 12q13, and less frequently in connection with aberrations elsewhere in the karyotype (Heim et al., 1988). More than half the fibromyomatous tumors of the uterus that have been studied also show clonal chromosome aberrations, in many cases involving rearrangement of 12q, but in other tumors involving rearrangements of chromosome 14 or chromosome 7 (Boghosian et al., 1988; Vanni et al., 1989; Nilbert and Heim, 1990). For these two lesions, the lipoma and uterine fibroid, evolution to malignancy or sarcomatous degeneration is extremely infrequent. An interpretation that the

TABLE IV
CHROMOSOME ABERRATIONS IN BENIGN PROLIFERATIONS

Tumor-specific aberrations

Benign tumors	Chromosome aberration
Meningioma	-22
Lipoma	$12q13-14$
Uterine leiomyoma	rearr(12q)
Parotid adenoma	rearr(8)(q12)
Colonic adenoma	$+8; 12q-$
Ovarian adenoma	$+12$
Warthin tumor	$-4, \pm 5$

Occasional reports

Lesion	Chromosome aberration
Nasal papilloma	46,XY,t(13)/46,XY,t(11;?)
Follicular thyroid adenoma	46,XY,t(10;19)
Angiomyolipomas	$+7; -13$; del(6),del(21)
Dysplastic nevi	$-9(9p-)$
Carcinoid of lung	$+7$
Hamartoma	t(15;19)
Hamartoma (endometrial polyp)	inv(12)
Cavernous hemangioma/angiosarcoma	$-Y, +5$
Renal lymphangioma	$-X, i(7q)$
Cold agglutinin disease	$+3, +12$
Atheromatous plaque	$+7$

clonal aberrations observed in more than 50% of the almost ubiquitous lipomatous and fibroid tumors is prognostic of evolution to malignant lesions is extremely unlikely.

The occasional reports of clonal aberrations in angiomyolipoma, endometrial polypoid hamartoma, etc. (see Table IV) are particularly disturbing in that these lesions, to many pathologists, do not represent true neoplasias but should be interpreted as developmental arrests that represent aberrant differentiation and have relatively poor proliferative potential. To add to the concern about these observations are recent reports of trisomy 7 in normal lung (Lee *et al.*, 1987), brain (Heim *et al.*, 1989a), and kidney (Kovacs and Brusa, 1989), adjacent to tumor. It has been known for some time that normal tissues may give rise to clonally aberrant cells in culture (Harnden *et al.*, 1976; Benn, 1977) and that cells of normal tissue origin acquire cytogenetic abnormalities when or before becoming immortal in culture (e.g., Soule *et al.*, 1990).

The complex relationships at issue can be well illustrated by examination of thyroid tumors. Tumors of the thyroid are desirable subjects for cytogenetic study because some are remarkably well differentiated and their ultimate prognosis is unpredictable. No sharp morphologic criteria exist to separate tumors of widely differing biologic potential; the distinction between benign and malignant follicular tumors is particularly difficult. Quantitative DNA determinations have not provided helpful markers. The few tumors that have been analyzed yield a confusing picture. Of 8 follicular tumors, 7 were diploid and 1 was marked by a t(10;19) in all cells (Bartnitzke *et al.*, 1989). Bondeson and co-workers (1989) studied 17 neoplasms, 9 adenomas, and 8 malignant tumors, 6 of which had metastasized. Four of the adenomas were chromosomally aberrant to some extent; two oxyphil adenomas, one with a stemline karyotype of $53,XX, + X, + X, + 4, + 5, + 7, + 7, + 12$ without structural anomaly, and the other with a normal stemline and a sideline clone marked by $51,XX, + 4, + 7, + 7, + 9, + 18$. Two adenomas showed structural rearrangements, one with a complex abnormal stemline and the other with a nonconstitutional marker in a clonal sideline. One of the medullary carcinomas showed a normal diploid stemline, as well as a clone with $47,XX, + 8$. Four of the 5 papillary carcinomas were diploid and the fifth showed a structural aberration involving chromosomes 2 and 15. Thus, both the frequency and extent of cytogenetic aberration were greater in the benign than the malignant tumors. The tumor origin of the cultured cells was supported by flow cytometry and by immunocytochemical demonstration of keratin.

In addition, medullary thyroid tumors are part of a complex of inherited neoplasia, based on a dominant gene whose chromosomal location on 10q is known, and an oncogene associated with human papillary thyroid carcinoma has been localized to the same region (Donghi *et al.*, 1989). Nevertheless, study of eight medullary carcinomas did not reveal deletion, marker participation, or preferential aneusomy involving chromosome 10 (Wurster-Hill *et al.*, 1990). Instead, the most common finding was that tumors were characterized by the normal diploid pattern with some tendency to random chromosome loss. The differentiated identity of the cultured cells was demonstrated by calcitonin production.

In summary, there is evidence that some chromosome aberrations are not clearly related to malignant evolution, that they are extremely common in some forms of benign neoplasm, that they may also characterize aberrant, nonneoplastic tissue proliferation and, finally, that the chromosomal normality of nontumor tissues may also be in question. On the other hand, the evidence supporting lack of karyotypic aberration in some tumors has also become stronger. In any event, it is clear that the easy assumption that the finding of chromosome aberrations justifies a malignant diagnosis can no longer be upheld.

E. METHODS AND LIMITATIONS (CELL CULTURE)

A major problem associated with this and similar studies is that much of the analysis of chromosome aberrations in solid tumors is based upon cells that have been cultured for variable periods of time. The ability to analyze tumor material directly, or even within a day or two, is limited because solid tumors do not, in general, divide rapidly, and the number of cells that enter metaphase is small. In addition, there are major problems in disaggregation of cells from solid tumors. Solid-tumor preparations, whether direct or from culture, often contain normal diploid metaphases. Whereas these may represent stromal or inflammatory cells, it is difficult, in many instances, to rule out the possibility that the diploid cells represent a component of the tumor-cell population. Similarly, the abnormal metaphases that are observed in direct tumor analyses may not represent the main population existing within the tumor. Instead, they may have resulted from pro-longed mitotic arrest, some inducible because of chromosome aberrations that could interfere with completion of cell division. Many other problems afflict interpretations of chromosome aberrations from cultured tumors. Selection in culture may be affected by the source of the tumor material, the methods of transport and disaggregation, and the methods of primary culture. Often selective agents are used in culture to facilitate growth of tumor cells and to prevent contamination by normal cell elements (for review, see Wolman *et al.*, 1988b). Emergence of new aberrations with time in culture has been noted frequently. However, despite these and other substantial disadvantages, cytogenetic analysis derived from cultured cells is often the only source of any pertinent information.

Solid-tumor cytogenetic analysis is at an early stage of development; even those laboratories that perform such studies usually do so as a research endeavor rather than a clinical service. Detailed recording of every step of the process is essential. Patient data collection is critical; the source of the tumor, the speed and nature of transport media to the laboratory, the methods of disaggregation, pathologic correlation, and the methods of processing or culture, all must be carefully tabulated. Concurrence of cytogenetic, histochemical, and molecular studies is urged whenever feasible. Collaborative studies of flow-cytometric analysis on either the fresh or fixed tumor may be of great value in assessing the significance of cytogenetic results.

The initial handling of samples should include assessment of viability; gross evidence of hemorrhage, infarction, or contamination should be noted and vital dye exclusion is a useful measure of cell preservation. Solid tumors are subjected to disaggregation methods, of which the most common are mechanical mincing or enzymic (trypsin-collagenase). Attempts at direct karyotypic analysis, while highly desirable, are not always feasible. Limitations imposed by the amount, cellularity, and viability of the specimen and its baseline mitotic rate will determine the yield of metaphases from direct analysis. The use of monolayer versus suspension growth can also select for specific types of tumors or subpopulations. The use of feeder layers, substrate modification by coating with extracellular matrix, or three-dimensional growth in agar or on floating collagen gels are just a few of the possibilities. Multiple harvests after differing periods in culture are recommended. The number of cells studied should be modified depending upon the observed uniformity or heterogeneity within the tumor or cells in culture.

IV. Biomarkers of Exposure

Many of the agents that cause chromosome breakage (clastogens) in mammalian cells are also known to be carcinogenic; these include ionizing radiation and many alkylating chemicals. Acceptance of a relationship between the ability of an exogenous agent to cause chromosome damage and its ability to cause cancer is widely prevalent and has led to recommendations for a variety of chromosomal tests to be used as screens or monitors for human exposure to mutagenic or carcinogenic agents. When such tests are applied to human populations, however, it must be remembered that the results may provide evidence of exposure and increased risk to the population, but not to the individual, regardless of individual test results. This approach forms the basis for assessment of radiation genotoxicity; the incidence of dicentric chromosome formation is regarded as a biologic dosimeter of exposure (Dolphin and Lloyd, 1974). Although this form of monitoring cannot provide a measure of risk to the individual, it does indicate reliably that the agent of exposure has passed many physiological and cytological barriers and has interacted with cellular DNA. The induction of sister chromatid exchanges (SCE) is an alternative tool for chromosome studies that examines DNA replication and has been widely utilized as a measure of exposure to genotoxic agents and predictor of adverse health effects. It is still not clear whether SCE occur in the course of normal DNA duplication or are a consequence of the exposure to BrdU (or other nucleotide substitutes) necessary for their demonstration.

Further justification for the assumed causal relationship between clastogens and cancer derives from observations of the higher frequency of chromosome abnormalities in leukemic patients with history of exposure to occupational mutagens (Mitelman *et al.*, 1981) and also in those treated with cytotoxic drugs for previous malignant conditions (Crane *et al.*, 1989; Narod and Dube, 1989; Golomb *et al.*, 1982; Rowley *et al.*, 1981). Moreover, in these *secondary* leukemias, specific involvement of certain chromosomes is noted, particularly with loss or rearrangement of 5q and 7q (LeBeau *et al.*, 1986; Narod and Dube,

1989). There is also some question as to the association of the t(8;21) of AML M2 with prior environmental exposures. A contributing effect of cigarette smoking on survival in CML has also been suggested (Archambaud *et al.*, 1989).

Aberrations resulting from genotoxic exposure are usually identified and tabulated in terms of chromosomal breakage and rearrangement, although numerical anomalies are also recorded, because the former more often show a dose-dependent response. Major limitations of this basis for evaluation of exposures are, first, that open breaks and chromosomal fragments resulting from interaction with chemicals are likely to be lost or repaired within the next or successive cell cycles. Therefore, persistent damage is representative of only a small fraction of the damage originally incurred. Second, the baseline rate of chromosome aberrations is low (less than 3% in most laboratories, based on routine diagnostic testing of peripheral blood lymphocytes); reliable identification of even a doubling of aberration frequency would require analysis of large numbers of cells.

SCE analysis has several advantages over more traditional methods of assessment of chromosome damage. The baseline level of SCE is approximately 5 to 10 per cell, depending on conditions of culture, and analysis consists of a simple counting of exchanges rather than the tabulation of many different kinds of aberrations. The SCE method, therefore, can be far more sensitive in detecting small effects and is easier to perform. For many types of mutagens and clastogens, and particularly for the alkylating agents, there is fairly good correspondence between induction of SCE and induction of chromosome aberrations or point mutations. Thus, the spectrum of induced lesions is to some extent agent-dependent. Moreover, the persistence of SCE-inducing lesions varies with the DNA-damaging agent, its mode of chemical action, and probably with the cell-cycle state at time of exposure.

No consistent differences in baseline SCE frequencies have been demonstrated convincingly in cancer cells or in individuals predisposed to develop cancer, other than those with Bloom's syndrome. The high *spontaneous* SCE rate in that condition is presumably linked to the underlying genetic defect in DNA replication or repair. Smoking history has been associated with elevation of the baseline frequency of SCE in well-controlled human population studies (Soper *et al.*, 1984). Exposure to cytostatic agents can result in marked increases in SCE in patients and significant increases in the oncology nurses whose exposures are much less (Sorsa *et al.*, 1982). Monitoring of workers exposed to ethylene oxide indicated the persistence of elevated SCE levels for years after the last known occupational exposure (Stolley *et al.*, 1984), but the consequences of the exposure and its biological effects are still unknown. In summary, SCE studies are preferable to traditional chromosome analysis because of simplicity of performance and greater sensitivity when the class of agent is known to induce SCE (X-ray and radiomimetic compounds being relatively poor inducers). However, the presumption of health risk is considerably less well documented in relation to SCE than is true for chromosome aberrations.

Fragile sites have been identified at fixed locations within the karyotype that are susceptible to induction of gaps and breaks upon exposure to eliciting conditions in culture. Several fragile sites are uniquely associated with particular chemical inducers. Translocation breakpoints of some malignancies are at or near known fragile sites (LeBeau and Rowley, 1984, Hecht, 1988), and it has been suggested that fragile-site expression is more common in cancer patients than controls and that fragile-site evaluation could serve as a marker for cancer-prone individuals (Sutherland and Hecht, 1985). Several recent studies have shown that constitutional fragile sites are no more likely to be expressed in tumor-bearing than in normal individuals (Green *et al.*, 1988; Rao *et al.*, 1988; Kampmann *et al.*, 1990). Some of the associations that have been observed (Glover *et al.*, 1988) may reflect only the frequency with which certain fragile sites are expressed.

V. New and Emerging Tools for Diagnosis

A. Interphase Cytogenetics

The recent development of tools for nonisotopic *in situ* hybridization of chromosomes will permit study of large and hitherto inaccessible populations of tumor cells that are not in metaphase. These tools will enable us to examine critical questions pertaining to chromosome instability and heterogeneity. Equally important, the probes may be applied simultaneous with markers for cell differentiation, cell turnover, or even specific markers of malignancy, so that more direct and population-based assessment of chromosome patterns in whole tumors will be possible. Two advances formed the basis for accessibility to interphase study: the introduction into DNA of modified bases that react with fluorescent or histochemical labels permitting light-microscopic analysis, and the recognition that the satellite highly repetitive DNAs show minor differences unique to individual chromosomes. The targets of these probes are the centromeric regions of human chromosomes, rich in repetitive DNA. In fixed and stained preparations, the number of target sites per nucleus corresponds to the copy number of the particular chromosome. In addition to addressing important issues in cancer cytogenetics, other valuable applications of the technique include rapid sex determination and detection of specific aneuploidy in prenatal samples.

Probes for satellite-specific identification of individual chromosomes are already commercially available, and several experimental studies attest to their value in cancer genetics. The new centromere-specific probes have been applied to detection of aneuploidy in tumor-cell populations in interphase as well as metaphase (Cremer *et al., 1988*). Such probes also can react with structurally altered chromosomes to demonstrate component contributions to recombinant marker formation. In that context they have been used for detection of multiple copies of a chromosome arm (1q) (Pequignot *et al., 1989*). They can be applied to the identification of aberrations of tumor cells extracted from paraffin-embedded material (Emmerich *et al., 1989*), as well as to cell suspensions and aspirates. They have particular utility for study of epithelial tumors, such as breast, that are not easily amenable to conventional cytogenetic assessment and for which there is discrepancy between results from direct harvest and cultured tumors. Probes for chromosome 18 and the X were utilized to demonstrate aneuploidy and heterogeneity in breast cancers (Devilee *et al., 1988*). More recently, in combination with BRDU uptake, centromere-specific probes illustrated not only heterogeneity of chromosome composition but also that in some breast cancers proliferation was selectively associated with the chromosomally aberrant cells (Waldman *et al., 1990*).

Another detection method is based on *chromosome-painting* probes (Pinkel *et al., 1988*). When a substantial number of genes has been mapped to a particular chromosome at varying positions along its axis, then a mixture or *cocktail* of the known genes and sequences can be combined as probes. When used together with an appropriate linked-fluorescent label, then the entire chromosome appears painted with the label. The combined attachment of a few hundred such probes is sufficient for easy visualization of whole chromosomes. Applications of this technique to detection of specific aneuploidy (Fuscoe *et al., 1989*; Lichter *et al., 1988*) and to identification of translocations (for which it should be far more powerful than the centromeric probes) (Pinkel *et al., 1988*), have been illustrated in a few reports, but the method is still beset by technical and interpretive difficulties.

B. DUAL MARKERS

Another area still in its infancy is that which seeks to apply markers of tissue differentiation to cells in metaphase. Although the problem of associating an abnormal metaphase with specific identifiers of cell lineage may be obviated to some extent by the advent of interphase cytogenetics, the resolution of specific aberrations by this means is very limited. An alternative approach that has met with some success has employed phenotyping of mitotic cells by labeling with monoclonal antibodies. B- and T-cell antibodies have been used to investigate the origin of lymphocyte subpopulations and of Reed-Sternberg cells from Hodgkin's lesions in karyotypic preparations (Teerenhovi *et al., 1986, 1988*). Although the method is not optimal for cytogenetic preparation, it does permit limited identification of aberrations. With refinement and improvement of techniques, this approach could have broad application to determination of tissue specificity and stage of maturation, depending on the availability of appropriate monoclonal antibodies.

VI. Conclusions

Chromosome studies have gained broad acceptance as important, practical, and sometimes critical determinants in the diagnosis and patient management of leukemic proliferations. The specificity of the chromosome aberrations in hematopoietic disorders, related either to differentiation pathways or to general properties of tumor cells, has been reinforced by new information from molecular biology. However, the principles that cells of malignant tumors are genetically and chromosomally abnormal, and that those tumors are clonal in origin, appear less generally valid for solid tumors than they are for the leukemias. The more prevalent tumors remain poorly described cytogenetically, and specificity of chromosome change rarely appears true for all tumors of a specific histologic classification or for all cells within a tumor. Some solid tumors, particularly those of squamous epithelium, are clearly characterized by cytogenetically unrelated clones. The existence of cytogenetically unrelated clones may indicate that broader and more frequent tumor-initiating events have occurred in a particular tissue; this interpretation is buttressed by a growing appreciation of the frequency of nonclonal aneuploid cells. An alternate possibility, that the tumor stem cell is diploid and genetically unstable, is supported by many observations of diploid cells in cultures derived from breast, prostate, and other, mainly glandular, epithelial tumors, in addition to some leukemias. The apparently normal diploid tumors should be highly informative tumors when examined with molecular tools; because they display a more limited array of genetic damage overall, their molecular aberrations are more likely to relate to critical events early in tumorigenesis. The observations of clonal cytogenetic aberrations in nonmalignant neoplastic lesions, and even in some nonneoplastic tissues, pose a different challenge. We must learn to be cautious in attributing a malignant diagnosis to a lesion based largely on the finding of cytogenetic aberration. It is possible that the stability of the genome is less reliable than has been taken for granted in karyotypic as in other (immunologic) respects.

Major questions must be addressed in tumor cytogenetics. We do not understand when and for what cell types chromosome changes are either necessary or specific for either tumor initiation or tumor progression. Relationships among hyperplasias, benign neoplasias, and malignant neoplasias, and the role of chromosome studies in helping us to define these proliferative states, are poorly appreciated for most tissue lineages. Although their importance is paramount, the genetic basis for chromosome instability and for the chromosomal heterogeneity that is characteristic of tumors, and that may be responsible for other biological aspects of tumor heterogeneity and tumor progression, is largely unknown and difficult to address.

Acknowledgment

Support from the Levy-Stone Program in Cancer Cytogenetics is gratefully acknowledged.

References

Archambaud, E., Maupas, J., Lecluze-Palazzolo, C., Fiere, D., and Viala, J. J. (1989). Influence of cigarette smoking on the presentation and course of chronic myelogenous leukemia. *Cancer* **63,** 2060–2065.

Arthur, D. C., Berger, R., Golomb, H. M., Swansbury, G. J., Reeves, B. R., Alimenta, G., Van Den Berghe, H., Bloomfield, C. D., de la Chapelle, A., Dewald, G. W., Garson, O. M., Hagemeijer, A., Kaneko, Y., Mitelman, F., Pierre, R. V., Ruutu, T., Sakurai, M., Lawler, S. D., and Rowley, J. D. (1989). The clinical significance of karyotype in acute myelogenous leukemia. *Cancer Genet. Cytogenet.* **40,** 203–216.

Bakhshi, A., Jensen, J. P., Goldman, P., Wright, J. J., McBride, O. W., Epstein, A. L., and Korsmeyer, S. J. (1985). Cloning the chromosomal breakpoint of t(14;18) human lymphomas clustering around JH on chromosome 14 and near a transcriptional unit on 18. *Cell* **41,** 899–906.

Bartnitzke, S., Herrmann, E. M., Lobeck, H., Zuschneid, W., Neuhaus, P., and Bullerdiek, J. (1989). Cytogenetic findings on eight follicular thyroid adenomas including one with a t (10;19). *Cancer Genet. Cytogenet.* **39,** 65–68.

Benn, P. A. (1977). Population kinetics of chromosomally abnormal human fibroblast subpopulations. *Cytogenet. Cell Genet.* **19,** 136–145.

Biedler, J. L., and Spengler, B. A. (1976). Metaphase chromosome anomaly: Association with drug resistance and cell-specific products. *Science* **191,** 185–187.

Bigner, S. H., Mark, K., and Bigner, D. D. (1990). Cytogenetics of human brain tumors. *Cancer Genet. Cytogenet.* **47,** 141–154.

Bloomfield, C. D., Arthur, D. C., Frizzera, G., Levine, E. G., Peterson, B. A., and Gajl-Peczalska, K. J. (1983). Nonrandom chromosome abnormalities in lymphoma. *Cancer Res.* **43,** 2975–2984.

Bodmer, W. F., Bailey, C. J., Bodmer, J., Bussey, H. J. R., Ellis, A., Gorman, P., Lucibello, F. C., Murday, V. A., Rider, S. H., Scambler, P., Sheer, D., Solomon, E., and Spurr, N. K. (1987). Localization of the gene for familial adenomatous polyposis on chromosome 5. *Nature* **328,** 614–616.

Boghosian, L., Dal Cin, P., and Sandberg, A. A. (1988). An interstitial deletion of chromosome 7 may characterize subgroups of uterine leiomyoma. *Cancer Genet. Cytogenet.* **34,** 207–208.

Bondeson, L., Bengtsson, A., Bondeson, A., Dahlenfors, R., Grimelius, L., Wedell, B., and Mark, J. (1989). Chromosome studies in thyroid neoplasia. *Cancer* **64,** 680–685.

Boveri, T., Fisher, J., (1914) Zur Frage der Entstehung Maligner Tumoren. English translation: Boveri, M. (1929). "The Origin of Malignant Tumors." Williams and Wilkins, Baltimore.

Bridge, J. A., Bridge, R. S., Borek, D. A., Shaffer, B., and Norris, C. W. (1988). Translocation t (X;18) in orofacial synovial sarcoma. *Cancer* **62,** 935–937.

Brodeur, G. M., Hayes, P. A., and Green, A. A. (1987). Consistent N-myc copy number in simultaneous or consecutive neuroblastoma samples from sixty individual patients. *Cancer Res.* **47,** 4248–4253.

Brothman, A. R., Peehl, D. M., Ankita, P. M., and McNeal, J. E. (1990). Frequency and pattern of karyotypic abnormalities in human prostate cancer. *Cancer Res.* **50,** 3795–3803.

Cavenee, W. K., Dryja, T. P., and Phillips, R. A. (1983). Expression of recessive alleles by chromosomal mechanisms in retinoblastoma. *Nature* **305,** 779–784.

Chen, R. T. (1988). SK-UT-1B, a human tumorigenic diploid cell line. *Cancer Genet. Cytogenet.* **33,** 77–81.

Costa, A., Silverstrini, G., Del Bino, G., and Motta, R. (1987). Implications of disaggregation procedures on biological representation of human solid tumours. *Cell Tissue Kinet.* **20,** 171–180.

Crane, M. M., Keating, M. J., Trujillo, J. M., Labarthe, D. R., and Frankowski, R. (1989). Environmental exposures in cytogenetically defined subsets of acute nonlymphocytic leukemia. *J.A.M.A.* **262,** 634–39.

Cremer, T., Tesin, D., Hopman, A. H. N., and Manuelidis, L. (1988). Rapid interphase and metaphase assessment of specific chromosomal changes in neurectodermal tumor cells by *in situ* hybridization with chemically modified DNA probes. *Exp. Cell Res.* **176,** 199–220.

Croce, C. M., Shander, M., Martinis, J., Cicurol, L., D'Ancona, G. G., Dolby, T. W., and Koprowski, H. (1982). Chromosomal location of the genes for human immunoglobin heavy chains *Proc. Natl. Acad. Sci. U.S.A.* **76,** 3416–3419.

Croce, C. M. (1987). Role of chromosomal translocations in human neoplasia. *Cell* **49,** 155–156.

Dahlin, D. C., and Beabout, J. W. (1971). Dedifferentiation of low-grade chondrosarcomas. *Cancer* **28,** 461–466.

Dalla-Favera, R., Bregni, M., Erikson, J., Patterson, D., Gallo, R. C., and Croce, C. M. (1982). The human c-MYC oncogene is located on the region of chromosome 8 which is translocated in Burkitt's lymphoma cells. *Proc. Natl. Acad. Sci. U.S.A.* **79,** 7824–7827.

Dao, D. D., Schroeder, W. T., Chao, L. Y., Kikuchi, H., Strong, L. C., Riccardi, V. M., Pathak, S., Nichols, W. W., Lewis, W. H., and Saunders, G. F. (1987). Genetic mechanisms of tumor-specific loss of 11p DNA sequences in Wilms' tumor. *Am. J. Hum. Genet.* **41,** 202–217.

Devilee, P., Thierry, R. F., Kievits, T., Kolluri, R., Hopman, A. H. N., Willard, H. F., Pearson, P. L., and Cornelisse, C. J., (1988). Detection of chromosome aneuploidy in interphase nuclei from human primary breast tumors using chromosome-specific repetitive DNA probes. *Cancer Res.* **48,** 5825–5830.

Dolphin, G. W., and Lloyd, D. C. (1974). The significance of radiation-induced chromosome abnormalities in radiological protection. *J. Med. Genet.* **11,** 181–189.

Donghi, R., Sozzi. G., Pierotti, M. A., Biunno, I., Miozzo, M., Fusco, A., Grieco, M., Santoro, M., Vecchio, G., Spurr, N. K., and Della Porta, G. (1989). The oncogene associated with human papillary thyroid carcinoma (PTC) is assigned to chromosome 10 q11-q12 in the same region as multiple endocrine neoplasia type 2A (MEN2A). *Oncogene* **4,** 521–523.

Emmerich, P., Jauch, A., Hofmann, M. C., Cremer, T., and Walt, H. (1989). Interphase cytogenetics in paraffin-embedded sections from human testicular germ-cell tumor xenografts and in corresponding cultured cells. *Lab. Invest.* **61,** 235–242.

Fifth International Workshop on chromosomes in leukemia–lymphoma. (1987). *Blood* **5,** 1554–1564.

Fourth International Workshop on chromosomes in leukemia. (1984). A prospective study of acute nonlymphocytic leukemia. *Cancer Genet. Cytogenet.* **11,** 249–360.

Furth, J., and Furth, O. B. (1936). Neoplastic diseases produced in mice by general irradiation with X-rays. *Am. J. Cancer* **28,** 54–65.

Fuscoe, J. C., Collins, C. C., Pinkel, D., and Gray, J. W. (1989). An efficient method for selecting unique-sequence clones from DNA libraries and its application: Fluorescent staining of human chromosome 21 using *in situ* hybridization. *Genomics* **5,** 100–109.

Geleick, D., Muller, H., Matter, A., Torhorst, J., and Regenass, U. (1990). Cytogenetics of breast cancer. *Cancer Genet. Cytogenet.* **46,** 217–229.

Gerbault-Seureau, M., Vielh, P., Zafrani, B., Salmon, R., and Dutrillaux, B. (1987). Cytogenetic study of twelve human near-diploid breast cancers with chromosomal changes. *Ann. Genet. Paris* **30**, 138–145.

Glover, T. W., Coyle-Morris, J. F., Li, F. P., Brown, R. S., Berger, C. S., Gemmill, R. M., and Hecht, F. (1988). *Cancer Genet. Cytogenet.* **31**, 69–74.

Golomb, H. M., Alimena,G., Rowley, J. D., Vardiman, J. W., Testa, J. R., and Sovik, C. (1982). Correlation of occupation and karyotype in adults with acute nonlymphocytic leukemia. *Blood* **60**, 404–411.

Green, R. J., Phillips, D. L., Chen, T. L., Reidy, J. A., and Ragab, A. H. (1988). Effects of folate in culture medium on common fragile sites in lymphocyte chromosomes from normal and leukemic children. *Hum. Genet.* **81**, 9–12.

Harnden, D. G., Benn, P. A., Oxford, J. M., Taylor, A. M. R., and Webb, T. P. (1976). Cytogenetically marked clones in human fibroblasts cultured from normal subjects. *Somat. Cell Genet.* **2**, 55–62.

Hecht, F. (1988). The fragile-site hypothesis of cancer. *Cancer Genet. Cytogenet.* **31**, 119–124.

Heim, S., and Mitelman, F. (1989c). Cytogenetically unrelated clones in hematological neoplasms. *Leukemia* **3**, 6–8.

Heim, S., Mandahl, N., Jin, Y., Stromblad, S., Lindstrom, E., Salford, L. G., and Mitelman, F. (1989a). Trisomy 7 and sex chromosome loss in human brain tissue. *Cytogenet. Cell Genet.* **52**, 136–138.

Heim, S., Mandahl, N., Rydholm, A., Willen, H., and Mitelman, F. (1988). Different karyotypic features characterize different clinico-pathologic subgroups of benign lipogenic tumors. *Int. J. Cancer* **42**, 863–867.

Heim, S., Mertens, F., Jin, Y., Mandahl, N., Johansson, B., Biorklund, A., Wennerberg, J., Jonsson, N., and Mitelman, F. (1989b). Diverse chromosome abnormalities in squamous cell carcinomas of the skin. *Cancer Genet. Cytogenet.* **39**, 69–76.

Henry, I., Grandjouan, S., and Couillin, P. (1989). Tumor-specific loss of 11p15.5 alleles in del 11p13 Wilms' tumor and in familial adrenocortical carcinoma. *Proc. Nat. Acad. Sci. U.S.A.* **86**, 3247–3251.

Herrera, L., Kakati, S., Gibas, L., Pietrzak, E., and Sandberg, A. A. (1986). Brief clinical report: Gardner syndrom in a man with an interstitial deletion of 5q. *Am. J. Med. Genet.* **25**, 473–6.

Kampmann, T., Schmidt, A., Rudiger, H. W., Tan, T. L., and Passarge, E. (1990). No difference in expression of chromosomal fragile sites in patients with solid malignant tumours and normal controls. *Genes Chromosomes & Cancer* **2**, 44–47.

Karlsson, I., Mandahl, N., Heim, S., Rydholm, A., Willen, H., and Mitelman, F. (1988). Complex chromosome rearrangements in an extraabdominal desmoid tumor. *Cancer Genet. Cytogenet.* **34**, 241–45.

Keating, M. J., Cork, A., Broach, Y., Smith, T., Walters, R. S., McCredie, K. B., Trujillo, J., and Freireich, E. J. (1987). Toward a clinically relevant cytogenetic classification of acute myelogenous leukemia. *Leuk. Res.* **11**, 119–133.

Kerbel, R. S., Waghorne, C., Korczak, B., Lagarde, A., and Breitman, M. L. (1988). Clonal dominance of primary tumors by metastatic cells; genetic analysis and biological implications. *Cancer Surv.* **7**, 594–629.

Kirsch, I. R., Morton, C. C., Nakahara, K., and Leder, P. (1982). Human immunoglobulin heavy-chain genes map to a region of translocations in malignant B lymphocytes. *Science* **216**, 301–303.

Klein, G., and Klein, E. (1985). Myc/Ig juxtaposition by chromosomal translocations: Some new insights, puzzles, and paradoxes. *Immunology Today* **6**, 208–215.

Kobayashi, H., Kaneko, Y., Maseki, N., and Sakurai, M. (1990). Karyotypically unrelated clones in acute leukemias and myelodysplastic syndromes. *Cancer Genet. Cytogenet.* **47**, 171–178.

Kovacs, G. and Brusa, P. (1989). Clonal chromosome aberrations in normal kidney tissue from patients with renal cell carcinoma. *Cancer Genet. Cytogenet.* **37**, 289–290.

Kurzrock, R., Gutterman, J. U., and Talpaz, M. (1988). The molecular genetics of Philadelphia chromosome–positive leukemias. *N. Engl. J. Med.* **319**, 990–998.

LeBeau, M. M., Albain, K. S., Larson, R. A., Vardiman, J. W., Davis, E. M., Blough, R. R., Golomb, G. M., and Rowley, J. D. (1986). Clinical and cytogenetic correlations in 63 patients with therapy-related myelodysplastic syndromes and acute nonlymphocytic leukemia: Further evidence for characteristic abnormalities of chromosomes no. 5 and 7. *J. Clin. Oncol.* **4**, 325–345.

LeBeau, M. M., and Rowley, J. D. (1984). Heritable fragile sites in cancer. *Nature* **308**, 607–608.

Lee, J. S., Pathak, S., and Hopwood, V. (1987). Involvement of chromosome 7 in primary lung cancer and nonmalignant normal lung tissue. *Cancer Res.* **47**, 6349–6352.

Leppert, M., Dobbs, M., Scambler, P., O'Connell, P., Wakamura, Y., Stauffer, D., Woodward, S., Burt, R., Hughes, J., Gardner, E., Lathrop, M., Wasmuth, J., Lalouel, J. M., and White, R. (1987). The gene for familial polyposis coli maps to the long arm of chromosome 5. *Science* **238**, 1411–1413.

Leung, W. Y., Schwartz, P. E., Ng, H. T., and Yang Feng, T. L. (1990). Trisomy 12 in benign fibroma and granulosa cell tumor of the ovary. *Gyn. Onc.* **38**, 28–32.

Lichter, P., Cremer, T., Tang, C. C., Watkins, P. C., Manuelidis, L., and Ward, D. C. (1988). Rapid detection of human chromosome 21 aberrations by *in situ* hybridization. *Proc. Natl. Acad. Sci. U.S.A.* **85**, 9664–9668.

Limon, J., Mrozek, K., Nedoszytko, B., Babinska, M., Jaskiewicz, J., Kopacz, A., Zoltowska, A., and Borowska-Lehman, J. (1989). Cytogenetic findings in two synovial sarcomas. *Cancer Genet. Cytogenet.* **38**, 215–222.

Mitelman, F. (1988). "Catalog of Chromosome Aberrations in Cancer." Third Ed. Alan R. Liss, New York.

Mitelman, F., Nilsson, P. G., Brandt, L., Alimena, G., Gastaldi, R., and Dallapiccola, B. (1981). Chromosome pattern, occupation, and clinical features in patients with acute nonlymphocytic leukemia. *Cancer Genet. Cytogenet.* **4**, 197–214.

Mohamed, A., Dan, M., and Wolman, S. R. (1990). Megakaryoblastic leukemia (M7); are chromosome 21 alterations specific? *Proc. Am. Assoc. Cancer Res.* **31**, 161.

Muller, H. J. (1928). Measurement of gene mutation rate in *Drosophila*, its high variability, and its dependence upon temperature. *Genetics* **13**, 279–357.

Narod, S., and Dube, I. D. (1989). Occupational history and involvement of chromosomes 5 and 7 in acute nonlymphocytic leukemia. *Cancer Genet. Cytogenet.* **38**, 261–69.

National Research Council, Advisory Committee on the Biological Effects of Ionizing Radiations (1980). The Effects on Populations of Exposure to Low Levels of Ionizing Radiation, pp. 135–471. National Academy of Sciences, Washington.

Nilbert, M., and Heim, S. (1990). Uterine leiomyoma cytogenetics. *Genes Chromosomes, and Cancer* **2**, 3–13.

Nowell, P. C., and Hungerford, D. A. (1960). A minute chromosome in human chronic granulocytic leukemia. *Science* **132**, 1497.

Pejovic, T., Heim, S., Mandahl, N., Elmfors, B., Floderus, U. M., Furgyik, S., Helm, G., Willen, H., and Mitelman, F. (1990). Trisomy 12 is a consistent chromosomal abberration in benign ovarian tumors. *Genes, Chromosomes, and Cancer* **2**, 48–52.

Pequignot, E. V., Jeanpierre, M., Dutrillaux, A. M., Seureau, M. G., Muleris, M., and Dutrillaux, B. (1989). Detection of 1q polysomy in interphase nuclei of human solid tumors with a biotinylated probe. *Hum. Genet.* **81**, 311–314.

Pinkel, D., Landegent, J., Collins, C., Fuscoe, J., Segraves, R., Lucas, J., and Gray, J. (1988). Fluorescence *in situ* hybridization with human chromosome-specific libraries: Detection of trisomy 21 and translations of chromosome 4. *Proc. Natl. Acad. Sci. U.S.A.* **85**, 9138–9142.

Potluri, V. R., Helson, L., Elsworth, R. M., Reid, T., and Gilbert, F. (1986). Chromosomal abnormalities in human retinoblastoma, a review. *Cancer* **58**, 663–671.

Rao, P., Heerema, N. A., and Palmer, C. G. (1988). Expression of fragile sites in childhood acute lymphoblastic leukemia patients and normal controls. *Hum. Genet.* **79**, 329–334.

Reeve, A. E., Sih, S. A., Raizis, A. M., and Feinberg, A. P. (1989). Loss of allelic heterozygosity at a second locus on chromosome 11 in sporadic Wilms' tumor cells. *Mol. Cell. Biol.* **9**, 1799–1803.

Rowley, J. D., Golomb, H. M., and Vardiman, J. W. (1981). Nonrandom chromosome abnormalities in acute leukemia and dysmyelopoietic syndromes in patients with previously treated malignant disease. *Blood* **58**, 759–767.

Shapiro, J. R., Yung, W. K. A., and Shapiro, W. R. (1981). Isolation, karyotype, and clonal growth of heterogeneous subpopulations of human malignant gliomas. *Cancer Res.* **41**, 2349–2359.

Smith, H. S., Liotta, L. A., Hancock, M. C., Wolman, S. R., and Hackett, A. J. (1985). Invasiveness and ploidy of human mammary carcinomas in short-term culture. *Proc. Natl. Acad. Sci. U.S.A.* **82**, 1805–1809.

Solis, V., Pritchard, J., and Cowell, J. K. (1988). Cytogenetic changes in Wilms' tumors. *Cancer Genet. Cytogenet.* **34**, 223–234.

Soper, K., Stolley, P., Galloway, S., Smith, J., Nichols, W., and Wolman, S. R. (1984). Sources of variation in sister chromatid exchange for control subjects. *Mutat. Res.* **129**, 77–88.

Sorsa, M., Norppa, H., and Vainio, H. (1982). Induction of sister chromatid exchanges among nurses handling cytostatic drugs. *In* (B. A. Bridges, B. E. Butterworth, and I. B. Weinstein, eds.), "Banbury Report 13: Indicators of Genotoxic Exposure," p.p. 341–354. Cold Spring Harbor Laboratory, Cold Spring Harbor, New York.

Soule, H. D., Maloney, T. M., Wolman, S. R., Peterson, W. D., Brenz, R., McGrath, C. M., Russo, J., Pauley, R. J., Jones, R. F., and Brooks, S. C. (1990). Isolation and characterization of a spontaneously immortalized human breast epithelial cell line, MCF-10. *Cancer Res.* **50**, 6075–6086.

Stark, G. R., Debatisse, M., Giulotto, E., and Wahl, G. M. (1989). Recent progress in understanding mechanisms of mammalian DNA amplification. *Cell* **57**, 901–908.

Stolley, P. D., Soper, K. A., Galloway, S. M., Nichols, W., Norman, S. A., and Wolman, S. R. (1984). Sister chromatid exchanges in association with occupational exposure to ethylene oxide. *Mutat. Res.* **129** (1) 89–102.

Sutherland, G. R., and Hecht, F. (1985). "Fragile Sites on Human Chromosomes. Oxford Monographs on Medical Genetics No. 13." Osford University Press, New York.

Taub, R., Kirsch, F., Morton, C., Lenoir, G., Swan, D., Tronick, S., Aaronson, S., and Leder, P. (1982). Translocation of the c-MYC- gene into the immunoglobulin heavy-chain locus in human Burkitt's lymphoma and murine plasmacytoma cells. *Proc. Natl. Acad. Sci. U.S.A.* **79**, 7837–7841.

Teerenhovi, L., Lindholm, C., Pakkala, A., Franssila, K., Stein, H., and Knuutila, S. (1988). Unique display of a pathologic karyotype in Hodgkin's disease by Reed-Sternberg cells. *Cancer Genet. Cytogenet.* **34**, 305–311.

Teerenhovi, L., Wasenius, V. M., Franssila, K., Keinanen, M., and Knuutila, S. (1986). A method for analysis of cell morphology, banded karyotype, and immunoperoxidase identification of lymphocyte subset on the same cell. *Am. J. Clin. Path.* **85**, 602–604.

Teyssier, J. R. (1989). The chromosomal analysis of human solid tumors. *Cancer Genet. Cytogenet.* **37**, 103–125.

Third International Workshop on chromosomes in leukemia. (1981). *Cancer Genet. Cytogenet.* **4**, 96–142.

Tsujimoto, Y., Jaffe, E., Cossman, J., Gorham, J., Nowell, P. C., and Croce, C. M. (1985). Clustering of breakpoints on chromosome 11 in human B-cell neoplasms with the E (11;14) translocation. *Nature* **315**(6017), 340–343.

Vanni, R., Nieddu, M., Paoli, R., and Lecca, U. (1989). Uterine leiomyoma cytogenetics. I. Rearrangements of chromosome 12. *Cancer Genet. Cytogenet.* **37**, 61–64.

Vogelstein, B., Fearon, E., Hamilton, S., Kern, S., Preisinger, A., Leppert, M., Nakamura, Y., White, R., Smits, A., and Bos, J. (1988). Genetic alterations during colorectal-tumor development. *N. Engl. J. Med.* **319**(9), 525–532.

Waldman, F. M., Balasz, M., Pinkel, D., and Gray, J. (1990). Heterogeneous proliferation and chromosome-specific aneusomy in primary breast cancer cells. *Proc. Am. Assoc. Cancer Res.* **31** (149), 26.

Wolman, S. R., Camuto, P. M., and Perle, M. A. (1988b). Cytogenetic diversity in primary human tumors. *J. Cell. Biochem.* **36**, 147–156.

Wolman, S. R., Camuto, P. M., Eisenberg, A. J., Feiner, H. D., and Greco, M. A. (1990). Wilms' tumor: A search for the critical lesion. *Hum. Pathol.* **21**, 715–721.

Wolman, S. R., Smith, H. S., Stampfer, M., and Hackett, A. J. (1985). Growth of diploid cells from breast cancers. *Cancer Genet. Cytogenet.* **16**, 49–64.

Wolman, S. R., and Henderson, A. S. (1989). Chromosomal aberrations as markers of oncogene amplification. *Hum. Pathol.* **20**, 308–315.

Wolman, S. R., Camuto, P. M., Golimbu, M., and Schinella, R. (1988a). Cytogenetic, flow cytometric, and ultrastructural studies of twenty-nine nonfamilial human renal carcinomas. *Cancer Res.* **48**, 2890–2897.

Wurster-Hill, D. H., Brown, F., Park, J. P., and Gibson, S. H. (1988). Cytogenetic studies in Dupytren's contracture. *Am. J. Hum. Genet.* **43**, 285–292.

Wurster-Hill, D. H., Pettengill, O. S., Noll, W. W., Gibson, S. H., and Brinck-Johnsen, T. (1990). Hypodiploid, pseudodiploid, and normal karyotypes prevail in cytogenetic studies of medullary carcinomas of the thyroid and metastatic tissues. *Cancer Genet. Cytogenet.* **47**, 227–241.

Yunis, J. (1981). New chromosome techniques in the study of human neoplasia. *Hum. Pathol.* **12**, 540–549.

Zalupski, M. M., Ensley, J. F., Ryan, J., Selvaggi, S., Baker, L. H., and Wolman, S. R. (1990). A common cytogenetic abnormality and DNA content alterations in dedifferentiated chondrosarcoma. *Cancer* **66**, 1176–1182.

Zhang, R., Wiley, J., Howard, S. P., Meisner, L. F., and Gould, M. N. (1989). Rare clonal karyotypic variants in primary cultures of human breast carcinoma cells. *Cancer Res.* **49**, 444–449.

Index

A

abl, 395
  translocated in chronic myelogenous
    leukemia, 395
Acute lymphoblastic leukemia (ALL)
  chromosomal aberrations, 403–404
  cytogenetics, difficult to band, 403
Acute myeloid leukemia (AML)
  chromosomal aberrations, 397–403
  loss of p53, 382–383
Acute nonlymphocytic leukemia (ANLL)
  chromosomal aberrations, 399–400
Acute promyelocytic leukemia (APL)
  loss of p53, 382
Adenovirus E1a gene product, 13
Adherence of malignant cells
  inhibition of adherence, 128–130
    proteolytic fragments
      fibronectin, 128, 130
      laminin, 128, 130
    specific for endothelial cells, 126
Adhesion molecules
  neoplastic cells, 127
  related to oncogene products, 5, 6, 15
Adhesion promoting molecules, 100, 127
Adjuvant therapy, 75
Adrenal cancer
  P-glycoprotein expression, 342
Adrenal cortex
  P-glycoprotein expression, 341
Adriamycin
  inhibitor of protein kinase C, 33
AIDS-related tumors
  some multiclonal, 409
Allelic deletions, *see also* Chromosomal
    alterations
  affect prognosis, 7
Anti-oncogenes, *see* Tumor-suppressor genes
Aminoacridines
  inhibitors of protein kinase C, 33

Androgens
  affect glutathione transferase activity, 189
Angiogenesis, 136
Angiomyolipomas
  chromosomal aberrations, 413
Antisense oligonucleotides, 157
Arginine-glycine-asparagine (RGD), 129–130,
    165
Arginine-glycine-asparagine-serine (RGDS),
    104, 111, 115, 117–119
Aryl hydrocarbon hydroxylase receptor, 235
Aspartate transcarbamylase
  estrogens induce in mammary carcinoma cell
    lines, 231
Astrocytoma, 4
  loss of heterozygosity, 10
  pyruvate kinase, 319–320
Atheromatous plaque
  chromosomal aberrations, 413
ATP-dependent transporters, 348–350
Autocrine growth factors, 156, 168
Azidopine
  photoaffinity labeling with, 356–359

B

B72.3 MAb to sialyl Tn, 300–302
Basal tumors of skin, 409
Basic fibroblast growth factor
  made by melanoma, 157
  required by cultured melanocytes, 153
bcl-1
  located at 11q13, 404
bcl-2
  located at 18q21, 404
bcr gene
  on chromosome 22, 395
  site of translocation in chronic myelogenous
    leukemia, 395
Beckwith-Wiedemann syndrome
  tumor suppressor loci, 4

427

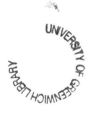